ORTHODONTICS – BASIC ASPECTS AND CLINICAL CONSIDERATIONS

Edited by **Farid Bourzgui**

INTECHOPEN.COM

Orthodontics – Basic Aspects and Clinical Considerations
Edited by Farid Bourzgui

Published by InTech
Janeza Trdine 9, 51000 Rijeka, Croatia

Edition 2014

Publishing Process Manager Ana Skalamera

Technical Editor Teodora Smiljanic

Cover Designer InTech Design Team

Additional hard copies can be obtained from orders@intechopen.com

Orthodontics – Basic Aspects and Clinical Considerations, Edited by Farid Bourzgui
p. cm.
ISBN 978-953-51-0143-7

Contents

Preface

One of the biggest challenges facing practitioners nowadays is offering quality dental care while demonstrating clinical *competence,* and comprehensive and *compassionate* patient *care*. Therefore, training and refreshing of knowledge are absolute necessities that contribute to successful clinical patient care.

The acquisition of new ideas is dependent on reading. As Nietzsche put in his book *Beyond Good and Evil* (1886) "Naturally in order to practice reading as an art, one thing above all is necessary, which nowadays has been thoroughly unlearned, for which one must almost be a cow and at any rate not a "modern man", namely rumination". Such reading should be selective, meeting well-defined objectives, with a critical understanding of the medical and scientific information.

Access to information and the demystification of knowledge are the currency of this century despite the efforts exerted by some retention. Production's "open source" plays and will continue to play a very important role in sharing and disseminating knowledge and expertise. The present book embodies such a state of mind.

The book reflects the ideas of nineteen academic and research experts from different countries. It provides an overview of the state-of-the-art, outlines the experts' knowledge and their efforts to provide readers with quality content explaining new directions and emerging trends in Orthodontics. The book should be of great value to both orthodontic practitioners and to students in orthodontics, who will find learning resources in connection with their fields of study. This will help them to acquire valid knowledge and excellent clinical skills.

Last but not at least, I would like to express my deep gratitude to the editorial team and colleagues who have contributed, one way or another, to the fulfilment of this work.

Farid Bourzgui
Faculty of Dentistry, University of Hassan II Ain Chok
Morocco

Part 1

Epidemiology and Prevention

1

Orthodontic Treatment Need: An Epidemiological Approach

Carlos Bellot-Arcís, José María Montiel-Company and José Manuel Almerich-Silla
Stomatology Department, University of Valencia
Spain

1. Introduction

The main aim of orthodontic treatment is to correct malocclusion, in order, whenever possible, to achieve functionally appropriate occlusion and optimum dental and facial aesthetics. To understand what malocclusion is, first we need to define its antonyms, in other words, what is meant by normal occlusion and ideal occlusion. Normal occlusion can be said to be that which meets certain predefined standards.

Edward Hartley Angle (1899) took the first permanent molars as the reference point and established the precise relations between the two dental arches that could be considered "norm-occlusion". "Normal occlusion" was thus defined as a concrete goal that the orthodontist should aim for in order to achieve a structural, functional and aesthetic norm (Canut, 1988). Since Angle's days, normal occlusion and ideal occlusion have been treated as synonyms in orthodontics, giving rise to both semantic and treatment difficulties. Nevertheless, from the statistical point of view the term "normal" implies a certain variation around the mean, while "ideal" implies a concept of perfection as the hypothetical aim (Bravo, 2003).

The occlusal norms that all orthodontists, over many years of professional practice, had borne in mind when deciding their clinical objectives were set out by Andrews (1972) in an article describing the six keys to normal occlusion. He later changed the adjective "normal" occlusion to "optimal" occlusion, arguing that he had used the word "normal" in the sense of optimal or ideal, as was often the case in the 1970s, and that normal occlusion was more correctly called "non-optimal occlusion".

"Orthodontic treatment need" can be defined as the degree to which a person needs orthodontic treatment because of certain features of his or her malocclusion, the functional, dental health or aesthetic impairment it occasions and the negative psychological and social repercussions to which it gives rise.

Throughout the history of orthodontics, there have been authors who have considered that malocclusion can lead to other problems, such as functional problems, temporomandibular dysfunction, and a greater propensity to trauma, caries, or periodontal disease. However, nowadays it is not so evident that these processes or diseases constitute indications for orthodontic treatment. Generally speaking, the psychological and social implications of poor dentofacial aesthetics can be more serious than the biological problems, and in clinical trials, strong correlations have been found between dental aesthetics, treatment need and the severity of the malocclusion (Lewis et al., 1982). Hamdam (2004) concluded that 40% of the patients who underwent orthodontic treatment had been the butt of jokes because of their teeth. However, there was no association between the degree of orthodontic treatment need measured by an objective index (IOTN DHC) and the need perceived by the patients. Kiekens et al. (2006) concluded that what the patients hope for from orthodontic treatment is an improvement in their dentofacial aesthetics and, as a result, greater social acceptance and higher self-esteem. Because of this, in recent decades orthodontists have been increasingly directing their treatments towards improving facial aesthetics.

Strictly speaking, malocclusion is not an illness but an occlusal relationship that lies within the bounds of all the possible occlusal relationships. Deciding the exact point at which a specific malocclusion should be treated remains an open question among orthodontists and the subject of considerable debate in the literature, as owing to its nature, reaching a general consensus is proving really complicated.

The WHO (World Health Organization) defines health as "a state of complete physical, mental and social well-being and not merely the absence of disease or infirmity". Consequently, a person cannot be considered completely healthy if a malocclusion prevents him or her from attaining this state of complete well-being, whether for physical (functional impairment) or psycho-social reasons (serious impairment of self-esteem or dentofacial aesthetics).

Disease does not always entail the absence of well-being, and even when well-being is absent this depends to a large extent on the patient's psychological state and personal and cultural principles and values. While clinical indices are concerned to measure the "disease", a purely biological concept, as objectively as possible, the indices that attempt to measure and determine "health" are very subjective, as health is a more psychological or sociological concept (Bernabé & Flores-Mir, 2006).

It should be emphasized that there is a lack of agreement on what is or is not considered malocclusion, and even greater disagreement when determining the orthodontic treatment need. However, enormous progress in this direction has been made in recent years, with important areas of consensus being reached among the specialists concerning specific situations in which orthodontic treatment should be recommended. The rapid development of indices to measure malocclusion and orthodontic treatment need have unquestionably contributed to these advances.

2. Using indices to measure malocclusion

2.1 Definition of "index"

Indices are quantitative assessment tools, employing continuous or numbered scales of malocclusion for epidemiological purposes and for a number of administrative applications.

An orthodontic treatment need index assigns a specific score to each malocclusion feature according to that feature's relative contribution to the overall severity of the malocclusion.

Each occlusal feature measured by a particular index is assigned a quantitative value or specific weight based on personal clinical concepts, consensus among specialists, reviews of the literature, social and administrative needs or scientific studies designed specifically for this purpose, hence the great variety of very different indices for recording malocclusion, which can have many uses.

Occlusal indices decide the need for treatment from the point of view of the orthodontist but tend to ignore the patients' own perceptions of their malocclusion and the repercussions it has in their daily lives, not only from a functional point of view but also on their looks, which undoubtedly have an effect on their social relationships. The traditional indices do not give any type of information on how the malocclusion affects the patients' lives from the psychosocial or functional point of view. These aspects seem to have become particularly important in recent years (Kok et al., 2004).

2.2 History, evolution, classification and properties of treatment need indices

Attempts to classify dentofacial disharmony date back to the beginning of the 19th century, to authors such as Joseph Fox (1776-1816), Christophe François Delabarre (1784-1862), Jean Nicolas Marjolin (1780-1850), Friedrich Christoph Kneisel (1797-1847) or Georg Carabelli (1787-1842). It was not until 1899, however, that Edward Hartley Angle (1855-1930) developed a clear, simple, practical classification that became universally accepted and used. Nonetheless, this index has evident limitations from the epidemiological point of view.

Angle's classification has been followed by many others. That of Lischer (1912) was similar but introduced the terms neutrocclusion (Angle Class I), mesiocclusion (Angle Class III) and distocclusion (Angle Class II). Simon (1922) proposed a classification that sets out the relation between the dental arches by reference to the three anatomical planes, based on different points on the skull. Dewey and Anderson (1942) published a book in which they extended Angle's classification to include five types of Class I malocclusion and three types of Class III malocclusion, known as the Dewey-Anderson Modification. The classification of Ackerman and Proffit (1969) was intended to overcome Angle's main weaknesses; however, it is more of a diagnostic procedure for listing the problems in each case of malocclusion in order to assist the clinician in drawing up a treatment plan.

All the methods described so far are qualitative and serve to describe and classify a patient's malocclusion. However, countries that have health services which offer orthodontic treatment have developed and applied a series of quantitative methods (malocclusion indices) to detect the severity and treatment need of each case, in an attempt to define the priority of some cases over others objectively and thus rationalize their public expenditure.

Tang and Wei (1993) reviewed the literature and summarized the evolution of methods for recording malocclusion in recent decades. They concluded that the trend in both qualitative and quantitative methods has changed, as initially researchers did not define the signs of malocclusion before recording them, chose the variables arbitrarily and recorded the data according to a criterion of all or nothing. This has now changed and a study of the progress in occlusal recording methods shows that they are increasingly accurate, reliable and scientifically-based, and consequently their detection of the problems possesses greater validity.

According to Richmond et al. (1997), an orthodontic index should consist of a numerical scale obtained by considering specific features of the malocclusion, making it possible to determine certain parameters such as treatment need or the severity of malocclusion in an objective way.

In 1966 the World Health Organization (WHO) defined the three characteristics that an index should possess: reliability, validity and validity over time.

There is wide agreement that an orthodontic treatment need index should possess the following characteristics:

- **Validity:** an index is said to be valid if it measures what it aims to measure. If a problem exists, it must detect it exactly and without error. In other words, it must identify the patients with the most detrimental malocclusions or those who would most benefit from treatment.
- **Objectivity:** the index design must attempt as far as possible to exclude examiner subjectivity.
- **Reliability (accuracy or reproducibility):** this is the degree of match between the results obtained when an index is applied to the same sample by different examiners or by the same examiner on different occasions.
- **Simplicity:** it must be able to be used by non-specialists. It must be capable of distinguishing between benign malocclusions that do not require treatment and more serious cases that need to be treated by a specialist.
- **Flexibility:** an index must be easily modified over time in the light of new research, discoveries or considerations.
- **Appropriate assessment of the aesthetic component of the malocclusion.**

Prahl-Andersen (1978) described the features that in his opinion an orthodontic treatment need index should possess. He emphasized that an index should not establish treatment priorities solely on the basis of the severity of the malocclusion and the functional problems that it could entail. It should also assess the degree to which the malocclusion occasions aesthetic impairment. In the medical field, a person's health should be judged on three criteria: objective signs (the orthodontist's diagnosis), subjective symptoms (the patient must recognize the problem) and social sufficiency (social attitudes).

Shaw et al. (1995) highlighted the following uses of the indices:

- Classifying, planning and promoting treatment standards.
- Assisting dentists and pediatric dentists to identify patients with orthodontic treatment need.
- Identifying patient prognoses and obtaining the patients' informed consent, informing them of the risks and treatment stability in both severe and borderline cases.
- Assessing the difficulty of the treatment that a particular patient must follow.
- Assessing the results of the treatment.

Throughout the history of orthodontics, indices have been developed to record malocclusions. Abdullah and Rock (2001) considered that most of them must have been developed with the following aims:

- To classify malocclusions in order to allow and facilitate communication between professionals.
- To compile a database to facilitate epidemiological studies.
- To classify cases according to the complexity of their treatment.
- To determine treatment needs and priorities.
- To identify the aesthetic aspects that affect treatment need.

It must not be forgotten that orthodontic treatment need indices, or at least most of them, are designed to determine treatment priority, in other words, to choose the potential patients who will most benefit from orthodontic treatment in a particular health service system.

In Europe, occlusal indices to estimate treatment need have been being used successfully since the end of the 1980s. The indices employed have generally been those developed by european authors but there has been no unanimity as regards which method to employ.

The controversy that surrounds orthodontic treatment need indices is such that in the United States, in 1969 the American Orthodontic Society adopted and recommended the *Salzmann Index* for estimating the treatment needs of the population but withdrew its recommendation in 1985 and currently does not recognize any index as more suitable than any other for this purpose (Parker, 1998).

Many very different indices have been developed to classify and group malocclusions according to severity or level of treatment need.

3. Principal treatment need indices

The *Malalignment Index* was developed by Van Kirk (1959) because he considered that there was no way of classifying patients objectively according to their tooth or bone malalignment. In this index, each tooth is given a score between 0 and 2 depending on its degree of rotation or displacement compared to the ideal position in the dental arch.

The state of New York started its Dental Rehabilitation Program in 1945 and one of the main problems was to select the patients who would receive orthodontic treatment. As a result, Draker (1960) developed and published *Handicapping Labio-lingual Deviation* (HLD) with the aim of determining orthodontic treatment need. This index assesses 7 criteria (displacement, crowding, overjet, increased overbite, open bite, anterior crossbite and ectopic eruptions) exclusively in the anterior sector, and also takes malformations into account. It can be applied both to models and to examinations of the mouth. When the scores for all the criteria total over 13, the subject is considered to present a physical malocclusion that needs treatment.

The *Treatment Priority Index* (TPI) was developed by Grainger (1967). This index is based on an assessment of ten occlusal features measured in a representative sample of 375 children of 12 years of age, of Anglo-Saxon origin, all without previous orthodontic treatment. The children were examined directly by orthodontic specialists. The patient is considered to need treatment when the scores for the ten occlusal features total over 4.5. A further eleventh feature is only considered in special cases (cleft palate or dysmorphism caused by traumatic injury) in which treatment is a priority. TPI has been used in many studies and although the results have not always been regular, it has proved to give high intra-examiner and inter-examiner reproducibility and reasonably good validity. However, it requires a certain degree of knowledge and experience on the part of the examiner.

Howitt et al. (1967) developed one of the first indices to consider the aesthetic aspects of malocclusion: the *Eastman Esthetic Index* (EEI). In spite of its innovation in measuring the degree of aesthetic impact associated with the malocclusion, it has not achieved such widespread use as other indices.

Salzmann (1967) was one of the first authors to be truly concerned about the patients' own perception of their malocclusion and about the impact and importance of orthodontics, and even of malocclusion, in society. As a result, he published the *Handicapping Malocclusion Assessment Record* (HMAR) index (Salzmann, 1968). The aim was to assess the patients' orthodontic treatment need, classifying the individuals examined according to the level of severity of the problem. This is considered an index with high reproducibility, as it does not use millimetrical measurements but concerns itself with determining functional problems that genuinely constitute an obstacle to the maintenance of oral health and interfere with the patients' proper development owing to their effect on dentofacial aesthetics, mandibular function or speech.

Summers (1971) published the *Occlusal Index* after observing the lack of consensus among orthodontic specialists. This index attempts to classify individuals as objectively as possible and presents clearly epidemiological characteristics. It measures nine occlusal features. Its main distinguishing feature is that it takes the patient's age into account.

Bjork et al. (1964) developed a method with clearly defined variables that can be recorded with good inter-examiner agreement. Based on this method, in 1969 a group of scientists from the World Dental Federation (FDI) Commission on Classification and Statistics of Oral Conditions-Measures of Occlusal Traits (COCSTC-MOT) analyzed the problem of determining occlusal status and developing recording systems for epidemiological purposes. The *Method for Measuring Occlusal Traits* was subsequently developed. This was adopted in 1972 by the FDI (1973) and modified by COCSTC-MOT in collaboration with the WHO, giving rise in 1979 to the final version of the "WHO/FDI Basic Method for Recording of Malocclusion", published in the Bulletin of the WHO (1979). The basic aims of this method, which follows clearly defined criteria, are to determine the prevalence of malocclusion and estimate the treatment needs of the population as a basis for planning orthodontic services.

The *Dental Aesthetic Index* (DAI) created by Cons et al. (1986), is unlike other indices in that the authors based it on the public's perception of dental aesthetics. This index has been used very successfully in numerous studies to assess the prevalence of malocclusion and the orthodontic treatment needs of different population groups. It will be discussed in greater detail in the next section.

The *Index of Orthodontic Treatment Need* (IOTN) described by Brook and Shaw (1989) has achieved widespread recognition both nationally and internationally as an objective method for determining treatment need. This index classifies the patients according to both the degree to which the malocclusion affects their stomatognathic system and their aesthetic perception of their own malocclusion, with the aim of identifying which patients would benefit most from orthodontic treatment (Uçüncü & Ertugay, 2001). A more detailed description is given in section 5.

The *Peer Assessment Rating* (PAR) is a more recent index, developed in Europe in 1992 by Richmond et al. (1992). In their article, the authors explained that it would be very helpful for orthodontists to have an index which would enable them to assess the results on completing the treatment. They considered that the indices developed up to that point lacked sufficient reproducibility and validity. The PAR makes it possible to compare the success of orthodontic treatments and also to predict the severity of cases. To develop this rating, 10 orthodontic specialists assessed 200 models and assigned a value to each of the 11 occlusal features they considered indispensable for evaluating the severity of a malocclusion. The total PAR score is the sum of each of the values of the different occlusal features. The success of a treatment is tested by measuring the PAR index before and after treatment and calculating the difference between the scores. The validity of the study was confirmed by another in which 74 dentists examined 272 dental models and assessed their deviation from the ideal on a scale of 1 to 9. They also calculated the PAR score for each of the models. The correlation between the professionals' opinion and the PAR score was r=0.74, showing that this index is a good predictor of subjective clinical assessment. Subsequently, its validity has also been corroborated by other authors (McGorray et al., 1999).

The latest index reported in the literature is the *Index of Complexity, Outcome and Need* (ICON) developed in 2000 by Daniels and Richmond (2002). Its aim is to bring assessment of need and of the results of orthodontic treatment together in a single index. Its development drew on 97 orthodontists from different countries who gave their subjective opinion of the treatment need, complexity of the treatment and improvement following treatment of 240 initial models and 98 treated models. The criteria employed are the five occlusal features that predicted the expert group's opinion and the IOTN AC (IOTN aesthetic component). Cut-off points were analyzed to determine at what point the index gave an accurate prediction of the specialists' decisions. Good results were obtained for accuracy (85%), sensitivity (85.2%) and specificity (84.4%).

4. Dental Aesthetic Index (DAI)

Cons et al. (1986) described and explained the Dental Aesthetic Index (DAI). The distinctive feature of the DAI is that it is an orthodontic index which relates the clinical and aesthetic components mathematically to produce a single score. It is based on the SASOC (Social Acceptability Scale of Occlusal Conditions) developed earlier by the same authors (Jenny et al., 1980).

The authors wanted to achieve a different index that would be based on the public's perception of dental aesthetics. This was determined through an evaluation of 200 photographs of different occlusal configurations. The 200 cases were chosen, by a random process, from a larger sample of 1337 study models used in a previous study. The 1337 models represented a population of half a million schoolchildren aged between 15 and 18 years from the state of New York. The 200 photographs employed as stimuli for the assessment of dental aesthetics were chosen through a process that ensured that even the most extreme cases were represented. Approximately 2000 adolescents and adults took part in rating the aesthetics of the 200 photographs, each of which showed the models' occlusion in front and side views. The presence and measurement of 49 occlusal features selected by an international committee as being those it was important to consider when developing an orthodontic index were taken into account for each photograph.

Regression analysis was employed to relate the public's assessment of dental aesthetics to the anatomical measurements of the occlusal features that were present in each photograph. This led to the choice of ten occlusal features as the most important ones to take into account in an orthodontic index, insofar as each of them affected the structures of the mouth and influenced dental aesthetics.

This study provided a statistical basis for establishing the value of the regression coefficients used for the ten occlusal features finally chosen for the regression calculations.

All the variables were adjusted in a linear regression model and a predictive equation called the DAI equation was obtained. In the DAI equation, the score for each of the ten DAI components is multiplied by its respective regression coefficient (weighting), the values are added together and a constant, 13, is added to the total. The result of this operation is the DAI score. The DAI equation is as follows:

Σ (DAI Component X Regression Coefficient) + 13

In the DAI equation the regression coefficients are usually rounded off, making it less precise but easier to apply, especially in epidemiological studies. The actual and rounded regression coefficients and constant are shown in Table 1.

The way to measure the ten DAI components correctly is as follows:

1. Number of missing visible teeth (incisors, canines, and premolars in the maxillary and mandibular arches). These are only taken into account if they affect the dental aesthetics, so if the space is closed, if eruption of the permanent tooth is expected or if the missing tooth has been replaced by a dental prosthesis, they should not be counted as missing visible teeth.
2. Assessment of crowding in the incisal segments. The aim is to calculate the existing crowding in the upper anterior and lower anterior sextants. The crowding discrepancy is not measured numerically but only as being present or absent. As a result the score will be 0 if there is no crowding, 1 if there is maxillary or mandibular crowding or 2 if the crowding affects both jaws.
3. Assessment of spacing in the incisal segments. In this case the space between the canines is greater than that required to accommodate the four incisors in a correct alignment. If one or more incisors has a proximal surface without interdental contact, the incisal segment is recorded as spaced. The score will be 0 if there is no spacing, 1 if there is maxillary or mandibular spacing or 2 if the spacing affects both jaws.
4. Measurement of any midline diastema in millimeters. Diastema is a very important occlusal feature from an aesthetic point of view. The midline diastema is defined as the space in millimeters between the two central permanent maxillary incisors when the points of contact are in their normal position.

5. Largest anterior irregularity on the maxilla in millimeters. The largest irregularity, again in millimeters, is measured according to the degree of vestibular-lingual displacement of each tooth in the anterior area of the maxillary arch. As the real crowding discrepancy cannot be measured in terms of millimeters of crowding without taking plaster models, which is not feasible in an epidemiological study, the largest irregularity encountered is recorded.
6. Largest anterior irregularity on the mandible in millimeters. The largest anterior irregularity is measured in millimeters, as for the maxilla.
7. Measurement of anterior maxillary overjet in millimeters. The distance from the labio-incisal edge of the upper incisor to the vestibular surface of the lower incisor. A WHO-type periodontal probe held parallel to the occlusal plane is employed for this measurement.
8. Measurement of anterior mandibular overjet in millimeters. The distance from the incisal edge of the most prominent lower incisor to the labial surface of the corresponding upper incisor.
9. Measurement of vertical anterior openbite. This measures the vertical space between the upper and lower incisors in millimeters.
10. Assessment of anteroposterior molar relation; largest deviation from normal either left or right. The score will be 0 if the occlusal relation is Angle Class I, 1 if the mesial or distal deviation is less than one full cusp and 2 if the mesial or distal deviation is one full cusp or more.

	Regression Coefficients	
DAI components	**Actual weights**	**Rounded weights**
1. Number of missing visible teeth (incisors, canines, and premolars in the maxillary and mandibular arches).	5.76	6
2. Assessment of crowding in the incisal segments: 0 = no segments crowded;1 = 1 segment crowded; 2 = 2 segments crowded.	1.15	1
3. Assessment of spacing in the incisal segments: 0 = no segments spaced;1 = 1 segment spaced; 2 = 2 segments spaced.	1.31	1
4. Measurement of any midline diastema in mm.	3.13	3
5. Largest anterior irregularity on the maxilla in mm.	1.34	1
6. Largest anterior irregularity on the mandible in mm.	0.75	1
7. Measurement of anterior maxillary overjet in mm.	1.62	2
8. Measurement of anterior mandibular overjet in mm.	3.68	4
9. Measurement of vertical anterior openbite in mm.	3.69	4
10. Assessment of anteroposterior molar relation; largest deviation from normal either left or right, 0 = normal, 1 = 1/2 cusp either mesial or distal, 2 = 1 full cusp or more either mesial or distal.	2.69	3
CONSTANT	13.36	13

Table 1. Components of the DAI regression equation and their actual and rounded regression coefficients (weights).

Although the DAI was developed for permanent teeth, it can easily be adapted for mixed dentition by simply ignoring missing permanent teeth if these are expected to erupt during the normal time range.

Once the patient's score has been calculated, it can be located on a scale in order to determine its position in relation to the dental aesthetics that are socially most acceptable and least acceptable. The higher the DAI score, the further the occlusal relation is from socially accepted dental aesthetics and the more easily it can be detrimental to the patient.

The DAI has ranges of scores to determine the severity of the malocclusion. A DAI score of 25 or less represents normal occlusion or slight malocclusion. Scores between 26 and 30 indicate moderate malocclusion with questionable treatment need. From 31 to 35, the malocclusion is more serious and treatment is recommended. Scores of 36 or more show severe malocclusion for which treatment is definitely needed.

As mentioned above, although the DAI scale offers these ranges to determine treatment need the scores can be placed on a continuous scale. The continuous scale makes the DAI sufficiently sensitive to differentiate between cases with a greater or lesser need within the same degree of severity. The cutoff points to decide which malocclusions should be treated by the public health services can be modified in view of the available resources.

One of the advantages of the DAI is that it can be obtained in barely 2 minutes, without X-rays, through an oral examination carried out by a trained dental assistant.

DAI components	Component x R. weight	Total
1. Number of missing visible teeth (incisors, canines, and premolars in the maxillary and mandibular arches).	1 missing tooth x 6	6
2. Assessment of crowding in the incisal segments: 0 = no segments crowded;1 = 1 segment crowded; 2 = 2 segments crowded.	1 segment x 1	1
3. Assessment of spacing in the incisal segments: 0 = no segments spaced;1 = 1 segment spaced; 2 = 2 segments spaced.	0 segments x 1	0
4. Measurement of any midline diastema in mm.	0 mm x 3	0
5. Largest anterior irregularity on the maxilla in mm.	3 mm x 1	3
6. Largest anterior irregularity on the mandible in mm.	2 mm x 1	2
7. Measurement of anterior maxillary overjet in mm.	5 mm x 2	10
8. Measurement of anterior mandibular overjet in mm.	0 mm x 4	0
9. Measurement of vertical anterior openbite in mm.	0 mm x 4	0
10. Assessment of anteroposterior molar relation; largest deviation from normal either left or right, 0 = normal, 1 = 1/2 cusp either mesial or distal, 2 = 1 full cusp or more either mesial or distal.	2 (full cusp) x 3	6
Constant		13
DAI score		41

Table 2. This hypothetical case illustrates how the DAI is calculated with the rounded coefficients.

The score for the hypothetical case in Table 2 is 41, which would place the patient in the "orthodontic treatment needed" category.

4.1 Validity and reliability of the DAI

While developing the DAI and after their studies and subsequent publications, Jenny et al. (1993) considered that one of its characteristics was its high degree of validity.

The authors (Jenny & Cons, 1996) tested the reliability of the DAI when measured by trained assistants and found very high intra-class correlation. Although deep overbites that damage the soft tissues are not scored numerically in the DAI, these and other severe congenital conditions are easily recognized by trained personnel, who can refer such cases to orthodontic specialists.

The same authors found that while the acceptability of particular physical features of faces varied widely between different racial and cultural groups, that of dental characteristics remained far more constant among different cultures. This has made it possible to employ the DAI to assess malocclusions in different regions and countries, where it has shown itself to be a quick, simple, reliable index with a high level of validity.

A comparison of an evaluation of 1337 models by orthodontists with the results of the DAI found 88% agreement (Cons et al., 1986). In a prospective study conducted in Australia it was found that a DAI score that indicated treatment need was a good predictor of future orthodontic treatment (Lobb et al., 1994).

One important aspect of the DAI is that it can be measured by trained dental assistants, and this prior screening of the malocclusion severity levels from which patients can be treated reduces the number of first visits by orthodontists employed in public programs.

Numerous studies have suggested that the DAI can be applied universally without any need for modification or adaptation, allowing it to be used independently of the sample in which the study was conducted (Baca-Garcia et al., 2004).

Also, nowadays, the DAI has been included in the latest WHO oral health survey update (1997). The WHO's recommendation of this method for assessing dentofacial anomalies is a major step in its dissemination as a universal method for evaluating malocclusions.

5. IOTN (Index of Orthodontic Treatment Need)

Peter Brook and William Shaw (1989) developed the Orthodontic Treatment Priority (OTP) index, which they later called the IOTN. It was based on a combination of the SCAN or Standardized Continuum of Aesthetic Need (Evans & Shaw, 1987) and the index employed by the Swedish Dental Health Board. The IOTN was subsequently modified by Richmond et al. (1992) and Lunn et al. (1993).

The IOTN consists of two separate components, the aesthetic component (AC) and the dental health component (DHC). It is a method that attempts to determine the degree of malocclusion of a particular patient and that patient's perception of his or her own malocclusion. The novel feature of the IOTN compared to other indices was that it was the first to include a sociopsychological indicator of treatment need.

The two components are analyzed separately and while they cannot be unified to give a single score, they can be combined to classify the patient as needing or not needing orthodontic treatment.

From the start, the authors wanted their index to have two separate components, one to assess the aesthetic impact of the malocclusion and another for the present or potential dental health and functional indications. They also wanted each occlusal feature that contributes to the greater or lesser longevity of the stomatognathic system to be precisely defined, with easily detected and measured levels of severity and cutoff points between them.

Owing to the difficulty in determining the relative contribution of each feature to dental health, the index has to be flexible so that it can be adapted in the light of future research and discoveries.

5.1 The DHC (Dental Health Component) of the IOTN

The DHC (Dental Health Component) is the clinical or dental health component of the IOTN. It is the result of a modification of the index used by the Swedish Dental Health Board (Linder-Aronson, 1974).

The salient feature of this component of the IOTN is that it classifies patients into five distinct grades with clear cutoff points between each, defined according to the occlusal features of each patient and the contribution of each feature to the longevity of the stomatognathic system. In other words, it classifies the occlusal findings that represent the greatest threat to good oral health and function into different grades. Also, it can be obtained directly from examination of the patient or from study models.

One of the main features of this index is that it is not cumulative: it only takes into account the most severe occlusal feature and classifies the patient directly into the appropriate grade. In the same way, it largely ignores the cumulative effect of less severe occlusal features and, consequently, can undervalue certain malocclusions in some individuals.

The DHC has five grades, from Grade 1 (no need for treatment) to Grade 5 (very great need for treatment).

Index of Orthodontic Treatment Need Dental Health Component (IOTN DHC), (Brook & Shaw, 1989).

Grade 5 (Very great)

- Defects of cleft lip and palate and other craniofacial anomalies.
- Increased overjet greater than 9 mm.
- Reverse overjet greater than 3.5 mm with reported masticatory and speech difficulties.
- Impeded eruption of teeth (with exception of third molars) due to crowding displacement, the presence of supernumerary teeth, retained deciduous teeth, and any pathological cause.
- Extensive hypodontia with restorative implications (more than one tooth missing in any quadrant) requiring pre-restorative orthodontics.

Grade 4 (Great)

- Increased overjet greater than 6 mm but less than or equal to 9 mm.

- Reverse overjet greater than 3.5 mm with no reported masticatory or speech difficulties.
- Reverse overjet greater than 1 mm but less than or equal to 3.5 mm with reported masticatory or speech difficulties.
- Anterior or posterior crossbites with greater than 2 mm displacement between retruded contact position and intercuspal position.
- Posterior lingual crossbite with no functional occlusal contact in one or both buccal segments.
- Severe displacement of teeth greater than 4 mm.
- Extreme lateral or anterior open bite greater than 4 mm.
- Increased and complete overbite causing notable indentations on the palate or labial gingivae.
- Less extensive hypodontia requiring prerestorative orthodontics or orthodontic space closure to obviate the need for a prosthesis (not more than 1 tooth missing in any quadrant).

Grade 3 (moderate)

- Increased overjet greater than 3.5 mm but less than or equal to 6 mm with incompetent lips at rest.
- Reverse overjet greater than 1 mm but less than or equal to 3.5 mm.
- Increased and complete overbite with gingival contact but without indentations or signs of trauma.
- Anterior or posterior crossbites with less than or equal to 2 mm but greater than 1 mm discrepancy between retruded contact position and intercuspal position.
- Moderate lateral or anterior open bite greater than 2 mm but less than or equal to 4 mm.
- Moderate displacement of teeth greater than 2 mm but less than or equal to 4 mm.

Grade 2 (little)

- Increased overjet greater than 3.5 mm but less than or equal to 6 mm with lips competent at rest.
- Reverse overjet greater than 0 mm but less than or equal to 1 mm.
- Increased overbite greater than 3.5 mm with no gingival contact.
- Anterior or posterior crossbite with less than or equal to 1 mm displacement between retruded contact position and intercuspal position.
- Small lateral or anterior open bites greater than 1 mm but less than or equal to 2 mm.
- Prenormal or postnormal occlusions with no other anomalies.
- Mild displacement oh teeth greater than 1 mm but less than or equal to 2 mm.

Grade 1 (None)

- Other variations in occlusion including displacement less than or equal to 1 mm.

Lunn et al. (1993) conducted a study to assess the use of the IOTN. They concluded that this index is a very valid tool for public administration purposes but suggested the need for certain modifications to make it quicker and easier to use.

Their suggestions included reducing the number of IOTN DHC grades to three in order to improve its reliability. These proposals were accepted by the Manchester team that had developed the IOTN.

- DHC 1-2 Little or no need for treatment
- DHC 3 Moderate need for treatment
- DHC 4-5 Great need for treatment

These modifications make it much easier to determine the treatment need of a population.

Burden et al. (2001) then proposed a further modification specifically for epidemiological studies, reducing the number of grades to two to make the IOTN DHC easier to use and to increase its validity and reliability.

- DHC 1-2-3 No need for treatment
- DHC 4-5 Need for treatment

They also decided to use the acronym MOCDO (Missing teeth, Overjet, Crossbites, Displacement of contact points, Overbite) to speed up the process and select the patients that need treatment.

This simplifies training and use. According to this modification, those with the following conditions need treatment:

- M (missing teeth): Hypodontia requiring prerestorative orthodontics or space closure. Impeded eruption of teeth. The presence of supernumerary teeth or retained deciduous teeth.
- O (overjet): Overjet greater than 6 millimeters. Reverse overjet greater than 3.5 millimeters without masticatory or speech difficulties. Reverse overjet greater than 1 millimeter but less than or equal to 3.5 millimeters with masticatory or speech difficulties.
- C (crossbites): Anterior or posterior crossbites with more than 2 millimeters displacement between retruded contact position and maximum intercuspal position.
- D (Displacement of contact points): Displacement of contact points greater than 4 millimeters.
- O (Overbite): Lateral or anterior open bite greater than 4 millimeters. Deep overbite causing gingival or palatal traumatic injury.

For the reasons mentioned above this modified IOTN is recommended for epidemiological studies, although it is not useful for administrative purposes because, having only two grades, the patients cannot be classified on a scale of malocclusion severity, so it is more difficult to adjust the resources to the needs.

5.2 The AC (Aesthetic Component) of the IOTN

Since one of the main reasons for undergoing orthodontic treatment is aesthetic, it was considered that the aesthetic component ought to be represented in a diagnostic tool or an index (Alkhatib et al., 2005) and that the patients' perception of their own malocclusion needed to be taken into account.

The aesthetic component (AC) employs the SCAN Index (Evans & Shaw, 1987). It consists of an illustrated scale showing ten grades of dental aesthetics and is employed to determine each patient's aesthetic perception of his or her own malocclusion. To design this index, 1000 intraoral photographs of 12-year-old children were collected and placed in order after a lengthy study (Brook & Shaw, 1989). The photographs were rated by six non-dental judges. The result was a scale of ten black and white photographs showing different levels of dental attractiveness, ranging from photograph 1, the most aesthetic, to number 10, the least aesthetic (Uçüncü & Ertugay, 2001).

The patient has to look at his or her mouth in a mirror and identify it with one of the ten photographs in the scale. In this way, each patient's perception of his or her malocclusion can be observed.

To make the IOTN quicker and easier to use and improve its reliability, Lunn et al. (1993) proposed reducing the number of IOTN AC grades from 10 to 3. These proposals were accepted by the Manchester team that had developed the IOTN.

- AC 1-4 Little or no need for treatment
- AC 5-7 Moderate need for treatment
- AC 8-10 Great need for treatment

Nowadays, for practical and epidemiological purposes only two grades are considered: patients who identify with photographs 1 to 7 do not need treatment, while those who identify with photographs 8 to 10 do need treatment. It should be pointed out that in most cases, almost no patients identify their own teeth with the great orthodontic treatment need group (photographs 8-10). It is also considered to be no easy task for patients to decide which of the 10 photographs most resemble their own teeth, especially when they are very young.

In practice, the two components of the IOTN are determined separately and an individual is considered to need treatment if the IOTN DHC grade is 4 or 5 or the IOTN AC is in the grades 8-10 group. In either of these two situations the child needs orthodontic treatment for either dental health reasons (DHC) or for exclusively aesthetic reasons (AC). However, according to the modified IOTN developed by Burden et al. (2001), when this is employed in epidemiological studies both components are required, in other words, DHC grades 4-5 and AC grades 8-10.

5.3 Validity and reliability of the IOTN

When designing and testing the IOTN, Brook and Shaw (1989) observed that the reproducibility of this index was particularly good when measured under suitable conditions, and slightly less good when measured, for example, in schools.

Richmond et al. (1995) confirmed the validity and reliability of the IOTN in a study in which 74 dentists and orthodontists assessed the treatment need of a total of 256 models of orthodontic patients representing all types of malocclusion. The Spearman coefficient for the aesthetic component was 0.84 and that of the dental health component was 0.64.

Brook and Shaw claim good intra- and inter-examiner reproducibility when the IOTN AC is assessed by a dentist. However, according to Holmes (1992), the patients' perception tends to be more optimistic than that of the professionals. Nevertheless, the use of the IOTN AC has been the subject of some controversy in recent years. This is because of the lack of correlation between the dental health component (DHC) and the aesthetic component (AC), as found by Soh and Sandham (2004) in a study of an adult Asian population and by Hassan (2006) in a region of Saudi Arabia. Also, some authors such as Svedström-Oristo et al. (2009) have described certain problems when asking patients, both children and young adults, to identify their mouths with one of the 10 photographs employed as stimuli.

According to Alkhatib et al. (2005), the IOTN is not only valid and reliable but is also sensitive to the needs of patients and accepted both by the patients themselves and by the professionals who employ it. Hamdam (2004) confirmed the validity and reliability of the IOTN. Mandall et al. (2000) and Birkeland et al. (1996) concluded that it is a reproducible and reliable index.

A recent study by Johansson and Follin (2009) showed that the clinical criterion employed by 272 Swedish orthodontists was in good agreement with the results of the IOTN DHC. The main differences were found in IOTN grade 3, as the orthodontists considered most of the malocclusions in this grade to be in need of treatment.

However, O'Brien et al. (1993) found large differences in the choice of the different grades of need in both the DHC and the AC. Turbill et al. (1996) concluded that the IOTN is essentially an epidemiological index that has limitations when assessing the treatment needs of individual patients.

The IOTN is currently employed in the United Kingdom for prioritizing public orthodontic care services. Its reliability and validity have been extensively proved, it is simple and easy to use, and it is also one of the most-often cited indices in the literature.

6. The epidemiology of treatment need

Appropriate assessment and measurement of malocclusions is essential in epidemiological studies in order to ascertain the prevalence and incidence of occlusal alterations among the population. There are certainly many indices and measures for assessing malocclusion, but the DAI and the IOTN are the best known and most widely used owing to their manageability and proven validity.

Tables 3 and 4 show a number of malocclusion prevalence studies conducted since the year of publication of each of these indices up to the present.

On examining the main studies it will be seen that both the DAI and the IOTN have been used to a greater extent in cross-sectional studies with large samples, generally randomly selected, although it will be observed that they meet the requirements for epidemiological or prevalence studies. While the IOTN is used to a greater extent in Europe, The DAI is employed to a similar extent throughout the world, though least in Europe. However, whereas the IOTN is employed more in child/adolescent populations, the DAI is more often employed in adolescent/adult ones.

As noted above, comparison between the different studies is very complicated. The first reason is that they employ different methods and their data collection criteria are sometimes not sufficiently well explained. Examination of the studies shows that they use different indices, so although they measure the same condition (malocclusion prevalence or treatment need), they do not measure it in the same way or consider the same occlusal features. Obviously, also, the different studies were conducted in different populations, with differing sample sizes, ages and geographical origins. For all these reasons, it is posible to make comparisons but prudence is required when drawing conclusions. Epidemiological studies of malocclusion prevalence and orthodontic treatment need in large, representative samples continue to be necessary in order to effect more rigorous comparisons.

Authors (publication year)	Country	n	Age	DHC(4-5)	AC(8-10)
Brook and Shaw (1989)	United Kingdom	222	11-12	32.7%	5.4%
So and Tang (1993)	Hong Kong	100	19-20	53%	-
So and Tang (1993)	China	100	20	52%	-
Burden and Holmes (1994)	United Kingdom	874 955	11-12	31% 32%	12% 8.5%
Tuominen et al. (1995)	Finland	89	16-19	11.2%	-
Tang and So (1995)	Hong Kong	105	18-22	54.2%	-
Birkeland et al. (1996)	Norway	359	11	26.1%	9%
Otuyemi et al. (1997)	Nigeria	704	12-18	12.6%	-
Riedmann and Berg (1999)	Germany	88	20	60.2%	60%
Tickle et al. (1999)	United Kingdom	7888	14	26.2%	-
Cooper et al. (2000)	United Kingdom	142	19	21%	12.8%
Kerosuo et al. (2000)	Finland	281	18-19	15%	0%
Cooper et al. (2000)	United Kingdom	314	11	34%	4%
Johnson et al. (2000)	New Zealand	294	10	31.3%	3.8%
Mandall et al. (2000)	United Kingdom	434	14-15	18%	6%
Uçüncü y Ertugay (2001)	Turkey	250	11-14	38.8%	4.8%
Abdullah and Rock (2001)	Malaysia	5112	12-13	30%	-
Hamdam (2001)	Jordan	320	14-17	28	-
Hunt et al. (2002)	United Kingdom	215	17-43	-	2.8%
De Olivera and Sheiham (2003)	Brazil	1675	15-16	22%	-
Klages et al. (2004)	Germany	148	18-30	-	0%
Flores-Mir et al. (2004)	Canada	329	18-20	-	2%
Soh and Sandham (2004)	Singapore	339	17-22	50.1 %	29.2%
Kerosuo et al. (2004)	Kuwait	139	14-18	28.1%	1.4%
Abu Alhaija et al. (2004)	Jordan	1002	12-14	34%	-
Tausche et al. (2004)	Germany	1975	6-8	26.2%	21.5%
Mugonzibwa et al. (2004)	Tanzania	386	9-18	22%	11%
Hamdam (2004)	Jordan	103	15	71%	16.7%
Kerosuo et al. (2004)	Kuwait	139	14-18	28%	2%
Hlonga et al. (2004)	Tanzania	643	15-16	3-13%	-
Soh et al. (2005)	Singapore	339	17-22	50.1%	29.2%
Alkhatib et al. (2005)	United Kingdom	3500	12-14	15%	2.1%
Mandall et al. (2005)	United Kingdom	525	11-12	44.8%	2.7%
Klages et al. (2006)	Germany	194	18-30	-	8.8%

Authors (publication year)	Country	n	Age	DHC(4-5)	AC(8-10)
Bernabé and Flores-Mir (2006b)	Peru	281	16-25	29.9%	1.8%
Hassan (2006)	Saudi Arabia	743	17-24	71.6%	16.1%
Souames et al. (2006)	France	511	9-12	21.3%	7%
Chestnutt et al. (2006)	United Kingdom	2595 2142	12 15	35% 21%	- -
Nobile et al. (2007)	Italy	1000	11-15	59.5%	3.2%
Ngom et al. (2007)	Senegal	665	12-13	42.6%	3.3%
Manzanera et al. (2009)	Spain	665	12 15-16	21.8% 17.1%	4.4% 2.4%
Svedström-Oristo et al. (2009)	Finland	434	16-25	-	2%
Puertes-Fernández et al. (2010)	Algeria	248	12	18.1%	13.7%
Hassan and Amin (2010)	Saudi Arabia	366	21-25	29.2%	-

Table 3. Studies of different populations using the IOTN (DHC/AC)

Authors (publication year)	Country	n	Age	Treatment Need (≥31)
Estioko et al. (1994)	Australia	268	12-16	24.1%
Katoh et al. (1998)	Japan Taiwan	1029 176	15-29 18-24	30.1% 25.9%
Otuyemi et al. (1999)	Nigeria	703	12-18	9.2%
Johnson et al. (2000)	New Zealand	294	10	55.4%
Chi et al. (2000)	New Zealand	150	10	47%
Abdullah and Rock (2001)	Malaysia	5112	12-13	24.1%
Esa et al. (2001)	Malaysia	1519	12-13	24.1%
Onyeaso et al. (2003)	Nigeria	64	16-45	48.4%
Baca-García et al. (2004)	Spain	744	14-20	21.1%
Onyeaso (2004)	Nigeria	136	6-18	50%
Onyeaso (2005)	Nigeria	577	12-17	22.7%
van Wyk and Drummond (2005)	South Africa	6142	12	31%
Frazão and Narvai (2006)	Brazil	13801	12-18	18%
Bernabé and Flores-Mir (2006a)	Peru	267	16-25	32.6%
Marques et al. (2007)	Brazil	600	13-15	53.3%
Hamamci et al. (2009)	Turkey	841	17-26	21.5%
Manzanera et al. (2010)	Spain	655	12 15-16	21.2% 16.1%
Puertes-Fernández et al. (2010)	Algeria	248	12	13.2%

Table 4. Studies of different populations using the DAI

7. Conclusions

Many very different indices have been developed for classifying malocclusions according to their severity or level of treatment need. Although a certain consensus has been reached on the features that the ideal index should possess, controversy continues over which should be used for this purpose.

Evidently, patients often seek orthodontic treatment but present considerable variations in malocclusion. The wide range of situations between ideal occlusion and very severe malocclusion make it very difficult to establish the precise limits of what should and should not be considered treatment need. Consequently, ascertaining the real malocclusion prevalence and establishing reliable comparisons concerning their frequency in different populations is by no means simple. Also, as there is also no unanimous criterion for deciding what to consider malocclusion, its real frequency cannot be established.

In this chapter we have presented a large number of orthodontic treatment need indices. However, the two indices that are currently most often used for epidemiological studies are the DAI and the IOTN. Hlonga et al. (2004) and Liu et al. (2011) have observed a significant correlation between the two indices. Nevertheless, high correlation does not necessarily imply high agreement (Manzanera et al., 2010). In epidemiological studies this is not a particularly important problem because both are valid methods for determining the orthodontic treatment need of a population, but when they are applied in individual cases, the choice of DAI or IOTN will lead to the appearance of both false negatives and false positives.

Comparison of these two indices finds similarities and differences. Both comprise two components, one anatomical and the other aesthetic, both measure occlusion features proposed by experts and both attempt to identify the individuals with the greatest treatment need in public programs. Although most of the features they measure are identical, each feature is rated differently in the two indices. The advantage of the DAI is that the aesthetic perception is linked to the anatomical assessment through regression analysis to produce a single score, whereas the IOTN has two components that cannot be unified. Also, the DAI offers a continuous scoring system, so it can classify different degrees of malocclusion within each of the pre-established levels. The IOTN cannot establish a continuous order within each grade, so it is more complicated to use for public health programs. In the DAI, unlike the IOTN, the occlusal features examined are different according to whether it is the primary dentition, mixed dentition or permanent dentition that is being measured, and since its design is more suitable for permanent teeth, it leads to the use of more than one epidemiological index.

It would appear, agreeing with some other authors, that DAI is more useful for administrative purposes, in other words, when the budget is limited and the patients must be placed in strict order of severity in order to give priority to those in most need of treatment. This is possible because the DAI scale is continuous, whereas the IOTN makes not distinctions within grades. The IOTN, however, being easily and quickly obtained, is more effective in epidemiological studies, to determine the percentage of the population in need of treatment without establishing priorities.

The great value that society sets on aesthetics nowadays, the importance that patients themselves ascribe to their malocclusions and the extent to which their condition affects their quality of life must not be forgotten. In recent years particular attention has been paid to surveys that attempt to measure the way in which malocclusion affects a person's quality of life; these include studies by De Baets et al. (2011), Liu et al. (2011) and Agou et al. (2011). Such surveys should be employed in decision-making as complementary tools to the different orthodontic treatment need indices.

8. References

Abdullah, M.S. & Rock, W.P. (2001). Assessment of orthodontic treatment need in 5,112 Malaysian children using the IOTN and DAI indices. *Community Dent Health*, Vol.18, No.4, pp. 242-248.

Abu Alhaija, E.S.; Al-Nimri, K.S. & Al-Khateeb, S.N. (2004). Orthodontic treatment need and demand in 12-14-year-old north Jordanian school children. *Eur J Orthod*, Vol.26, No.3, pp. 261-263.

Ackerman, J.L. & Proffit, W.R. (1969). Characteristics of malocclusion: a modern approach to classification and diagnosis. *Am J Orthod*, Vol.56, No.5, pp. 443-454.

Agou, S.; Locker, D.; Muirhead, V.; Tompson, B. & Streiner, D.L. (2011). Does psychological well-being influence oral-health-related quality of life reports in children receiving orthodontic treatment?. *Am J Orthod Dentofacial Orthop*, Vol.139, No.3, pp. 369-377.

Alkhatib, M.N.; Bedi, R.; Foster, C.; Jopanputra, P. & Allan, S. (2005). Ethnic variations in orthodontic treatment need in London schoolchildren. *BMC Oral Health*, 27;5:8.

Angle, E.H. (1899). Classification of malocclusion. *Dent Cosmos*, Vol.41, pp. 248-264.

Andrews, L.F. (1972). The six keys to normal occlusion. *Am J Orthod*, Vol.62, pp.296-309.

Baca-Garcia, A.; Bravo, M.; Baca, P.; Baca, A. & Junco, P. (2004). Malocclusions and orthodontic treatment needs in a group of Spanish adolescents using the Dental Aesthetic Index. *Int Dent J*, Vol.54, no.3, pp. 138-142.

Bernabé, E.; Flores-Mir, C. (2006a). Orthodontic treatment need in Peruvian young adults evaluated through dental aesthetic index. *Angle Orthod*, Vol.76, No.3, pp. 417-421.

Bernabé, E. & Flores-Mir, C. (2006b). Normative and self-perceived orthodontic treatment need of a Peruvian university population. *Head Face Med*, 3;2:22.

Birkeland, K.; Boe, O.E. & Wisth, P.J. (1996). Orthodontic concern among 11-year-old children and their parents compared with orthodontic treatment need assessed by index of orthodontic treatment need. *Am J Orthod Dentofacial Orthop*, Vol.110, No.2, pp. 197-205.

Björk, A.; Krebs A.A. & Solow, B. (1964). A method for epidemiological registration of malocclusion. *Acta Odontol Scand*, Vol.35, pp. 161-165.

Bravo, L.A. (2003). Naturaleza de la maloclusión y justificación del tratamiento ortodóncico, In: Manual de Ortodoncia, Bravo, L.A., pp. (25-52), Editorial Síntesis, Madrid.

Brook, P.H. & Shaw, W.C. (1989). The development of an index of orthodontic treatment priority. Europ J Orthod, Vol.11, pp. 309-320.

Burden, D.J. & Holmes, A. (1994). The need for orthodontic treatment in the child population of the United Kingdom. *Eur J Orthod*, Vol.16, No.5, pp.395-399.

Burden, D.J.; Pine, C.M. & Burnside, G. (2001). Modified IOTN: an orthodontic treatment need index for use in oral health surveys. *Community Dent Oral Epidemiol*, Vol.29, pp. 220-225.

Canut, J.A. (2 Ed.). (1988). Concepto de ortodoncia, In: *Ortodoncia clínica y terapéutica*, Canut, J.A., pp. (1-16), Masson, Barcelona.

Chestnutt, I.G.; Burden, D.J.; Steele, J.G.; Pitts, N.B.; Nuttall, N.M. & Morris, A.J. (2006). The orthodontic condition of children in the United Kingdom, 2003. *Br Dent J*, Vol.200, No.11, pp. 609-612.

Chi, J.; Johnson, M. & Harkness, M. (2000). Age changes in orthodontic treatment need: a longitudinal study of 10- and 13-year-old children, using the Dental Aesthetic Index. *Aust Orthod J*, Vol.16, No.3, pp. 150-156.

Cons, N.C.; Jenny, J. & Kohout, F.J. (1986). DAI: The Dental Aesthetic Index. Iowa City, Iowa: College of Dentistry, University of Iowa.

Cooper, S.; Mandall, N.A.; DiBiase, D. & Shaw, W.C. (2000). The reliability of the Index of Orthodontic Treatment Need over time. *J Orthod*, Vol.27, No.1, pp. 47-53.

Daniels, C. & Richmond, S. (2000). The development of the index of complexity, outcome and need (ICON). *J Orthod*, Vol. 27, No.2, pp. 149-162.

De Oliveira, C.M. & Sheiham, A. (2003). The relationship between normative orthodontic treatment need and oral health-related quality of life. *Community Dent Oral Epidemiol*, Vol.31, No.6, pp. 426-436.

De Baets, E.; Lambrechts, H.; Lemiere, J.; Diya, L. & Willems, G. (2011). Impact of self-esteem on the relationship between orthodontic treatment need and oral health-related quality of life in 11- to 16-year-old children. *Eur J Orthod*, [Epub ahead of print].

Draker, H.L. (1960). Handicapping labio-lingual deviation: A proposed index for public health purposes. *Am J Orthod*, Vol.46, pp. 295-305.

Dewey, M. & Anderson G.M. (6 Ed.). (1942). *Practical Orthodontics*, C.V. Mosby Company, St. Louis, Missouri.

Esa, R.; Razak, I.A. & Allister, J.H. (2001). Epidemiology of malocclusion and orthodontic treatment need of 12-13-year-old Malaysian schoolchildren. *Community Dent Health*, Vol.18, No.1, pp. 31-36.

Estioko, L.J.; Wright, F.A. & Morgan, M.V. (1994). Orthodontic treatment need of secondary schoolchildren in Heidelberg, Victoria: an epidemiologic study using the Dental Aesthetic Index. *Community Dent Health*, Vol.11, No.3, pp. 147-151.

Evans, M.R. & Shaw, W.C. (1987). Preliminary evaluation of an illustrated scale for rating dental attractiveness. *Eur J Orthod*, Vol.9, pp. 314-318.

Federation Dentaire Internationale (1973). A method for measuring occlusal traits, commission on classification and statistics for oral conditions. Working Group 2 on dentofacial anomalies, 1969-1972. *Int Dent J*, Vol.23, pp. 530-537.

Flores-Mir, C.; Major, P.W. & Salazar, F.R. (2004). Self-perceived orthodontic treatment need evaluated through 3 scales in a university population. *J Orthod*; Vol.31, No.4, pp. 329-334.

Frazão, P. & Narvai, P.C. (2006). Socio-environmental factors associated with dental occlusion in adolescents. *Am J Orthod Dentofacial Orthop*, Vol.129, No.6, pp. 809-816.

Grainger, R.M. (1967). Orthodontic Treatment priority index. *Vital Health Stat;* Vol.2, pp. 1-49.

Hamamci, N.; Başaran, G. & Uysal, E. (2009). Dental Aesthetic Index scores and perception of personal dental appearance among Turkish university students. *Eur J Orthod,* Vol.31, No.2, pp. 168-173.

Hamdan, A.M. (2001). Orthodontic treatment need in Jordanian school children. *Community Dent Health,* Vol.18, No.3, pp. 177-180.

Hamdan, A.M. (2004). The relationship between patient, parent and clinician perceived need and normative orthodontic treatment need. *Eur J Orthod,* Vol.26, No.3, pp. 265-271.

Hassan, A.H. (2006). Orthodontic treatment needs in the western region of Saudi Arabia: a research report. *Head Face Med,* 18;2:2.

Hassan, A.H. & Amin, Hel-S. (2010). Association of orthodontic treatment needs and oral health-related quality of life in young adults. *Am J Orthod Dentofacial Orthop,* Vol.137, No.1, pp. 42-47.

Hlongwa, P.; Beane, R.A.; Seedat, A.K. & Owen, C.P. (2004). Orthodontic treatment needs: comparison of two indices. *SADJ,* Vol.59, No.10, pp. 421-424.

Howitt, J.W.; Stricker, G. & Henderson, R. (1967). Eastman Esthetic Index. *N Y State Dent J,* Vol.33, No.4, pp. 215-220.

Hunt, O.; Hepper, P.; Johnston, C.; Stevenson, M. & Burden, D. (2002). The Aesthetic Component of the Index of Orthodontic Treatment Need validated against lay opinion. *Eur J Orthod,* Vol.24, No.1, pp. 53-59.

Jenny, J.; Cons, N.C.; Kohout, F.J. & Frazier, P.J. (1980). Test of a method to determine socially acceptable occlusal conditions. *Community Dent Oral Epidemiol,* Vol.8, No.8, pp. 424-433.

Jenny, J.; Cons, N.C.; Kohout, F.J. & Jakobsen, J. (1993). Predicting handicapping malocclusion using the Dental Aesthetic Index (DAI). *Int Dent J,* Vol.43, pp. 128-132.

Jenny, J. & Cons, N.C. (1996). Establishing malocclusion severity levels on the Dental Aesthetic Index (DAI) scale. *Australian Dent J,* Vol.41, pp. 43-46.

Johansson, A.M. & Follin, M.E. (2009). Evaluation of the Dental Health Component, of the Index of Orthodontic Treatment Need, by Swedish orthodontists. *Eur J Orthod,* Vol.31, No.2, pp. 184-188.

Johnson, M.; Harkness, M.; Crowther, P. & Herbison, P. (2000). A comparison of two methods of assessing orthodontic treatment need in the mixed dentition: DAI and IOTN. *Aust Orthod J,* Vol.16, No.2, pp. 82-87.

Katoh, Y.; Ansai, T. & Takehar, T. (1998). A comparison of DAI scores and characteristics of occlusal traits in three ethnic groups of Asian origin. *Int Dent J,* Vol.48, pp. 405-411.

Kerosuo, H.; Kerosuo, E., Niemi, M. & Simola, H. (2000). The need for treatment and satisfaction with dental appearance among young Finnish adults with and without a history of orthodontic treatment. *J Orofac Orthop,* Vol.61, No.5, pp. 330-340.

Kerosuo, H.; Al Enezi, S.; Kerosuo, E. & Abdulkarim, E. (2004). Association between normative and self-perceived orthodontic treat- ment need among Arab high school students. *Am J Orthod Dentofacial Orthop*, Vol.125, pp. 373-378.

Klages, U.; Bruckner, A. & Zentner, A. (2004). Dental aesthetics, self-awareness, and oral health-related quality of life in young adults. *Eur J Orthod*, Vol.26, No.5, pp. 507-514.

Klages, U.; Claus, N.; Wehrbein, H. & Zentner, A. (2006). Development of a questionnaire for assessment of the psychosocial impact of dental aesthetics in young adults. *Eur J Orthod*, Vol.28, No.2, pp. 103-111.

Kiekens, R.M.; Maltha, J.C.; van't Hof, M.A. & Kuijpers-Jagtman, A.M. (2006). Objective measures as indicators for facial esthetics in white adolescents. *Angle Orthod*, Vol.76, No.4, pp. 551-556.

Kok, Y.V.; Mageson, P.; Harradine, N.W. & Sprod, A.J. (2004). Comparing a quality of life measure and the Aesthetic Component of the Index of Orthodontic Treatment Need (IOTN) in assessing orthodontic treatment need and concern. *J Orthod*, Vol.31, No.4, pp. 312-318.

Lewis, E.A.; Albino, J.E.; Cunat, J.J. & Tudesco, L.A. (1982). Reliability and validity of clinical assessments of malocclusion. *Am J Orthod*, Vol.81, pp. 473-477.

Linder-Aronson, S. (1974). Orthodontics in the Swedish Public Dental Health System. Transactions of the European Orthodontic Society 233-240.

Liu, Z.; McGrath, C. & Hagg, U. (2011). Associations between orthodontic treatment need and oral health-related quality of life hmong young adults: does it dependo on how toy assess them? *Community Dent Oral Epidemiol*, Vol.39, pp. 137-144.

Lischer, B.E. (1912). Principles and methods of orthodontics. Lea & Febiger. Filadelfia, Pensilvannia.

Lobb, W.K.; Ismail, A.I.; Andrews, C.L. & Spracklin, T.E. (1994). Evaluation of orthodontic treatment using Dental Aesthetic Index. *Am J Othod Dentofac Othop*, Vol.106, No.1, pp. 70-75.

Lunn, H.; Richmond, S. & Mitropoulos, C. (1993). The use of the index of Orthodontic Treatment Need (IOTN) as a public health tool: a pilot study. *Community Dent Health*, Vol.10, pp. 111-121.

Mandall, N.A.; McCord, J.F.; Blinkhorn, A.S.; Worthington, H.V. & O'Brien, K.D. (2000). Perceived aesthetic impact of malocclusion and oral self-perceptions in 14-15-year-old Asian and Caucasian children in greater Manchester. *Eur J Orthod*, Vol.22, No.2, pp. 175-183.

Mandall, N.A.; Wright, J.; Conboy, F.; Kay, E., Harvey, L. & O'Brien, K.D. (2005). Index of orthodontic treatment need as a predictor of orthodontic treatment uptake. *Am J Orthod Dentofacial Orthop*, Vol.128, No.6, pp. 703-707.

Manzanera, D.; Montiel-Company, J.M.; Almerich-Silla, J.M. & Gandía, J.L. (2009). Orthodontic treatment need in Spanish schoolchildren: an epidemiological study using the Index of Orthodontic Treatment Need. *Eur J Orthod*, Vol.31, No.2, pp. 180-183.

Manzanera, D.; Montiel-Company, J.M.; Almerich-Silla, J.M. & Gandía, J.L. (2010). Diagnostic agreement in the assessment of orthodontic treatment need using the Dental Aesthetic Index and the Index of Orthodontic Treatment Need. *Eur J Orthod*, Vol.32, No.2, pp.193-198.

Marques, C.R.; Couto, G.B.; Orestes Cardoso, S. (2007). Assessment of orthodontic treatment needs in Brazilian schoolchildren according to the Dental Aesthetic Index (DAI). *Community Dent Health*, Vol.24, No.3, pp. 145-148.

McGorray, S.P.; Wheeler, T.T.; Keeling, S.D.; Yurkiewicz, L.; Taylor, M.G. & King, G.J. (1999). Evaluation of orthodontists´ perception of treatment need and the peer assessment rating (PAR) index. *The Angle Orthodontist*, Vol.69, No.4, pp. 325-333.

Mugonzibwa, E.A.; Kuijpers-Jagtman, A.M.; Van 't Hof, M.A. & Kikwilu, E.N. (2004). Perceptions of dental attractiveness and orthodontic treatment need among Tanzanian children. *Am J Orthod Dentofacial Orthop*, Vol. 125, No.4, pp. 426-433.

Nobile, C.G.; Pavia, M.; Fortunato, L. & Angelillo, I.F. (2007). Prevalence and factors related to malocclusion and orthodontic treatment need in children and adolescents in Italy. *Eur J Public Health*, Vol.17, No.6, pp. 637-641.

Ngom, P.I.; Diagne, F.; Dieye, F.; Diop-Ba, K. & Thiam, F. (2007). Orthodontic treatment need and demand in Senegalese school children aged 12-13 years. An appraisal using IOTN and ICON. *Angle Orthod*, Vol.77, No.2, pp. 323-330.

O´Brien, K.D.; Shaw, W.C. & Roberts, C.T. (1993). The use of occlusal indices in assessing the provision of orthodontic treatment by the hospital orthodontic service of England and Wales. *Br J Orthod*, Vol.20, pp.25-35.

Onyeaso, C.O.; Arowojolu, M.O. & Taiwo, J.O. (2003). Periodontal status of orthodontic patients and the relationship between dental aesthetic index and community periodontal index of treatment need. *Am J Orthod Dentofacial Orthop*, Vol.124, No.6, pp. 714-720.

Onyeaso, C.O. (2004). Orthodontic treatment need of Nigerian outpatients assessed with the Dental Aesthetic Index. *Aust Orthod J*, Vol.20, No.1, pp. 19-23.

Onyeaso, C.O. & Sanu, O.O. (2005). Perception of personal dental appearance in Nigerian adolescents. *Am J Orthod Dentofacial Orthop*, Vol.127, No.6, pp. 700-706.

Otuyemi, O.D.; Ugboko, V.I.; Adekoya-Sofowora, C.A. & Ndukwe, K.C. (1997). Unmet orthodontic treatment need in rural Nigerian adolescents. *Community Dent Oral Epidemiol*, Vol.25, No.5, pp. 363-366.

Otuyemi, O.D.; Ogunyinka, A.; Dosumu, O.; Cons, N.C. & Jenny, J. (1999). Malocclusion and orthodontic treatment need of secondary school students in Nigeria according to the dental aesthetic index (DAI). *Int Dent J*; Vol.49, No.4, pp. 203-210.

Parker, W.S. (1998). The HLD index and the index question. *Am J Orthod Dentofacial Orthop*; Vol.114, pp. 134-141.

Prahl-Andersen, B. (1978). The need for orthodontic treatment. *Angle Orthod*; Vol.48, No1. pp. 1-9.

Puertes-Fernández, N.; Montiel-Company, J.M.; Almerich-Silla, J.M. & Manzanera, D. (2010). Orthodontic treatment need in a 12-year-old population in the Western Sahara. *Eur J Orthod*, [Epub ahead of print].

Richmond, S.; Shaw, W.C.; O'Brien, K.D.; Buchanan, I.B.; Jones, R.; Stephens, C.D.; Roberts, C.T. & Andrews, M. (1992). The development of the PAR Index (Peer Assessment Rating): reliability and validity. *Europ J Orthod*, Vol.14, No.2, pp. 125-139.

Richmond, S.; Shaw, W.C.; O'Brien, K.D.; Buchanan, I.B.; Stephens, C.D.; Andrews, M. & Roberts, C.T. (1995). The relationship between the index of orthodontic treatment need and consensus opinion of a panel of 74 dentists. *Br Dent J*, Vol.178, pp. 370-374.

Richmond, S.; Daniels, C.P.; Fox, N. & Wright, J. (1997). The professional perception of orthodontic treatment complexity. *Br Dent J*, Vol.183, No.10, pp. 371-375.

Riedmann, T. & Berg, R. (1999). Retrospective evaluation of the outcome of orthodontic treatment in adults. *J Orofac Orthop*, Vol.60, No.2, pp. 108-123.

Souames, M.; Bassigny, F.; Zenati, N.; Riordan, P.J. & Boy-Lefevre, M.L. (2006). Orthodontic treatment need in French schoolchildren: an epidemiological study using the Index of Orthodontic Treatment Need. *Eur J Orthod*, Vol.28, No.6, pp. 605-609.

Summers, C.J. (1971). The occlusal index: a system for identifying and scoring occlusal disorders. *Am J Orthod*, Vol.59, No.6, pp. 552-567.

Salzmann, J.A. (1967). Orthodontics and society. *Am J Orthod*; Vol.53, No.10, pp. 783-785.

Shaw, W.C.; Richmond, S. & O'Brien, K.D. (1995). The use of occlusal indices: A European perspective. *Am J Orthod Dentofac Orthop*, Vol.107, pp. 1-10.

Simon, P. (1922). Grundzuge einer systematischen diagnostik der gebiss-anomalien. Meusser. Berlín.

So, L.L. & Tang, E.L. (1993). A comparative study using the Occlusal Index and the Index of Orthodontic Treatment Need. *Angle Orthod*, Vol 63, No.1, pp. 57-64.

Soh, J. & Sandham, A. (2004). Orthodontic treatment need in Asian adult males. *Angle Orthod*, Vol.74, No.6, pp. 769-773.

Soh, J.; Sandham, A. & Chan, Y.H. (2005). Malocclusion severity in Asian men in relation to malocclusion type and orthodontic treatment need. *Am J Orthod Dentofacial Orthop*; Vol.128, No.5, pp. 648-652.

Svedström-Oristo, A.L.; Pietilä, T.; Pietilä, I.; Vahlberg, T.; Alanen, P. & Varrela, J. (2009). Acceptability of dental appearance in a group of Finnish 16- to 25-year-olds. *Angle Orthod*, Vol.79, No.3, pp. 479-483.

Tang, E.L.K. & Wei, S.N.Y. (1993). Recording and measuring malocclusion: a review of the literature. *Am J Orthod Dentofac Orthop*, Vol.103, pp. 344-351.

Tang, E.L. & So, L.L. (1995). Correlation of orthodontic treatment demand with treatment need assessed using two indices. *Angle Orthod*, Vol.65, No.6, pp. 443-450.

Tausche, E., Luck, O. & Harzer, W. (2004). Prevalence of malocclusions in the early mixed dentition and orthodontic treatment need. *Eur J Orthod*, Vol.26, No.3, pp. 237-244.

Tickle, M.; Kay, E.J. & Bearn, D. (1999). Socio-economic status and orthodontic treatment need. *Community Dent Oral Epidemiol*, Vol.27, No.6, pp. 413-418.

Tuominen, M.L.; Nystrom, M. & Tuominen, R.J. (1995). Subjective and objective orthodontic treatment need among orthodontically treated and untreated Finnsih adolescents. *Community Dent Oral Epidemiol*, Vol.23, pp. 286-290.

Turbill, E.A.; Richmond, S. & Wright, J.L. (1996). Assessment of General Dental Services orthodontic standards: the Dental Practice Board´s gradings compared to PAR and IOTN. *Br J Orthod*, Vol.23, pp. 211-220.

Uçüncü, N. & Ertugay, E. (2001). The use of the Index of Orthodontic Treatment need (IOTN) in a school population and referred population. *J Orthod*, Vol.28, No.1, pp. 45-52.

Van Kirk, L.E. (1959). Assessment of malocclusion in population groups. *Am J Public Health Nations Health*, Vol.49, pp. 1157-1163.

Van Wyk, P.J. & Drummond, R.J. (2005). Orthodontic status and treatment need of 12-year-old children in South Africa using the Dental Aesthetic Index. *SADJ*; Vol.60, No.8, pp. 334-336.

WHO (1979). Basic method for recording occlusal traits. WHO Bull;57(6):955-61.

WHO (1997). Health Surveys. Basic Methods. Ed. 3 Geneve: World Health Organization.

2

3D Facial Soft Tissue Changes Due to Orthodontic Tooth Movement

R.A. Al-Sanea[1], B. Kusnoto[2] and C.A. Evans[2]
[1]*Department of Dentistry-Central Region,*
National Guards Health Affairs
[2]*Department of Orthodontics,*
University of Illinois at Chicago
[1]*Kingdom of Saudi Arabia*
[2]*USA*

1. Introduction

Two-dimensional (2D) geometric morphometric analysis is the predominant basis for assessment of changes in facial structures resulting from orthodontic or orthognathic surgical treatment. Linear, angular and proportional 2D measurements of the profile are used to assess changes that take place in the three-dimensional (3D) facial soft tissues. However, these methods give little information about frontal soft tissue changes following treatment. Since patients tend to assess their appearance from frontal and three-quarter profile views, measurement of orthodontic outcomes only in the sagittal view as recorded in 2D lateral cephalograms or profile photographs may not be sufficiently informative. Cone Beam Computerized Tomography (CBCT) as well as 3D surface laser head scans offer better frontal and three-quarter profile data for diagnosis, treatment planning and patient education purposes. However, these 3D methods result in large computer files that require large virtual memory and storage media. Moreover, due to lack of normative 3D databases, the 3D images produced can only provide descriptive rather than geometric data of clinical significance. This chapter outlines the current methods used for morphometric assessment of facial soft tissues and their applications and limitations in the field of orthodontics. A simple and accurate method for the assessment of 3D changes occurring in facial soft tissues due to orthodontic tooth movement is explained. Finally, volumetric changes occurring after orthodontic tooth movement due to soft tissue profile advancement or soft tissue profile retraction are outlined.

2. Two-dimensional morphometrics of facial soft tissues

2.1 Two-dimensional imaging

Frontal and lateral photographs and anthropometric measurements along with lateral and frontal cephalometrics are considered the standard records for diagnosis and treatment planning in orthodontic treatment. Two-dimensional geometric morphometrics such as linear, angular and proportional measurements are used to assess changes that take place in facial soft tissues. Research including frontal and lateral photographs has shown that some soft tissue measurements tend to be more reliable than others. In general, frontal measurements are more reliable than lateral ones, and linear measurements are more reliable than angular measurements. Measurements that include subnasale, pogonion, and gnathion tend to be less reliable. Despite the fact that much of the reported evidence in the scientific literature is built around two-dimensional measurements, a substantial amount of information is lacking because:

a. Three-dimensional structures are represented by a set of two-dimensional coordinates. Subject/film/focus geometric relationship could lead to size magnification, distortion, vertical and horizontal displacement in relation to imaging source.
b. Patients tend to assess their appearance from frontal and three-quarter profile views; measurement of orthodontic outcomes only in the sagittal view as recorded in 2D lateral cephalograms or profile photographs may not be sufficiently informative. An example of that would be surgical orthognathic patients who can relate to malar region changes or mandibular angle and soft tissue chin changes rather than lip profile and incisor position.
c. For pre-treatment consultation or education sessions, and for discussion purposes, patients tend to describe the soft tissue of the face pointing at vermillion border and philtrum of lips and soft tissue facial folds rather than describing landmarks and linear measurements (Figure 1). The facial folds are skin folds or lines that become accentuated with facial expressions. The most significant factors that contribute to the prominence of the folds are excess skin, skin thinning, excess cheek fat, and ptosis of cheek fat. Many research studies are conducted in the field of plastic and cosmetic surgery on changes that take place in the facial folds with aging and with weight loss or weight gain. Since orthodontic tooth movement contributes to soft tissue profile advancement or retraction, in other words thinning or thickening of soft tissue around the lips as a result of tooth movement, then it would be only practical to borrow these terms for the purpose of patient education and treatment planning in the field of orthodontics.

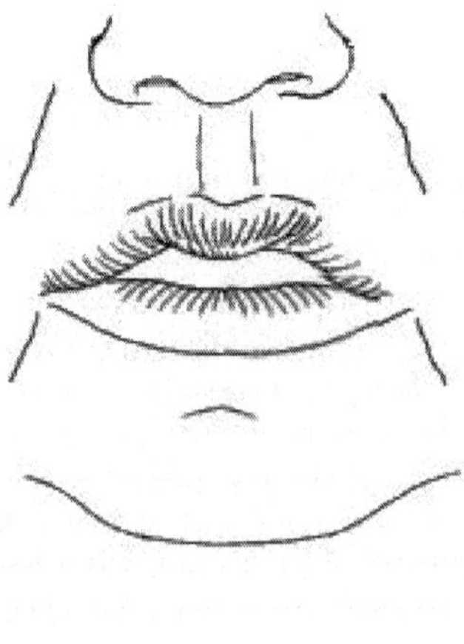

Fig. 1. Facial folds.

2.2 Two-dimensional morphometric analysis of facial soft tissues

When superimposing different faces, a limited number of labeled points on each face, e.g., the tip of the nose, corner of the eye and less prominent points on the cheek must be located precisely (Farkas, 1987). Linear and angular measurements between the landmarks provide useful measurements for comparison. The number of reported manually labeled landmarks varies, but usually ranges from 50 to 300 as shown in Figure 2 (O'Toole et al., 1999; Clement & Marks, 2005). Only a correct alignment of all these points allows acceptable comparison between faces, intermediate morphs, a convincing mapping of motion data from the reference or initial treatment image into final treatment image.

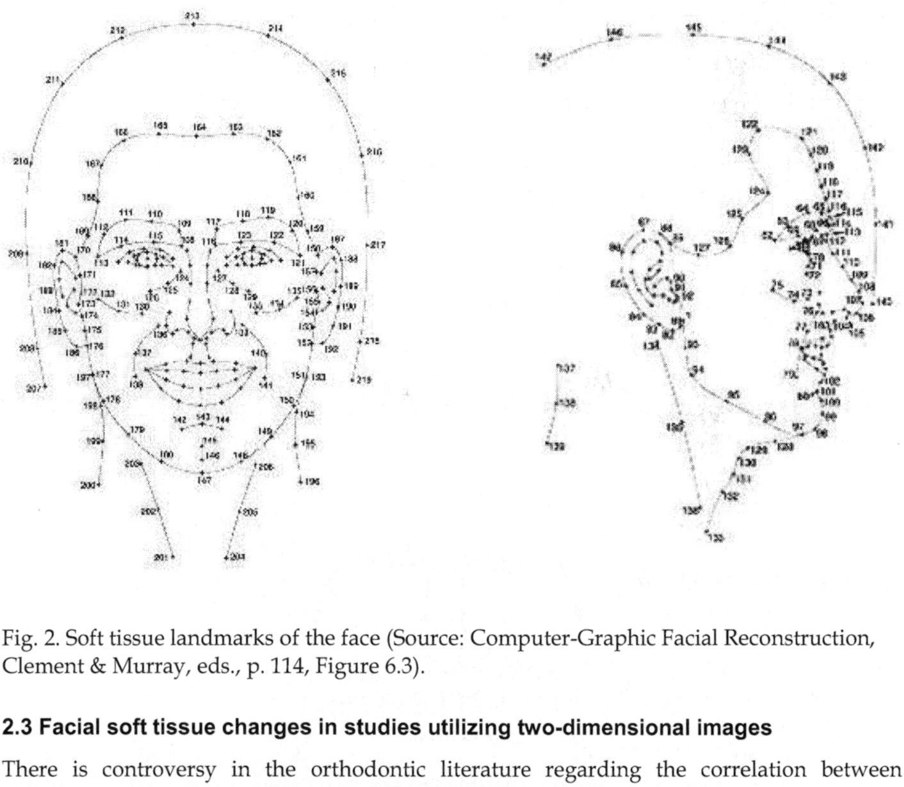

Fig. 2. Soft tissue landmarks of the face (Source: Computer-Graphic Facial Reconstruction, Clement & Murray, eds., p. 114, Figure 6.3).

2.3 Facial soft tissue changes in studies utilizing two-dimensional images

There is controversy in the orthodontic literature regarding the correlation between craniofacial skeletal and soft-tissue profile form (Denis & Speidel, 1987; Bloom, 1961; Burke, 1983; Savara, 1965). For instance, although stereophotogrammetric (Savara, 1965; Burke, 1983; Peck & Peck, 1995), computed tomographic (Marsh & Vannier, 1983; Moss et al., 1987) and cephalometric studies (Riedel, 1950; Tweed, 1944) have indicated soft-tissue profile form is markedly influenced by orthodontic tooth movement and or orthognathic surgery, other studies have suggested the relative independence of the facial soft tissues on the underlying skeletal form (Finnoy et al., 1987; Wisth, 1974).

In an attempt to determine the effects of orthodontic treatment on the soft tissue profile of the lips, several studies were conducted to quantify and to predict the relationship between incisor retraction and lip retraction (Bloom, 1961; Rudee, 1964; Garner, 1974; Roos, 1977; Wisth, 1974; Hershey, 1972). With the exception of one study that found a predictable amount of soft tissue changes in response to incisor retraction (Bloom, 1961) the majority of the studies on both growing and non-growing subjects concluded that the large individual variation prevents the accurate prediction of lip response to incisor retraction in any given person.

Some studies pointed that lip structure seems to have an influence on lip response to incisor retraction. Oliver found that patients with thin lips or a high lip strain displayed a significant correlation between incisor retraction and lip retraction, whereas patients with thick lips or low lip strain displayed no such correlation (Oliver, 1982). In addition, Wisth (1974) found that lip response, as a proportion of incisor retraction, decreased as the amount of incisor retraction increased. This seems to indicate that the lips have some inherent support.

Al-Mesad (1998) studied soft tissue changes in extraction and non-extraction orthodontic patients and found that for the most part, the drape of the upper and lower lips was highly correlated to the changes in both upper and lower incisors. Changes in position of upper and lower incisors were found to influence the final position of upper and lower lips after orthodontic treatment in the total sample for both extraction and non-extraction samples. For every millimeter change in the upper incisor tip in the non-extraction group, approximately 0.2 mm of changes in the upper lip and 0.9 mm in the lower lip occurred. Greater changes were observed in individuals with thin upper and lower lips (0.8 mm changes for the upper lip with only 0.6 mm changes for the lower lip).

Bishara et al. (1995) used standardized facial photographs to compare the soft tissue profile changes in persons with Class II, division 1 malocclusions who were treated with either an extraction or non-extraction treatment modalities. The found that: (1) After treatment the upper and lower lips were retracted significantly more in the extraction group compared with the non-extraction group. These differences persisted into retention; (2) Upper lip length increased more among subjects who were treated without extractions; (3) Upper vermilion height in male subjects and the upper and lower vermilion heights in female subjects increased among subjects who were treated without extractions and decreased among subjects who were treated with four first premolar extractions; (4) Nasolabial angle became significantly more obtuse among the female subjects who were treated with four first premolar extractions (Bishara et al., 1995). Similar findings were noted by Kocadereli (2002). On the other hand, Charles Tweed (1944) firmly stated that non-extraction approach would place the teeth in an unstable position in the basal bone leading to unacceptable relapse afterwards.

Paquette et al. (1992) looked at 'borderline' extraction/non-extraction cases 14.5 years out of retention and found that in the long term, the non-extraction patients had profiles that were 2 mm fuller. A similar study (Luppanapornlarp & Johnston, 1993) looked at carefully selected and defined first premolar-extraction cases and non-extraction cases over the same post-retention time frame. The results indicated that the extraction of first premolars tended to flatten the profile by 2-3 mm when compared with non-extraction treatment. Interestingly, the non-extraction patients had the more concave faces post-treatment and this challenges the concept of extractions as part of orthodontic treatment 'dishing the face'. The ability to predict from post-treatment lateral photographs, whether individuals had been treated with or without extractions has been investigated (Boley et al., 1998) The findings indicated a correct response in only 54% of cases - just greater than pure chance.

In a sample of forty adult patients who underwent orthodontic treatment that resulted in either soft tissue profile retraction or soft tissue profile advancement, Al-Sanea, Kusnoto and Evans (Al-Sanea, 2007) studied linear changes occuring in cephalometric soft tissue landmarks: Sn, A, UL, LL, B. Patient selection was based on the following criteria: availability of pre-treatment and post-treatment lateral cephalometric radiographs; availability of acceptable clarity pre-treatment and post-treatment frontal and lateral photographs with lips closed or slightly touching without strain and the patient's head properly oriented in the three planes of space; and absence of facial hair, eye glasses or jewelry. The following criteria were added as part of the study design to minimize undesirable soft tissue facial changes:

1. Any patient with lip incompetence of more than 2 millimeters was excluded as this interfered later on with the morphing procedure in FaceGen™ Modeller 3.1 (Singular Inversions, Toronto, ON, Canada, 2005).
2. Diminished growth with a minimum pre-treatment age of sixteen years for females and eighteen years for males.
3. Absence of craniofacial anomalies or significant skeletal discrepancy.
4. Treatment modalities included fixed appliance therapy with no orthognathic surgical treatment involved in any case.
5. No measurable weight gain or weight loss changes instead of treatment related soft tissue change as determined from interzygomatic width and submental soft tissue which were compared between the pre-treatment and post-treatment frontal photographs after image resizing is carried out in Adobe Photoshop™ software (Adobe System Inc., San Jose, CA, 2005).

In all 2D landmark measurements (Figure 3), a negative soft tissue change was observed in the soft tissue profile retraction group. The opposite was observed in the group that showed advancement of the soft tissue profile. In the profile retraction group, change was the greatest in the upper lip and lower lips (-1.68 and –1.58 mm). Similarly, the most change in the profile advancement group was observed in upper and lower lip and Sn (0.73, 0.85 and 0.86) (Table 1).

In this sample of patients, the overall soft tissue change in the profile retraction group was significantly greater in comparison to the change reported in the profile advancement group in all 2D landmarks ($p<0.05$). The highest difference in 2D measurements between the two groups was noted in the upper and lower lip (2.40 and 2.42 mms) followed by change at SfB (1.95 mm), followed by change at Sn (1.75 mm) and SfA (1.36 mm). Lack of change at SfA in the soft tissue profile advancement group was the reason why change at SfA was the lowest in comparison to other 2D measurements (Table 2).

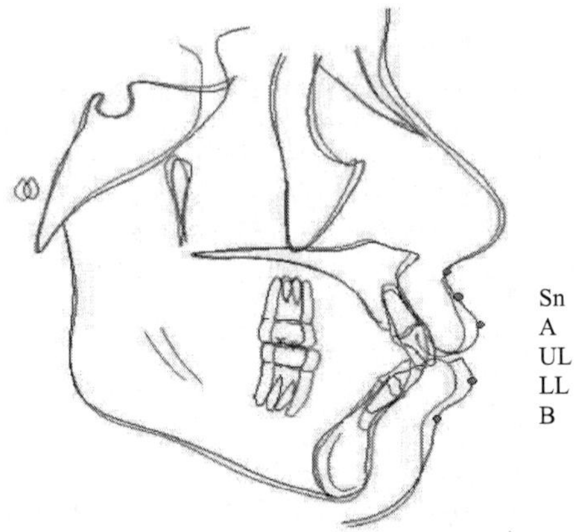

Fig. 3. 2D landmarks of soft tissue profile.

Retraction Group			Advancement Group		
Measurements	N	Mean ± SD (mm)	Measurements	N	Mean ± SD (mm)
2D-Sn	20	-0.89 ± 1.58	2D-Sn	20	0.86 ± 1.65
2D-SfA	20	-0.78 ± 2.14	2D-SfA	20	0.58 ± 1.96
2D-UL	20	-1.68 ± 1.80	2D-UL	20	0.73 ± 2.38
2D-LL	20	-1.58 ± 2.44	2D-LL	20	0.85 ± 2.63
2D-SfB	20	-1.30 ± 2.09	2D-SfB	20	0.65 ± 2.24

* $p \leq 0.05$

Table 1. Means and standard deviations for linear horizontal changes in the soft tissue profile groups.

Measurements	Mean Difference (mm)	Student t -value	p-value*
2D-Sn	-1.75	-3.42	0.001
2D-SfA	-1.36	-2.09	0.044
2D-UL	-2.40	-3.60	0.001
2D-LL	-2.42	-3.02	0.004
2D-SfB	-1.95	-2.84	0.007

* $p \leq 0.05$

Table 2. Comparison of 2D measurements of soft tissue profile retraction and advancement groups.

3. Three-dimensional morphometrics of facial soft tissues

3.1 Three-dimensional facial models

The goal of imaging in medicine and dentistry has been to display a patient's anatomic truth. Until now, imaging technology has been largely confined to two dimensions. The development of a 3D digital model of a patient's anatomy would greatly improve our ability to determine different treatment options, to monitor changes over time (the fourth dimension), to predict and display final treatment results, and to measure treatment outcomes more accurately. Lately, computer graphic head modeling has gained wide popularity in the field of plastic and orthognathic surgery for the prediction and simulation of treatment effects. The technique offers great advantages in surgical planning and the prediction of facial deformation. Furthermore, three-dimensional modeling of patient anatomy allows for engineering principles to be applied to such areas as local and general stress analysis of the stomatognathic system, analysis of asymmetry and how it may affect function, TMJ loading and occlusal forces, and reconstruction in oral and maxillofacial surgery. Finally, functional studies on dynamic 3D models will help us to understand the dynamic relationship of the anatomy which orthodontists and maxillofacial surgeons affect everyday in their practices (Quintero et al., 1999; Moss &Linney, 1990; Hatcher & Dial, 1999, Harrell et al., 2002).

3.1.1 Directly acquired three-dimensional facial models

Three-dimensional facial models "3D Facial Model" can be defined as three-dimensional coordinate data of facial soft tissues (Figure 4). Facial models can be acquired directly in 3D format utilizing computed tomograms (CT), including cone-beam tomography, magnetic resonance imaging (MRI), digital radiography, and digital ultrasound. Those techniques involve the use of ionizing radiation with varying degree, and can produce facial models with surface as well as deep data, depending on degree of segmentation.

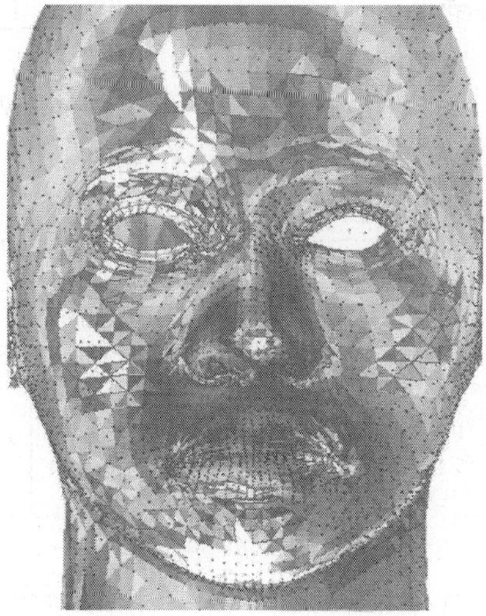

Fig. 4. Three-dimensional facial model.

Other direct techniques for producing 3D facial models, that do not involve the use of ionizing radiation, include stereophotogrammetry and simultaneous image capture from more than one camera source. This approach can produce only surface data or a "3D shell of the face." All of the above mentioned allow for the volumetric registration of the hard and or soft tissue of the craniofacial structures and the face with adequate resolution. The end result is a 3D facial model that can be easily viewed on a computer monitor. However, all the techniques generate huge files that require large virtual memory and storage media.

3.1.2 Manually reconstructed three-dimensional facial models

Facial Models can be reconstructed into 3D format utilizing a variety of 2D or 3D images that are calibrated and merged into a 3D "digital replica" of anatomy. Surface laser scanning can produce multiple 3D images from different angles with a spatial resolution of 0.5 mm (Figure 5). Those images can be manually stitched together, utilizing the scanner software, into a 3D facial model. Similarly, multiple 2D images taken at different views can also be used to construct 3D facial models. In both cases, texture data can be mapped on to the 3D surface which produces a photorealistic 3D model. The main draw back in these settings is that post-processing of the acquired data can significantly alter the dimensions and appearance, particularly with over smoothing. While there have been numerous reports on the use of 3D facial images in evaluation of facial soft tissue changes following orthognathic surgery, these approaches and systems have not been critically validated. The task of validation of these systems for facial imaging is difficult due to the multitude of variables in post-processing and the conditions of image acquisition in the clinic.

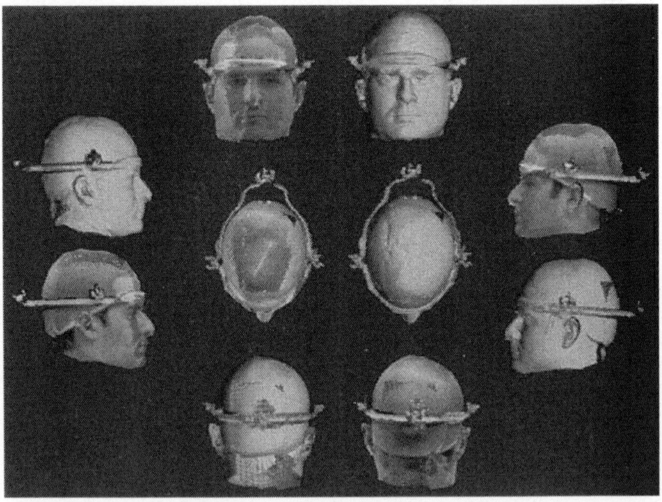

Fig. 5. Different surface laser scans before stitching into one 3D head model. (Source: Computer-Graphic Facial Reconstruction, Clement & Murray, eds., p. 234, Figure 12.9).

Furthermore, all systems suffer from potential for patient movement and alterations of facial expression between the multiple views needed to construct a 3D model of the face. Laser-based systems are a safety concern. While these systems are deemed safe for use with adults, the United State Food and Drug Administration (FDA) has no statement on the safety of laser systems in children, who constitute a majority of the orthodontic and craniofacial treatment group. The light-based imaging systems generally lack the precision of the laser-based systems and suffer from image artifacts due to skin tone, color and reflectance. Additionally, the majority of 3D imaging systems utilize frontal and three-quarter facial views to produce a facial model; however this approach does not provide sufficiently accurate representations of the facial profile. The "profile" view generated from these systems is not a true view of the facial profile, as one would have with a camera positioned from the patient's profile. The generated "profile" can be distorted by several millimeters and lack detail of specific features, especially in the lower face and lips. This deficiency is a significant setback because much of our knowledge of growth and development and treatment outcomes is based upon the profile view.

3.1.3 Mathematically reconstructed three-dimensional facial models

This process involves the use of a framework of anthropometric measurements and texture information that characterize faces in a data set of 3D head scans. Principal Component Analysis (PCA), which is a powerful statistical technique that has found application in fields such as face recognition and image compression where the luxury of graphical representation is not available, can be utilized to analyze patterns of similarities and differences in this data set. After finding patterns in the data, anthropometric measurements and texture information act as geometric constraints for morphing a prototype (i.e., average) 3D facial model. This avarage is then registered on the 2D image and mathematically mapped into a 3D model of the face. A hierarchial algorithm is applied to adjust the model parameters for an optimal 3D reconstruction of the target image. Some imaging software utilize robust mathematical registration and algorithmic methods for the automatic mapping or simulation of faces with varying degree of accuracy depending on the amount of detailed information obtained from the date set. In applying the method to several images of a person, and when more detailed statistics (such as covariance information or exact distributions) are included, the 3D reconstructions can reach almost the quality of laser scans (Blanz & Vetter, 1999). The herarchial modeling technique utilized in software Facegen™ Modeller 3.5 (Singular Inversions, 2009) would serve as a practical, accurate and user friendly interface for the mathematical reconstruction of 3D facial models from readily available 2D images of orthodontic treatments and growth studies.

3.2 Three-dimensional morphometric analysis of facial soft tissue

Many studies were conducted on the evaluation of facial soft tissues utilizing 3D facial models of orthognathic surgical cases. Regardless whether the facial model was a true capture or a reconstructed one, several factors are impeding our understanding of 3D soft tissue changes in the orthodontic/orthognathic field:

- Lack of normative 3D craniofacial databases that are age-, gender-, race-specific for reference purposes in diagnosis and treatment planning.
- Lack of 3D data of facial changes during growth, maturation, and aging.
- Superimposition methods that do not work: Two-dimensional measurements rely solely on manual annotation with landmarks. This procedure is time-consuming and subject to

error in 3D facial models. Three-dimensional models require sophisticated registration mathematics for analysis. The combined robust mathematics in the Euclidean Distance Matrix Analysis (EDMA) and Dense Correspondence Algorithm (DCA) serve as reliable registration methods for 3D models. However, further sophisticated mechanisms such as Thin Spline Plate Analysis (TSP) and Finite Element Analysis (FEA) need to be utilized for comparison of 3D changes between pre treatment and post treatment models.

- The 3D images before, during and after processing require computer processers with large virtual memories, not to mention the large storage and back up needed.

3D Facial Model	Acquired	Manually reconstructed	Mathematically reconstructed
Pros	True replica Of surface anatomy. Deep data as well in Cone Beam CT	Almost true replica of surface anatomy	Surface anatomy with quality similar to surface laser scans, utilizes readily available 2D images, inexpensive method, user friendly, no radiation or laser use
Cons	Radiation exposure in CBCT, light based systems produce image artifacts and potential for patient movement while image capture	Stitching required, over smoothening, computer manipulation, laser use poses safety concerns, potential for patient movement while image capture	Not true capture, Computer manipulation required

Table 3. A comparison between the three different modes of acquisition of 3D facial models.

3.2.1 Three-dimensional methods of registration

3.2.1.1 Euclidean distance matrix analysis (EDMA)

In general, the distance between points and in a Euclidean space is given by Weisstein (Weisstein, 1999)

$$d = |x - y| = \sqrt{\sum_{i=1}^{x'} |x_i - y_i|^2}$$

To explain the method of EDMA, let's represent an object by M (K X D) matrix where K is number of landmarks in the object and D is the dimensions, in which these landmarks lie, i.e., a landmark coordinate system (Lele & Richtsmeire, 1991; Lele & Cole, 1995). The form of an object as represented by this collection of landmark coordinates is that characteristic which remains invariant under the group of transformation consisting of rotation (spinning the object on an axis), reflection and translation (moving the object within a given coordinate system). The invariant condition is when the Difference M1, M2 = Diff (M1 R1+1t1, M2 R2+1t2) for any choice of rotation parameters R1, R2 and translation parameters t1, t2. A collection of all K X D matrices that can be obtained by rotation, reflection and translation of M is called an orbit. Under definition of form all matrices in the same orbit represent exactly the same form.

Any object with K landmarks in D dimensions can be represented in an invariant fashion using the vector of distances between all possible pairs of landmarks. This is called the form matrix (Lele & Richtsmeier, 1991). In the Euclidean Distance Matrix Analysis (EDMA) for any two objects with K landmarks, we end up with two form matrices i.e., the vectors of all possible pair wise distances for each one of the objects. One particular description that has been used to outline the difference between these two objects is the vector of the ratios of the corresponding differences, i.e., the form difference matrix (Lele and Richtsmeier, 1991; Lele & Cole, 1995). The important property of this description is that it only depends on the orbits to which the two forms belong, not on the exact locations along these orbits. This overcomes the problem of the lack of the coordinate system for location of change.

3.2.1.2 Finite Element Analysis (FEA)

Three-dimensional face models are described from a mathematical point of view by a huge number of polygons, forming something like a mesh. The nodes of the mesh are the vertices of the polygons. Finite-element scaling analysis can be used to depict clinical changes in terms of allometry (size-related shape-change), and the change in form between an initial configuration and a target configuration can be viewed as a continuous deformation from the initial form, which can be quantified based on major and minor strains (principal strains). If the two strains are equal, the change in form is characterized by a simple increase or decrease in size. However, if one of the principal strains changes in a greater proportion, both size and shape are transformed. The product of the strains indicates a change in size if the result is not equal to 1. For example, a product >1 indicates an increase in size (measured from the base of the mesh of the initial form) equal to the remainder; 1.30 indicates a 30% increase in volume (positive allometry). Similarly, a product of 0.65 indicates a 35% decrease in volume (negative allometry). The products and ratios can be resolved for individual landmarks within the configuration and these can be made linear using a log-linear scale. For ease of interpretation, a pseudocolour-coded scale can be used to provide a graphic display of change in size, as shown in Figure 6 (Singh et al., 2006).

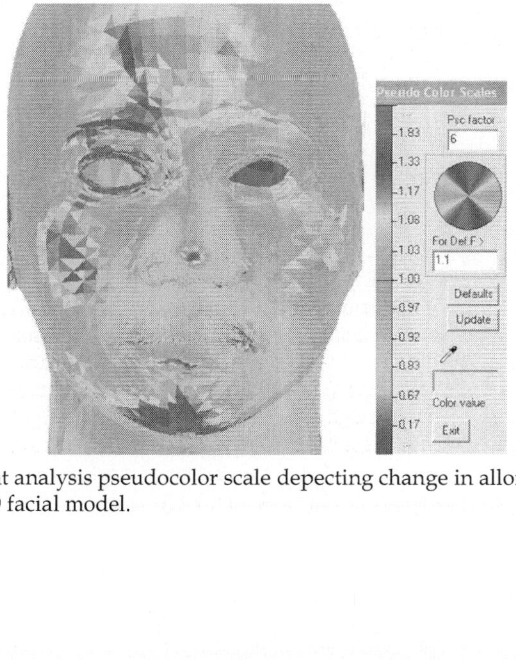

Fig. 6. Finite element analysis pseudocolor scale depecting change in allometry between initial and target 3D facial model.

3.2.1.3 Thin Plate Spline analysis (TPS)

Suppose that all of the specimen landmarks, in the initial stage, are embedded into a thin, 2D, non-deformed, elastic plate. Due to transformation, landmarks will migrate to other new positions (final stage), so the thin-plate will be distorted, that is, all of the points belonging to the thin-plate will be relocated or dragged by landmark movements. TPS is applied to the comparison of forms as a regression mechanism with the requirement that bending energy or smoothness function is minimized. Applying finite element algorithms, it's possible to define an Area Factor, a Deformation Factor and a Principal Axis Direction for any point in the plate after deformation.

3.2.1.4 Dense Correspondence Algorithm (DCA)

For three-dimensional morphometric comparisons of pre-treatment and post-treatment head models, comparisons cannot be carried out unless the models are homologous (having equal number of nodes). Based on the closest point algorithm, the post-treatment meshes will utilize the landmarks from the pre-treatment head model as the basic mesh for the dense correspondence procedure when comparing the pre- to post-treatment head model of the same patient. In the closest point algorithm principle, the two models are aligned utilizing the digitized surface landmarks. The new position of the target vertices that lie in-between the landmarks of the post-treatment model are determined using the Euclidean Distance Matrix Analysis (EDMA) approach. This way the points in the reassembled post-treatment mesh have a one-to-one correspondence with those of the pre-treatment mesh. Finally Thin-Plate Spline analysis is applied. As a result, all of the forms will have the same quantity of nodes, which enables comparison later on (Hutton et al., 2001).

Care should be taken in specifying the greatest distance between homologous landmarks while alignment of the head models. If the distance between a generic landmark of the basic mesh (pre-treatment model) and the surface of any non-basic mesh (post-treatment model) is greater than the parameter specified, then the landmark is definitively discarded.

3.3 Facial soft tissue changes in studies utilizing three-dimensional images

Ismail and Moss (2002) prospectively compared the 2D and the 3D effects on the face of extraction and non-extraction orthodontic treatment in patients with skeletal Class I patterns. They showed, based on cephalometric values, that the nasolabial angle was larger in the extraction group, while the vermilion boarder of the upper lip was forward in comparison to the extraction group at the end of treatment. Differential geometrics and surface shape analysis showed that for the two treatment modalities in the current study, there was a significant difference in the changes in upper lip thickness. The reduction in upper lip thickness in the extraction group was accompanied by a decrease in exposed vermilion. The converse was true for the non-extraction group, which showed an increase in upper lip thickness in the study. Furthermore, the non-extraction group had more convex cheeks and chins by the end of treatment compared to the extraction group. They also pointed an increased concavity of the labiomental fold region by the end of treatment in the extraction group. Faces in the extraction group became relatively more protrusive with treatment. The surface shape analysis technique showed that the cheeks were flatter in the none-extraction group at the start of treatment, but this reversed with time. In the extraction group, the concavity of the labiomental fold increased, while the non-extraction group showed no change in this area.

In a geometric morphometric study on changes in the soft tissue facial profile following orthodontics, Singh et al. (2005) reported a statistically significant difference in the premaxillary region with the non-extraction group being relatively larger in that region by 25%. For the non-extraction group after treatment, localized increases in relative size in the naso-maxillary region size of 25% ($p < 0.01$) were present. For the extraction group after treatment, a non-significant reduction in relative size of 15% was localized in the putative bicuspid area.

Studies that used FEA to analyze the effect of extraction and non-extraction orthodontic treatment mostly used lateral cephalometrics. Finite elements were constructed using anatomical landmarks in lateral cephalometrics as vertices of the triangular elements and then analysis was carried out as the deformational change needed to produce the final cephalometric radiograph (Lavelle & Carvalho, 1989; Singh et al., 2005). The technique is good as it portrays the change as the amount of strain required to produce the final image. However, the technique utilizes two-dimensional images to portray three-dimensional structures. Therefore, those studies inherit the same limitations associated with studies of two-dimensional data.

Other studies used surface shape analysis to report changes in the face after orthodontic treatment (Ismail & Moss, 2002). They used 3D surface laser scans and compared faces after extraction and non-extraction orthodontic treatment. The experimental design involved description of the shape of the surfaces (i.e., saddle, spherical, dome, ridge, etc). The comparison was carried out mainly to detect how the surface changed in either shape or area. The technique might be useful in terms of comparing three-dimensional data on its own. However, much of our knowledge in growth and development and treatment results are derived from two dimensional landmark measurements of two dimensional radiographs and photographs.

4. Morphometric analysis of three-dimensional facial models generated utilizing two-dimensional photographs

Much of our knowledge of treatment outcomes and growth and development of facial soft tissues is based on the frontal and profile photographs of patients. It would be greatly advantagous if these readily available images can be data mined into 3D facial models. A simple and accurate technique for the generation of 3D facial models from sets of 2D readily available pre treatment and post treatment photographs is proposed by Al-Sanea, Kusnoto and Evans (Al-Sanea, 2007).

The pretreatment and post-treatment images for each patient are resized by creating a duplicate layer of the post-treatment image in a contrasting balance, and then adjusting the opacity of the created layer to 60-70%. Later on the post-treatment image layer is overlaid on top of the pretreatment image and its size adjusted until a perfect fit on the eyes is achieved.

Three-dimensional head models were constructed using FaceGen™ Modeller 3.1 and 3.5 (Singular Inversions Inc., Toronto, ON, Canada, 2005 and 2009) from the resized frontal and lateral photographs of the same patients where the 2D cephalometric analysis was carried out. Following the recommendations of the software, 11 surface landmarks were digitized on the frontal photographs and 7 landmarks on the lateral photograph. The surface landmark locations suggested by the software are in accordance with facial soft tissue landmarks definitions outlined by Farkas (1987). After landmark digitization the software computes the average face and the mode of variation in its own dataset based on the age, gender, race, and symmetry information specified to it by the operator. Based on this information the software predicts and produces an average head that can be morphed into the patient's head. During the morphing procedure, the software calculates the texture and geometric information in the image and modifies the 3D model accordingly. The three-dimensional image produced is saved in two formats (Facegen: Fg) and (VRML. 97).

A pre-treatment and a post-treatment model were generated for each patient. Computer graphic facial analysis was carried out for those models in each patient using Morphostudio™ 3.02.39 (Orthovisage, New York, NY, 2005). First, twelve surface landmarks are digitized on the face of the model (Figure 7) in order to apply the dense correspondence algorithm. The dense correspondence algorithm transforms vertices in the 3D models into homologous landmarks that are easily compared. For consistency and reliability, the surface landmarks were selected in accordance with the surface landmarks already used to generate the 3D model in Facegen™.

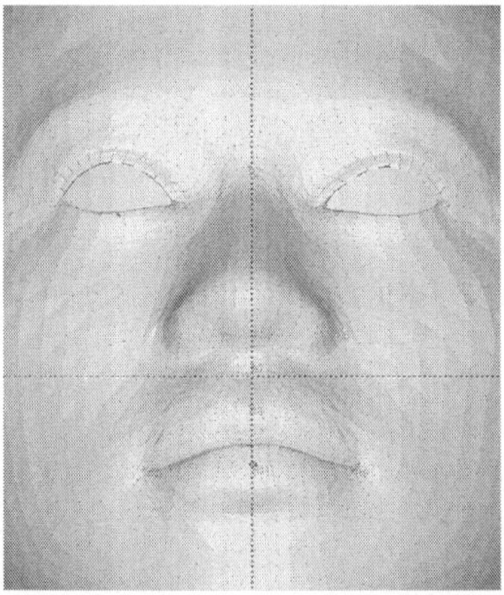

Fig. 7. Landmarks used to generate 3D head model in Facegen™ software as well as apply the dense correspondence algorithm function in Morphostudio™.

The percentage of volume deformation in the post-treatment model (as measured from the base of the mesh of the pretreatment model) was reported through the Finite Element Analysis function of the Morphostudio™ 3.02.39 (Orthovisage, New York, NY, 2005).[30] This is represented in the color-coded graphic display in the software (Figure 6). A total of thirty-four pseudocolor scale measurements were recorded from the surface of the 3D model at different nodes around the lips (Figure 8).

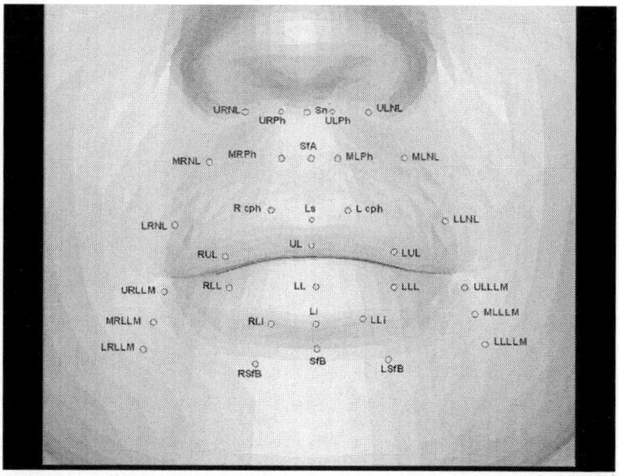

Fig. 8. Landmark areas where psudocolor scale measurements were recorded.

Since the deformation was expressed over a large area around the lips, point measurements at single nodes were not effective. Multiple measurements had to be recorded at different regions around the lips and averaged together in order to report the average volumetric deformation occurring in that region (Figure 9). Measurements were analyzed to determine changes in the soft tissue of the face following orthodontic treatment that resulted in soft tissue profile retraction or soft tissue profile advancement.

As shown in Figure 8, four lateral measurements were recorded on the same horizontal level of Sn at both the nasolabial fold and the philtrum of the upper lip. These measurements were labeled as upper right and left nasolabial fold (URNL, ULNL) and upper right and left philtrum (URPh, ULPh) respectively. Four lateral measurements were recorded on the same horizontal level of SfA on the nasolabial fold and the philtrum of the upper lip. Those measurements were the middle right and left nasolabial and the middle right and left philtrum (MRNL, MLNL, and MRPh, MLPh respectively). Two lateral measurements were also recorded at the junction of the nasolabial fold and the upper lip (lower right nasolabial and lower left nasolabial- LRNL and LLNL). Three measurements were recorded for the upper lip vermillion boarder in the areas of labiale superius (ls) and crista philtri landmark (cph). Three measurements were recorded on the convex surface of the upper lip, two on each side and one in the middle (RUL, MUL, LUL). The same was for the lower lip, two measurements were recorded on each side of the convex surface and one middle measurement was taken (RLL, MLL, LLL). Three measurements right, left and middle were recorded on the lower lip vermilion border (Rli, Mli, Lli). Two measurements were recorded on the labiomental folds on each side of SfB (RSfB, LSfB). Two measurements (URLLM, ULLLM) were recorded on the lateral labiomental folds and fall at the junction of the lateral labiomental folds and the lower lip. Two other measurements on the lateral labiomental folds were recorded and fell on the same horizontal level of Rli, Mli, Lli (MRLLM, MLLLM). Two measurements (RSfB, LSfB) were recorded on the lateral labiomental folds and fell on the same horizontal level of SfB.

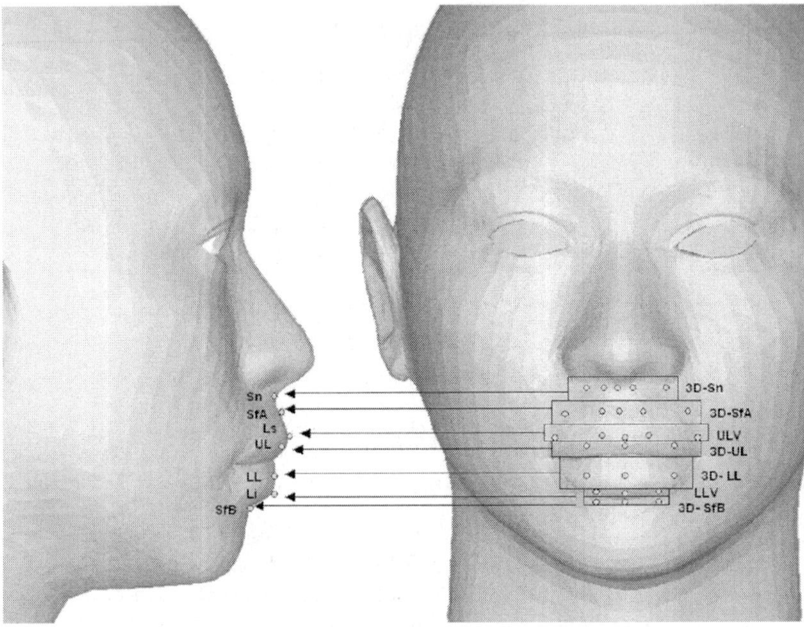

Fig. 9. Averaged 3D measurements.

The percentages of volumetric change were calculated by averaging each five pseudocolor scale measurements on the same horizontal level of each reference landmark. These values were used to report the mean percentage of 3D volumetric change at areas of Sn, SfA, UL, LL, SfB. The averaging procedure for these landmarks is shown in Figure 9.

Furthermore, bilateral measurements at the folds of the face were also averaged. Three bilateral measurements on the right and left nasolabial folds were averaged together denoting change at the nasolabial folds (Right nasolabial fold measurements: URNL, MRNL, LRNL and left nasolabial measurements: ULNL, MLNL, LLNL). All nine measurement enclosed within the philtrum of the upper lip were averaged together (URPh, Sn, ULPh, MRPh, SfA, MLPh, LRPh, Ls, LLPh). Three bilateral vertical measurements on the lateral labiomental folds were averaged together denoting change at the lateral labniomental folds (Right lateral labiomental fold measurements: URLLM, MRLLM, LRLLM and left labiomental fold measurements: ULLLM, MLLLM, LLLLM). These averaged measurements are shown in Figure 10.

Reliability of the FEA method was obtained by recording pseudocolor scale values on different time points for six randomly selected patients and estimating the pair wise correlations among these pseudoscale values. Two-tailed sample Student t-test was calculated to compare the mean measurements in soft tissue profile retraction and soft tissue profile advancement groups at 0.05 level of significance.

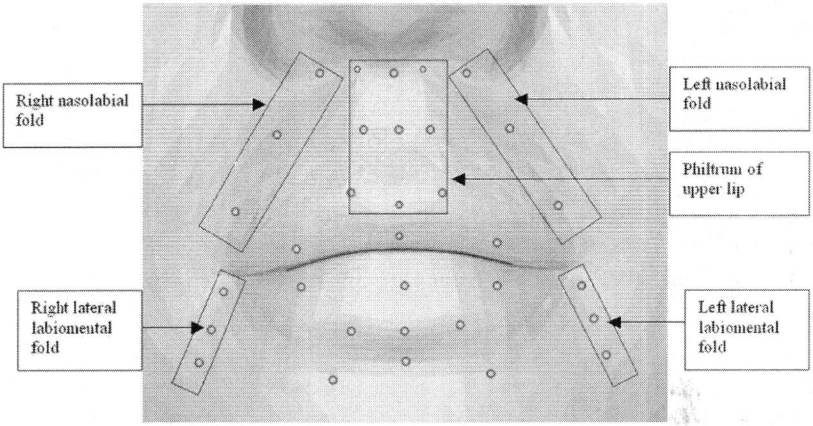

Fig. 10. Average measurements at the folds of the face.

The percentages of volumetric deformation of the surface nodes from the base of the pre-treatment mesh were calculated by averaging the five pseudocolor scale measurements on the same horizontal level of each reference landmark; leading to the mean percentage of volumetric change at areas of Sn, SfA, UL, LL, SfB. Change was the greatest in upper and lower lip measurements in both profile retraction and profile advancement groups. Change in the profile retraction group was the greatest at the upper lip vermilion border (3D-UV), which was 12.47 %. In the soft tissue profile advancement group however, change was greatest at the vermilion border of the lower lip (7.09%). The greatest difference in 3D measurements between the two groups was noted in the vermilion boarder of the upper lip at 15.71% (Tables 4 and 5).

Groups		Retraction	Advancement
Measurements	N	Mean ± SD (%)	Mean ± SD (%)
3D-Sn	20	-7.72 ± 9.51	5.80 ± 9.48
3D-SfA	20	-10.99 ± 7.02	-0.30 ± 12.82
3D-LL	20	-9.92 ± 20.41	4.29 ± 22.91
3D-UL	20	-6.59 ± 14.83	2.00 ± 10.17
3D-LV	20	-2.59 ± 14.65	7.09 ± 17.59
3D-UV	20	-12.47 ± 9.41	3.23 ± 10.81
3D-SfB	20	-8.69 ± 13.49	5.16 ± 10.28

$p \leq 0.05$

Table 4. Means and standard deviations for the percentage of volume deformation in the soft tissue profile groups.

Measurements	Mean Difference	Student t-value	p- value*
3D-Sn	-13.51	-4.50	0.000
3D-SfA	-10.69	-3.27	0.003
3D-UL	-8.56	-2.13	0.040
3D-LL	-14.21	-2.07	0.045
3D-LV	-9.69	-1.89	0.066
3D-UV	-15.71	-4.90	0.000
3D-SfB	-13.86	-3.65	0.001

* $p \leq 0.05$

Table 5. Comparison of 3D measurements of soft tissue profile retraction and advancement groups.

Statistically significant differences were found between soft tissue profile retraction and soft tissue profile advancement groups in the percentage of volume deformation at the facial folds regions. The greatest difference between soft tissue profile retraction and soft tissue profile advancement was noted at the Philtrum (Ph) Where the difference was -12.02 and 2.78 respectively while the Lowest difference was at 3D-LLM (-3.36 and 1.71 respectively)

Results are outlined in Table 6.

Groups		Retraction	Advancement
Measurements	N	Mean ± SD	Mean ± SD
3D-NL	20	-5.32 ± 8.11	3.82 ± 9.55
3D-Ph	20	-12.02 ± 0.86	2.78 ± 10.82
3D-LLM	20	-3.36 ± 1.16	1.71 ± 11.09

Table 6. Means and standard deviation for the percentage volume deformation at the facial folds on the soft tissue profile (%).

5. Correlation between two-dimensional and three-dimensional measurements

Current orthodontic research reports linear 2D or volumetric 3D changes in the facial soft tissues without establishing a relationship between 2D and 3D measurements. Knowing this relationship could enable clinicians to use 2D measurements as a routine tool to determine the behavior of the soft tissue of the face in the three planes of space. This can serve as a useful guide in diagnosis, treatment planning/ prediction and patient communication.

In an attempt to study the relationship between 3D morphologic measurements of soft tissue change following orthodontic treatment and the corresponding two-dimensional change, we (Al-Sanea, Kusnoto and Evans) tested the hypothesis that there is significant correlation between 3D morphologic measurements and 2D morphologic measurements of facial soft tissue change following orthodontic treatment in the same regions of the face in the same patient.

5.1 Correlation measurements between two-dimensional and three-dimensional changes in the soft tissue profile retraction group

Pearson correlation coefficient was calculated to determine the relationship between two-dimensional and three-dimensional measurements in the soft tissue profile retraction group at (0.05) level of significance. No statistically significant correlation existed between two-dimensional and three-dimensional measurements. The p values of the correlation ranged between (0.084- 0.661). Table 7 shows the Pearson Correlation values while scatter diagrams are represented in Figure 11-15.

Measurements	Number	ρ	Significance
2D-Sn and 3D- Sn	20	-0.173	NS
2D-SfA and 3D-SfA	20	0.212	NS
2D-UL and 3D-UL	20	-0.136	NS
2D-LL and 3D-LL	20	0.396	NS
2D-SfB and 3D-SfB	20	-0.104	NS

NS: Statistically non significant
*P value is statistically significant at 0.05

Table 7. Correlation measurements between two-dimensional and three dimensional changes in the soft tissue profile retraction group.

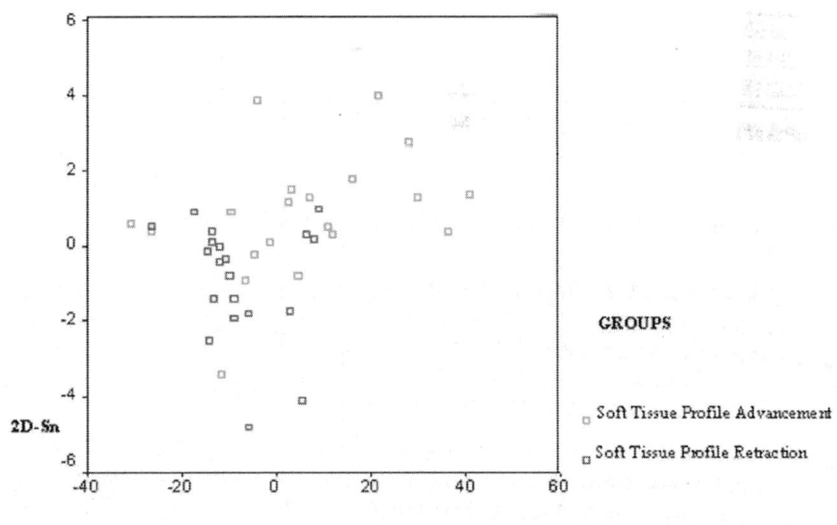

Fig. 11. Scatter diagram of correlation between 2D-Sn and 3D-Sn values.

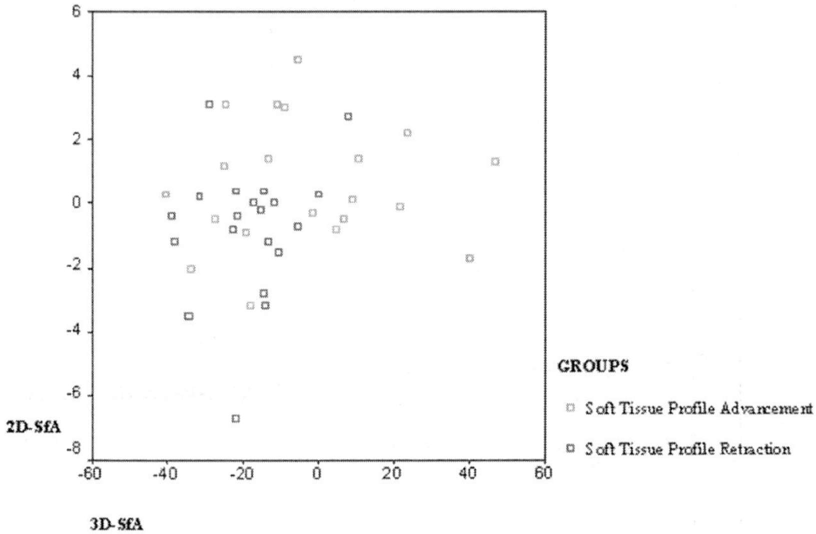

Fig. 12. Scatter diagram of correlation between 2D-SfA and 3D- SfA.

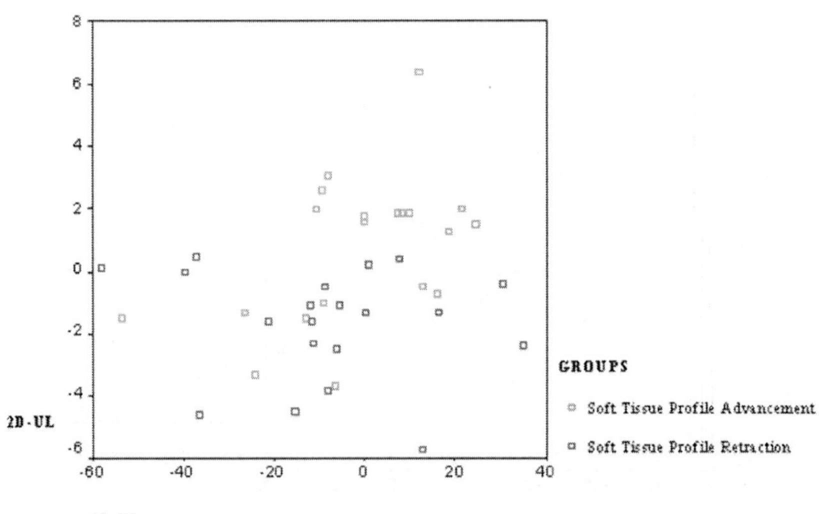

Fig. 13. Scatter diagram of correlation between 2D-UL and 3D- UL.

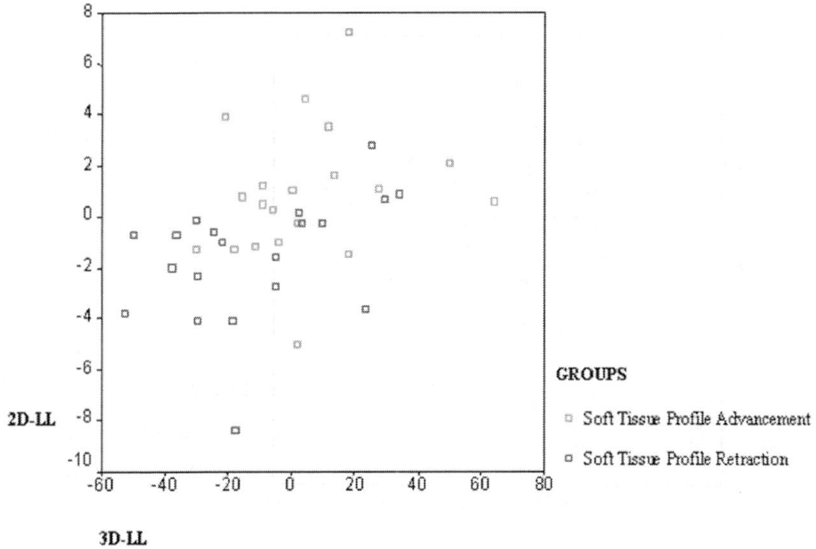

Fig. 14. Scatter diagram of correlation between 2D-LL and 3D-LL.

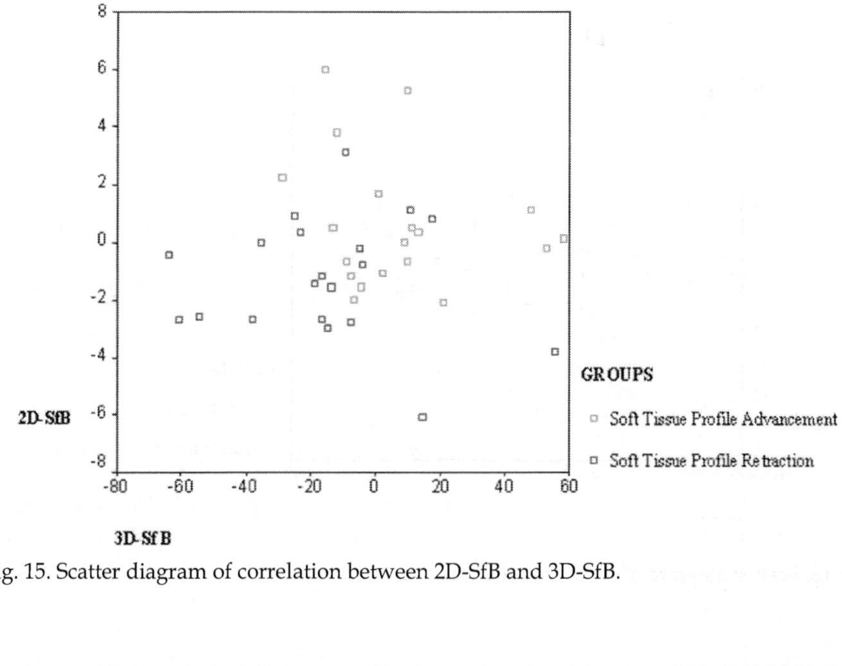

Fig. 15. Scatter diagram of correlation between 2D-SfB and 3D-SfB.

5.2 Correlation measurements between two-dimensional and three dimensional changes in the soft tissue profile advancement group

Pearson correlation coefficient was calculated to determine the relationship between two-dimensional and three-dimensional measurements in the soft tissue profile advancement group at (0.05) level of significance. No statistically significant correlation existed between two-dimensional and three-dimensional measurements except in the upper lip values (2D-UL and 3D-UL) where the p value was 0.033. The p values of the correlation in the rest of the measurements ranged between (0.116-0.917). The Pearson Correlation values and the scatter diagrams are shown in Table 8 and Figures 11-15 respectively.

Measurements	Number	ρ	Significance
2D-Sn and 3D- Sn	20	0.363	NS
2D-SfA and 3D-SfA	20	0.025	NS
2D-UL and 3D-UL	20	0.477*	S
2D-LL and 3D-LL	20	0.212	NS
2D-SfB and 3D-SfB	20	-0.207	NS

NS: Statistically non significant
*P value is statistically significant at 0.05

Table 8. Correlation measurements between two-dimensional and three dimensional changes in the soft tissue profile advancement group.

6. References

Al-Mesad, S. (1998). Soft Tissue Changes in White and Black Orthodontic Populations. Master's Thesis A447, University of Illinois at Chicago, Chicago, pp. 1-68.

Al-Sanea, R. (2007). Three Dimensional Morphometric Analysis of Facial Soft Tissue Changes Following Orthodontic Treatment. M.S. dissertation, University of Illinois at Chicago, United States - Illinois, Dissertations & Theses @ CIC Institutions, (Publication No. AAT 1449189), pp. 1-91, ISBN 9780549284208

Bishara, S.E.; Cummins, D.M. & Jakobsen, J.R. (1995). A Computer Assisted Photogrammetric Analysis of Soft Tissue Changes After Orthodontic Treatment, Part II: Results. *American Journal of Orthodontics and Dentofacial Orthopedics*, Vol.108, No.1, (July 1995), pp 38-47, ISSN 0889-5406

Blanz, V. & Vetter, T. (1999). A Morphable Model for the Synthesis of 3D Faces. *SIGGRAPH' 99 Conference Proceedings*, pp. 187-194, ISSN 0097-8930

Bloom, L.A. (1961). Perioral Profile Changes in Orthodontic Treatment. *American Journal of Orthodontics and Dentofacial Orthopedics*, 47:371, 1961, ISSN 0889-5406

Boley, J.C.; Pontier, J.P.; Smith, S. & Fulbright, M. (1998). Facial Changes in Extraction and Non-Extraction Patients. *Angle Orthodontist*, Vol.68, No.6, (December 1998), pp. 539-546, ISSN 0003-3219

Burke, P. (1983). Stereophotogrammetic Measurement of Change in Soft Tissue Following Surgery. *British Dental Journal*, Vol.155, No.11, (December 1983), pp. 373-379, ISSN 00007-0610

Clement, J.G. & Marks, M.K., eds. (2005) Computer-Graphic Facial Reconstruction . Amsterdam and Boston, Elsevier Academic Press, 2005, pp. 1-390, ISBN 0124730515

DeCarlo, D.; Metaxas, D. & Stone, M. (1998). An Anthropometric Face Model Using Variational Techniques. *SIGGRAPH' 98 Conference Proceedings,* pp. 67-74, ISSN 0097-8930

Denis, K.L. & Speidel, T.M. (1987). Comparison of the Three Methods of Profile Change Prediction in the Adult Orthodontic Patient. *American Journal of Orthodontics and Dentofacial Orthopedics,* Vol.92, No.5, (November 1987), pp. 376-402, ISSN 0889-5406

Farkas, L.G: (1987). Anthropometric Facial Proportions. Springfield, Charles C. Thomas Publisher, ISBN 0398052611

FaceGen™. (2005, 2009) Singular Inversions © 2005, 2009. Vancouver, British Columbia, Canada.

Finnoy, J.P.; Wisth, P.J. & Boe, O.E. (1987). Changes in Soft Tissue Profile During and After Orthodontic Treatment. *European Journal of Orthodontics,* Vol.9, No.1, (February 1987), pp. 68- 78, ISSN 0141-5387

Garner, L.D. (1974). Soft Tissue Changes Concurrent With Orthodontic Tooth Movement. *American Journal of Orthodontics and Dentofacial Orthopedics,* Vol.66, No.4, (October 1974), pp. 357–377, ISSN 0889-5406

Harrell, W.; Hatcher, D. & Bolt, R. (2002). In Search of Anatomic Truth: 3D Digital Patient Modeling and the Future of Orthodontics, *American Journal of Orthodontics and Dentofacial Orthopedics,* Vol.122, No.3, (September 2002), pp. 125-130, ISSN 0889-5406

Hatcher, D.C. & Dial, C. (1999). Dental Imaging Centers. *Journal of the California Dental Association,* Vol.27, No.12, (December 1999), pp. 953-9, ISSN 1043-2256

Hershey, H.G. (1972). Incisor Tooth Retraction and Subsequent Profile Change in Postadolescent Female Patients. *American Journal of Orthodontics and Dentofacial Orthopedics,* Vol.61, No.1, (January 1972), pp. 45–54, ISSN 0889-5406

Hutton, T.J.; Buxton, B.F.; Hammond, P. & Potts, H.W.W. (2003). IEEE Transactions on Medical Imaging. 22, 2003.

Ismail, S.F. & Moss, J.P. (2002). The Three-Dimensional Effects of Orthodontic Treatment on the Facial Soft Tissues - a Preliminary Study. *British Dental Journal,* Vol.192, No.2, (January 2002), pp. 104 108, ISSN 0007-0610

Kocadereli, I. (2002). Changes in Soft Tissue Profile After Orthodontic Treatment With and Without Extractions. *American Journal of Orthodontics and Dentofacial Orthopedics,* Vol.122. No.1, (July 2002), pp. 67-72, ISSN 0889-5406.

Lavelle, C.L., Carvalho, R.S.: An Evaluation of the Changes in Soft-Tissue Profile Form Induced by Orthodontic Therapy. *American Journal of Orthodontics and Dentofacial Orthopedics,* Vol.96, No.6, (December, 1989), pp. 467-476, ISSN 0889-5406

Lele, S. & Richtsmeire, J.T. (1991). Euclidean Distance Matrix Analysis: a Coordinate-Free Approach for Comparing Biological Shapes Using Landmark Data. *American Journal of Physical Anthropology,* Vol.86, No.3, (November 1991), pp. 415-427, ISSN 0002-9483

Lele, S. & Cole, T.M. (1995). Euclidean Distance Matrix Analysis: a Statistical Review. In: Current Issues in Statistical Shape Analysis, Eds. Mardia, K.K.V. & Gill, C.A., Leeds University Press, pp. 49-53, ISBN 0853161615

Luppanapornlarp, S. & Johnston, L.E. Jr. (1993). The Effects of Premolar-Extraction: a Long-Term Comparison of Outcomes in "Clear-Cut" Extraction and Nonextraction Class II Patients. *Angle Orthodontist,* Vol.64, No.4, (Winter 1993), pp. 257-272, ISSN 0003-3219

Marsh, J.L. & Vannier, M.V. (1983). The "Third Dimension" in Craniofacial Surgery. *Plastic and Reconstructive Surgery*, Vol.71, No.6, (June 1983), pp. 759-767, ISSN 0032-1052

Moss, J.P.; Linney, A.D.; Grindrod, S.R.; Ridge, S.R. & Clifton, J.S. (1987). Three-Dimensional Visualization of the Face and Skull Using Computerized Tomography and Laser Scaling Techniques. *American Journal of Orthodontics and Dentofacial Orthopedics*, Vol.94, No.4, (November 1987), pp. 247-253, ISSN 0089-5406

Moss, J.P. & Linney, A.D. (1990). The Prediction of Facial Aesthetics. *The New York State Dental Journal*, Vol.56, No.6, (June-July 1990), pp. 44-46, ISSN 0028-7571

Oliver, B.M. (1982). The Influence of Lip Thickness and Strain on Upper Lip Response to Incisor Retraction. *American Journal of Orthodontics and Dentofacial Orthopedics*, Vo.82, No.2, (August 1982), pp. 141–148, ISSN 0889-5406

O'Toole, A.J.; Vetter, T. & Blanz, V. (1999). Three-Dimensional Shape and Two-Dimensional Surface Reflectance Contributions to Face Recognition: An Application of Three-Dimensional Morphing. *Vision Research*, Vol.39, No.18, (September 1999), pp. 3145-3155, ISSN 0042-6989

Paquette, D.E.; Beattie, J.R. & Johnston, L.E. Jr. (1992). A Long-Term Comparison of Nonextraction and Premolar Extraction Edgewise Therapy in "Borderline" Class II Oatients. *American Journal of Orthodontics and Dentofacial Orthopedics*, Vol.102, No.1, (July 1992), pp. 1-14, ISSN 0889-5406

Peck, S. & Peck, L. (1995). Selected Aspects of the Art and Science of Facial Esthetics. *Seminars in Orthodontics*, Vol.1, No.1, (June 1995) pp. 105-126, ISSN 1073-8746

Quintero, J.C.; Trosien, A.; Hatcher D. & Kapila S. (1999). Craniofacial Imaging in Orthodontics: Historical Perspective, Current Status, and Future Developments. *Angle Orthodontist*, Vol.69, No.6, (December 1999), pp. 491-506, ISSN 0003-3219

Riedel, R.A. (1950). Esthetics and Its Relation to Orthodontic Therapy. *Angle Orthodontist*, Vol.20, No.3, (July 1950), pp. 168-78, ISSN 0003-3219

Roos, N. (1977). Soft Tissue Changes in Class II Treatment. *American Journal of Orthodontics and Dentofacial Orthopedics*, Vol.72, No.2, (August 1977), pp. 165-175, ISSN 0889-5406

Rudee, D.A. (1964). Proportional Profile Changes Concurrent With Orthodontic Therapy. *American Journal of Orthodontics and Dentofacial Orthopedics*, Vol.50, No.6, (June 1964), pp. 421-434, ISSN 0889-5406

Savara, B.S. (1965). Applications of Photogrammetry for Quantitative Study of Tooth and Face Morphology. *American Journal of Physical Anthropology*, Vol.23, No.4, (December 1965), pp. 427-434, ISSN 0002-9483

Singh, G.D.; Maldonado, L. & Thind, B.S. (2004-2005). Changes in the Soft Tissue Facial Profile Following Orthodontic Extractions: a Geometric Morphometric Study. *The Functional Orthodontist*, Vol.22, No.1, (Winter 2004-Spring 2005), pp. 34-38, 40, ISSN 8756-3150

Tweed, C. H. (1944). Indications for the Extraction of Teeth in Orthodontic Procedure. *American Journal of Orthodontics and Oral Surgery*, Vol.30, No.8, (August 1944), pp. 405-428, ISSN 0096-6347

Weisstein, E.W. (1999). Distance. From: *MathWorld--A Wolfram Web Resource*. http://mathworld.wolfram.com/Distance.html, 1999.

Wisth, P.J. (1974). Soft Tissue Response to Upper Incisor Retraction in Boys. *British Journal of Orthodontics*, Vol.1, No.5, (October 1974), pp. 199–204, ISSN 0301-228X

3

Are the Orthodontic Basis Wrong? Revisiting Two of the Keys to Normal Oclusion (Crown Inclination and Crown Angulation) in the Andrews Series

C. Jiménez-Caro[1,2], F. de Carlos[1,2], A.A. Suárez[1,3], J.A. Vega[4] and J. Cobo[1,2]

[1]Instituto Asturiano de Odontología, Oviedo
[2]Departamento de Cirugía y Especialidades Médico-Quirúrgicas (sección de Odontología), Universidad de Oviedo
[3]Departamento de Construcción e Ingeniería de la Fabricación (Sección de Ingeniería Mecánica), Universidad de Oviedo
[4]Departamento de Morfología y Biología Celular, Universidad de Oviedo
Spain

1. Introduction

In the second half of the last century, Lawrence F. Andrews studied a series of 120 casts, of non-orthodontic subjects with ideal patterns of dental occlusion, and established "*The six keys to normal occlusion*". These were the basis to program the tooth movement directly on the bracket and not in wire bending, and were also the origin of the straight-wire, or preadjusted, appliance of current use in orthodontics. However, until now, the postulates of Andrews never have been contrasted using the scientific method and a proper statistical analysis. Moreover, some orthodontists have the suspect that the criteria of Andrews are not universal and applicable to the whole population since he do not distinguished age-dependent changes, ethnical group, sex, or left-right asymmetry. The critical analysis of the Andrews' work is the goal of this Chapter, but we have centered our efforts in the date related to Crown angulation (the mesiodistal "tip") and Crown inclination (labiolingual or buccolingual inclination) which are of capital importance to perform accurately functional and aesthetic orthodontic treatments.

2. Background: Historical context

The use of the fixed appliance in orthodontic is directly linked to the proposal and guides of Edward H. Angle to move the teeth to the so-called "occlusion line", defined as "*the line, shape and position, must be teeth in balance if there is a normal occlusion*". Angle described in detail the relationships between maxillary and mandible, and maxillary-mandible and teeth, and especially the teeth among them, in order to achieve an ideal occlusion (Angle, 1929b; see the Special Edition of 1981).

These recommendations required the designing of special devices for three-dimensional control of teeth in order to reach the occlusion line and allow teeth to be correctly aligned in both the maxillary and mandible. Furthermore, according to Angle the alignment of the teeth, both crown and root, would result in the expansion of both the maxillary and mandible arches. This was also one of the main objectives to design the Angle's devices. Nevertheless, these postulates are still under discussion (Canut, 2000; Peck, 2008).

In 1887, Angle developed the "E" arch appliance formed by a thick gold wire placed for labial and some stainless steel tape on the first molar adjusted at pressure. This type of arch expanded both maxillary and mandible arches sagittally and transversely, and allowed a movement of simple inclination of the crown through a few ligatures that surrounded the tooth and conformed to the arch.

In the early 20th century with the development of metallurgy emerged the possibility of banding all the teeth and welding devices for the control of rotations. In 1910, Angle introduced the first appliance with individual tooth action and fullbanding, the so-called "pin and tube appliance", which welded small vertical tubes in the bands to introduce a stem attached to the wire. This device facilitated the labiolingual as mesiodistal expansion of the maxillary, and its drawback was the requirement for adjustment and accuracy in addition to the skill by the clinician (Bravo, 2007). Unfortunately one of the problems posed by this device was its inestability (Graber and Vanarsdall, 1994). Later, in 1916, Angle designed a bracket, called "ribbon arch appliance wire-band", containing a rectangular wire fixed by a few pins and placing the wider side on the tooth. This device properly controlled the labiolingual as well as vertical placement of teeth, by facilitating the correction of giroversions. However, it was difficult to place on the cusp and the looseness of the wire in the slot prevented mesiodistal control. Another substantial contribution of Angle was the frontal slot bracket, as opposed to the ribbon arch appliance of vertical opening, which featured great advantages, especially the ease to introduce the wire and the possibility to control the premolars and the adjustment of mesiodistal movement. In 1926 he presented the "bracket 447" with a horizontal slot .022 "x.028" which served to introduce a rectangular wire of the same thickness through the more narrow are, i.e. edgewise. It was made in gold and was called "soft bracket", as it opened easily and distorting (see for a review the Special Edition of Angle's work, 1981).

Over the basis of this model Steiner developed the "bracket 452" (hard bracket), more resistant to deformation which allowed to control teeth movement at the three levels through bends as tip, torque and in-out. This would become the prototype of the contemporary brackets.

Previously to the emergence of the straight wire, Angle already proposed to place the brackets to mesial or distal from the teeth to help to correct teeth rotations (Angle, 1929a), and a posterior angulation of the brackets to get proper root movements (see Meyer and Nelson, 1978). Later, Lewis (1950) joined segments ("arms") linked to the brackets, in contact with the wires for controlling rotations. Thereafter, Holdaway (1952) proposed that the buccal aspect of the brackets could be angulated depending on the degree of severity of the malocclusion. Twenty years later the original idea of Lewis, with some modifications, was adapted by Gottlieb et al. (1972). On the other hand Jarabak and Fizell (1963) minted the well-known phrase "*building treatment into the appliance*" which proposed to incorporate angles within the bracket, and these authors presented at the meeting of the American Association of Orthodontist in 1960 the first bracket model combining crown angulation and crown inclination (Wahl, 2008).

All together the work of all these authors consisted in eliminating bends in the wire to be incorporated into the bracket. All this led to the evolution of the bracket of edgewise to the bracket of straight wire incorporating the information in the slot of the bracket (Figure 1).

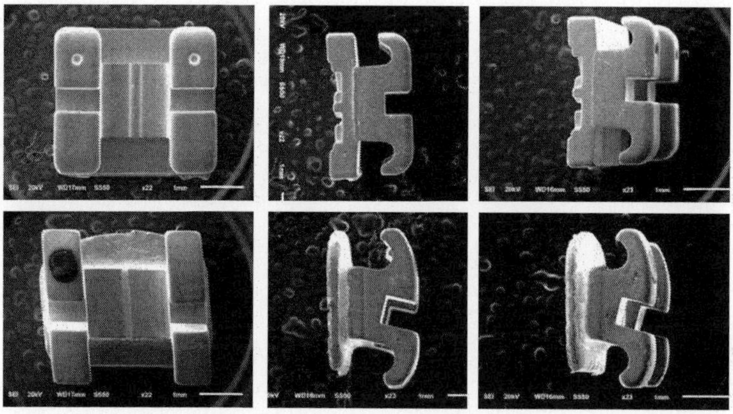

Fig. 1. Top line: Scanning electron microscopy of one bracket of standard edgewise appliance from a frontal (A), lateral (B), and oblique (C) view. Bottom line: Scanning electron microscopy of one straight wire bracket from a frontal (D), lateral (E), and oblique (F) view. The absence of information in the slot of the bracket of standard edgewise appliance in comparison with the bracket of the straight-wire appliance can be observed.

2.1 The work of L.F. Andrews

From 1960 Andrews published a series of five studies, which resulted in the development of a new concept for the orthodontic treatment: the straight wire appliance.

The **First study** had as purpose the completion of a thesis for obtaining the certification of the American Board of Orthodontics. It consisted of the static analysis of the occlusion in post-orthodontic treatment casts. He found that there were features common to all them: absence of rotations in the incisors, no cross-bites, and Class I molar relationship of Angle, except in cases of extractions in a single maxillary. However, other parameters were not common at all. He deduced that the optimal positioning of the teeth should sustain in studies of optimal natural dentures (see Andrews, 1989).

In order to perform the **Second study**, Andrews selected 120 casts of non-orthodontic, untreated, patients with supposedly ideal occlusions, from which arose a few assumptions that should determine the occlusal objectives after orthodontic treatment. The compilation of the cases was carried out between 1960 and 1964 with the help of various Orthodontists, among them Brodie (Andrews, 1989). These casts have in common, in addition to lack of orthodontic treatment, a correct teeth alignment and positioning as well as a seemingly an "excellent" occlusion. The concept was, in essence, that if it is know what is right it can identify and quantify what's wrong in a direct and methodical manner. Over the casts Andrews conducted a series of marks: the facial axis (axial) of the clinical crowns, the most prominent portion of incisors, canines and pre-molars, as well as the projection of the medial groove in molars, and the midpoint of the height of each clinical crown.

In the **Third study** he described six characteristics that were always present in the 120 casts. These features would be referred to as *"The six keys to normal occlusion"* and were published in 1972 in the American Journal of Orthodontics (Andrews, 1972). The "Six Keys" would assess the occlusal situation without using measuring instruments, as in the keys II and III (referring to the crown angulation and crown inclination, respectively), Andrews do not use units but simply the positive or negative sign (he used terms such as lightly positive, generally negative, etc). According to Andrews the "Six Keys" are interdependent components of the structural system of optimal occlusion and serve as a basis to assess the occlusion.

They consisted of a series of significant characteristics shared by all of the non-orthodontic normal teeth, and were the following: specific molar relationship (key I), crown angulation (the angulation or mesiodistal "tip" of the long axis of the crown: Key II), crown inclination (the labiolingual or buccolingual inclination of the long axis of the crown: Key III), no rotations (key IV), absence of spaces (key V), and the occlusal plane (key VI). In the own Andrews words *"The six keys to normal occlusion contribute individually and collectively to the total scheme of occlusion and, therefore, are viewed as essential to successful orthodontic treatment"*.

The 120 casts analyzed by Andrews showed similarities in values of crown angulation, crown inclination, shape, and size for the different types of teeth. But this was not enough for the design of the new device. Therefore, in a further study attempted to determine the shape, size and position of each tooth in the arch.

For the **Fourth study**, Andrews made new measurements over the 120 casts (see Andrews, 1989). The measurements made in this case were: the determination of the bracket area for each teeth, vertical crown contour, crown angulation, crown inclination, offset of maxillary molars, horizontal crown contour, crown facial prominence and depth of the curve of Spee. So, he doubled the 120 casts and removed the occlusal halves of the crown. On these surfaces he defined a line that joins the portion more vestibular of contact points and the most prominent portions of each clinical crown. He denominated this line as the embrasure line. The values obtained were incorporated into the design of the bracket to eliminate the first order bends. These measurements, except bracket size and curve of Spee, were averaged for each tooth type, and the results served as norms for the design of the new appliance: the straight-wire. After describing outcomes, Andrews concludes that the study reveals essential data on the position (with the exception of the inclination of the incisors), morphology and relative vestibular prominence of each tooth in the arch. The differences in the inclination of the incisors were attributed to disharmonies between the maxillary bones.

The **Fifth**, and final, **study** consisted of comparison of 1156 casts post-treatment in terms of occlusion, with the 120 casts from non-treated subjects with optimal occlusion. This study was focused to the design of a new device able to include the "six keys". The conclusion was that very few of the analyzed casts presented all the "six keys" (Andrews, 1976a). Therefore, he considered necessary the establishment of some premises of treatment, including common objectives, coupled with a new device. The straight wire appliance of Andrews was the first completely pre-adjusted orthodontic appliance. It was designed for the treatment of cases without extraction with one less than 5° ANB, avoiding the need for bends in the wire. As the closure of the spaces after premolar extractions produces undesirable side effects (rotation, inclination), Andrews subsequently introduced different brackets for cases with extractions. Moreover, when designing their brackets, Andrews differentiated between treatments in which the translation of teeth is necessary and that no, the so-called brackets of translation and standard brackets (Andrews, 1976c, 1989). In a short time the new straight-wire appliance was adopted by the American universities and most of the orthodontists (Andrews, 1976b, 1989). Some year later (Roth, 1976, 1987), designed brackets with information at the three levels, varying the characteristics described by Andrews. He developed the second generation of preprogrammed brackets, increasing the crown inclination in the canines up to 13° to achieve the "best functional occlusion".

The third generation of brackets was developed by McLaughlin, Bennett and Trevisi (MBT™, McLaughlin et al., 1997; see also McLaughlin and Bennett, 1989). It is based on light forces and sliding mechanics maintaining the advantages of the prescriptions of Andrews and Roth, but eliminating certain limitations.

The introduction of straight-wire appliance in orthodontics led to a great controversy initially, but soon was accepted by all American orthodontic companies since it easily consent to control dental positions with the placement of brackets. Since then, others have developed new appliances, also fully programmed pre-adjusted (see for a review and references Proffit et al., 2008).

3. The Andrew's series: The values for crown angulation and crown inclination revisited

The first step of our work was to collect the individual values for crown angulation and crown inclination contained in the text and annex from Andrews' book "Straight-Wire, The Concept and Appliance" (Andrews, 1989), confirm that the descriptive statistical are exact, and apply to them a descriptive statistical analysis using the actual current methods.

When we try to validate the Andrews' statistical design the following questions and methodological troubles emerge when analyze the series of 120 casts that are the basis of the Andrews' work:

1. The origin of the sample: the author does not indicate how was selected the sample and what were the selection criteria;
2. The type of clustering of the data: he reports data from 240 casts instead of 120, because he evaluated together teeth from left and right side without checking whether or not there are differences between hemi-arch;
3. The variability between the data in the same group: the data are presented as a tabulation of centralization and dispersion of the maxillary and mandibular angles measures as did Andrews, with 240 data as if they were separate measures.

Therefore, our second step was the verification of the validity of the Andrew's design by contrast of hypothesis. It was carried out a Student t test of paired data to know whether or not there are significant differences in the crown angulation and crown inclination between the right and left hemi-arch with respect of their average values. The null hypothesis was that there are no significant differences in the crown angulation or crown inclination of teeth with respect to the side ($p \geq 0.05$) and the study hypothesis was that there are significant differences in the crown angulation or crown inclination of teeth with respect to the side ($p \leq 0.05$).

Descriptive statistics in the Andrew's series

Surprisingly, several errors in the basic descriptive statistics (count, average, standard deviation, minimum and maximum values) were detected for crown angulation but not for crown inclination (Tables 1 and 2). Thus, there is an error between the source (single) data and statistic results appearing in his publication. Moreover, in comparing these basic descriptive statistics with those obtained by us, applying the some probes on the Andrews data, it can be observed again that do not match for crown angulation (Table 1). Thus, there is an error between the source (single) data and statistic results appearing in his publication, and the statistics are no well calculated.

	Maxillary			**Mandible**		
Tooth	n	Range min/max	mean±SD	n	Range min/max	mean±SD
Andrews data/Our data						
1L+1R	240	-3/9	3.59±1.65	240	-4/3	0.53±1.29
1L+1R	240	-3/9	3.59±**1.70**	240	-4/3	0.53±1.29
2L+2R	240	**-2**/15	**8.04**±2.80	240	-5/3	0.38±1.47
2L+2R	240	-26/15	**7.90±3.53**	240	-5/3	0.38±1.48
3L+3R	239	**1**/17	**8.40**±2.97	240	-11/12	2.48±3.28
3L+3R	240	0/17	**8.13±3.21**	240	-11/12	2.48±3.29
4L+4R	240	-2/**12**	**2.65**±1.69	240	-10/10	1.28±1.90
4L+4R	240	-2/14	**2.90±2.29**	240	-10/10	1.28±1.90
5L+5R	240	0/12	**2.82**±1.52	240	-5/7	1.54±1.35
5L+5R	240	0/12	**2.86±1.54**	240	-5/7	1.54±1.36
6L+6R	240	-7/16	**5.73**±1.90	240	-2/6	2.03±1.14
6L+6R	240	-7/16	**5.69±1.97**	240	-2/6	2.03±1.14

Table 1. **Crown angulation**. Basic descriptive statistics of Andrews' data after revisited by us (black), and after the descriptive statistical study we have carried out (red). Values are expressed in degrees, and the observed differences are highlighted in bold.

	Maxillary			**Mandible**		
Tooth	n	Range min/max	mean±SD	n	Range min/max	mean±SD
Andrews data/Our data						
1L+1R	240	-7/15	6.11±3.97	240	-17/16	-1.71±5.79
1L+1R	240	-7/15	6.11±3.98	240	-17/16	-1.71±5.80
2L+2R	240	-6/17	4.42±4.38	239	-19/15	-3.24±5.37
2L+2R	240	-6/17	4,42±4.39	240	-19/15	-3.24±5.38
3L+3R	240	-17/10	-7.25±4.21	239	-26/2	-12.73±4.65
3L+3R	240	-17/10	-7.25±4.22	239	-26/2	-12.73±4.66
4L+4R	240	-20/5	-8.47±4.02	240	-35/-1	-18.95±4.96
4L+4R	240	-20/5	-8.47±4.03	239	-35/-1	-18.95±4.97
5L+5R	240	-20/3	-8.78±4.13	240	-45/-8	-23.63±5.58
5L+5R	240	-20/3	-8.78±4.14	240	-45/-8	-23.63±5.60
6L+6R	240	-25/2	-11.53±3.91	240	-55/-9	-30.67±5.90
6L+6R	240	-25/2	-11.53±3.92	240	-55/-9	-30.67±5.91

Table 2. **Crown inclination**. Basic descriptive statistics of Andrews' data after revisited by us (black), and after the descriptive statistical study we have carried out (red). Values are expressed in degrees, and the observed differences are highlighted in bold.

As Andrews considered the data together then we analyzed if there are differences between left and right teeth. For crown angulation, in comparing the average values of the right side and the left side differences were found to be significant ($p<0.05$) for all maxillary and mandibular teeth, except for the lower central incisor (Table 3). On the other hand, the comparison of mean averages for crown inclination of the right and left sides significant differences ($p<0.05$) were found for all upper teeth, except for the canines and first premolars, and for all lower teeth expect for both central and lateral incisors (Table 4).

	Maxillary			Mandible		
Tooth	t	fd	p	t	df	p value
1	3.00	119	**0.003**	1.11	119	0.270
2	5.71	119	**0.000**	-1.98	119	**0.050**
3	2.39	118	**0.013**	-2.62	119	**0.010**
4	2.30	119	**0.023**	-2.52	119	**0.013**
5	2.11	119	**0.037**	-3.86	119	**0.000**
6	2.79	119	**0.006**	-3.97	119	**0.000**

df: degrees of freedom

Table 3. **Crown angulation**. Student t test for crown angulation of right vs left arch. Significant differences are highlighted in bold.

	Maxillary			Mandible		
Tooth	t	fd	p	t	df	p values
1	4.00	119	**0.000**	0.11	119	0.909
2	4.95	119	**0.000**	-0.56	119	0.830
3	-1.22	119	0.223	-3.37	118	**0.008**
4	0.65	119	0.518	-4.60	118	**0.00**
5	2.34	119	**0.021**	-5.12	119	**0.000**
6	2.99	119	**0.003**	-6.56	119	**0.000**

df: degrees of freedom

Table 4. **Crown inclination**. Student t test for crown inclination for right vs left arch. Significant differences are highlighted in bold.

These results consent to affirm that significant differences exists between the right and left sides of each arch, for the angulation of crown for all the teeth of the upper arch, and for the majority of the lower arch. Regarding the crown inclination significant differences do not occur in all the maxillary and mandibular teeth but all show any difference.

3.1 Descriptive statistics of separate hemi-arch

Since significant differences between the right and left hemi-arch were found in the Andrews' series we decided to perform and basic descriptive statistical analysis of both crown angulation and crown inclination in each hemi-arch separately. At a value of the confidence interval 95% the standard deviation shows very high values in some teeth, and the variable dispersion is therefore very broad.

In the upper maxillary the greater homogeneity in crown angulation was found for the central incisor, the second premolar and first molar (Table 5; Fig. 2A). The mandible crown angulation shows a more homogeneous behavior, except for the canine (Table 5; Fig. 2B). The presence of outlier values implies a high variability, and so at a confidence interval 95% wider than would be desirable (Figs. 3A and 3C, and Figs. 3B and 3D).

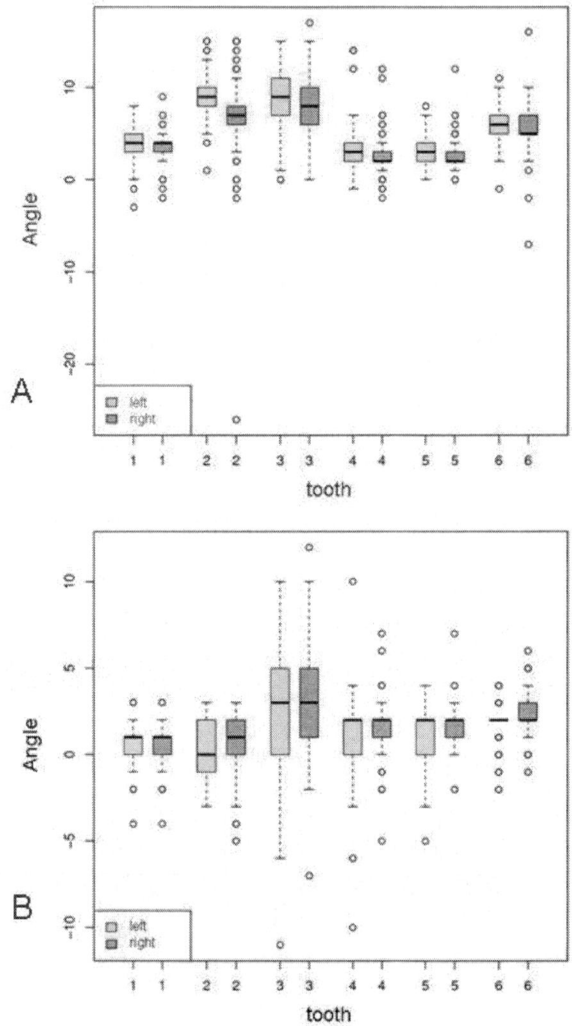

Fig. 2. Box-plot representation of the maxillary crown angulation (A) and mandibular crown angulation (B) of the data from the Andrews' series.

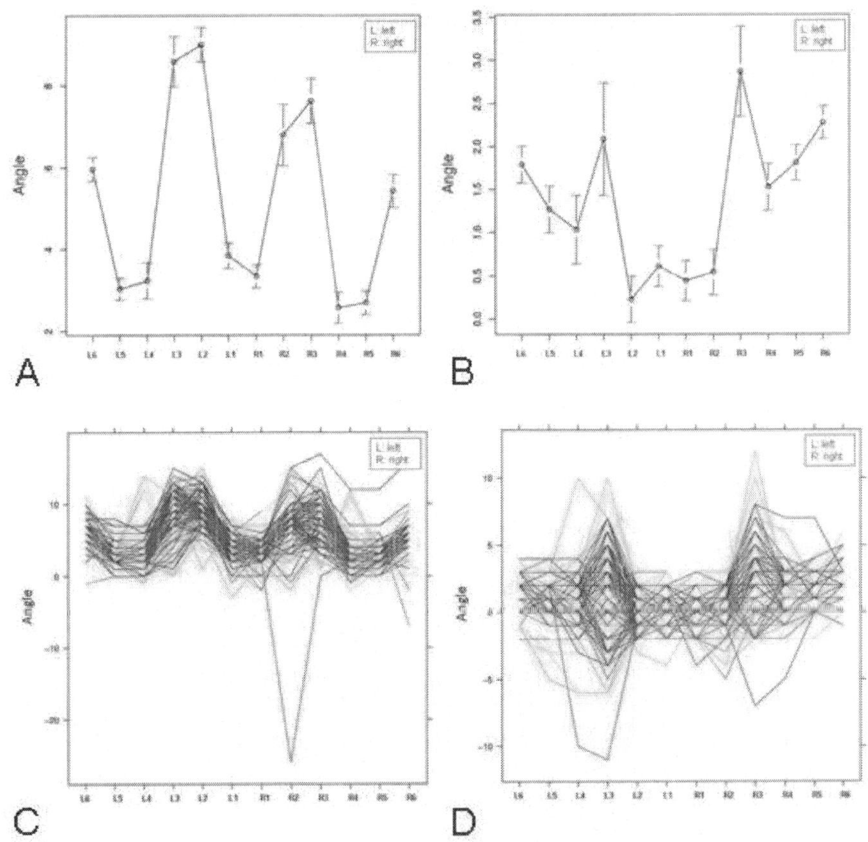

Fig. 3. Mean values of confidence interval 95% and profiles of the maxillary crown angulation (A,C) and mandibular crown angulation (B,D) of the data from the Andrews' series.

Tooth		n	mean±SD	range of confidence interval
Right hemi-arch				
1R	upper	120	3.42±1.56	3.06 - 3.62
	lower	120	0.44±1.28	0.21 - 0.67
2R	upper	120	6.79±2.85	6.04 - 7.54
	lower	120	0.54±1.46	0.28 - 0.81
3R	upper	119	7.61±2.95	7.07 - 8.16
	lower	120	2.87±2.89	2.34 - 3.39
4R	upper	120	2.57±2.13	2.19 - 2.96
	lower	120	1.52±1.51	1.25 - 1.80
5R	upper	120	2.69±1.55	2.40 - 2.98
	lower	120	1.81±1.13	1.60 - 2.01
6R	upper	120	5.42±2.12	5.01 - 5.82
	lower	120	2.27±1.04	2.09 - 2.46
Left hemi-arch				
1R	upper	120	3.84±1.70	3.53 - 4.15
	lower	120	0.61±1.30	0.37 - 0.84
2R	upper	120	9.00±2.33	8.58 - 9.42
	lower	120	0.54±1.48	0.28 - 0.81
3R	upper	120	8.58±3.37	7.97 - 9.20
	lower	120	2.87±3.61	2.34 - 3.39
4R	upper	120	3.23±2.43	2.80 - 3.67
	lower	120	1.52±2.20	1.25 - 1.80
5R	upper	120	3.03±1.47	2.77 - 3.30
	lower	120	1.81±1.50	1.60 - 2.01
6R	upper	120	5.96±1.62	5.66 - 6.25
	lower	120	2.27±1.19	2.09 - 2.46

Table 5. **Crown angulation**. Basic descriptive statistics of Andrews' data for hemi-arch after revisited by us. Values are expressed in degrees.

The results for crown inclination are reflected in table 6, and Figures 4A and 4B, which show that the variability of the data is very similar for all teeth. The mandible data presented a top-down performance in terms of average values of the central incisor to the first molar. The study of confidence intervals 95% shows differences between the teeth and the side. In general, the profiles of the subjects were similar for both the maxillary and mandibular teeth (Figs. 5A and 5C, and Figs. 5B and 5D).

Tooth		n	mean±SD	range of confidence interval
Right hemi-arch				
1R	upper	120	5.76±4.01	-2.76 – -0.67
	lower	120	-1.71±5.77	0.21 – 0.67
2R	upper	120	3.83±4.43	3.03 – 4.63
	lower	120	-3.25±5.60	-4.26 – -2.24
3R	upper	120	-7.02±4.52	-7.84 – -6.21
	lower	119	-12.19±4.28	-12.96 – -11.42
4R	upper	120	-8.57±4.11	-9.31 – -7.82
	lower	119	-18.12±4.95	-19.01 – -17.22
5R	upper	120	-9.17±4.23	-9.93 – -8.40
	lower	120	-22.49±5.46	-23.48 – -21.50
6R	upper	120	-12.0±4.08	-12.73 – -11.26
	lower	120	-29.4±5.75	-30.44 – -28.36
Left hemi-arch				
1R	upper	120	6.47±3.94	5.75 – 7.18
	lower	120	-1.70±5.85	-2.76 – -0.64
2R	upper	120	5.00±4.28	4.23 – 5.77
	lower	120	-3.21±5.15	-4.14 – -2.28
3R	upper	120	-7.47±3.90	-8.17 – -6.76
	lower	120	-13.17±5.01	-14.09 – -12.24
4R	upper	120	-8.37±3.96	-9.09 – -7.66
	lower	120	-19.78±4.87	-20.66 – -18.90
5R	upper	120	-8.39±4.01	-9.12 – -7.66
	lower	120	-24.77±5.81	-25.76 – -23.77
6R	upper	120	-11.07±3.71	-11.74 – -10.39
	lower	120	-31.93±8.02	-32.98 – -30.88

Table 6. **Crown inclination.** Basic descriptive statistics of Andrews' data for hemi-arch after revisited by us. Values are expressed in degrees.

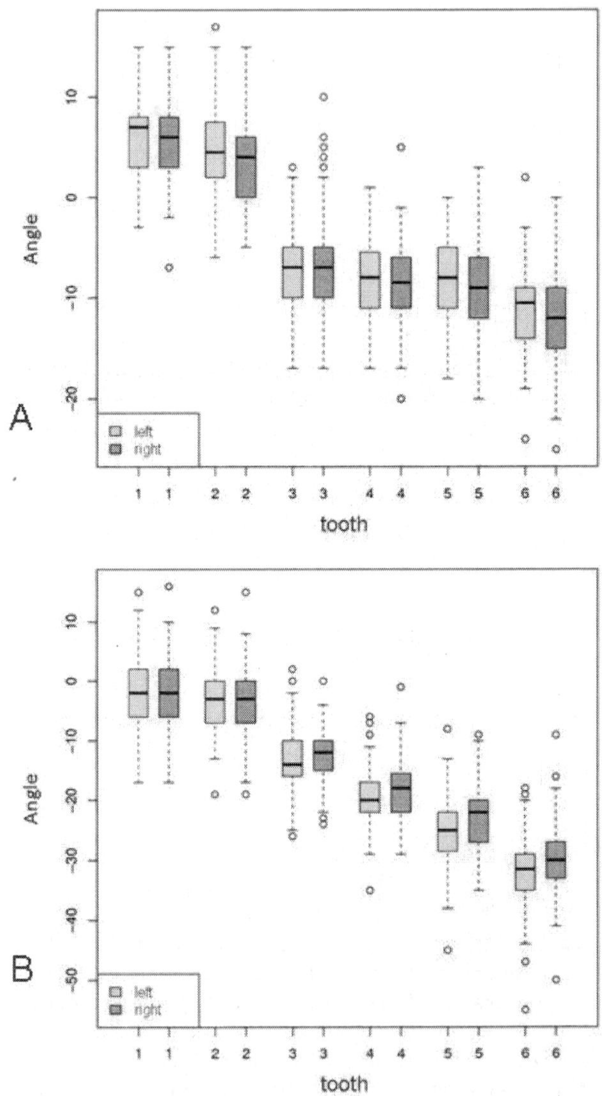

Fig. 4. Box-plot representation of the maxillary crown inclination (A) and mandibular crown inclination (B) of the data from the Andrews' series.

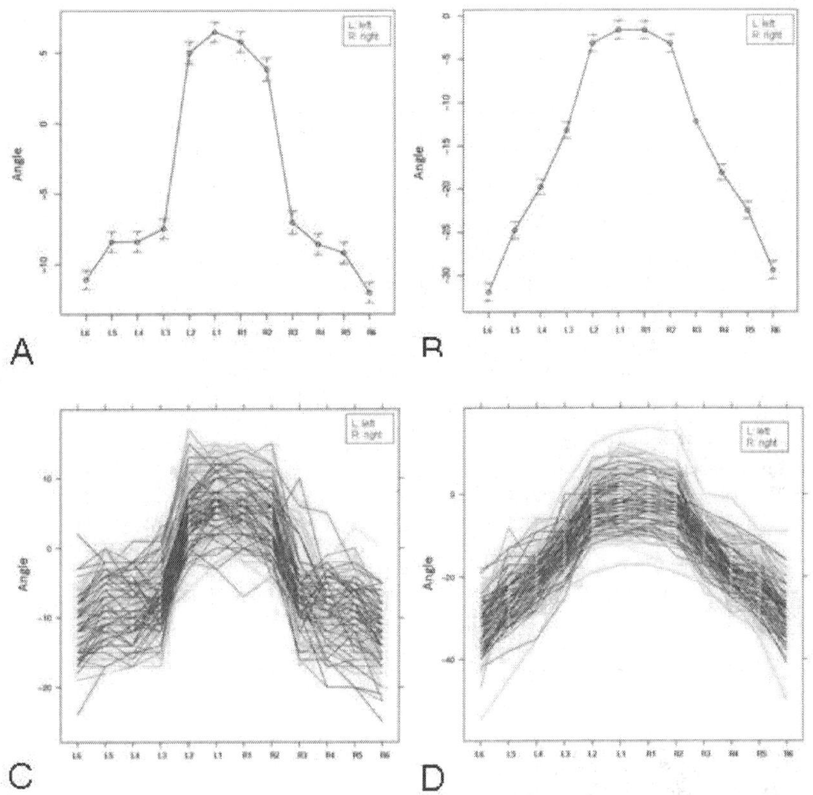

Fig. 5. Mean values of confidence interval 95% and profiles of the maxillary crown inclination (A,C) and mandibular crown inclination (B,D) of the data from the Andrews' series.

3.2 Critical comments to the Andrews' work

After the analysis of the data published by Andrews (1989) in his book *Straight-Wire, The Concept and Appliance* the first thing that draws attention is that the author annex provide data relating to 240 casts instead of 120, which are those said to have studied. This may be due to the fact that the author carried out two measurements by subject (left and right) in each arch, and then globalize the data into a single; but Andrews does not clarify this fact. Is this right? The statistical study we have performed on the Andrews' data shows that there are significant differences between left and right for crown angulation and crown inclination for most of the upper teeth, and form the lower teeth for crown angulation of the lateral incisor to the first molar, and for crown inclination in the canine, premolars and first molar. Therefore, it seems evident that the data from the Andrews study cannot be grouped, and it is necessary to work with each hemi-arch separately and perform the descriptive and comparative analysis for each one of them. From these results the following question arises: it should be necessary use different brackets on left and right side of each patient?

Another surprising finding of our review of the Andrews' data was that the results presented in terms of basic descriptive statistic not always coincide with those from the sources. These errors can be due to erroneous data sheets records or that have been made evil the descriptive analysis.

The Andrews' results are expressed as average values, and the standard deviation was occasionally elevated, thus reflecting a significant dispersion of the sample values. For example, the following measurements for crown angulation (mean±standard deviation, range: minimal-maximal) in the first premolar realize this: upper 2.65°±1.69°, -2.0° to +12°; lower: 2.90°±2.29°, -2° to +14°. The ranges show the enormous variation of values. If in cases of optimal occlusions the crown angulation of this tooth vary between -2° and 12°, take as reference a value of 2.65° in orthodontic appliances does not seems logical.

It would also be desirable that Andrews had studied the type of the data distribution in the sample, and the author seems to assume that the distribution is symmetric, but in the light of the results presented here, it is unlikely to be so. In fact, the normality test indicates that the distribution is not normal in all cases.

The listing of all the individual data of the sample is a sign of honesty by the author, and reflects the statistical methodology of the 1970s. But at the same time it allows us to appreciate their low methodological rigor, in the light of current knowledge when presenting the conclusions as a definitive response to a widely discussed problem. Thus, it is difficult to understand why the orthodontists from around the world have continued to put the brackets using as a reference the average values of the measurements made on 120 casts without rigorous selection criteria. In our casts, as well as in those from other groups (Roth, 1987; Martínez-Asúnsolo and Plasencia, 2004; Zanelato et al., 2004), the findings of Andrews for the crown angulation and inclinations were not confirmed.

Therefore, the Andrews study in terms of design, include the following shortcomings: definition of the characteristics of the sample, the exact criteria of selection of the subjects included in the sample, the absence of a descriptive statistic that analyze the way of the distribution of the data (if distribution is markedly asymmetrical, would be preferable to choose the mean than the average as a measure of central tendency), the type of sampling, and sample size calculation. In the Andrews study the sample size is adequate (240 measurements from 120 casts). Nevertheless, to work with greater precision, for example 0.5 mm, the sample should be higher.

On the other hand, the development of the work of Andrews also suffers from some defects. In this kind of studies it is necessary to assess their reproducibility or reliability, both intra-observer and inter-observed. It is not aware that the Andrews work has been performed by several observers, and therefore it must be we assumed that the measurements were carried out by Andrews himself or by another individual. Still, in any case Andrews should be repeated, at least once more, all measures in the same models and to analyze the reliability between measurements. Also, as quantitative variables, the degree of reliability should have been studied through the appropriate statistical tests: Bradley-Blackwood, correlation coefficient, tor the Student t test for paired samples. The errors we have detected in the

Andrews work are surely sufficient to raise necessary a reassessment of the theories of the straight wire. The real debate must be focused on whether the recommendations of Andrews for the crown angulation an inclination may continue to be used for the creation, development and industrialization of orthodontic appliances to serve for the entire population. The tooth size (Agenter et al., 2009; Lee et al., 2011), the place of each teeth in each side hemi-arch, the gender, and the ethnic group (Naranjilla and Rudzki-Janson, 2005) should be considered in the development of future orthodontic appliances.

4. Concluding remarks

While Andrews work is thorough and interesting for its time, it has enough limitations of design or execution to be considered actually as the foundations for the use of an appliance with universal angulation and inclination. Furthermore, we have not found one sufficient material and methodology description in the of Andrews' work to reproduce it accurately. In fact a number of errors in the results of basic descriptive statistics were detected in the Andrews' series. This could be due to errors is the data sheet, or to errors in calculating descriptive statistics.

On the other hand, it cannot be included in a common sample data from measurements obtained from the right and left sides of the maxillary and the mandible as Andrews, given that there are significant differences between the average values of both sides. Therefore it does not seem appropriate to use average angle and tilt values without specifying the side of the arch which belongs to the tooth. Considering the large standard deviations observed in values from the Andrews' series the values of both inclination and angulation cannot be standardized. The variations in the values of angulation and inclination reported by different authors would be sufficient to raise the need for a re-evaluation of the theories of the straight-wire appliance in orthodontics.

5. References

Agenter MK, Harris EF, Blair RN. 2009. Influence of tooth crown size on malocclusion. Am J Orthod Dentofacial Orthop 136:795-804.

Andrews LF. 1972. The six keys to normal occlusion. Am J Orthod 62: 296-309.

Andrews LF. 1976a. The diagnostic system: occlusal analysis. Dent Clin North Am 20:671-690.

Andrews LF. 1976b. The straight-wire appliance archform, wire bending & an experiment. J Clin Orthod. 10:581-588.

Andrews. LF. 1976c. The straight-wire appliance. Extraction brackets and classification of treatment. J Clin Orthod 10:360-377.

Andrews LF. 1989. Straight Wire. The concept and appliance. San Diego, L.A.: Wells Company.

Angle EH. 1929a. The latest and best in orthodontic mechanism. Dental Cosmos 71: 164-173.

Angle EH. 1929b. The latest and best in orthodontic mechanism. Dental Cosmos 71:260-720.

Angle EH. 1981. Treatment of malocclusion of the teeth. Special Edition. Ed. The Classics of Dentistry Library. Birmingham Alabama Division of Gryphon Editions Ltd., pp. 198-262.

Bravo LA. 2007. Manual de Ortodoncia. Madrid Ed. Síntesis S.A., pp. 372-375. (Spanish text)

Canut JA. 2000. Ortodoncia clínica y terapéutica. 2ª edición. 2000. Barcelona Ed. Masson S.A., pp. 18-21. (Spanish text)

Gottlieb EL, Wildman AJ, Lang HM, Lee IF, Struch EC Jr. 1972. The Edgelok bracket. J Clin Orthod 6:613-623.

Graber TM, Vanarsdall RL Jr. 1994. Orthodontics Currents Principles and Techniques. 2ª edición. St. Louis, Missouri. Ed Mosby-YearBook Inc., pp. 627-635.

Holdaway RA. 1952. Bracket angulation as applied to the edgewise appliance. Angle Orthod 22:227-236.

Jarabak JR, Fizell JA. 1963. Technique and treatment with the light-wire appliance. Sant Louis, Missouri. Mosby.

Lee SJ, Ahn SJ, Lim WH, Lee S, Lim J, Park HJ. 2011. Variation of the intermaxillary tooth-size relationship in normal occlusion. Eur J Orthod 33:9-14.

Lewis PD. 1950. Space closure in extraction cases. Am J Orthod 36: 172-191.

McLaughlin RP, Bennett JC. 1989. The transition from standard edgewise to preadjusted appliance systems. J Clin Orthod 23:142-153.

McLaughlin R, Bennett J, Trevisi H. 1997. A clinical review of the MBT orthodontic treatment program. Orthod Perspec 4:3-15.

Martinez-Asúnsolo P, Plasencia E. 2004. Las 6 llaves de la oclusión de Andrews en 32 modelos con oclusiones ideales no tratadas. Rev Esp Ortod 34:235-244 (Spanish text)

Meyer M, Nelson G. 1978. Preajusted edgewise appliances: Theory and practice. Am J Orthod 73:485-498.

Naranjilla MA, Rudzki-Janson I. 2005. Cephalometric features of fi lipinos with class I occlusion according to the Munich analysis. Angle Orthod 75:63-68.

Peck S. 2008. So what's new? Arch expansion again. Angle Orthod 78:574-575.

Proffitt WR, Fields HW, Sarver DM. 2008. Ortodoncia Contemporánea. 4ª edición. Elsevier España 2008 Barcelona (Spanish Edition)

Roth RH. 1976. Five year clinical evaluation of the Andrews straight-wire appliance. J Clin Orthod 10:836-850.

Roth RH. 1987. The straight-wire appliance 17 years later. J Clin Orthod 21:632-642.

Wahl N. 2008. Orthodontics in 3 millenia. Chapter 16: Late 20th-century fixed appliances. Am J Orthod Dentofacial Orthop 134: 827-830.

Zanelato RC, Grossi AT, Mandetta S. 2004. Individualización de torque para los caninos en aparatos preajustados. Rev Ortodon Dental Press 3:39-55.

4

The Importance and Possibilities of Proper Oral Hygiene in Orthodontic Patients

Melinda Madléna
Semmelweis University
Hungary

1. Introduction

The number of orthodontic treatments has been increased nowdays (Silva & Kang, 2001; Thilander et al., 2001; Ciuffolo et al., 2005; Mtaya et al, 2009; Bittencourt & Machado, 2010). The most important motivation for orthodontic treatment is to achieve an improvement in appearance and the fact that in connection with this change some psychological problems could be decreased. These factors are contributed not only to the position but the esthetic appearance of the tooth itself. In some cases orthodontic treatments can attribute to caries preventive intervention, when tooth movements may reduce crowding or other anomalies, thus can contribute to the effectiveness of proper oral hygiene. On the other hand, orthodontic treatments may cause or aggravate plaque accumulation and in this way the development of caries and periodontal diseases which are basically caused by dental plaque. It is suggested that the information about both benefits and risks of orthodontic treatment should be sheared with potential patients.

This chapter explaines the relationships between orthodontic anomalies and orthodontic treatments and dental plaque induced diseases, delineates how to determinate the risk of the orthodontic treatment causing dental caries and periodontal diseases. The third part of this chapter summarizes the possibilities to avoid and reduce these effects using different modern equipments, techniques and adjuvants.

2. Relations between orthodontic anomalies / orthodontic treatment and dental plaque induced diseases

2.1 Associations of the orthodontic anomalies with dental caries

It is wellknown for a long time that in some orthodontic cases patients have greater difficulties in maintaining proper oral hygiene (Katz, 1978; Miller & Hobson, 1961). In spite of this, some authors published no correlation between positional anomalies and the caries prevalence. Helm and Petersen (1989a) examined 176 adolescents aged 13-19 years and re-examined them after 20 years in order to detect any relationship between malocclusion and caries, found no association between malocclusion traits and caries prevalence. Other authors published the relationship between the dental caries and the presence of certain malocclusions concerning oral hygiene (e.g. crowding) (Gábris et al., 2006; Nobile et al., 2007; Mtaya et al, 2009). Stahl & Grabowski (2004) reported no positive correlation between prevalence of caries and any malocclusion in primary teeth but in their study significant parallelism in prevalence of malocclusion and caries was found for posterior cross-bite and mandibular overjet in children with mixed dentition.

2.2 Associations of the orthodontic anomalies with periodontal parameters concerning oral hygiene

The accumulation of plaque can cause gingival redness, bleeding, edema, changes in gingival morphology, reduced tissue adaptation to the teeth, an increase in the flow of gingival crevicular fluid and other clinical signs of inflammation (Figure 1). Maloccluded teeth can be associated with periodontal diseases because of the physically hampered proper oral hygiene.

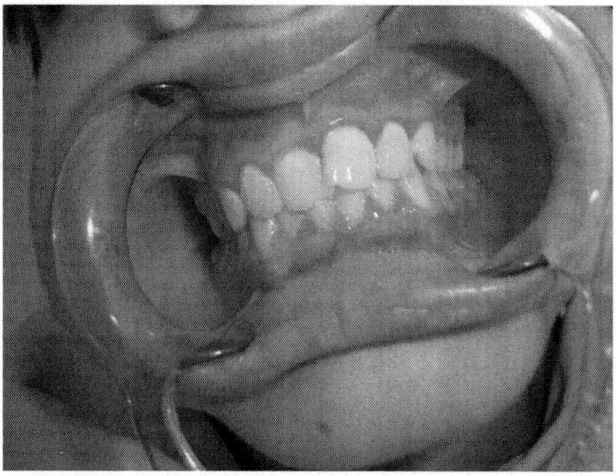

Fig. 1. Crowded frontal teeth with large amount of plaque.

In case of this anomaly the oral hygiene is harmful, the plaque elimination needs more time and special method. The picture shows a gingivitis as a consequence of the lack of proper oral hygiene.

According to the oral hygiene the most important basic symptom which can show more serious periodontal problems is gingival bleeding on probing (Geiger, 2001). The presence of a positive correlation between malocclusion (e.g. crowding, when the removal of plaque is difficult) and periodontal health has been described by Helm and Petersen (1989b) and Gábris et al. (2006), but on the contrary other studies found no association between amount of plaque or periodontal parameters and malocclusion (including crowding and spacing) (Geiger et al., 1974; Katz, 1978; Buckley, 1980). Other results had been published by Geiger (2001) found the possible associations between certain malocclusions (eg. anterior overjet and overbite, crossbite etc.) and periodontal problems, but these cases probably are not really in connection with oral hygiene.

2.3 Plaque accumulation concerning removable and fixed orthodontic appliances

The great plaque accumulation on different dental materials has been wellknown for a long time. From these points of view, we also consider removable appliances. In case of removable appliances, the resin base has microporosity. The greater accumulation of plaque on dental materials than on natural enamel is also wellknown (Skjörland, 1973). This is an increase in microorganisms which can provide an increased risk of carious lesions theoretically. Thus basically the orthodontic treatment with removable appliance causes an additional problem for the oral environment. The surface of the removable appliance will be coated within a short time mainly with streptococci and gram negative and positive rods (Bickel & Geering, 1982). According to the results of Batoni et al. (2001) the use of removable appliances may lead to the creation of new retentive areas and surfaces, which favour the local adherence and growths of streptococcus mutans. However, Schlagenhauf et al. (1989) found that the increase in number of streptococcus mutans was not significant in patients having removable orthodontic appliance comparing to those who weared fixed appliance.

The plaque accumulation is promoted by the physical constituton of different parts of fixed appliance, but there are some other factors having a great importance on plaque accumulation. In the oral cavity all of the tooth surfaces are exposed and rapidly covered by salivary proteins causing different effects (interactions between material, pellicle and bacteria). As a part of fixed appliances, orthodontic bands can cause a gingiva inflammation (Huser et al., 1990). Plaque accumulates particularly beneath bands from which some cement has been washed out adjacent to adhesive retention elements (Gwinnett & Cheen, 1979; Mizrahi, 1982). Plaque is found predominantly cervically to brackets under the arch wires. The scores of different periodontal parameters (Plaque Index, Gingival Bleeding Index) and proportion of spirochetes were found higher for banded molars than for molars with brackets (Boyd & Baumrind, 1992; Freundorfer et al. 1993). The loss of attachment is the highest approximally, particularly in adults, because the margins of band are frequently located subgingivally at approximal sites. In this way band with subgingival margins can promote the higher accumulation of the amount of plaque and contribute to development of gingivitis or periodontitis. In case of periodontitis besides the inflammation of gingiva the loss of connective tissue attachment (wich is irreversible change) also can be seen in the periodontium. In these situations gram negative and anaerobic microrganisms (Porphyromonas gingivalis, Prevotella intermedia, Actinomyces) are disproportionally present along the subgingival band margins (Diamanti-Kpioti et al., 1987) which are frequently associated with further periodontal problems. Beside of this, there is an increased number of spirochetes, mobile rods and fusiform organisms. Gingival hyperplasia may also occure and this complicates the oral hygiene and the dental treatment procedures (Figure 2.)

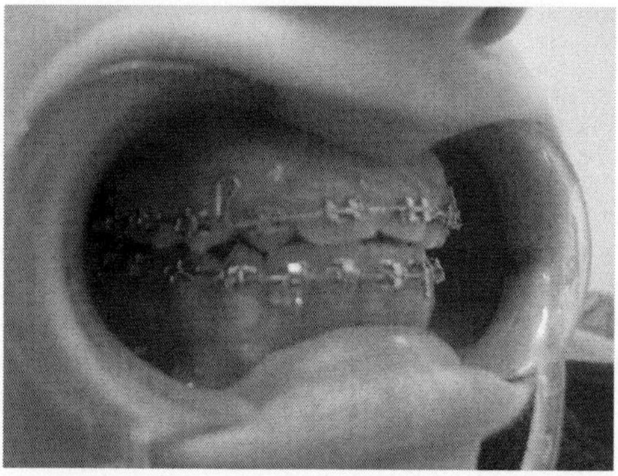

Fig. 2. Gingival hyperplasia in patient undergoing orthodontic treatment with fixed appliance.

The situation is caused by neglected oral hygiene, which complicate the treatment and oral hygienic procedures.

It has ben published that the elements of fixed orthodontic appliance can change the biologic balance in the oral cavity (Figure 3.).

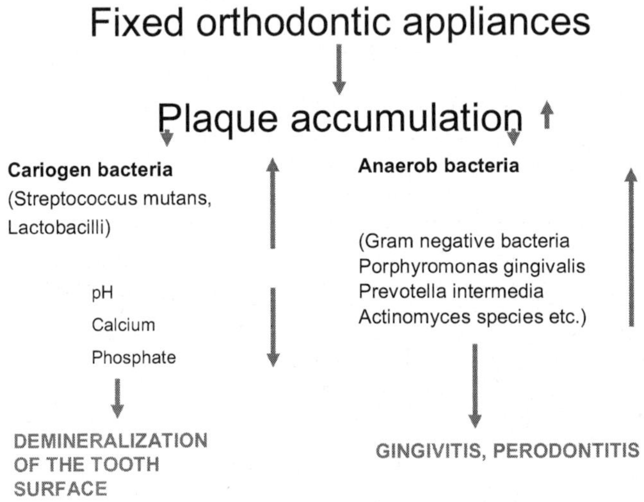

Fig. 3. Risk of treatment with fixed orthodontic appliances.

Plaque in patients with fixed orthodontic appliance has a lower pH than in non-orthodontic patients (Gwinnett & Cheen, 1979). There is a rapid shift in the composition of the bacterial flora, especially there is an increase in the levels of acidogenic bacteria (streptococcus mutans, lactobacilli), which leads to a decrease in pH. As the pH drop reaches the level of critical value (pH 5.5), the demineralization-remineralization balance is pushed toward mineral loss and demineralization/decalcification.

2.3.1 Decalcification of enamel caused by dental plaque accumulation (white spot lesions) during orthodontic treatment with fixed appliances

The first clinical evidence of the demineralization is the white spot lesion (WSL), which potentially can become a cavitated carious lesion extending even into the dentin (Featherstone, 2003; Featherstone et al, 2007). White spot lesions are nonfluoridated opacities having a more defined shape and are well differentiated from sorrounding enamel which are often located in the middle of the tooth (Sangamesh & Amitabh, 2011). The WSL has been defined as „subsurface enamel porosity from carious demineralization" presenting itself as a „milky white opacity" when located on smooth surfaces (Nicholson, 2006). Beside of that fact that WSL is a first step to destruction of the teeth, this enamel demineralization associated with fixed orthodontic appliances means an other significant clinical problem for the orthodontists (Ogaard, 1989; Bishara & Ostby, 20008). Because of the plaque accumulation on typical places, without proper oral hygiene, during or after the orthodontic treatment demineralization (white spot lesions) can be observed at these above mentioned plaque retention sites and the location of possible carious lesions are changed compared to the situation without orthodontic appliances (Muhler, 1970). The white spot lesions are predominantly appeare on the lower and upper premolars, first molars, maxillary and mandibular lateral inciors and lower canines as a change of tooth structure around the brackets basis or between the brackets/bands and gingival margin in the cervical region and middle third of the teeth, under the orthodontic wires (Ogaard, 2008). The frequency of WSL in orthodontically treated patients were in order lateral incisors, canines, first premolars, 2nd premolars, central incisors (Ogaard, 1989; Chapman et al., 2010). An other previous study showed similar results except those finding that the maxillary central incisors had a greater frequency of WSLs than did the maxillary second premolars (Gorelick et al., 1982). No significant differences were found in WSL incidence and prevalence between the right and left sides of the maxilla and mandible (Gorelick et al., 1982; Ogaard, 1989).

Evaluation of white spot lesions can be performed by macroscopic methods (clinical examination, photographic examination, optical nonfluorescent and fluorescent methods), microscopic methods (orthodontic caries models) and research methods (assessing different preventive agents) (Benson, 2008). The detected prevalence depends on the analytic methods. The highest prevalence of demineralization was detected by quantitative light induced fluorescence method which is much more sensitive than the simple direct visualization (Boersma, 2005). Inspector's unique analysis software is available to determinate the demineralization (Amaechi, 2009). Sound tooth tissue will show up glowing brightly without reflections, demineralised areas generally have a diffuse outline and are darker at the center which distinguishes them from stains and discoloration.

According to the study of Gorelick et al. (1982) the incidence of white spot formation in patients treated with fixed orthodontic appliances was nearly 50% compared to 24% in an untreated control group. In the literature great variations have been published (from 2 - to 97% of the patients) for WSL prevalence associated with orthodontic treatment (Zachrisson and Zachrisson, 1971; Gorelick et al., 1982; Mizrahi, 1982; Artun & Brobakken, 1986; Geiger et al., 1988; Ogaard, 1989, Mitchell, 1992). Although orthodontic patients had significantly more WSLs than non-orthodontic patients but in this stage generally were not registered as caries, requiring restorative treatment (Ogaard et al., 2004). However in some cases, the development of these lesions could be such rapid that it requiers rapid debonding and treatment procedures. It can be occured already within 4 weeks (Ogaard et al., 1988). Carious lesions may appear after debonding in association with bonded retainer also. Earlier studies showed increased caries frequency and higher prevalence of caries and also fillings in persons treated with fixed orthodontic appliances, but most of the further investigations did not confirm this statement which could be in connection with the higher motivation of the patients and the widespread possibility of oral hygiene regimens (Ingerwall, 1962; Zachrisson & Zachrisson, 1971; Hollender & Ronnerman, 1978; Southard et al., 1986; Ogaard, 1989). Muhler (1970) published that the orthodontic treatment without proper oral prophylaxis resulted in an increased incidence of caries which was significantly reduced after an appropriate prophylaxis. According to the study of Zachrisson & Zachrisson (1971) in case of cooperative patients with proper oral hygiene dental caries is a relatively minor problem and the number of new cavities is relatively low but it is contributed by different factors. For example, beside of the individual susceptibility, it has to be considered that generally the patients aged 6-10 years and during an early period of adolescents are in active caries phase, the number of new cavities may increase rapidly during fixed orthodontic treatment in these cases. The publicated incidence and prevalence of WSL can vary by sex. Although Ogaard (1989) found no significant difference between genders, most of the studies published it. According to the study of Zachrisson & Zachrisson (1971), girls had better caries index scores, (and also better periodontal indices) than boys during orthodontic treatment. In spite of these findings, Gorelick et al. (1982) found that females have higher incidence in WSL prevalence, while Boersma (2005) and Al Maaltah et al. (2011) published higher incidence of WSL in male. Chapmen et al. (2010) published a higher incidence of WSLs and also the more severe demineralization in males compared with female patients. It can be in connection with those results of some authors that female patients have been shown to have a greater interest in oral health, they had better oral health and tend to brush and floss their teeth more frequently (Kuusela et al., 1996; Sakki et al., 1998; Ostberg et al., 1999). Chapmen et al. (2010) published that early age at start of fixed appliance treatment, inadequate oral hygiene before the treatment, many treatment appointments with poor oral hygiene were associated with greater incidence and severity of WSLs. Al Maaltah et al. (2011) published that patients with WSLs were significantly younger and more likely to have diseased first molars.

Classification of white spot lesions can be found in a modification of material in publication of Nyvad et al. (1999):

White spot stage 1. Inactive caries (intact surface):

Surface of enamel is white, brown or black. It is glossy with no loss of luster; feels smooth and hard when the tip of the probe is gently moved across the surface. No clinically detectable loss of enamel. Smooth surface lesion typically located away from the gingival margin.

White spot stage 2. Inactive caries (surface discontinuity):

Surface enamel is white, brown or black. It is glossy with no loss of luster; feels smooth and hard when the tip of the probe is gently moved across the surface. Localized surface defects (microcavity) could be found in enamel only. No undermined enamel or softened floor detectable with the explorer.

When on the surface there are cavitated lesion, enamel/dentin cavity easily visible with naked eye, surface cavity feels hard on gentle probing and appears shiney. There is no pulpal involvement.

3. Determination of the risk causing dental caries and periodontal diseases during orthodontic treatment

It is wellknown that because of the great possibility for the increased plaque accumulation orthodontic patients who are treated with fixed appliance, mainly generally belong to a potentially higher risk group. So a list of risk factors should be recorded for orthodontic patients to identify those persons who need special preventive interventions. Orthodontic treatment may be hazardous for those patients who have no motivaton, no proper supervision or preventive programme. To notice the increased plaque accumulation, it is important for both patients and clinicians to prevent tooth decay, gingival or periodontal problems and tooth discoloration that could compromise the esthetic of smile and well being of the patients. The key for this is represented by dental plaque.

3.1 Identification of dental plaque

Dental plaque is „the soft tenaciosus material found on tooth surfaces which is not readily removed by rinsing with water" (Axelsson, 2000) (Figure 4.).

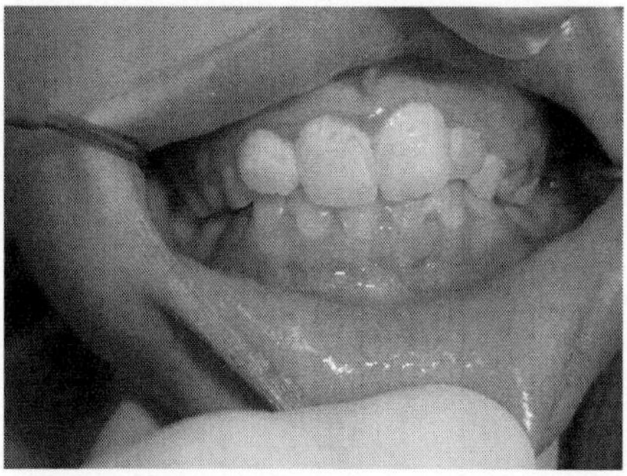

Fig. 4. Unstained dental plaque on the labial dental surfaces, on the cervical regions of the frontal teeth.

In this patient the consequences of the large amount of plaque (decalcification, gingivitis) are also seen.

In some cases the identification of plaque can be hard with the naked eye because it could have a whitish colour, similarly to the teeth. The plaque amount and localization can be determined by different methods. The simpliest way to scrape the tooth surface with a periodontal probe. Special test tablets containing red or blue dye can be used to stain the plaque. One tablet is chewed thoroughly, moving the mixture of saliva and dye over the teeth and gums for approximately 30 seconds. Then the mouth is rinsed with water and teeth are checked to identify the stained unremoved plaque. The disadvantage of these tablets that may cause a temporary pink or blue color of lips, cheeks, mouth or tongue. (Figure 5.). An other method is using plaque fluorescence. A special fluorescent solution is swirled around the mouth. After that the mouth is rinsed gently with water and the teeth and gums can be checked with an ultraviolet light. The plaque will be coloured in a brillant orange-yellow. This method does not leave stains on other tissues in the mouth.

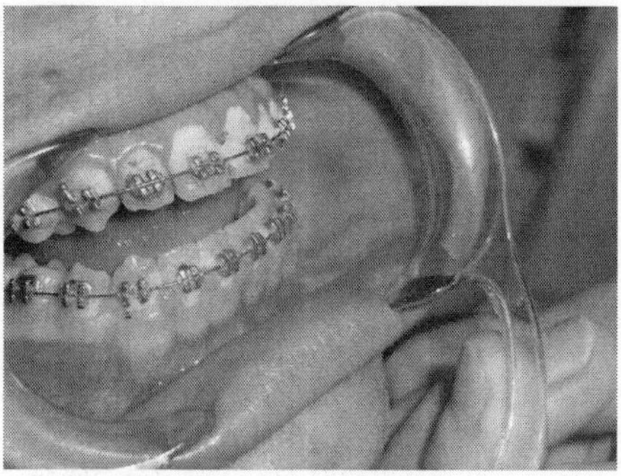

Fig. 5. The situation after plaque staining with tablets.

The method cause a temporary discoloration on the bucca or the tongue. Matured and fresh plaque can be seen in different colors. More blue plaque coloration means inproper oral hygiene

Some types of plaque staining products can differentiate between the cariogenic and noncariogenic plaque with different colors (Figure 5.). Acid producing ability of a plaque sample and its cariogenic potential can be determined. Non-cariogenic samples turn green or yellow, while cariogenic plaque samples turn red or orange after sucrose challenge from the solution. Some products contain a neutralising solution (e.g. Plaque Indicator Kit from the GC) which can be used for education of the patients, eg. regarding the protective actions of the saliva and a disclosing gel for the demonstration of plaque. The composition of plaque changes in time, which allows pathogenic bacteria to be active on the tooth surface. Using a special disclosing gel, a more than 48 hours old (matured) plaque and a fresh plaque can be seen in two different colours (blue, redish-pink).

The Inspektor QLF-D BiLuminator™ is a sophisticated device for assessment and monitoring of oral hygiene in the dental surgery. The QLF-D BiLuminator software supports easy acquisition of image pairs and orders them automatically on a visit-patient basis. Plaque and calculus show up brightly red in the QLF -image made by this equipment (Figure 6.). Only those plaque will be seen that has been present for some time (> 1 day).

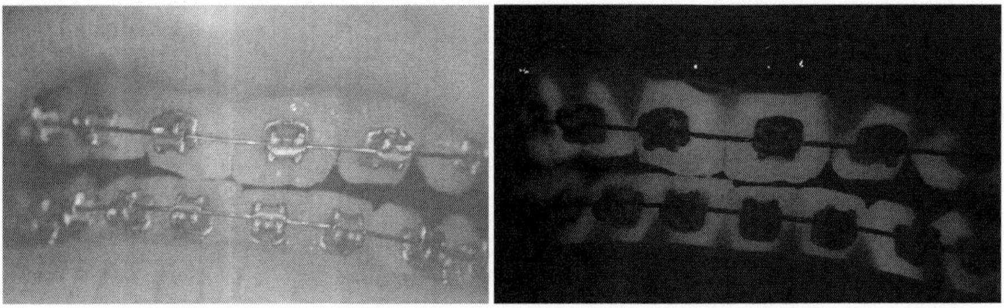

Fig. 6. White light and QLF image of teeth with orthodontic brackets (publication of the pictures with permission of Inspektor Research System BV, Netherlands).

The BiLuminator™ can be tremendous help to prevent any damage that may follow the placement of orthodontic brackets. By regularly inspecting teeth it can be ensured that teeth are well cleaned before the brackets are placed and mature plaque will not seen during the orthodontic treatment (Amaechi, 2009).

3.1.1 Measurement of plaque amount

There are a lot indices for the measurement of plaque amount, among them the index of Silness and Löe (1964) which is very easy to use, is one of the most frequently used in clinical practice. The Plaque Accumulation Rate Index (PFRI) performed by Axelsson (1991), based on the amount of disclosed plaque which is freely accumulated in the 24 hours following professional mechanical tooth cleaning (during which period subjects refrain from all oral hygiene practices. For the PFRI a five point scale was constructed (Figure 7.). There are positive correlations between the scores of PFRI and e.g. gingival bleeding, Plaque Index, level of streptococcus mutans, caries prevalence etc. (Axelsson, 2000).

Plaque Formation Rate Index (PFRI) (Axelsson, 1991)

- Score 1: 1 to 10% of surfaces affected: very low
- Score 2: 11 to 20% of surfaces affected: low
- Score 3: 21 to 30% of surfaces affected: moderate
- Score 4: 31 to 40% of surfaces affected: high
- Score 5: more than 40% of surfaces affected: very high

Fig. 7. The scores of Plaque Formation Rate Index by Axelsson (1991).

3.2 Microbiological and clinical parameters for determination of caries risk

As caries is a multicausal disease, it is not optimal to examine just one etiological factor for the general prognosis. Caries risk assessment models involve a combination of factors including diet, fluoride exposure, a susceptible host, microflora which all can interplay with a variety of social, cultural and behavioural factors (Featherstone, 2003; Nicolau et al., 2003).

The combination of clinical and microbiological findings increases the sensitivity of caries prognosis to almost 100% (Kneist et al., 1998; Krasse, 1988). New carious lesions will develop if high bacterial counts have been recorded, thus the evaluation of microbiological data is also recommended before the starting of orthodontic treatment, because the caries risk tends to increase dramatically in patients with high bacterial counts after the placement of brackets, due to the difficulties in performing adequate oral hygiene (Kristofferson et al., 1985).

The risk of caries can be determined by other different testing procedures, these are based on determination of quality and quantity of saliva.

3.2.1 Microbiological parameters

In a regular dental practice the „chairside tests" are very easy to apply for determination of cariogen bacteria and salivary parameters. These tests are available since the begining of 1970s years. Using these products allows semiquantitative evaluation of mutans streptococci in saliva or plaque and lactobacilli in saliva (Larmas, 1975; Jensen & Bratthall, 1989).

Earlier test systems (Dentocult SM, Dentocult LB from Orion Diagnostica, Cariescreen SM from APO Diagnostics, Caries Check SM and Caries Check LB from Hain Diagnostika) needed relatively complicated laboratory working procedures. The newer type of Dentocult tests allows simplier technical work but they work on the same basis.

3.2.1.1 Estimation of mutans streptococci

The basis of the determination of streptococcus mutans is represented by a basic method of Dentocult SM test could be used for estimation of mutans streptococci. Originally it has been developed by Jensen & Bratthall (1989), but this Dentocult SM (Strip Mutans) is a newer development of the spatula method of Köhler & Bratthall (1979). The test is based on those facts that adhesing of mutans streptococci can be experienced not only to tooth surface but to wooden or plastic spatulas and removable devices also and on the ability of mutans streptococci to grow on hard surfaces and use of a selective broth (high sucrose concentration in combination with bacitracin). The test result shows the risk of caries depending on the level of mutans streptococci CFU (Colony Forming Units/ml) in saliva or in dental plaque, but the result has to be interpreted in relation to the number of the teeth in the mouth (Zickert et al., 1982). An other type of the available simple and accurate chairside test is „Saliva - Check mutans" from the GC, which detects the patients level of streptococcus mutans in 15 minutes only. For this test there is no need for incubator (in contrast with the previously mentioned product) or any other devices. High accuracy is possible as the test strip containes 2 monoclonal antibodies that selectively detect only the streptococcus mutans species, meaning no other bacteria modify the results.

3.2.1.2 Estimation of lactobacilli

The other organisms that can be associated with caries are lactobacilli. Althoug probably they don't play a primary role in the etiology of caries, lactobacilli can be important from the viewpoint of caries activity (Socransky, 1968). Based on different studies the presence of lactobacilli reflects only high consumption of carbohydrates and therefore it is an indirect test for caries (Klock & Krasse, 1979; Crossner, 1981). On the other hand the test provides information about the activity of existing carious lesions (high levels of lactobacilli show an incresed carious activity which can lead to early treatment of the lesions).

For the estimation of lactobacilli can be used a method of dip slide test (Larmas, 1975). The applied selective lactobacillus agar which supports the grows of the acid forming and acid resistant lactobacilli (mainly Lactobacillus casei). The dip slide has to be placed into the transport tube and incubated for four days at 37 °C (99 °F). Estimation of lactobacilli, similarly to mutans streptococci, can be performed by comparing the result to the chart. For the evaluation the number of the colonies means the relevant information. Because of different incubation times for the various test vials and the short shelf life of the mutans streptococci tests, further efforts have been made for optimize the tests in accordance with the practical viewpoints.

3.2.1.3 CRT bacteria test for combined determination of cariogenic bacteria

The prognosis for caries risk is more certain in those case when mutans streptococci and lactobacillus tests are combined (Stecksen-Blicks, 1985). CRT Bacteria (Vivadent, Shaan, Lichtenstein) (Figure 8.) is a test which is available for the evaluation of the level both important oral microorganisms by means of selective agars as previously described.

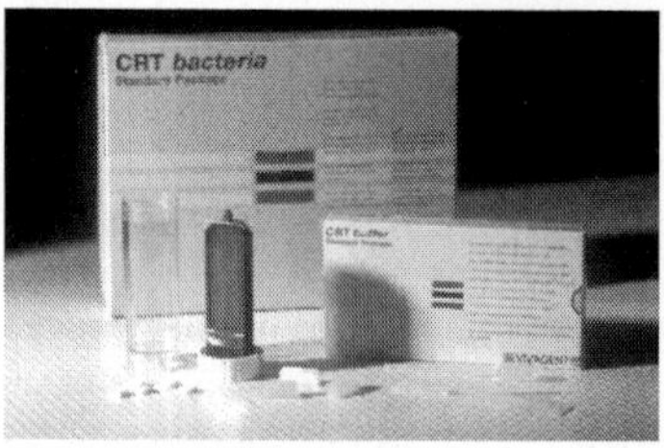

Fig. 8. CRT Bacteria test.

This test give a possibility for the determining mutans streptococci and lactobacilli at the same time, during the evaluation of caries risk.

Performing the clinical procedures, after two days incubation at 37 °C (99 °F) can be detected and evaluated for both mutans streptococci and lactobacilli. Leaving CRT bacteria in the incubator for more than 48 hours for any reason, it will not cause any change in bacterial count. The test sample can be stored in the refrigerator for up to two weeks without any changes.

Evaluation of the CRT bacteria test (with the model chart): higher values than 10^5 CFU/mL of mutans streptococci in saliva indicate a high risk (Krasse, 1988; Anderson et al., 1993). CRT bacteria test can be applied to check the effectiveness of different antimicrobial treatment of the risk patients. The modification of the above presented procedure gives a possibility for the determination of mutans streptococci not only in saliva but in dental plaque also, but applying this saliva based method, the examination of incubated plaque samples provides only a semiquantitative evaluation of the microorganisms (Kneist et al., 1998). This measure is indicated to monitor the the edges around brackets in orthodontic patients.

The tests are contraindicated after treatment with previous antibiotic treatment (within the previous two weeks) or after the use of antibacterial rinsing solution (the waiting time at least 12 hours).

All tests are very easy to use, can be applied to demonstrate the proper oral hygiene and to check the effects of motivation, generally less expensive than conventional microbiological methods (Newbrun et al., 1984) and do not need specially trained personnel. These are important diagnostic tools for dentists who strive to maintain oral health of their patients.

Presently the trends towards using simple, quick tests which can demonstrate the results clearly (without any other special equipments like e.g. incubator) for the patients in a short time. These tests are based on various methods: e.g. monoclonal antibodies are employed in Saliva Check Mutans from GC, Clinpo ™ Cario L-Pop ™ from 3M need local measurement of acid production for assessment. This last test was used in a 12 month follow up cohort study to evaluate the association between having a high score on this test and caries occurance in young patients undergoing orthodontic treatment (Chaussain et al., 2010). More studies are needed for the evaluation because of basic method of these tests not yet fully matured in terms of their sensitivity and handling properties.

3.2.2 Assessment of salivary factors

Salivary factors are in closed connection with caries risk. Determination of salivary enzymes and ions is difficult in the everyday practice, but measurement of salivary flow rate (the volume of saliva during a given period of time) or salivary buffer capacity can be performed relatively easily.

3.2.2.1 Salivary flow rate

It is wellknown for a long time that in patients with xerostomia the caries rate is increased. So the measurement of this factor must be of interest to evaluate the potentially high risk groups of orthodontic patients. The flow rate can be established easily without any special equipments. The saliva has to be collected in calibrated tube (tube for the lactobacillus test can be used to measure the salivary flow rate as well) (Figure 9.). Secretion rate should be determined for resting saliva and paraffin stimulated saliva. The values for the determination are shown in the Table 1.

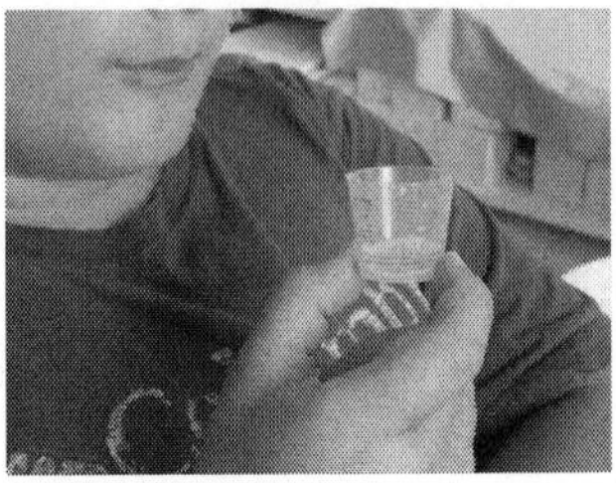

Fig. 9. Collecting saliva in a calibrated container.

For determining the risk of caries the dentist should measure the salivary secretation rate.

For the adults stimulated salivary flow rate is less than 0.7 ml/min is considered low, while higher than 1.0 mL/min is considered normal. In case of women the salivary flow rate is generally slightly lower than in men (similarly to the children when compared with the adolescents).

Secretion rate (ml/min)	Very low	Low	Normal
Resting saliva	< 0.1	0.1 - 0.25	0.25-0.35 (mean 0.30)
Stimulated saliva	< 0.7	0.7 - 1	1 – 3 (mean 2)

Table 1. Classification of salivary secretion rate for resting and paraffin-stimulated whole saliva (Axelsson, 2000).

The results could be affected by different drug intake (e.g. antihistamines, neuroleptic or antihypertensive agents).

3.2.2.2 Buffer capacity

Buffering capacity of saliva ensures the pH level and ability for remineralization. The threshold is *under 4* when the process of caries can become faster. For the evaluation can be easily used e.g. Dentobuff strip test also from the Vivadent. A disposable syringe is used to place a single drop paraffin stimulated saliva on a test strip. After about five minutes the color change on the pH indicator strip is compared with the color chart provided. Similar possibility for measuring buffering capacity is Saliva Check Buffer from the GC.

Although it can be important information, the determination of buffer capacity, similarly to the salivary flow rate, has only subordinate role in the reliable identification of patients at high caries risk. The buffer capacity test has greater value in those patients who have exposed root surfaces because exposed dentin is more sensitive to acid than the enamel (Heintze et al, 1999).

3.3 Determination and assessment of the risk of periodontal diseases

Development and progression of periodontitis basically depends on the interaction of periodontopathogenic bacteria and the host's immune defense system. Science has long sought a diagnostic procedure to predict the risk of periodontitis with determination of the attack and defense mechanisms. For the daily practice, clinical parameters are sufficient to identify patients with potential disease activity. Periodontal diseases are in tight connection with systemic diseases (eg. cardiovascular diseases, diabetes etc.), and there is an evidence that periodontitis associated bacteria or their tissue derived inflammatory mediators are transmitted eg. during pregnancy from mother to child (Genco, 1996; Herzberg & Meyer, 1996; Slavkin, 1997). There are some chairside test which can measure different parameteres associated with periodontitis development. However, it is not clear how these tests could be clinically significant. According to several recently published reviews, none of the available tests is capable identify with at least 80% accuracy those individuals who are at risk for periodontitis (Lang & Bragger, 1991; Jeffcoat et al., 1997). Therefore, clinical evaluation seems to be more useful to carry out periodontal diagnosis and assessment the risk. The dentist has to determine the following points (Heintze et al, 1999):

1. Does gingival bleeding appear on probing?
2. Do periodontal pockets exist and how deep are they?
3. Are alterations of periodontal bone apparent on radiographs (for this periapical, bitewing and panoramic pictures are needed)

3.3.1 Clinical measurements

Greater plaque accumulation, tendency for bleeding and increased pocket depth have been observed more frequently in orthodontic patients. Therefore, to examine these factors are necessary to determine and monitor a risk of periodontal disease concerning orthodontic treatment.

3.3.1.1 Gingival Bleeding Index

Gingival Bleeding Index published by Ainamo & Bay (1975) is very simply to use in orthodontic patients. The sulcus is probed carefully on the buccal and lingual surfaces with periodontal probe. It is useful to develop a specific system e.g. to proceed by quadrants. Probing begins on the buccal surface, proceeding from the distal to mesial surfaces, then on the lingual surface from the distal to mesial. Thus each tooth has four points of measurement: buccal, lingual, mesioproximal and distoproximal.

In patient with fixed appliance performing the probing can be more difficult due to bands and other attachments limiting access to the gingival margin (Figure 10.). Still, it is necessary to probe the gingival margin along its entire lengh to get valuable data and to perform adequate preventive interventions.

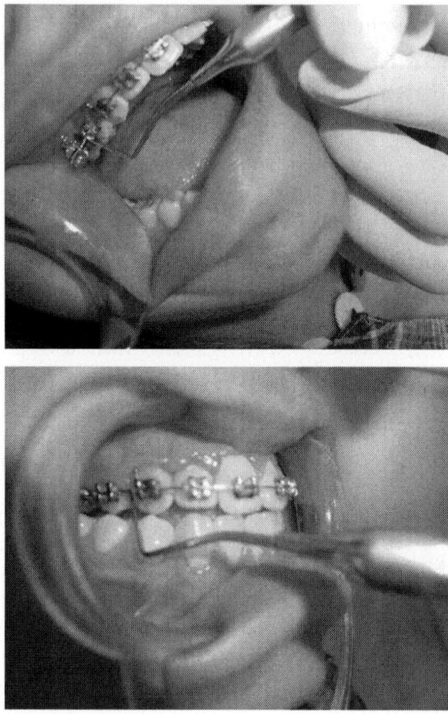

Fig. 10. Performing clinical measurements for the evaluation of periodontal conditions with a periodontal probe in orthodontic patients.

Although periodontal parameters are very important for the determination of the risk or the exist of periodontal diseases due to orthodontic treatment, sometimes it is difficult to perform because of different parts of the appliance.

3.3.1.2 Loss of attachment

The gingival sulcus is probed gently with a special periodontal probe. The depth of the gingival sulcus is considered maximally 0.5 mm deep in case of sound gingiva. In some orthodontic cases (mainly in adult patients) the measuring loss of attachment and its documentation are important, but measurement of attachment loss does not correlate with inflammatory activity of a pocket (Lang & Bragger, 1991).

3.3.2 RT-PCR (Reverse Transcription –Polymerase Chain Reaction)

One of the newest method is the RT-PCR. This is the most sensitive technique for mRNA detection and quantification currently available. It is a fully automated process and exact quantification of anaerob periodontopathogenic bacteria from a small sample of dental plaque. The advantages of this method are high specificity, high sensitivity and objectivity (Dharmaraj, 2011).

In addition to clinical and radiographic parameters and additional data provide information about the groups at higher risk for periodontitis (Fox, 1992). Patients are in higher risk in the following cases:

1. Heavy mokers
2. Diabetics
3. Patients with osteoporosis
4. Persons with inproper oral hygiene
5. Patients with previous periodontal disease
6. Elderly patients

The clinicians must identify susceptible patients and develop strategies to prevent loss of attachment and/or gingival recession. Each patient must be assessed individually for periodontal factors which mean for the patients high risk of developing periodontal disease during orthodontic treatment (Vanarsdall, 2000).

4. Possibilities to avoid or reduce the risk of caries and periodontal diseases concerning orthodontic treatment

Concerning the orthodontic treatment removable appliances do not cause significant plaque accumulation, while patients with fixed orthodontic appliances have a higher risk for increased plaque formation and with its harmful consequences for demineralization of the teeth and periodontal problems. Most of the lesions occure during fixed orthodontic treatment and appear mainly to be surface demineralization rather than a subsurface lesion. De-and remineralization processes are performed continuously. Sometimes the amount of remineralization can not totally overcome the amount of demineralization (Wilmot, 2008).

Longitudinal studies have shown the beneficial effects of recommendation to perform preventive measures during orthodontic treatment mainly in case of fixed appliances. Applying the possibilities, in these patients there was no clinically significant damage on either hard tissues of the teeth or periodontium (Boyd et al., 1989; Zachrisson & Zachrisson, 1971). Beside of the orthodontists, the general dentists and oral hygienists have a significant role in maintaining proper and effective oral hygiene of the patients undergoing orthodontic treatment with fixed appliances.

4.1 Patients with removable appliances

Although removable orthodontic appliances do not increases alone the absolute level of pathogenic microorganisms, but frequently provide more retention places for bacterial deposits (Figure 11.). In these cases the aim of oral hygienic procedures is the elimination of plaque from the appliance to prevent reinfection of the cleaned teeth. It is very difficult to keep the removable appliance totally free of plaque. Different cleaning methods are recommended mainly for home care. The orthodontist can suggest to clean with toothbrush and toothpaste (or soap) under running water or to clean the appliance in water bath containig a cleanser tablet. Both of them show some disadvantages: the combination of toothbrush-toothpaste cleaning is effective only on the easily accessable surfaces (Diedrich,

1989), while the use of self acting cleansing tablet allows just 2-3% of total deposits remaining on the appliances (Rabe et al., 1986). The antibacterial effectiveness of these tablet cleansers is doubtful and they can lead to obvious corrosion of the metal solder connections (Rabe et al.,1986). One more possibility for cleaning the removable appliances can be an ultrasonic bath, which is an expensive method and is not affordable for all patients wearing removable orthodontic appliances.

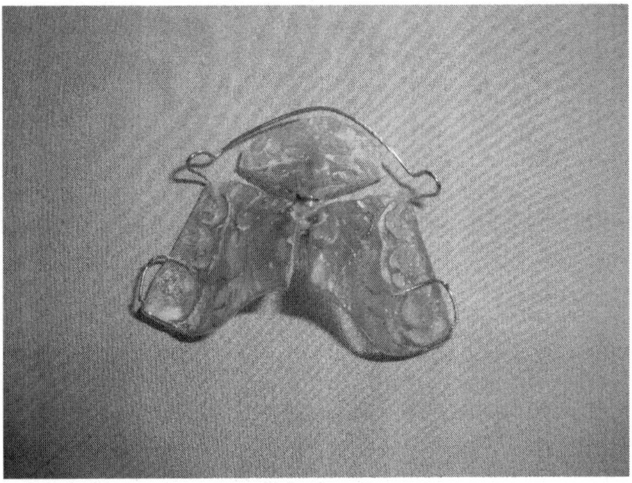

Fig. 11. Removable appliance with many retention sites and bacterial deposits.

In case of removable appliance it is necessary to clean the appliance to prevent reinfection of the cleaned teeth.

In the literature different materials are mentioned for reducing the level of pathogenic bacteria in the mouth. E.g. application of SRD (Slow Release Dosage) of chlorhexidine on the tooth surface showed a plaque reducing effect (Friedman et al., 1985), but other material with the same ingredient (e.g. Cervitec varnish) can be used effectively. Cervitec can successfully reduce cariogenic bacteria like mutans streptococci on different tooth surfaces, and promote the plaque reducing effect in the mouth (Huizinga et al., 1990; Petersson et al., 1991; Twetman & Petersson, 1997; Madléna et al., 2000). Slow release fluoride devices also can be used in case of high risk patients with removable appliances, although these products are preferred for patients treated with fixed appliances. Using slow fluoride release containing polymethyl metacrylate (Orthocryl Plus) ensures continuous low concentration of fluoride in saliva for more months which provides an optimal circumstance for the remineralization of initial carious lesions (Miethke & Newesely, 1988; Alacam et al., 1996). In case of patients using removable appliance to perform all dental and gingival treatment should be offered before the begining of the treatment.

4.2 Patients with fixed appliances

For the proper effects preventive actions and interventions should begin as early as possible, long before the active orthodontic therapy both in removable and fixed applience cases, but especially important for patients with fixed appliances.

There are three main categories should be considered concerning the preventive program for orthodontic patients: preventive actions and interventions *before, during and after* the active orthodontic treatment (Table 2.).

<table>
<tr><th>Before</th><th>During</th><th>After</th></tr>
<tr><td colspan="3">Motivation of the patients and oral hygienic training</td></tr>
<tr><td colspan="3">Control of oral hygiene</td></tr>
<tr><td colspan="3">Dietary counselling</td></tr>
<tr><td colspan="3">Professional tooth cleaning (repeatedly if it seems to be necessary)</td></tr>
<tr><td></td><td>Special oral hygienic instructions concerning the fixed orthodontic appliance</td><td></td></tr>
<tr><td rowspan="3"></td><td colspan="2">Use of fluorides</td></tr>
<tr><td>Chemical plaque control</td><td>Chemical plaque control in case of fixed retainer</td></tr>
<tr><td></td><td>Remineralization</td></tr>
</table>

Table 2. Preventive viewpoints before, during and after the active orthodontic treatment with fixed orthodontic appliance (Lundström et al., 1980; Hotz, 1982).

In all patients but especially in case of fixed appliance it is very important that all general dental and periodontal treatment should be completed *before* orthodontic treatment. It is compulsory to consult with the general dentist or any specialist to gain a statement that the patient is ready for orthodontic treatment. To prepare a written inform consent including the necessity of improved oral hygiene is also necessary before begining of the treatment. The oral condition has also to be recorded on the patient's chart and demonstrated with clinical photos.

Concerning the treatment, bonding of molars is better and ensures better possibilities to remove the plaque than banding, especially in adults. For the same reason it is suggested to use single arch wires, if the case allows and to remove excess composite around brackets (mainly from the gingival third). Theoretically use of fluoride containing orthodontic adhesives are preferable during orthodontic treatment and in case of fixed retainer. In vitro studies glass ionomer cements have demonstrated a more sustained fluoride release and evidence that these cements may reduce decalcification (Vorhies et al., 1998; Chung et al., 1999; Millett et al., 1999). At the same time, according to a systematic review, glass ionomer cement could be more effective than composite resin in preventing white spot formation, but still the scientific evidence is weak. The authors conclude that fluoride releasing bonding material for bonding brackets showed almost no demineralization-inhibiting effect (Derks et al., 2004).

Because of the limitation of successful bonding with glass ionomer adhesives, further investigations are needed for the recommendations on the usage of fluoride containing adhesives during fixed orthodontic treatment (Rogers et al., 2010). Uysal et al. (2011) conclude that using antibacterial monomer containing adhesive for bonding orthodontic brackets successfully inhibited caries incidence in vivo, the cariostatic effect was localized around the brackets and proved to be significant after 30 days.

Lingual appliances can cause extra difficulties in performing proper oral hygiene. The longer the treatment time with fixed appliance, the more time needed to maintain oral health in such a non-ideal circumstance. It is preferable to minimize the length of treatment with either conventionally or lingually placed fixed orthodontic appliance (e.g. by early corrections of skeletal and alignment problems in the mixed dentition with removable appliances). In addition a light cure sealant containing fluoride should also be advisable to be applied on the entire free surface, which can also be reapplied during the treatment (Frazier et al., 1996). Fluoride containing elastomeric chains also may reduce the degree of decalcification (Banks et al., 2000).

4.2.1 Motivation of the patients and oral hygienic training; control of oral hyiene

Before the orthodontic treatment it is very important to inform the patients about the importance of the improved oral hygiene concerning orthodontic treatment with fixed appliance and to explain the causes of caries and periodontal disease. The dentist can use any gingival indices and disclosure of the plaque for the patient to be motivated. The patients need proper information about the preventive possibilities concerning fixed orthodontic appliance after its application. It could be very useful to check the oral hygiene throught the complete orthodontic therapy. Beside of the use of fluoride containing toothpaste and brushing with conventional brushes also during the treatment at least twice a day, additional methods could be suggested helping to improve oral hygiene. Recording and documentation of the improvement in oral hygiene in the patient's chart is also necessary. Although motivation and oral hygiene training represent the most important points before the orthodontic treatment, it can be repeated as frequently as it is needed not only before but during the active orthodontic treatment as well. *After finishing the orthodontic treatment* the orthodontist also has to advice the patients to maintain proper oral hygienic habits.

4.2.2 Oral hygienic training methods

It is a possibility and a responsibility of the orthodontists to involve their patients in a systemic program for the prevention of caries and periodontal diseases focusing on mechanical removal of plaque and elimination of pathogen microorganisms. Because of tooth cleaning is much more difficult in patients undergoing orthodontic therapy with fixed appliance, patients and orthodontists/dentists or specially trained personnel require much efforts and time to show the possibilities of proper oral hygiene. Ask the patients to demonstrate the efficiency of brushing at each regular visit until they have mastered the technique.

The patients can use both hand or electric tooth brushes with short head, soft and rounded bristle end, but they can apply special orthodontic brushes (eg. when middle row of bristles is shorter than the outer row) and have to ask other special equipments also (eg. floss, interdental brushes, etc.) (Figure 12.). The patients may be instructed in the modified Bass technique. It is also important to let the toothbrush air-dried for 24 hours between uses. Tooth cleaning requires at least 10 minutes for patients. Approximal surfaces could be cleaned properly with dental floss. Interdental brushes and Superfloss must be used for the proper oral hygiene not only on the approximal surfaces but the tooth surfaces around the bracket and band margins as well (Heintze et al., 1999; Boyd, 2001).

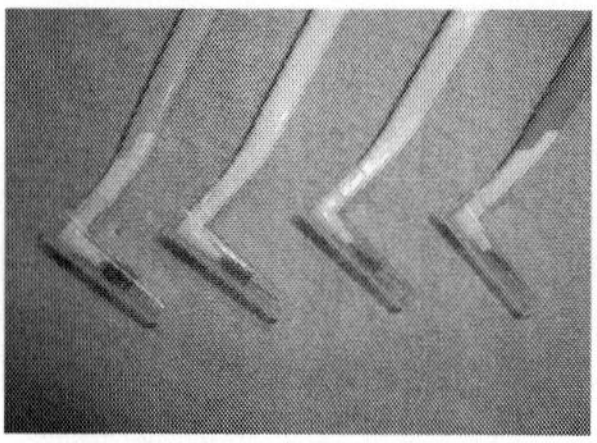

Fig. 12. Special brushes for orthodontic patients.

During the orthodontic treatment with fixed appliance it is necessary to suggest special equipments for the proper oral hygiene and to check the effectiveness of them.

4.2.3 Control of oral hygiene

During the active treatment patients should evaluate their teeth (and appliances) and determine these are whether clean or not. Regular recall examinations are necessary but the intervals between the recall examinations depend on the initial conditions. At the recall examinations during both the active treatment phase and the retention period regularly should perform the determination of caries risk (mutans streptococci and lactobacilli counts) and the evaluation of the condition of gingiva.

During the retention phase, removable retainers mean lower risk because these appliances allow an easier tooth cleaning procedure. The attached fixed retainers represent plaque retentive sites in the mouth, although these appliances are believed not to lead to initial carious lesions or periodontal problems if properly fabricated (Artun, 1984; Gorelick et al., 1982). Further advantage of removable devices is that they could be used as carriers of medicaments to provide more intensive prophylaxis.

4.2.4 Dietary counselling

Sugar is not a single causative factor of dental caries but it can appear as an important external modifying risk factor in this process. Due to this reason the dental personnel have to ask the patients about their nutritional habits, optimally using a questionnaire. It is very important to know the average frequency of intake of any types of the cariogenic foods (Axelsson, 1999).

The dietary control is in close connection with microbiologic evaluations. As high salivary levels of lactobacilli indicate a high sugar intake and a low pH in the oral cavity, the lactobacillus test is useful for the objective supplement to the dietary questionnaire (Axelsson, 1999). Sugar intake can be assessed eg. from a 24 hour recall questionnaire. For caries prevention and control the following dietary recommendations should be performed for the patients according to Axelsson (1999):

1. The first meal of the day (breakfast), should be a balanced composition of dairy products, grains and fruit eg. yogurt and muesli, fresh fruit and vegetables. It is not the same as the commercial continental breakfast containing mainly fat, sugar and water which causes rapid swings in blood sugar levels stimulating a high frequency of sugar intake all day.
2. The total number of meals, including all, should be limited to about four.
3. Sticky, sugar containing products should be eliminated. Sugarless sweets containing sugar substitutes (xylitol, sorbitol, aspartam etc.) should be used.
4. In each meal, fiber rich products that stimulate chewing and salivary flow should be included.
5. Selected individuals with extremely high risk of development of caries should clean all surfaces just before each meal, to limit the drop in pH during and immediately after the meal.

4.2.5 Professional tooth cleaning

Professional tooth cleaning represents a basic method and means professional removal of all deposits from the teeth by dentist, dental hygienist or specially trained nurses. For the proximal surfaces dental floss must be used (and fissures must be sealed if indicated). Calculus (mineralized plaque) can be removed with manual or ultrasonic scalers, after it the teeth should be polished. A complete professional tooth cleaning should be performed before the active orthodontic treatment and at the appointments of control examinations.

4.2.6 Use of fluorides

A correlation between reduced caries prevalence and natural fluoride content of drinking water was published firstly by Dean (1938). Saliva usually contains a low amount of fluoride (Twetman et al., 1999). The importance of fluoridation is basic to maintain the health of teeth, particularly in the prevention of caries and remineralization of incipient carious lesions. A report published by the WHO (1994) and a review article by Rolla et al. (1991) state that the use of fluoridated tooth paste had led to a significant decrease in the incidence of caries in the industrialized countries. The ability of fluoride to retard or prevent the development of dental caries appears to involve several mechanisms including a reduction in the acid solubility of enamel, promotion of enamel remineralization, inhibition of glucose uptake and utilization by acidogenic bacteria. Demineralization refers to the loss of minerals (mainly calcium and phosphate ions) from the tooth structure due to the acidic and cariogenic challenge. Fluoride can help to prevent the mineral loss. When the pH drops below approximately 5.5, calcium ions are dissolved from the enamel and bond with fluoride ions forming a calcium fluoride (CaF_2) layer (Rolla & Saxegaard, 1990). CaF_2 is insoluble in the saliva and remains on the teeth for months (Dijkman et al., 1983). The CaF_2 layer functions as a pH controlled fluoride reservoir and is the most important supplier of free fluoride ions during the cariogen challenge (Fischer et al., 1995). Fluoride uptake and release of the enamel are strongly dependent on the duration of contact with the fluoridated agent (Ten Cate & Arends, 1980; Chen et al., 1985). With an appropriate fluoride formulation, incipient lesions could be reduced in size or even be repaired (Tranaeus et al., 2001).

Research suggests that topical fluorides might also decrease decalcification during orthodontic treatment (Geiger et al., 1988; Shannon & West, 1979; Benson et al., 2004; Derks et al., 2004; Chadwick et al., 2005; Sudjalim et al, 2006). Daily use of fluoride toothpaste, in combination with specific oral hygienic instructions, is recommended as the basis of caries and periodontal prophylaxis programme. Although fluoride concentration in different products may vary, below 0.1% in a dentifrice is not recommended for orthodontic patients (Ogaard et al., 2004). There are a number of locally applicable agents to improve maintain proper oral hygiene. The most important aim with the fluoridated dental care products first of all to strengthen of enamel against to caries, enhance the remineralization, protection against demineralization and improve or ensure gingival health. Beside of the toothpaste, fluoridated agents are included in different forms of gels, mouthrinses, varnishes and other products.

Topical fluoride may be applied by professional personnel in dental office or by patients at home. Using other local fluoridaton's method, a balance should be maintain between the prevention of dental caries and minimising the risk of dental mottling (Oulis et al., 2009). Generally, dentifrice alone is ineffective in preventing development of lesions (O'Reilly & Featherstone, 1987).

4.2.6.1 Fluoride rinses

Relevant studies have shown that daily use of fluoride rinse during the orthodontic treatment can reduce the incidence of initial carious lesions. At the same time, relatively few of orthodontic patients rinsed daily with fluoride containing mouthrinses (Geiger et al., 1988).

It has been published that caries reduction with different mouthrinses was estimated 25-30 % (Geiger et al., 1988; Newbrun, 1992). Rinses generally contain 0.025 to 0.05 % sodium fluoride, 0.025 % amine fluoride, 0.01 % zinc fluoride or 0.025 % APF (Acidulated Phosphate Fluoride), but more highly concentrated solutions are recommended for patients with increased risk (Zachrisson, 1975). Patients in high caries risk such as orthodontic patients should use a daily rinse of eg. 0.05% sodium fluoride at home (Petersson, 1993). Fluoride containing mouthrinse can be used at a time that is different to any tooth brushing for an additive effect to fluoride toothpaste (Oulis et al., 2009) or after the toothbrushing to complete the fluoride intake.

4.2.6.2 Fluoride gels

Fluoride containing gels can be used on patients yearly or half-yearly in dental office or can be used regularly by the patient, at home. The application of fluoride gels can reduce the occurance of caries by 21-30 % (Marinho et al., 2002; Marthaler, 1988).

4.2.6.3 Fluor protector gel

The Fluor Protector Gel (Vivadent, Shaan, Liechtenstein) contains calcium (Ca), phosphate and 1450 ppm fluoride (F) forming a CaF_2 layer and a direct incorporation of Ca, fluoride and phosphate ions into the tooth enamel. CaF_2 preferably deposits on demineralized surfaces and this layer is additionally stabilised by phosphate ions (Rolla and Saxegaard, 1990), which are also contained in Fluor Protector Gel. If the pH falls into the acidic range, the calcium fluoride layer releases Ca and phosphate ions which are released into the saliva and form a depot. It will work against demineralization or can contribute to the formation of fluoro-apatite or fluoro-hydroxyl-apatite. This replacement of hydroxy ion by a fluoride ion in the hydroxy apatite ensures the tooth enamel with higher resistance to pH drops (Fischer et al., 1995).

The Fluor Protector Gel can either used by the dentist in the dental surgery or by the patients at home, in different ways. It can be used in place of toothpaste to brush the teeth, or in the evening, after cleaning the teeth with toothpaste, when Fluor Protector Gel can be additionally applied with the toothbrush. It is suggested for cleaning interdental spaces of natural dentition or fixed dental restorations etc.. It also can be used with a tray filled with gel inserting it once or twice daily, and leaving it in place for 10 minutes every occasion.

It is especially recommended in high risk patients undergoing orthodontic treatment with fixed appliances.

4.2.6.4 Stannous fluoride gel

Since the late 1970s, 0.4% stannous fluoride (SnF_2) gels have been widely used as therapeutic agents for number of common oral diseases and conditions, and promoted as the preferred preventive and treatment products (Hastreiter, 1989; Paraskevas & van der Weiden, 2006). It contains more than 90% available stannous ion (Sn^{2+}) which is useful againts either plaque accumulation or gingivitis.

4.2.6.5 Halitosis tooth and tongue gel, Amine fluoride gel (see below)

4.2.6.6 Amine fluoride/ amine and stannous fluoride containing products

The use of amine fluorides in dentistry was recommended firstly by Mühlemann et al. (1957). The beneficial effects of them are well known as protective agents against mainly caries and dental plaque accumulation (Schmid, 1983; Öhrn & Sanz, 2009). These products were used in the form of dentifrices, gels and fluids in various caries preventive programs and suggested as alternatives or adjunctives for systemic fluoridation. Clinical studies with amine fluorides can be divided into trials with dentifrice only, with gel only or combined use of these products similarly to the use of mouthrinse and/or toothpaste. Fluoride containing gels are recommended annually or semiannually in the dental office. By the patients' home use, it is suggested to brush once a week, after a regular toothbrusing. Gels contain high concentration of different types of fluorides. Gels containing amine fluoride (in 12 500 ppm concentration) (Elmex gel, Gaba Int. Ltd., Switzerland) are used mostly in Europe. The active ingredients of the clinically tested relatively new product (Halitosis tooth and tongue gel) (Gaba Int. Ltd., Switzerland) (Figure 13.) are amine fluoride/ stannous fluoride and zinc lactate). This gel protects against caries, cleans the teeth and tongue (by helping a special tongue cleaner) and even neutralizes odour-active compounds in the oral cavity. It is offered for adults and childrens above the age of 12 years. It is also very useful for orthodontic patients with fixed orthodontic appliances because of these appliances can cause oral malodour (Babacan et al., 2011). This product is available in the form as mouthrinse with 250 ppm fluoride content.

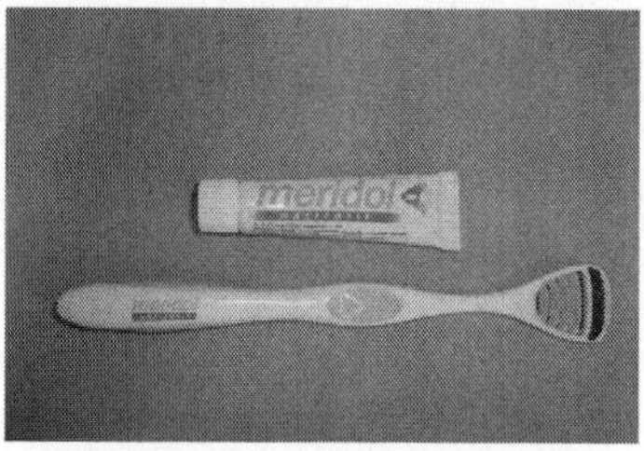

Fig. 13. Halitosis tooth and tongue gel and a tongue scraper.

This product is very useful for the patients undergoing orthodontic treatment.

Clinical trials with amine fluoride toothpaste, performed between 1968 and 1995 with a duration of 2.5-7 years, has reported reduction in mean DMFT/DMFS of between 7.1 and 35 % (Marthaler, 1968; 1974; Patz & Naujoks, 1970; Ringelberg et al., 1979; Cahen et al., 1982; Leous et al.,1995). Studies with amine fluoride gel between 1970 and 1989 with a duration of 1.5-7 years reported caries reductions of 31 - 53 % (Marthaler et al., 1970; Shern et al., 1976; Franke et al., 1977; Obersztyn & Kolwinski, 1984; Szőke & Kozma, 1989). In a 7-year clinical study using a combination of amine fluoride products a 43% reduction in DMFS mean values was found (Künzel et al., 1977). Madléna et al. (2002) published significant reduction in DMFS value (38 % including white spot lesions) and 34 % (not including white spot lesions) and a significant reduction in Plaque Index values with the combined use of amine fluoride containing toothpaste and gel in a high risk groups of adolescents. Márton et al. (2008) published beneficial effects of amine fluoride products.

The effects of Sn_2F or AmF/Sn_2F containing products on plaque accumulation were examined by many investigators (Øgaard et al., 1980; Bánóczy et al., 1989; Zimmermann et al., 1993; Mengel et al., 1996; Madléna et al., 2004; Gerardu et al., 2007). Madléna et al. (2009) proved the beneficial effects of amine fluoride /stannous fluoride containing products on periodontal parameters in patients treated with fixed orthodontic appliances. However, during a short term (four week-) examination period, there was no found significant difference between the groups using amine fluoride containing toothpaste only and the other group with combined use of toothpaste and mouthrinse containing the same ingredient. Although, at the same time numbers of streptococcus mutans and lactobacilli were reduced and level of periopathogen microorganisms also showed a very impressive decrease after even a four weeks use (Madléna et al., 2009; Nagy et al, 2010).

4.2.6.7 Fluoride varnishes

The development of fluoride varnishes started after the study of Mellberg et al. (1966). These authors found that considerable amounts of fluoride were released from enamel within the first 24 hours following the topical application of acidulated fluoride phosphate preparations. APF (Acidulated Phosphate Fluoride) increases the uptake of fluoride into the enamel because of its low pH. It is used mostly in the US. Schmid (1964) presented a topical fluoride method using a varnish with a high fluoride concentration. It was the Duraphat (Colgate Oral Pharmaceutical Inc., Canton, USA) which had the ability to adhere to tooth surfaces in the presence of saliva. Duraphat varnish consists of a natural resin (colophonium base with 5 % sodium fluoride (2.23 % F^-) dissolved in ethanol. It hardens the enamel in contact with saliva producing a temporary cover over the enamel. The patient is instructed to refrain from brushing for four hours after application (Retief et al, 1985; Staley 2008). The varnish also leaves calcium fluoride on the surface of the enamel in a CaF_2-like material that is less soluble and most likely leaches away from the surface through the pellicle (Dijkman & Arends, 1988). The other similar varnish system (Fluor protector) (Vivadent, Shaan, Liechtenstein) was introduced by Arends and Schuthof in 1975. Fluor protector contains 0.1 % F^- as difluorosilane dissolved in ethyl acetate and isoalylpropionate solution which has acidic properties. It is advisable that the patients avoid rinsing after application. Eating or brushing the teeth should also be avoided at least 45 minutes after the treatment. The differences can be found between the two varnishes are important in solvent, fluoride concentration, consistency, hardening time, colour, scent and taste. The varnishes coat the tooth surfaces as a thin layer that hardens a few minutes after application. The cost benefit ratio of fluoride varnishes is better then that of gels, and these products ensure the elimination the problem of compliance, as they are applied professionally (two to four times per year).

Beside of the above mentioned two types of fluoride varnish there are some other products. Duraflor (DenTrek, registered trademark of OMNI™ Preventive Care) is a 5 % NaF varnish containing xylitol and a bubble gum flavouring. Cavity shield contains 5% NaF in a neutral resin. The fluoride content is reported more uniform than that of Duraphat (Shen & Autio-Gold, 2002). The unit dose can be mixed easily and applied to teeth (Chu & Lo, 2006). Bifluorid 12 (Oceanwealth Horizon , (Voco), Düsseldorf, Germany) contains both NaF (2.7% F) and CaF_2 (2.9 % F). This combination of fluoride allows more fluoride deposit on the surface of demineralized enamel than NaF varnish alone (Attin et al., 1995).

Clinical studies showed beneficial effects of fluoride varnishes on caries reduction in both permanent and deciduous dentitions (Marinho, 2004). In the permanent dentition it was ranged from 20-70% compared to untreated controls (Petersson, 1975; de Bruyn & Arends, 1987), although it is very important to consider that clinical results are strongly influenced by different factors (e.g. caries prevalence, frequency of application of the varnish, caries risk etc.). Fluoride varnishes should be considered for use as a preventive adjunctive method to reduce demineralization adjacent to orthodontic brackets, especially in patients exhibiting pure compliance in oral hygiene and home fluoride use (Todd et al., 1999).

Advantages of fluoride varnishes are multiple: prolonged contact time acting as a slow release reservoir; these could be applied simply, quickly, easily; there is no need for widespread professional prophylaxis before the application of varnish because this procedure does not mean any additional effect, varnishes are safe, for even very young children. (Chu & Lo, 2006). Both parents and dentists prefer fluoride varnishes to fluoride gels (Warren et al., 2000). One disadvantage of Duraphat is its poor esthetic effect (a yellow film of varnish remains on the teeth for several hours after application) (Warren et al., 2000).

In a conclusion: there is moderate information is available on remineralization effectiveness of fluoride varnishes, but based on some investigations these could be offered for potential remineralization of the enamel (Castellano & Donly, 2004; Ogaard et al., 1984, 1996).

4.2.6.8 Slow release fluoride devices

Considering that intraoral levels of fluoride play a key role in the dynamics of dental caries, it has been suggested that the use of controlled and sustained delivery systems can be considered as a means of controlling dental caries incidence in high risk individuals (Mirth, 1980).

In a review of Pessan et al. (2008) there are three types of devices: Copolymer membrane device, Glass device, Hydroxyapatite Eudragit RS100 diffusion controlled F system. The third one is the newest type of slow release device, which consists of a mixture of hydroxyapatite, NaF and Eudragit RS100; it contains 18 mg NaF and intended to release 0.15 mg F/day. It was demonstrated that the use of this device is able to significantly increase salivary and urinary F concentration for at least 1 month (Altinova et al., 2005). These devices are effective in raising intraoral F concentrations at levels able to reduce enamel solubility, resulting in caries protective effect. The use of slow relesase devices have been shown to have a very favourable benefit regarding cost-effecitiveness ratios (Toumba, 1996). Slow release devices can show a high anticaries effect for patients in high caries risk (Featherstone, 2006). Beside of this, such a device would overcome compliance problems also. It may not eliminate all carious lesions, but would lead to dramatic reduction and in combination with antibacterial treatments could indeed eliminate caries in high risk individuals (Pessan et al., 2008).

4.2.7 Oral health care products for chemical plaque control

4.2.7.1 Chlorhexidine (CHX) containing products

Among chemical plaque control agents chlorhexidine digluconate has proven to be the most effective and safe. It seems to be the most important antimicrobial ingredient in dental products, which is available in forms of rinse, gel and varnish. Inspite of the side effects, experienced first of all with the mouthrinse, using of these products is considered as the best possibility to treat gingivitis.

4.2.7.1.1 Chlorhexidine mouthrinses

These types of clorhexidine containing products [(e.g. Corsodyl mouthrinses (GlaxoSmithKline, Brentford, UK)] are the most frequently used form in dentistry for patients with gingivitis and periodontitis and before or after surgical procedures. Professionally chlorhexidine solution could be used for irrigation the inflammed pockets. Anderson et al. (1997) published that use of CHX mouthrinse in addition to regular oral hygiene was effective in reducing plaque and gingivitis in adolescents undergoing orthodontic treatment. Ready to use 0.1 or 0.2 % mouthrinses are available. Löe et al. (1972) published that twice daily rinsing with an 0.2% CHX solution reduced the total bacterial count in saliva by 85-90%. In practice, it is offered for twice-daily use for a limited, 6 week term because of the side effects of this agent. These are the discoloration of the teeth, fillings and tongue, taste disturbances (hot and bitter) in the mouth. It can leave an unpleasant aftertaste and repeated use lead to an impaired sense of taste and desquamations.

Based on the available reviews, chlorhexidine rinses have not been highly effective in preventing caries or at least the clinical data are not convincing (Autio-Gold, 2008). Due to the current lack of long term clinical evidence for caries prevention and reported side effect, CHX rinses should not really be recommended for caries prevention. However, the use of gels, and varnishes should also be studied further on to have evidence-based recommendations for their clinical role in caries prevention (Autio-Gold, 2008).

4.2.7.1.2 Chlorhexidine gels

Treatment with gel seems to be more effective than treatment with mouthrinse because the gel adheres to the tooth surface for longer period. Emilson (1981) published that CHX containing gel inhibited the plaque formation on tooth surfaces, effected on Gram positive and Gram negative bacteria such as mutans streptococci. CHX containing gel (e.g. Corsodyl with 1% CHX) (GlaxoSmithKline, Brentford, UK) similarly to other gels can be applied with toothbrush or in a custom made tray. The use of tray is better because the gel can attach the tooth surface without dilution and it is not distributed on the mucosa. The CHX gel ensures significant reduction in mutans streptococci, at the same time the patient has no unpleasent sense of taste. The time tested ingredient CHX reduces the growth of harmful bacteria and yeast. So there are less plaque formed on the teeth or appliances and the inflammation of gum tissues subsides.

Because of the beneficial effects, CHX containing gel suggested to use with a special soft tray. This therapy delivered by a tray which is offered for only older children, adolescents or adults who are able to apply the gel and tray safety, otherwise the gel should be used with toothbrush or with cotton roll.

Clinical studies defined the caries inhibiting effect of CHX (Zickert et al., 1982). It was also published that the effect of CHX gel is increased with combined use of fluoride gel (Ostela & Tenovuo, 1990; Meurman, 1988). In addition to the antibacterial CHX (0.11%), Cervitec gel (Vivadent, Schaan, Liechtenstein) containing fluoride (900 ppm) which promotes remineralization and protects the teeth from caries. At the same time it is an effective antimicrobial product. Cervitec gel can be used with interdental brushes, with toothbrush, tray or it can be applied directly on the gum.

4.2.7.1.3 Chlorhexidine varnishes

During the past decade, varnishes for local delivery of antimicrobial agents have been developed and investigated in vitro and in vivo. The inhibitory effect of CHX on mutans streptococci or new carious lesions was confirmed with fixed orthodontic appliances (Lundström and Krasse, 1987; Madléna et al., 2000; Derks et al., 2004) (Figure 14.).

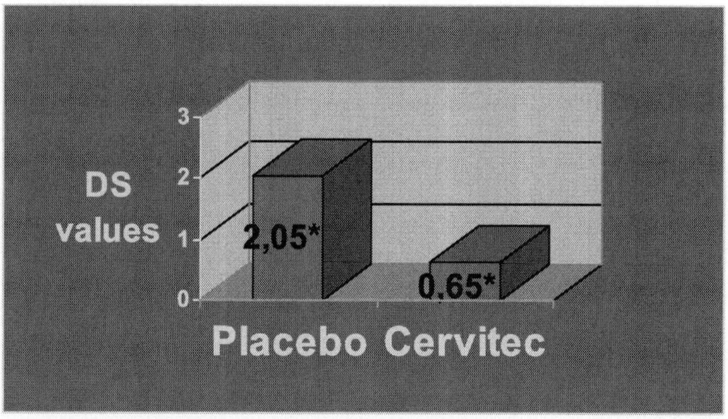

Fig. 14. The effect of chlorhexidine containing varnish (Cervitec) on newly developed carious lesions during orthodontic treatment (*$p<0.05$)
The number of the new carious lesions was significantly lower in the quadrants treated with Cervitec than in the quadrants treated with placebo (*$p<0.05$).(Madléna et al., 2000).

It has been concluded by a review that the most persistent reduction of mutans streptococci have been achived by chlorhexidine varnishes followed by gels and lastly mouthrinses (Autio-Gold, 2008). Cervitec plus is a newer, now available member of the „Cervitec family" (Vivadent, Shaan, Liechtenstein) containing chlorhexidine and thymol). Comparing three varnish systems (Chlorzoin, containing CHX 10% (Knowell Therapeutic Technologies, owned company Toronto, Canada), EC 40, containing CHX 40% (Biodent BV, Nijmegen, The Netherlands), Cervitec Plus, containing CHX 1%), a single application of a highly concentrated varnish (EC 40), is sufficient even with reduced contact time, whereas repeated applications and longer retention time required for varnishes with lower chlorhexidine concentration (Chlorzoin and Cervitec). All of the three varnish systems had a similar effect on mutans streptococci in the oral flora. However, none of these varnishes could maintain a significant suppression of mutans streptococci for a period of up to 6 months (repeated application is required for the effectiveness). Concerning the chlorhexidine containing varnishes there may be noticed some advers effects, similarly to other chlorhexidine containing products: staining of teeth and tongue, or taste disturbancies associated with accidental contact of CHX varnish with oral mucosa (Matthijs & Adriaens, 2002).

The most sensitive bacteria to chlorhexidine-thymol varnish (Cervitec plus) are Porphyromonas gingivalis and Aggregatibacter Actynomycetemcomitans. Therefore, chlorhexidine varnishes may be promising for the prevention of periodontal disease or as an adjunct to periodontal therapy (Petersson et al. 1992; Matthijs & Adriaens, 2002). Twetman and Petersson (1997) reported that a combined treatment with a chlorhexidine – thymol and a fluoride varnish resulted in a longer inhibiting effect on interdental plaque samples, than chlorhexidine-thymol varnish alone. The use of dental varnishes with antimicrobial properties might have potential benefits for patients with chronic gingival inflammation (Matthijs & Adriaens, 2002).

4.2.7.2 Other products

4.2.7.2.1 Essential oils containing products - Listerine (Johnson & Johnson, Maidenhead, UK)

Active ingredients of this oral rinse are essential oils (eucalyptol, thymol, menthol) for bactericid effect, contains methyl salicylate (against analgesia and inflammation) and alcohol (in which the active ingredients are diluted). It should be used as a rinse twice daily for 1 minute. As it does not contain any fluoride or its fluoride concentration is very low (in the newer products), has no effect on caries, but it has an antigingivitis effect According to a systematic review published by Van Leeuwen et al. (2011), in long term use, the standardized formulation of essential-oil mouthwas appeared to be a reliable alternative to chlorhexidine mouthwash with respect to parameters of gingival inflammation. Listerine toothpaste is not established as effective product against gingivitis (Boyd, 2001).

4.2.7.2.2 Triclosan-containing products - (Colgate total) (Colgate Palmolive Co. USA)

It is also an antigingivitis agent including good taste and supragingival calculus control (Volpe et al., 1996). Triclosan is available only in toothpaste (Colgate total) (Colgate Palmolive Co. USA), has an antibacterial effect and is often combined with zinc to increase the antiplaque effect. Thus, it may give potential benefits for orthodontic patients as a supplement to fluoride dentifrice during orthodontic treatment.

4.2.7.2.3 Hyaluronic acid containing products (Gengigel) (Ricefarma, Milano, Italy)

Hyaluronic acid is naturally occures as physiological constituent of connective tissue (especially in gingival mucosa). It ensures antioedematous and tissue repair functions, helps to perform an antiinflammatoric effect, so can be helpful during the orthodontic treatment with fixed appliances. The lack of hyaluronic acid is responsible for the continuation of the inflammatory condition. In these cases application of hyaluronic acid provides periodontal tissue with accelerated repair functions by preventing the deficiency of natural gingival hyaluronic acid and enhancing its effects.

The hyaluronic acid containing Gengigel can be available in forms gel, rinse and spray. Pistorius et al. (2002) published positive effects of Gengigel spray: this product ensured significant improvements in gingival parameters in case of gingivitis, after 7 days application. All Gengigel products are suggested to use in case of gingivitis, gingival bleeding, gingival pockets (also gingival recession, abrasion and other tissue trauma etc.), after the correct oral hygiene three to five times a day (after main meals) for 3-4 weeks, continuing until the symptomes have disappeared. Side effect has not been experienced with these products.

4.2.7.2.4 Antibiotics

Use of oral or systemic antibiotic therapy is indicated to eliminate specific pathogenic organisms. However, antibiotic therapy can never replace the mechanical removal of subgingival deposits and it should be only a supplemental, supportive therapy, similarly to the treatment of serious periodontal diseases, but this indication belongs to an experienced periodontist and should not be administrated routinly by an orthodontist.

4.3 Remineralization – Treatment of white spot lesions after removal of fixed appliance

4.3.1 Fluorides

Fluoride increses the initial rate of remineralization of early enamel lesions and slow down the progress of carious process by reacting with the minerals present in the surface of the lesion. Enamel can be remineralized with meticulous toothbrushing twice per day, with fluoridated dentifrice. Additional fluoride application can further enhance the remineralization process. This would include eg. fluoridated dentifrice with higher dose, fluoride rinses, topical fluoride gels, fluoride varnishes and professionally applied topical fluoride such as 2% sodium fluoride, 8% stannous fluoride and 1.23% acidulated phosphate fluoride (Donly & Sasa, 2008). At the same time it was published that when high doses of fluoride are used locally (mainly during the first few weeks after completed the orthodontic treatment), the arrested lesion stays the same size and frequently becomes unsightly and stained with organic debris which is esthetically not optimal on the labial surfaces (Ogaard et al., 2004; Willmot, 2008). To avoid arresting the lesion and obtunding the surface layer several authors recommended low dose fluoride applications to enhance subsurface remineralization It was published that 50 ppm fluoride mouthrinse had a higher efficiency for remineralization than control solution for regular mouthrinse containing 250 ppm (Linton, 1996; Lagerwij et al., 1997). In spite of these observations, Wilmot (2004) did not confirm the therapeutic effect of low fluoride (50 ppm) products and concluded that postorthodontic white spot lesions (WSL) reduced in size during the 6 months by approximately half of the original size, but there was no clinical advantage of using the low fluoride formulation of mouthrinse/toothpaste in this process comparing to those of using fluoride free products as a control. The mean size of the lesions reduced with time in both groups. A therapeutic effect (less than 30%) was non significant. Beside of the labial surfaces application of concentrated fluoride was suggested to prevent the progresson of the lesions. It has been also suggested that acid etching of fluoride treated lesions could facilitate remineralization of the lesions by oral fluids (Hicks et al., 1984).

4.3.2 Use of Casein Phosphopeptide-Amorphus Calcium Phosphate (CPP-ACP)

Enamel can also be remineralized with Casein Phosphopeptide-Amorphus Calcium Phosphate preparations. CPP-ACP is capable to be absorbed through the enamel surface and could affect the carious process (Reynolds, 1987) CPP-ACP system (the trade name is Recaldent™) which allows freely available calcium and phosphate ions to attach to enamel and reform into calcium phosphate crystals. The free calcium and phosphate ions released from the CPP-ACP and deposit into the enamel rods. The available types of these products: water based mousse, topical creme (these are the most frequently used forms) mouthrinses, sugarfree lozenges and chewing gum (which is not suggested for orthodontic patients).

As CPP-ACP is derived from milk casein, should not be used in patient with protein and or hydroxybenzoates allergy. Studies of the effects of CPP-ACP show a dose related increase in enamel remineralization (Sudjalim et al., 2006). These products have beneficial effects in reducing area of demineralized lesions after 4 weeks (Bröchner et al., 2011).

Using the mousse (GC Tooth Mousse) to treat post-orthodontic lesions, a thermoplastic retainer needs in which a pea sized amount of CPP-ACP mousse has been spread evenly.

After proper oral hygiene the patient places the mousse at night and wears the retainer throughout sleep. Flavouring helps to stimulate saliva flow rate which helps to rinse bacteria and food residues from the teeth and enhances the effectiveness of CPP ACP in the mouth.

The GC MI Paste Plus is a water based topical creme containing Recaldent ™ CPP-ACP and fluoride (900 ppm). It can be used on teeth at home when the patient apply the products with a tray (Figure 15.), similarly to the mousse or without a tray simply with clean finger or cotton tipped applicator and let it work for 3-5 minutes.

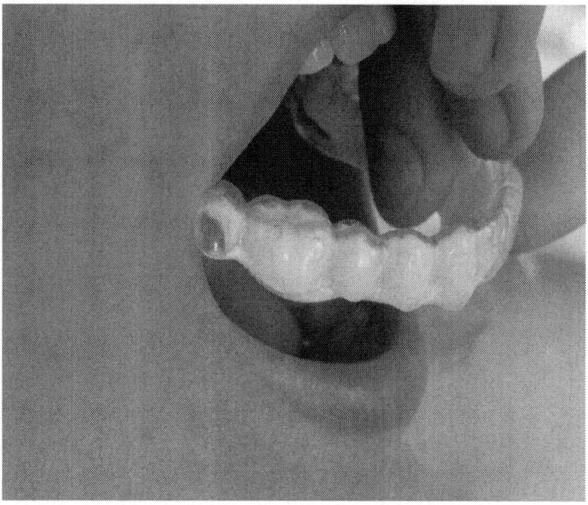

Fig. 15. Use of MI Paste Plus with a tray.

This material containing CPP ACP and fluoride can help in remineralization process e.g. after finishing the orthodontic treatment with fixed appliance

4.3.3 Microabrasion

Enamel microabrasion abrades the enamel surface, leaving a highly polished surface with Ca phosphate packed into the interprismatic enamel surface space. This highly polished enamel surface can then be bleached.

This method has been widely used for the removal of superficial non-carious enamel defects for which it can be use for example performing 18% hydrochloric acid and pumice technique (Welbury & Shaw, 1990; Rodd & Davidson, 1997). This method seems to be an effective treatment approach for cosmetic improvement of long-standing postorthodontic demineralized enamel lesions (Welbury & Carter, 1993; Croll & Bullock, 1994). Studies demonstrate that although microabrasion removes small amounts of the enamel surface, the new polished surface is less susceptible to bacterial colonization and demineralization than natural non abraded enamel (Segura et al., 1997 a,b).

Following the microabrasion technique, a 4 minute 2% sodium fluoride treatment is recommended. If the microbrasion technique could not ensure optimal esthetics and some whitened enamel is still remain, vital tooth bleaching can be considered (Donly & Sasa, 2008).

5. Conclusion

The number of orthodontic treatments among them the frequency of treatments with fixed appliances is increasing nowadays. In some cases orthodontic treatments mean caries preventive interventions when tooth movements may reliese crowding or other anomalies thus can contribute the effectiveness of proper oral hygiene. On the other hand these treatments may have causative effect on plaque induced oral diseases. For these patients effective preventive oral health care is needed and orthodontists have to be responsible for helping to keep proper oral hygiene in their patients.

The risk of caries can be determined by different tests (e.g. SM, LB chairside tests) or assessment of some salivary factors. Measurement of plaque has been found also very useful to determinate the risk of caries. The severity of periodontal diseases and the risk for these diseases can be determined by clinical measurements. Bleeding on probing remained the most certain clinical sign of periodontal inflammations. Chairside tests are available to measure different parameters associated with periodontitis, but presently there is no such a particular parameter or method predicting the possibility of periodontitis.

For prevention of caries and periodontal diseases clinicians should instruct the patients effectively to be able to perform proper oral hygiene. Regular removal of plaque and calculus at critical places can help a lot. Regular recalls, well constructed programs of regular professional oral hygiene can give great help for at-risk patients.

Beside of dietary counselling, to reduce cariogenic bacteria, use of professional and home care measures and techniques (cleaning instruments, fluoridated paste, restorative methods, application of fluoride and chlorhexidine containig materials, plaque disclosing products, special toothbrushes and other equipments etc.) could provide help.

Because of the increasing number of patients in need of orthodontic appliances, this chapter is important and useful not only for orthodontists, but general dentists or periodontists and dental students as well.

6. Acknowledgements

The author is greatfully acknowledge the review of the chapter by professor Gábor Nagy and excellent technical assistance of Ágnes Siki to find all necessary data of the references.

7. References

Ainamo, J. & Bay, I. (1975). Problems and proposals for recording gingivitis and plaque, *Int Dent J* 25(4): 229-235.

Alacam, A., Ulusu, T., Bodur, H., Oztas, N. & Oren, M. C. (1996). Salivary and urinary fluoride levels after 1-month use of fluoride-releasing removable appliances, *Caries Res* 30(3): 200-203.

Al Maaltah, E. F., Adeyemi, A. A., Higham, S. M., Pender, N. & Harrison, J. E. (2011). Factors affecting demineralization during orthodontic treatment: a post-hoc analysis of RCT recruits, *Am J Orthod Dentofacial Orthop* 139(2): 181-191.

Altinova, Y. B., Alacam, A., Aydin, A. & Sanisoglu, S. Y. (2005). Evaluation of a new intraoral controlled fluoride release device, *Caries Res* 39(3): 191-194.

Amaechi, B. T.(2009). Emerging technologies for diagnosis of dental caries: The road so far, *J Appl Phys* 105(10):an:102047

Anderson, G. B., Bowden, J., Morrison, E. C. & Caffesse, R, G. (1997). Clinical effects of chlorhexidine mouthwashes on patients undergoing orthodontic treatment, *Am J Orthod Dentofac Orthop* 111(6): 606-612.

Anderson, M. H., Bales, D .J. & Omnell, K. A. (1993). Modern management of dental caries: the cutting edge is not the dental bur, *J Am Dent Assoc* 124(6): 36-44.

Arends, J. & Schuthof, J. (1975). Fluoride content in human enamel after fluoride application and washing: An in vitro study, *Caries Res* 9(5): 363-372.

Artun, J. (1984). Caries and periodontal reactions associated with long-term use of different types of bonded lingual retainers, *Am J Orthod Dentofac Orthop* 86(2): 112-118.

Artun, J. & Brobakken, BO. (1986). Prevalence of carious white spots after orthodontic treatment with multibonded appliances, *Eur J Orthod* 8(4): 229-234.

Attin, T., Hartmann, O., Hilgers, R. D. & Hellwig, E. (1995). Fluoride retention of incipient enamel lesions after treatment with a calcium fluoride varnish in vivo, *Arch Oral Biol* 40(3): 169-174.

Autio-Gold, J. (2008). The role of chlorhexidine in caries prevention, *Oper Dent* 33(6): 710-716.

Axelsson, P. (1991). A four-point scale for selection of caries risk patients, based on salivary S. mutans levels and plaque formation rate index, In: *Risk Markers for Oral Diseases,* N. Johnson, (Ed), 158-170, Cambridge University Press, ISBN 9780521375634, London, England

Axelsson, P. (1999). Other caries preventive factors. Dietary control, In: *An introduction to risk prediction and preventive dentistry,* P. Axelsson (Ed.) 101-102, Quintessence Publishing Co Inc,. ISBN 0-86-715-361-X, Berlin, Germany

Axelsson, P. (2000). Etiologic factors involved in dental caries, In: *Diagnosis and Risk: Prediction of Dental Caries, P. Axelsson (Ed.)* 1-42, ISBN0-86715-362-8, Quintessence Publishing Co Inc., Chicago, USA

Babacan, H., Sokucu, O., Marakoglu, I., Ozdemir, H. & Nalcaci, R. (2011). Effect of fixed appliances on oral malodor, *Am J Orthod Dentofac Orthop* 139(3): 351-355.

Banks, P. A., Chadwick, S. M., Ascher-McDade, C. & Wright, J. L. (2000). Fluoride-releasing elastomerics - a prospective controlled clinical trial, *Eur J Orthod* 22(4): 401-407.

Banoczy, J., Szoke, J., Kertesz, P., Toth, Z., Zimmermann, P. & Gintner Z. (1989). Effect of amine fluoride stannous fluoride-containing toothpaste and mouth-rinsings on dental plaque, gingivitis, plaque and enamel f-accumulation, *Caries Res* 23(4): 284-288.

Batoni, G., Pardini, M., Giannotti, A., Ota, F., Giuca, M. R., Gabriele, M., Campa, M. & Senesi, S. (2001). Effect of removable orthodontic appliances on oral colonisation by mutans streptococci in children, *Eur J Oral Sci* 109(6): 388-392.

Benson, P. (2008). Evaluation of white spot lesions on teeth with orthodontic brackets, *Semin Orthod* 14(3): 200-208.

Benson P. E, Parkin N, Millett D. T, Dyer F. E, Vine, S. & Shah A. (2004). Fluorides for the prevention of white spots on teeth during fixed brace treatment, *Cochrane Database Syst Rev* (3): CD003809.

Bickel, M. & Geering, A. H. (1982). Zur bakteriellen Besiedelung der Prothesenbasis, *Schweiz Monatsschr Zahnheilkd* 92(9): 741-745.

Bishara, S. E. & Ostby, A. W. (2008). White spot lesions: formation, prevention, and treatment, *Semin Orthod* 14(3): 174-182.

Bittencourt, M. A. V. & Machado, A. W. (2010). An overview of the prevalence of malocclusion in 6 to 10 –year-old children in Brazil, *Dental Press Orthod* 15(6): 113-22.

Boersma, J. G., van der Veen, M. H., Lagerweij, M. D., Bokhout, B. & Prahl-Andersen, B. (2005). Caries prevalence measured with QLF after treatment with fixed orthodontic appliances: influencing factors, *Caries Res* 2005, 39(1): 41-47.

Boyd, R.L. (2001). Orthodontic consideration during orthodontic treatment, *In*: *Textbook of orthodontics*, Bishara S. E. (Ed.), 442-452, WB Saunders Company, ISBN 0-7216-8289-8, Philadelphia, USA

Boyd, R. L., Leggott, P. J., Quinn, R. S., Eakle, W. S. & Chambers, D. (1989). Periodontal implications of orthodontic treatment in adults with reduced or normal periodontal tissues versus those of adolescents, *Am J Orthod Dentofac Orthop* 96(3): 191-198.

Boyd, R. L. & Baumrind, S. (1992). Periodontal considerations in the use of bonds or bands on molars in adolescents and adults, *Angle Orthod* 62(2): 117-126.

Brochner, A., Christensen, C., Kristensen, B., Tranæus, S., Karlsson, L., Sonnesen, L. & Twetman, S. (2011). Treatment of post-orthodontic white spot lesions with casein phosphopeptide-stabilised amorphous calcium phosphate, *Clin Oral Investig* 15(3): 369-373.

Buckley, L. A. (1980). The relationships between irregular teeth, plaque, calculus and gingival disease. A study of 300 subjects, *Br Dent J* 148(3): 67-69.

Cahen, . M., Frank, R. M., Turlot, J. C. & Jung, M. T. (1982). Comparative unsupervised clinical-trial on caries inhibition effect of monofluorophosphate and amine fluoride dentifrices after 3 years in Strassbourg, France, *Community Dent Oral Epidemiol* 10(5): 238-241.

Castellano, J. B. & Donly, K. J. (2004). Potential remineralization of demineralized enamel after application of fluoride varnish, *Am J Dent* 17(6): 462-464.

Chadwick, B. L., Roy, J., Knox, J. & Treasure, E. T. (2005). The effect of topical fluorides on decalcification in patients with fixed orthodontic appliances: A systematic review, *Am J Orthod Dentofac Orthop* 128(5): 601-606.

Chapman, J. A., Roberts, W. E., Eckert, G. J., Kula, K. S. & González-Cabezas, C. (2010). Risk factors for incidence and severity of white spot lesions during treatment with fixed orthodontic appliances, *Am J Orthod Dentofacial Orthop* 138(2):188-194.

Chaussain, C., Opsahl Vital, S., Viallon, V., Vermelin, L., Haignere, C., Sixou, M. & Lasfargues. J. J. (2010). Interest in a new test for caries risk in adolescents undergoing orthodontic treatment, *Clin Oral Investig* 14(2): 177-185.

Chen, W. C., Zawacki, S. J., Nancollas, G. H. & White, D. J. (1985). Constant composition remineralisation of early carious lesions in bovine enamel, *J Dent Res* 64(Spec. iss.): 301-301.

Chu, C. H. & Lo, E. C. M. (2006). A review of sodium fluoride varnish, *General Dentistry* 54(4): 247-253.

Chung, C. H., Cuozzo, P. T. & Mante, F. K. (1999). Shear bond strength of a resin-reinforced glass ionomer cement: An in vitro comparative study, *Am J Orthod Dentofac Orthop* 115(1): 52-54.

Ciuffolo, F., Manzoli, L., D'Attilio, M., Tecco, S., Muratore, F., Festa, F. & Romano, F. (2005). Prevalence and distribution by gender of occlusal characteristics in a sample of Italian secondary school students: a cross-sectional study, *Eur J Orthod* 27(6): 601-606.

Croll, T. P. & Bullock, G. A. (1994). Enamel microabrasion for removal of smooth surface decalcification lesions, *J Clin Orthod* 28(6): 365-370.

Crossner, C. G. (1981). Salivary lactobacillus counts in the prediction of caries activity, *Community Dent Oral Epidemiol* 9(4): 182-190.

de Bruyn, H. & Arends, J. (1987). Fluoride varnishes--a review, *J Biol Buccale* 15(2): 71-82.

Dean, H. T. (1938). Endemic fluorosis and its relation to dental caries, *Public Health Rep* 53(33): 1443-1452.

Derks, A., Katsaros, C., Frencken, J. E., van't Hof, M. A. & Kuijpers-Jagtman, A. M. (2004). Caries-inhibiting effect of preventive measures during orthodontic treatment with fixed appliances. A systematic review, *Caries Res* 38(5): 413-420.

Dharmaraj, S. (2011). RT-PCR: The basics [Internet] Applied Biosystems [cited: 2011.08.22.] Available from: http://www.ambion.com/techlib/basics/rtpcr/index.html

Diamanti-Kipioti, A., Gusberti, F. A. & Lang, N. P. (1987). Clinical and microbiological effects of fixed orthodontic appliances, *J Clin Periodontol* 14(6): 326-333.

Diedrich P. (1989). Keimbesiedlung und verschiedene Reinigungsverfahren kieferorthopadischer Gerate, *Fortschr Kieferorthop* 50(3): 231-239.

Dijkman, A. G., de Boer, P. & Arends, J. (1983). In vivo investigation on the fluoride content in and on human enamel after topical applications, *Caries Res* 17(5): 392-402.

Dijkman, T. G. & Arends, J. (1988). The role of 'CaF2-like' material in topical fluoridation of enamel in situ, *Acta Odontol Scand* 46(6): 391-397.

Donly, K. J. & Sasa, I. S. (2008). Potential remineralization of postorthodontic demineralized enamel and the use of enamel microabrasion and bleaching for esthetics, *Semin Orthod* 14(3): 220-225.

Emilson, C. G. (1981). Effect of chlorhexidine gel treatment on streptococcus mutans population in human saliva and dental plaque, *Scand J Dent Res* 89(3): 239-246.

Featherstone, J. D. (2003). The caries balance: Contributing factors and early detection, *J Calif Dent Assoc* 31(2): 129-133.

Featherstone, J. D. B. (2006). Delivery challenges for fluoride, chlorhexidine and xylitol, *BMC Oral Health* 6 (SUPPLEMENTUM 1): S8

Featherstone, J. D., Domejean-Orliaguet, S., Jenson, L., Wolff, M. & Young, D. A. (2007). Caries risk assessment in practice for age 6 through adult, *J Calif Dent Assoc* 35(10): 703-713.

Fischer, C., Lussi, A. & Hotz, P. (1995). Kariostatische Wirkungsmechanismen der Fluoride. Eine Ubersicht, *Schweiz Monatsschr Zahnmed* 105(3): 311-317.

Franke, W., Kuenzel, W., Treide, A. & Bluethner, K. (1977). Karieshemmung durch aminfluorid nach 7 jahren kollektiv angeleiteter mundhygiene, *Stomat DDR* 27(1): 13-16

Frazier, M. C., Southard, T. E. & Doster, P. M. (1996). Prevention of enamel demineralization during orthodontic treatment: An in vitro study using pit and fissure sealants. *Am J Orthod Dentofac Orthop* 110(5): 459-465.

Freundorfer, A., Purucker, P. & Miethke, R.R. (1993). Kieferorthopädische Behandlungen können ohne professionelle Mundhygiene zu dauerhaften Veränderungen der subgingivalenPlaqueflora führen, *Prakt Kieferorthop* 7(3): 187-200.

Friedman, M., Harari, D., Raz, H., Golomb, G. & Brayer, L. (1985). Plaque inhibition by sustained-release of chlorhexidine from removable appliances, *J Dent Res* 64(11): 1319-1321.

Fox, C.H. (1992). New considerations in the prevalence of periodontal disease. New considerations in the prevalence of periodontal disease, *Curr Opin Dent* 2: 5-11.

Gabris, K., Marton, S. & Madlena, M. (2006). Prevalence of malocclusions in Hungarian adolescents, *Eur J Orthod* 28(5): 467-470.

Geiger, A. M. (2001). Malocclusion as an etiologic factor in periodontal disease: a retrospective essay, *Am J Orthod Dentofacial Orthop* 120(2): 112-115.

Geiger, A. M., Wasserman, B. H. & Turgeon, L. R. (1974). Relationship of occlusion and periodontal disease. 8. Relationship of crowding and spacing to periodontal destruction and gingival inflammation, *J Periodontol* 45(1): 43-49.

Geiger, A. M., Gorelick, L., Gwinnett, A. J. & Griswold, P. G. (1988). The effect of a fluoride program on white spot formation during orthodontic treatment, *Am J Orthod Dentofac Orthop* 93(1): 29-37.

Genco, R.J (1996). Current view of risk factors for periodontal diseases, *J Periodontol* 67 (10 Suppl): 1041-1049.

Gerardu, V. A. M., Buijs, M, van Loveren, C. & ten Cate, J. M. (2007). Plaque formation and lactic acid production after the use of amine fluoride/stannous fluoride mouthrinse, *Eur J Oral Sci* 115(2): 148-52.

Gorelick, L., Geiger, A. M. & Gwinnett, A. J. (1982). Incidence of white spot formation after bonding and banding, *Am J Orthod Dentofac Orthop* 81(2): 93-98.

Gwinnett, A. J. & Ceen, RF. (1979). Plaque distribution on bonded brackets - scanning microscope study, *Am J Orthod Dentofac Orthop* 75(6): 667-677.

Hastreiter RJ. (1989). Is 0.4% stannous fluoride gel an effective agent for the prevention of oral diseases, *J Am Dent Assoc* 118(2): 205-208.

Heintze, S. D., Jost-Brinkmann, P. G., Finke, C. & Miethke, R, R. (1999). *Oral health for the orthodontic patient,* 25-43, 111-128, Quinessence publishing Co Inc, ISBN 0-86715-295-8, Chicago, USA

Helm, S. & Petersen, P. E. (1989a). Causal relation between malocclusion and caries, *Acta Odontol Scand* 47(4): 217-221.

Helm, S. & Petersen, P. E. (1989b). Causal relation between malocclusion and periodontal health, *Acta Odontol Scand* 47(4): 223-228.

Herzberg, M. C. & Meyer, M. W. (1996). Effects of oral flora on platelets: possible consequences in cardiovascular disease, *J Periodontol* 67(10 Suppl): 1138-1142.

Hicks, M. J., Silverstone, L. M. & Flaitz, C. M. (1984). A scanning electron microscopic and polarized light microscopic study of acid-etching of caries-like lesions in human tooth enamel treated with sodium fluoride in vitro, *Arch Oral Biol* 29(10): 765-772.

Hollender, L. & Rönnerman, A. (1978). Proximal caries progression in connection with orthodontic treatment, Swed Dent J 2(5): 153-160.

Hotz, P. R. (1982). Prävention von Karies und Gingivitis bei der kieferorthopädischen Behandlung, Schweiz Monatsschr Zahnheilkd. 92(Spec No): 880-888.

Huizinga, E. D., Ruben, J. & Arends, J. (1990). Effect of an antimicrobial-containing varnish on root demineralization in situ, Caries Res 24(2): 130-132.

Huser, M. C,, Baehni, P. C. & Lang, R. (1990). Effects of orthodontic bands on microbiologic and clinical parameters, *Am J Orthod Dentofac Orthop* 97(3): 213-218.

Ingervall, B. (1962). The influence of orthodontic appliances on caries frequency, *Odontol Revy* 13(2): 175-190.

Jeffcoat, M.K. & McGuire, M. & Newman, M.G. (1997). Evidence-based periodontal treatment. Highlights from the 1996 World Workshop in Periodontics, *J Am Dent Assoc* 128(6): 713-724.

Jensen, B. & Bratthall, D. (1989). A new method for the estimation of mutans streptococci in human-saliva, *J Dent Res* 68(3): 468-471.

Katz, R. V. (1978). An epidemiologic study of the relationship between various states of occlusion and the pathological conditions of dental caries and periodontal disease, *J Dent Res* 57(3): 433-439.

Klock, B. & Krasse, B. (1979). Comparison between different methods for prediction of caries activity, *Scand J Dent Res* 87(2): 129-139.

Kneist, S., Laurisch, L., Heinrich-Weltzien, R. & Stosser, L. (1998). A modified mitis salivarius medium for a caries diagnostic test, *J Dent Res* 77(Spec. Issue B):970-970. an. 2712.

Kohler, B. & Bratthall, D. (1979). Practical method to facilitate estimation of streptococcus-mutans levels in saliva, *J Clin Microbiol* 9(5): 584-588.

Krasse, B. (1988). Biological factors as indicators of future caries, *Int Dent J* 38(4): 219-225.

Kristoffersson, K., Grondahl, HG. & Bratthall, D. (1985). The more streptococcus-mutans, the more caries on approximal surfaces, *J Dent Res* 64(1): 58-61.

Kuusela, S., Honkala, E. & Rimpelä, A. (1996). Toothbrushing frequency between the ages of 12 and 18 years - longitudinal prospective studies of Finnish adolescents, *Community Dent Health* 13(1): 34-39.

Künzel, W., Franke, W. & Treide, A. (1977). Klinisch-röntgenologische Parallelüberwachung einer Längsschnittstudie zum Nachweis der Karieshemmenden Effektivität 7 Jahre lokal angewandten Aminfluorids im Doppelblindtest, *Zahn Mund Kieferheilk* 65(6): 626-637.

Lagerweij, M. D., Damen, J. J. M. & Stookey, G. K. (1997). Remineralization of small enamel lesions by fluoride, *J Dent Res* 76 (Spec Issue): 22-22.

Lang, N. P. & Bragger, U. (1991). Periodontal diagnosis in the 1990s, *J Clin Periodontol* 18(6): 370-379.

Larmas, M. (1975). A new dip slide method for the counting of salivary lactobacilli, *Proc Finn Dent Soc* 71(2): 31-35.

Leous, P., Pakhomov, G. & Ramanathan, J. (1995). Effectiveness of toothbrushing with amine fluoride toothpaste in the prevention of caries and periodontal diseases among young adults, WHO, Geneva

Linton, J. L. (1996). Quantitative measurements of remineralization of incipient caries, *Am J Orthod Dentofac Orthop* 110(6): 590-597.

Loe, H., Von der Fehr, F. R. & Schiott, C. R. (1972). Inhibition of experimental caries by plaque prevention. the effect of chlorhexidine mouthrinses *Scand J Dent Res* 80(1): 1-9.

Lundstrom, F., Hamp, S. E. & Nyman, S. (1980). Systematic plaque control in children undergoing long-term orthodontic treatment, *Eur J Orthod* 2(1): 27-39.

Lundstrom, F., & Krasse, B. (1987). Streptococcus mutans and lactobacilli frequency in orthodontic patients; the effect of chlorhexidine treatments, *Eur J Orthod* 9(1): 109-116.

Madlena, M., Vitalyos, G., Marton, S. & Nagy, G. (2000). Effect of chlorhexidine varnish on bacterial levels in plaque and saliva during orthodontic treatment, *J Clin Dent* 11(2): 42-46.

Madlena, M., Nagy, G., Gabris, K., Marton, S., Keszthelyi G. & Banoczy, J. (2002). Effect of amine fluoride toothpaste and gel in high risk groups of Hungarian adolescents: Results of a longitudinal study, *Caries Res* 36(2): 142-146.

Madlena, M., Dombi, C., Gintner, Z. & Banoczy, J. (2004) Effect of amine fluoride/stannous fluoride toothpaste and mouthrinse on dental plaque accumulation and gingival health, *Oral Dis* 10(5): 294-297.

Madlena, M., Banoczy, J., Gotz, G., Szadeczky, B., Marton, S. & Nagy, G. (2009). Effects of Amine Fluoride/Stannous Fluoride Products on Plaque accumulation and Gingival Health in Orthodontic patients, *Caries Res* 43(3): 210-210. an. 86

Marinho, V. C., Higgins, J. P., Logan, S. & Sheiham, A. (2002). Fluoride varnishes for preventing dental caries in children and adolescents, *Cochrane Database Syst Rev (Online)* (3): CD002279

Marthaler, T. M. (1968). Caries-inhibition after seven years of unsupervised use of an amine fluoride dentifrice, *Br Dent J* 124(11): 510-515.

Marthaler, T. M. (1974). Caries-inhibition by an amine fluoride dentifrice results after 6 years in children with low caries activity, *Helv Odontol Acta* 18(Suppl 8): 35-44.

Marthaler, T. M. (1988). Clinical cariostatic effects of various fluoride methods and programs, In: *Fluoride in Dentistry,* Ekstrand, J., Fejerskov, O. & Silverstone, L. M. (Eds.), 252-275, Munksgaard, ISBN 9788716099624, Copenhagen, Denmark

Marthaler, T. M., Konig, K. G. & Muhlemann, H. R. (1970). The effect of a fluoride gel used for supervised toothbrushing 15 or 30 times per year, *Helv Odontol Acta* 14(2): 67-77.

Marton, S., Nagy, G., Gabris, K., Banoczy, J. & Madlena, M. (2008). Logistic regression analysis of oral health data in assessing the therapeutic value of amine fluoride containing products, *OHDMBSC* 7(4): 26-29.

Matthijs, S. & Adriaens, P. A. (2002). Chlorhexidine varnishes: a review, *J Clin Periodontol* 29(1): 1-8.

Mellberg, J. R., Laakso, P. V. & Nicholson, C. R. (1966). The acquisition and loss of fluoride by topically fluoridated human tooth enamel, *Arch Oral Biol* 11(12): 1213-1220.

Mengel, R., Wissing, E., Schmitz Habben, A. & Flores de Jacoby, L. (1996). Comparative study of plaque and gingivitis prevention by AmF/SnF2 and NaF - A clinical and microbiological 9-month study, *J Clin Periodontol* 23(4): 372-378.

Meurman, J. H. (1988). Ultrastructure, growth, and adherence of streptococcus mutans after treatment with chlorhexidine and fluoride, *Caries Res* 22(5): 283-287.

Miethke, R. R. & Newesely, H. (1988). Continuous fluoride release from removable appliances, *J Clin Orthod* 22(8): 490-491.

Miller, J. & Hobson, P. (1961). The relationship between malocclusion, oral cleanliness, gingival conditions and dental caries in school children, *Br Dent J* 111(2): 43-52.

Millett, D. T., Nunn, J. H., Welbury, R. R. & Gordon, P. H. (1999). Decalcification in relation to brackets bonded with glass ionomer cement or a resin adhesive, *Angle Orthod* 69(1): 65-70.

Mirth, D. B. (1980). The use of controlled and sustained release agents in dentistry: A review of applications for the control of dental caries, *Pharmacol Ther Dent* 5(3-4), 59-67.

Mitchell, L. (1992). Decalcification during orthodontic treatment with fixed appliances--an overview, *Br J Orthod* 19(3): 199-205.

Mizrahi, E. (1982). Enamel demineralization following orthodontic treatment, *Am J Orthod Dentofac Orthop* 82(1): 62-67.

Mtaya, M., Brudvik, P. & Astrom, A. N. (2009). Prevalence of malocclusion and its relationship with socio-demographic factors, dental caries, and oral hygiene in 12- to 14-year-old Tanzanian schoolchildren, *Eur J Orthod* 31(5): 467-476.

Muhler, J. C. (1970). Dental caries--orthodontic appliances--SnF_2, *J Dent Child* 37(3): 218-221.

Mühlemann, H. R., Schmid, H. S. & Konig, K. G. (1957) Enamel solubility reduction studies with inorganic and organic fluorides, *Helv Odont Acta* 1: 23–33.

Nagy, G., Banoczy, J., Gotz, G., Szadeczky, B., Marton, S. & Madlena, M. (2010). Effects of amine fluoride/stannous fluoride products on oral microflora in orthodontic patients, *Caries Res* 44(3): 200-200. n.73

Newbrun, E. (1992). Current regulations and recommendations concerning water fluoridation, fluoride supplements, and topical fluoride agents, *J Dent Res* 71(5), 1255-1265.

Newbrun, E., Matsukubo, T., Hoover, C. I., Graves, R. C., Brown, A. T., Disney, J. A. & Bohannan, H. M. (1984). Comparison of 2 screening-tests for streptococcus mutans and evaluation of their suitability for mass screenings and private-practice, *Community Dent Oral Epidemiol* 12(5): 325-331.

Nicholson, J. W. (2006). Biologic Considerations, In: *Fundamentals of Operative Denistry. A contemporary approach*, Summitt, J. B., Robbins, J. W., Hilton, T. J. & Schwartz, R. S. (Eds.), 2-4, Quintessence Publishing, ISBN: 978-0-86715-452-8, Chicago, USA

Nicolau, B., Marcenes, W., Bartley, M. & Sheiham, A. (2003). A life course approach to assessing causes of dental caries experience: The relationship between biological, behavioural, socio-econornic and psychological conditions and caries in adolescents, *Caries Res* 37(5): 319-326.

Nobile, C. G. A., Pavia, M., Fortunato, L. & Angelillo, I. F. (2007). Prevalence and factors related to malocclusion and orthodontic treatment need in children and adolescents in Italy, *Eur J Public Health* 17(6): 637-641.

Nyvad, B., Machiulskiene, V. & Baelum, V. (1999). Reliability of a new caries diagnostic system differentiating between active and inactive caries lesions, *Caries Res* 33(4): 252-260.

Obersztyn, A. & Kolwinski, K. (1984). Amine fluoride gel in a caries prophylaxis program for soldiers in Poland, *Community Dent Oral Epidemiol* 12(5): 288-291.

Ogaard, B. (1989). Prevalence of white spot lesions in 19-year-olds - a study on untreated and orthodontically treated persons 5 years after treatment, *Am J Orthod Dentofac Orthop* 96(5): 423-427.

Ogaard, B. (1989). Incidence of filled surfaces from 10-18 years of age in an orthodontically treated and untreated group in Norway, *Eur J Orthod* 11(2): 116-119.

Ogaard, B. (2008). White spot lesions during orthodontic treatment: Mechanisms and fluoride preventive aspects, *Semin Orthod* 14(3): 183-193.

Ogaard, B., Gjermo, P. & Rolla, G. (1980). Plaque-inhibiting effect in orthodontic patients of a dentifrice containing stannous fluoride, *Am J Orthod Dentofac Orthop* 78(3):266-272.

Ogaard, B., Rolla, G., & Helgeland, K. (1984). Fluoride retention in sound and demineralized enamel in vivo after treatment with a fluoride varnish (Duraphat), *Scand J Dent Res* 92(3): 190-197.

Ogaard, B., Rolla, G. & Arends, J. (1988). Orthodontic appliances and enamel demineralization. Part 1. Lesion development, *Am J Orthod Dentofac Ortop* 94(1): 68-73.

Ogaard, B., Duschner, H., Ruben, J. & Arends, J. (1996). Microradiography and confocal laser scanning microscopy applied to enamel lesions formed in vivo with and without fluoride varnish treatment, *Eur J Oral Sci* 104(4): 378-383.

Ogaard, B., Bishara, S. E. & Duschner, H. (2004). Enamel effects during bonding –debonding and treatment with fixed appliances, In: *Risk management in orthodontics: experts' guide to malpractice*, Graber, T. M., Eliades, T. & Atanasiou, A. (Eds.), 19-46, Quintessense Publishing Co, ISBN 0-86715-431-4, Chicago, USA

Öhrn K. & Sanz M. (2009). Prevention and therapeutic approach to gingival inflammation, *J Clin Periodontol* 36(Suppl. 1): 20-26.

O'Reilly, M. M. & Featherstone, J. D. B. (1987). Demineralization and remineralization around orthodontic appliances - an in vivo study, *Am J Orthod Dentofac Orthop* 92(1): 33-40.

Ostberg, A., Halling, A. & Lindblad, U. (1999). Gender differences in knowledge, attitude, behavior and perceived oral health among adolescents, *Acta Odontol Scand* 57(4): 231-236.

Ostela, I. & Tenovuo, J. (1990). Antibacterial activity of dental gels containing combinations of amine fluoride, stannous fluoride, and chlorhexidine against cariogenic bacteria, *Scand J Dent Res* 98(1): 1-7.

Oulis C. J. Raadal I. & Markus L, (2009). Guidelines on the use of fluoride in children: an EAPD policy document. European Academy of Paediatric Dentistry (2009). Guidelines on the use of fluoride in children: an EAPD policy document, *Eur Arch Paediatr Dent* 10(3): 129-35.

Patz, J. & Naujoks, R. (1970). Die kariesprophylaktische Wirkung einer aminfluoridhaltigen Zahnpaste bei Jugendlichen nach dreijahrigem unuberwachten Gebrauch, *Dtsch Zahnarztl Z* 25(6): 617-625.

Paraskevas S. & van der Weijden G. A. (2006). A review of the effects of stannous fluoride on gingivitis, *J Clin Periodontol* 33(1): 1-13.

Pessan, J. P., Al-Ibrahim, N. S., Buzalaf, M. A. R. & Toumba, K. J. (2008). Slow-release fluoride devices: A literature review, *J. Appl Oral Sci* 16(4): 238-246.

Petersson, L. G. (1975). *On topical application of fluorides and its inhibiting effect on caries* [Thesis]. University of Lund, Malmö

Petersson, L. G., Edwardsson, S. & Arends, J. (1992). Antimicrobial effect of a dental varnish, in vitro, *Swed Dent J* 16(5): 183-189.

Petersson, L. G. (1993). Fluoride mouthrinses and fluoride varnishes, Caries Res 27(1): 35-42.

Petersson, L. G., Maki, Y., Twetman, S. & Edwardsson, S. (1991). Mutans streptococci in saliva and interdental spaces after topical applications of an antibacterial varnish in schoolchildren, *Oral Microbiol Immunol* 6(5): 284-287.

Pistorius, A., Rockmann, P., Martin, M. & Willershausen B. (2002). Effectiveness of hyaluronic acid (Gengigel (R)) in the therapy of gingivitis, *J Dent Res* 81(Spec. Issue):A453 an: 3694.

Rabe, H., Miethke, RR. & Newesely, H. (1986). Gefüge und Festigkeit von Silberloten für die Kieferorthopädie nach Behandlung mit handelsüblichen "Zahnspangenreinigern", *Dtsch Zahnarztl Z* 41(7):714-719.

Retief, D. H., Harris, B. E. & Bradley, E. L. (1985). In vitro enamel fluoride uptake from topical fluoride agents, *Dent Materials* 1(3): 93-97.

Reynolds, E. C. (1987). The prevention of sub-surface demineralization of bovine enamel and change in plaque composition by casein in an intra-oral model, *J Dent Res* 66(6): 1120-1127.

Ringelberg, M. L., Webster, D. B., Dixon, D. O. & Lezotte, D. C. (1979). Caries-preventive effect of amine fluorides and inorganic fluorides in a mouthrinse or dentifrice after 30 months of use, *J Am Dent Assoc* 98(2): 202-208.

Rogers, S., Chadwick, B. & Treasure, E. (2010). Fluoride-containing orthodontic adhesives and decalcification in patients with fixed appliances: A systematic review, *Am J Orthod Dentofac Orthop* 138(4): 390.e1-8.

Rodd, H. D. & Davidson, L. E. (1997). The aesthetic management of severe dental fluorosis in the young patient, *Dent Update* 24(10): 408-411.

Rolla, G. & Saxegaard, E. (1990). Critical evaluation of the composition and use of topical fluorides, with emphasis on the role of calcium fluoride in caries inhibition, *J Dent Res* 69(SPEC. ISS. FEB.): 780-785.

Rolla, G., Ogaard, B. & Cruz, R. A. (1991). Clinical effect and mechanism of cariostatic action of fluoride-containing toothpastes: A review, *Int Dent J* 41(3): 171-174.

Sakki, T. K., Knuuttila, M. L. E. & Anttila, SS. (1998). Lifestyle, gender and occupational status as determinants of dental health behavior, *J Clin Periodontol* 25(7): 566-570.

Sangamesh, B. & Amitabh, K. (2011) Iatrogenic effects of orthodontic treatment - Review on white spot lesions, *IJSER* 2(5): 1-16.

Schlagenhauf, U., Tobien, P. & Engelfried, P. (1989). Der Einfluss kieferorthopädischer Behandlung auf Parameter des individuellen Kariesrisikos, *Dtsch Zahnarztl Z* 44(10): 758-760.

Schmid, H. F. (1964). Ein neues tauchieringsmittel mit besondres lang anhalten dem intensivem Fluoriderungseffekt, *Stoma* 17: 71–75.

Schmid H. (1983). Chemie und Oberflächenwirkungen der Aminfluoride, *Dtsch Zahnärztl Z*; 38 (Suppl. 1): S9-13.

Segura, A., Donly, K. J. & Wefel, J. S. (1997a). The effects of microabrasion on demineralization inhibition of enamel surfaces, *Quintessence Int* 28(7): 463-466.

Segura, A., Donly, K. J., Wefel, J. S. & Drake, D. (1997b). Effect of enamel microabrasion on bacterial colonization, *Am J Dent* 10(6): 272-274.

Shannon, I. L. & West, D. C. (1979). Prevention of decalcification in orthodontic patients by daily self-treatment with 0.4% SnF2 gel, *Pediatr Dent* 1(2): 101-102.

Shen, C. & Autio-Gold, J. (2002). Assessing fluoride concentration uniformity and fluoride release from three varnishes, *J Am Dent Assoc* 133(2): 176-182.

Shern, R. J., Duany, L. F., Senning, R. S. & Zinner, D. D. (1976). Clinical-study of an amine fluoride gel and acidulated phosphate fluoride gel, *Community Dent Oral Epidemiol* 4(4): 133-136.

Silva, R. G. & Kang, D. S. (2001). Prevalence of malocclusion among Latino adolescents, *Am J Orthod Dentofac Orthop* 119(3): 313-315.

Silness, J. & Loe, H. (1964). Periodontal disease in pregnancy. II. correlation between oral hygiene and periodontal condition, *Acta Odontol Scand* 22(1): 121-135.

Skjorland, K. K. (1973). Plaque accumulation on different dental filling materials, *Scand J Dent Res* 81(7): 538-542.

Socransky, S. S. (1968). Caries-susceptibility tests, *Ann NY Acad Sci* 153(1): 137-146.

Southard, T. E., Cohen, M. E., Ralls, S. A. & Rouse, L. A. (1986). Effects of fixed-appliance orthodontic treatment on DMF indices, *Am J Orthod Dentofac Orthop* 90 (2): 122-126.

Slavkin, H. C. (1997). First encounters: transmission of infectious oral diseases from mother to child, *J Am Dent Assoc* 128(6): 773-778.

Stahl, F. & Grabowski, R. (2004). Malocclusion and caries prevalence: is there a connection in the primary and mixed dentitions?, *Clin Oral Invest* 8(2): 86-90.

Staley, R. N. (2008). Effect of fluoride varnish on demineralization around orthodontic brackets, *Semin Orthod* 14(3): 194-199.

Stecksen-Blicks, C. (1985). Salivary counts of lactobacilli and streptococcus mutans in caries prediction, *Scand J Dent Res* 93(3): 204-212.

Sudjalim, T. R., Woods, M. G. & Manton, D. J. (2006). Prevention of white spot lesions in orthodontic practice: A contemporary review, *Aust Den J* 51(4): 284-289.

Szoke, J. & Kozma, M. (1989). Ergebnisse einer dreijährigen Untersuchung über Zähneputzen mit einem Aminfluorid-Gelee, *Oralprophylaxe* 11(4): 137-143.

Ten Cate, J. M. & Arends, J. (1980). Remineralization of artificial enamel lesions in vitro: III. A study of the deposition mechanism, *Caries Res* 14(6): 351-358.

Thilander, B., Pena, L., Infante, C., Parada, S. S. & De Mayorga, C. (2001). Prevalence of malocclusion and orthodontic treatment need in children and adolescents in Bogota, Colombia. An epidemiological study related to different stages of dental development, *Eur J Orthod* 23(2): 153-167.

Todd, M. A., Staley, R. N., Kanellis, M. J., Donly, K. J. & Wefel, J. S. (1999). Effect of a fluoride varnish on demineralization adjacent to orthodontic brackets, *Am J Ortod Dentofacial Ortop* 116(2): 159-167.

Toumba, K. J. (1996). *In vivo and in vitro evaluation of a slow release fluoride glass for prevention of dental caries in high risk children* [Thesis], University of Leeds, Leeds.

Tranæus, S., Al-Khateeb, S., Björkman, S., Twetman, S. & Angmar-Månsson, B. (2001). Application of quantitative light-induced fluorescence to monitor incipient lesions in caries-active children. A comparative study of remineralisation by fluoride varnish and professional cleaning, *Eur J Oral Sci* 109(2): 71-75.

Twetman, S. & Petersson, L. G. (1997). Effect of different chlorhexidine varnish regimens on mutans streptococci levels in interdental plaque and saliva, *Caries Res* 31(3): 189-193.

Twetman, S., Skold-Larsson, K. & Modeer, T. (1999). Fluoride concentration in whole saliva and separate gland secretions after topical treatment with three different fluoride varnishes, *Acta Odontol Scand* 57(5): 263-266.

Uysal, T., Amasyali, M., Ozcan, S., Koyuturk, A. E. & Sagdic, D. (2011). Effect of antibacterial monomer-containing adhesive on enamel demineralization around orthodontic brackets: an in-vivo study, *Am J Orthod Dentofac Orthop* 139(5): 650-656.

Vanarsdall, R. J.(2000). Periodontal/orthodontic interrelationships, In: *Orthodontics: Current principles and techniques* Graber, T. M. & Vanarsdall, R. .J. (Eds.), 801-838. Mosby Inc, (Third edition), ISBN 0-8151-9363-7, St Louis, USA

Van Leeuwen, M. P. C., Slot, D. E. & Van Der Weijden, G. A. (2011). Essential oils compared to chlorhexidine with respect to plaque and parameters of gingival inflammation: A systematic review, *J Periodontol* 82(2): 174-194.

Volpe, A. R., Petrone, M. E., De Vizio, W., Davies, R. M. & Proskin, H. M. (1996). A review of plaque, gingivitis, calculus and caries clinical efficacy studies with a fluoride dentifrice containing triclosan and PVM/MA copolymer, *J Clin Dent* 7(Suppl): S1-S14.

Vorhies, A. B., Donly, K. J., Staley, R. N. & Wefel, J. S. (1998). Enamel demineralization adjacent to orthodontic brackets bonded with hybrid glass ionomer cements: An in vitro study, *Am J Orthod Dentofac Orthop* 114(6): 668-674.

Warren, D. P., Henson, H. A. & Chan, J. T. (2000). Dental hygienist and patient comparisons of fluoride varnishes to fluoride gels, *J Dent Hyg* 74(2): 94-101.

Welbury, R. R. & Shaw, L. (1990). A simple technique for removal of mottling, opacities and pigmentation from enamel, *Dent Update* 17(4): 161-163.

Welbury, R. R. & Carter, N. E. (1993). The hydrochloric acid-pumice microabrasion technique in the treatment of post-orthodontic decalcification, *Br J Orthod* 20(3): 181-185.

WHO (1994). *Fluorides and oral health. Report of a WHO Expert Committee on Oral Health Status and Fluoride Use*, WHO, Genf: 1-37. ISBN: 92-4-120846-5

Willmot, D. (2008). White spot lesions after orthodontic treatment, *Semin Orthod* 14(3): 209-219.

Zachrisson, B. U. (1975). Fluoride application procedures in orthodontic practice, current concepts, *Angle Orthod* 45(1): 72-81.

Zachrisson, B. U. & Zachrisson, S. (1971). Caries incidence and oral hygiene during orthodontic treatment, *Scand J Dent Res* 79(6): 394-401.

Zachrisson, B. U. & Zachrisson, S. (1971). Caries incidence and orthodontic treatment with fixed appliances, *Scand J Dent Res* 79(3): 183-192.

Zahradnik, R. T. (1980). Effect of fluoride rinses upon in vitro enamel remineralization, *J Dent Res* 59(6): 1065-1066.

Zickert, I., Emilson, C. G. & Krasse, B. (1982). Effect of caries preventive measures in children highly infected with the bacterium streptococcus-mutans, *Arch Oral Biol* 27(10): 861-868.

Zimmermann, A., Flores de Jacoby, L. & Pan, P. (1993). Gingivitis, plaque accumulation and plaque composition under long-term use of meridol®, *J Clin Periodontol* 20(5): 346-351.

5

Other Applications of Photo Catalyst in Dental Treatments in Diverse Fields

Seung-Ho Ohk[1] and Hyeon-Shik Hwang[2]
[1]*Department of Oral Microbiology,*
[2]*Department of Orthodontics and Dental Science Research Institute, Chonnam National University*
Korea

1. Introduction

Photocatalysts do not make the light faster. The term 'photocatalyst' represents chemical substances that act as a catalyst when exposed to light. For several decades numerous studies have been published about photocatalyst in water treatment process and air pollution control. Among several photocatalysts, TiO_2 has been considered as the most useful and harmless substance. With the illumination of UV-A light, TiO_2 photocatalysts decompose organic compounds through oxidation, with hydroxyl radicals (HO·) being produced by the oxidation of water. Various methods have been introduced for the surface modification of orthodontic treatment devices. Among them, Sol-gel dip-coating, CVD and PE-CVD methods were applied to coat photocatalytic TiO_2 on the surface of orthodontic wires and brackets. The antibacterial activities of the surface-modified orthodontic wires and brackets were demonstrated on *Streptococcus mutans* and *Porphyromonas gingivalis.* Viable cell counts with dilution-agar plate method and spectrophotometry were carried out to evaluate the antibacterial effect of photocatalytic TiO_2. Besides the photocatalytic degradation of organic compounds, there are several unique characteristics of photocatalytic TiO_2 were reported. In virtue of those characteristics it can be used in various ways such as preventing air contamination, anti-fog glasses and anti-bacterial paints. Sometimes many useful points are considered as handicaps in other point of view and vice versa. For example, to show photocatalytic activity for the TiO_2, usually it needs illumination with wavelength of less than 380. However, this drawback could be, in turn, used as a useful tool to control the release of hydroxyl radical from water since there is not much of UV-A in normal sun light.

The definition of photocatalysts and basic mechanism of photocatalytic activity will be described in this chapter.

Application and evaluation methods of photocatalyst, antibacterial efficiency on oral pathogens and safety of photocatalyst will be mentioned also. With the advantage of photocatalytic TiO_2, safety, versatile applications and other important remarkable characteristics of photocatalytic TiO_2 will be described in this section.

2. What is photocatalyst?

2.1 Photochemical reaction

Does the 'photocatalyst' catalyze photo-reaction or catalyze reactions with the exposure of light? Literally, both of the meanings are correct. However, the later will be explained in this chapter.The term 'photocatalyst' represents chemical substance that act as a catalyst when exposed to light. 'Photocatalytic reaction' again can be classified as one of photo-reactions. The most popular example of photo-reaction is a photographic film. Although digital imaging technique is popular these days, one of the most excellent inventions was the development of photography. In a traditional way of taking photo, a target image was exposed to a roll of film installed in the dark space of camera. This photographic film is a sheet of plastic paper such as polyester, nitrocellulose or cellulose acetate coated with a light-sensitive silver bromide emulsion. When the emulsion is exposed to sufficient light, bromide ion (Br^-) produces brom-atom and electron (e^-). This electron, in turns, binds to silver ion (Ag^+) to make metallic silver, which blocks light and appears as the black part of film negative.

$$Br^- + [\text{light}] \rightarrow Br + e^-$$

$$Ag^+ + e^- \rightarrow Ag$$

In 1972, Honda and Fujishima have reported electrochemical decomposition of water (Fujishima & Honda, 1972). They have found that when platinum and titanium dioxide (TiO_2) were connected as cathode and anode, respectively, water is decomposed with a illumination of xenon lamp to make hydrogen and oxygen molecules (Fig.1).

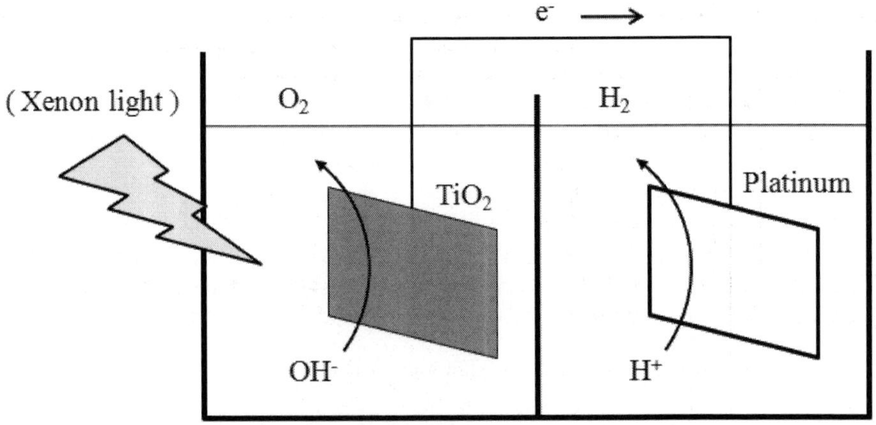

Fig. 1. Decomposition of water with photocatalytic TiO_2.

$$2H_2O + [\text{Light}, < 400\text{ nm}] + TiO_2 \rightarrow 2H + O_2$$

This is a coupled reaction of reduction ($4H^+ \rightarrow 2H_2$) and oxidation ($4OH^- \rightarrow O_2 + 2H_2O$) with four molecules of water ($4H_2O$, $4H^+ + 4OH^-$) producing hydrogen and oxygen molecules.

Titanium dioxide can absorb light energy of below 400 nm and emits electrons to catalyze the decomposition of water.

2.2 Photocatalytic TiO_2

Several substances have been known to have photocatalytic activities such as ZnO, Nb_2O_5, WO_3, SnO_2, ZrO_2, CdS, ZnS, CdSe, and GaP. One of the most important reason that titanium dioxide is widely used is that it is chemically stable in most of acid, base and organic solvents. In the contrary, ZnO has similar energy band and high photocatalytic activity. However, when it is illuminated with light in aqueous solution, it can be easily dissolved in water as a Zn^+ ion. It also can be easily melt with sulfuric acid or nitric acid. Therefore, ZnO cannot be used separately.

3. Surface modification of orthodontic treatment devices

3.1 Anodic oxidation

When metal or silicon plates are immersed in an appropriate electrolyte a fine and rigid thin oxidized film will form on the surfaces plates. Anodic oxidation of aluminum is commonly introduced for their (semi-) transparent, anti-corrosion characteristics. The film composed by anodic oxidation usually shows stable conductivity. Neutral or acidic electrolytes are commonly used for aluminum, but there are not many options for other metals. Several dental implants have used anodic oxidation method for the surface modification to enhance their bone integration efficiency (Schupbach *et al.*, 2005).

3.2 Sol-gel dip-coating method

Dip-coating method is the oldest and most commonly used technique in deposition of thin film. Jenaer Glaswerk Schott & Gen are the first who have filed a patent with dip-coating technique for silica film in 1939. Sol-gel coatings, on the other hand, are being studied and applied in a diverse way such as protective coatings, passivation layers, ferroelectrics, sensors and membranes. The sol-gel dip-coating method uses inorganic precursors in aqueous or organic solvents. Those precursors are hydrolyzed and condensed to form polymers. Solid substrates are usually taken out of coating bath vertically at a constant speed. While taken out of the bath, the substrate entrains the liquid. Along with the evaporation of the solvent, wedge shaped film is formed on the surface of substrate. A lot of researchers have used sol-gel dip-coating method to study the application of the photocatalytic TiO_2 (Dongare *et al.*, 2003; Lee *et al.*, 2004; Zainal *et al.*, 2005).

3.3 CVD (Chemical vapor deposition) and PE-CVD (Plasma enhanced-CVD) method

Chemical vapor deposition method is the most widely used technique in semiconductor industries. It can form thin films from different precursors onto a substrate. In a CVD technique, a substrate is exposed to multiple volatile precursors with an inert gaseous carrier at high temperature and pressure. Those volatile precursors react or decompose on the surface of desired substrates, which form a thin film. Since CVD is one of the most well studied, and set up techniques, it is good for mass production.

Plasma enhanced CVD (PE-CVD) is a more progressed and important technique in VLSI (Very-large-scale integration) and TFT (Thin film transistor) manufacturing. The most important advantage of PE-CVD is low process temperature, which enables lower the manufacturer's budget. It uses plasma energy instead of heat energy for the reaction between precursors and substrates. Due to the wide range of applications of photocatalytic TiO_2, much of studies have been reported with CVD and PE-CVD technique for the application (Giavaresi *et al.*, 2003; Gluszek *et al.*, 1997; Gonzalez-Elipe *et al.*, 2004; Mills *et al.*, 2002).

4. Antibiotic effect of photocatalytic TiO_2

After Fujishima and Honda (Fujishima & Honda, 1972) reported the photolytic effect of TiO_2 in 1972, a series of efforts have been carried out to apply in various ways. Among them Matsunaga *et al.* have first reported photocatalytic TiO_2 has antibacterial effect on *Lactobacillus acidophilus, Saccharomyces cerevisiae* and *Escherichia coli* (Matsunaga *et al.*, 1985). Since hydroxyl radical (HO•) became of interest in decomposing organic compounds, it is no wonder to try antibacterial effect on various microorganisms. It was well documented that chemical oxidation with hydroxyl radical has a high activity in degradation of organic compounds (Ireland & Valinieks, 1992). Accordingly, antibacterial effect of photocatalytic TiO_2 that could efficiently produce hydroxyl radical in aqueous solution with illumination of light was demonstrated. Major microorganisms that have tested with photocatalytic TiO_2 were listed in Table 1.

According to the early report presented by Ireland *et al.* *Escherichia coli* showed rapid cell death in a mixture with the anatase crystalline form of titanium dioxide (Ireland *et al.*, 1993). Cho *et al.* also explained correlation between HO• radicals and the rate of *E. coli* inactivation which indicates that the HO• radical is the primary oxidant species responsible for inactivating *E. coli* in the UV/TiO_2 process (Cho *et al.*, 2004). Effort to clarify the antibacterial effect of titanium plate by surface modifications has been also reported. Yoshinari *et al.* tried to modify the surface of titanium plate by ion implantation (Ca^+, N^+, and F^+), oxidation (anode oxidation, titania spraying), ion plating (TiN, alumina), and ion beam mixing (Ag, Sn, Zn, Pt) with Ar^+ (Yoshinari *et al.*, 2001). Among them they have reported that F^+-implanted specimens significantly inhibited the growth of both *Porphyromonas gingivalis* and *Actinobacillus actinomycetemcomitans*. However, this antibacterial effect might be caused by the formation of a metal fluoride complex on the surfaces.

Since orthodontic wires and brackets provide a sufficient habitat for oral infectious microorganisms, orthodontic patients might have a higher risk of contracting other dental diseases (Balenseifen & Madonia, 1970; Sakamaki & Bahn, 1968; Scheie *et al.*, 1984). Therefore, as well as the orthodontic patients, clinicians should pay attention to reduce the chances for oral microorganisms to adhere to the surfaces of teeth and orthodontic wires. Chun *et al.* have tried to apply photocatalytic TiO_2 to orthodontic wires (Chun *et al.*, 2007). They used sol-gel dip coating method to modify the surfaces of wires. Special device for efficient illumination of UV-light to TiO_2-coated orthodontic wires using quartz cylinder was designed and used for the adhesion assay (Fig. 2). Since *Streptococcus mutans* that causes dental caries can easily adhere to tooth surface or orthodontic devices attached to tooth surfaces anti-adhesion effect of photocatalytic TiO_2 was monitored. Modified surface of wires showed effectively reduced adhesion of bacterial cells. Surface modification with photocatalytic TiO_2 enabled orthodontic wires to have effective anti-adherent characteristics. Using Scanning electron microscope damaged bacterial cell surfaces could be observed when treated with TiO_2. Similar effect was observed in *Porphyromonas gingivalis,* which is known as one of the major pathogen of periodontitis.

	Species	References
Bacteria	*Escherichia coli*	(Cho *et al.*, 2004; Ireland *et al.*, 1993; Kuhn *et al.*, 2003; Matsunaga *et al.*, 1985; Salih, 2002)
	Lactobacillus acidophilus	(Matsunaga *et al.*, 1985)
	Saccharomyces cerevisiae	(Matsunaga *et al.*, 1985)
	Streptococcus mutans	(Chun *et al.*, 2007; Elsaka *et al.*, 2011)
	Porphyromonas gingivalis	(Chun *et al.*, 2007; Yoshinari *et al.*, 2001)
	Bacillus atrophaeus	(Muranyi *et al.*, 2010)
	Kocuria rhizophila	(Muranyi *et al.*, 2010)
	Pseudomonas aeruginosa	(Kuhn *et al.*, 2003)
	Staphylococcus aureus	(Kuhn *et al.*, 2003)
	Enterococcus faecium	(Kuhn *et al.*, 2003)
Fungi	*Aspergillus niger*	(Muranyi *et al.*, 2010)
Yeast	*Candida albicans*	(Kuhn *et al.*, 2003)
Viruses	Rota virus	(Sang *et al.*, 2007)
	Astrovirus	(Sang *et al.*, 2007)
	Feline calcivirus (FCV)	(Sang *et al.*, 2007)
	Bacteriophage	(Gerrity *et al.*, 2008; Liga *et al.*, 2011)
Prion	PrP^{SC}	(Paspaltsis *et al.*, 2006)

Table 1. Major microorganisms that have positive results with photocatalytic TiO_2.

Other than antibacterial effect, the efficacies of TiO_2 on viruses and prion have also demonstrated. Sang *et al.* have tested rotavirus, astrovirus, and feline calcivirus (FCV) to verify the inactivation effect of TiO_2 with irradiation of visible light (Sang *et al.*, 2007). According to the report, light activated TiO_2 could partially degrade dsRNA of the rotavirus particles. They have found that activated TiO_2 with illumination of light in aqueous solution produces a significant amount of reactive oxygen species such as superoxide anions (O_2^-) and hydroxyl radicals (•OH) after activation for 8, 16, and 24 hrs. Destruction of nucleic acid was also confirmed by Ashikaga *et al.* (Ashikaga *et al.*, 2000). Those reactive oxygen species affect not only nucleotides but also other organic compounds such as peptides or proteins. With this special features, Paspaltsis *et al.* have examined the photocatalytic TiO_2 to prion protein, which is known to cause transmissible spongiform encephalopathy (TSB) (Paspaltsis *et al.*, 2006). Inoculation of prion protein (PrP^{SC}) with a TiO_2/H_2O_2 treatment to Syrian hamsters showed higher survival rate than control group and retarded presentation of clinical symptom for 50 days later. Since prion is strongly resistant to commonly used conventional decontamination methods, they have presented photocatalytic TiO_2 as a potential disinfecting agent for liquid waste and TSE infectious agent.

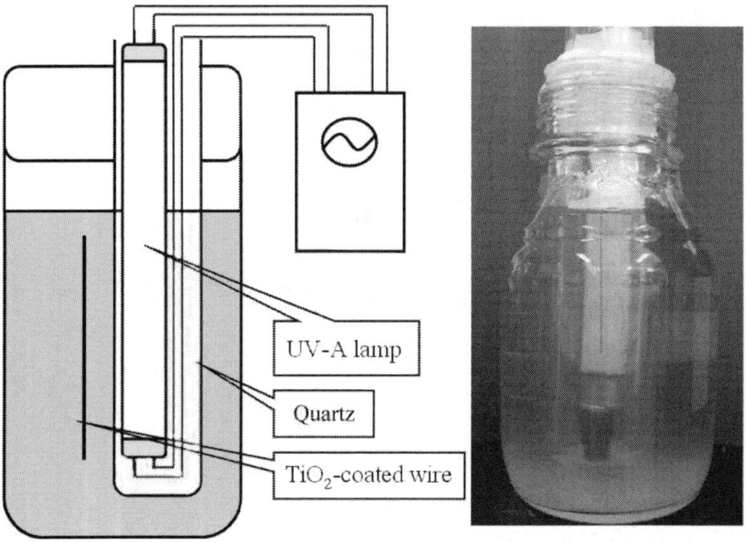

Fig. 2. Apparatus for the assay of anti-adhesion effect of TiO_2-coated orthodontic wire.

5. Other applications of photo catalyst in dental treatments

We are unconsciously in contact with diverse form of titanium dioxide these days. It is now commonly used in making papers, fabrics, toothpastes and wall paints. Photocatalytic TiO_2 has a broad spectrum of applications in virtue of its almighty capability of degrading almost every organic compounds. It has been realized that TiO_2 can absorb energy from light (usually UV light) and react with water molecules to produce reactive oxygen species.

One of the main focuses of applying photocatalytic TiO_2 was decontamination of polluted environments such as air cleaning system, decomposition of waste water. At the beginning of studies on the photocatalytic TiO_2, it was mainly applied to degrade highly toxic dyes from textile industries (Muneer *et al.*, 1997; Saquib & Muneer, 2003). However, its scope has been gradually expanded to various areas such as herbicides (Singh *et al.*, 2003) or pesticides (Daneshvar *et al.*, 2004) and other industrial waste water (Makino *et al.*, 2007).

Several companies producing ceramic tiles are using TiO_2 on the very surface of their products which is so-called self-cleaning tiles. Due to the ability to decompose organic molecules, these self-cleaning tiles can disinfect contamination of their surfaces by themselves only if there's a little portion of moisture and enough sun light. It might be very useful in hospitals, public restrooms, and household bathrooms. This unique advantage can be expanded to trivial devices used in most of clinics such as forceps, spatulas, scissors, and any rigid ceramic or metal surfaces to reduce the opportunity of cross infection.

Another useful aspect of TiO_2 is the hydrophilic property. Coating with photocatalytic TiO_2 layer on rigid ceramic or metal surfaces provides super-hydrophilic property that might dramatically reduce contact angle. Ohdaira *et al.* in Department of General Surgery, Jichi Medical Universitym Japan have designed special laparoscope that has antifogging effect (Ohdaira *et al.*, 2007). This property also can be applied to dental mirrors, bathroom mirrors, and car windows to impose antifogging characteristics.

6. Limitations and drawbacks of photocatalytic TiO_2

Even though photocatalytic TiO_2 has various utilities and potentials, still it has some limitations and drawbacks. It still needs improvements in reaction rate, broad spectrum of light source, specificity (or wide range of target) and stability. Several limitations and expected solutions are listed in Table 2. However, many of these are not solved yet.

Limitations	Solutions
Low reaction rate	Increasing surface area
Incomplete reaction	Fluid type reactor
Low efficiency	Increasing surface area
	Gas type reactor
Low specificity	Reactor design for specifically adsorption of target substances
Light source	Mixing with other inorganic compounds

Table 2. Several limitations of photocatalytic TiO_2.

6.1 Surface area

Since photocatalytic reaction occurs at the solid surface of TiO_2, it is very easy to separate substrates or products from photocatalyst. However substrates should be in contact with photocatalyst, which causes relatively low reaction rate and less homogeneity compared to other reactions such as gas-gas, or liquid-gas reactions. The first way to manage this problem is to increase surface area of the catalysts and the way to increase surface area is to reduce the particle sizes. Some solid catalysts are used in a unique three dimensional structure such as 'honey comb structure' to increase surface area. However it is not suitable for the photocatalytic TiO_2 because it needs illumination of UV or day light to activate. Therefore making round shaped particles and reduction in size may be the only way to increase surface area. Average diameter of commonly used TiO_2 ranges from 20 nm to 0.5 µm. Ultrafine particles of even below 10 nm of diameter are now developed and used in some fields. The average surface area of some ultrafine particle is reduced down to 7 nm which has about 300 m^2/g of surface area. Photocatalytic activity of this particle is 2 - 4 times higher than the particle that has 50 m^2/g of surface area. The activity did not increase as much as the surface area because ultrafine particles usually can aggregate each other. But there is no reason not to use ultrafine particles if it shows higher activity even though increasing fold of activity is not high as that of surface area.

6.2 Crystalline forms

Titanium dioxide forms three kinds of crystals: those are rutile, anatase, and brookite (Fig. 3). It is usually said that anatase crystal has higher photocatalytic activity than others. Depending on the crystalline type, binding structure of T-O and characteristics of crystal surface varies of course. However, the reason is unclear until now. Anatase crystal of TiO_2 can be formed between 400 – 500 °C and transformed to rutile at more than 900 °C.

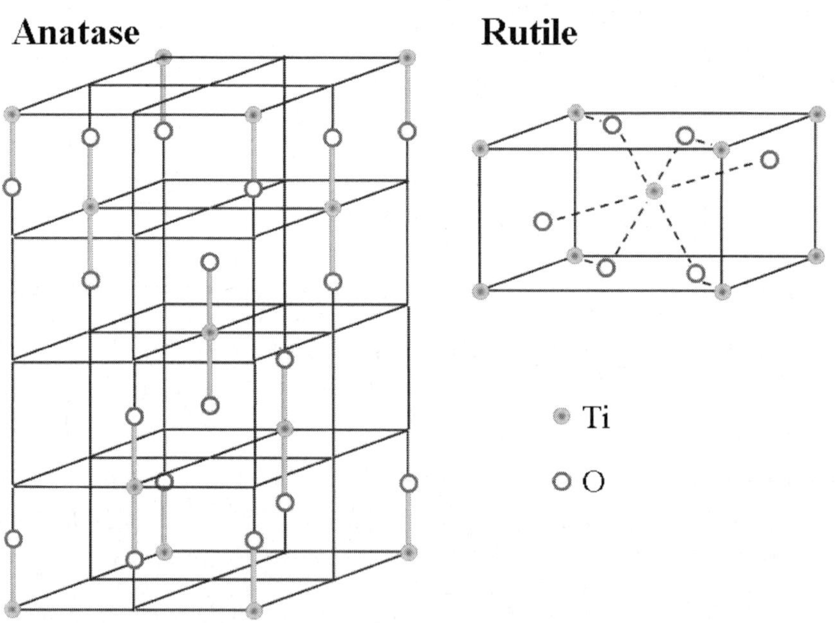

Fig. 3. Anatase and rutile forms of crystalline TiO_2.

6.3 Light sources

As the term 'photo-' represents, illumination of light is essential for the photocatalytic TiO_2 to get catalytic activity. It is the most important limitation in designing reactors with photocatalytic TiO_2. Even worse is the fact that most of photocatalytic TiO_2 can only utilize UV rather than visible light. It may not be a drawback of TiO_2, if any devices or reactors use natural sun light as a light source. However, in the view point of energy efficiency, if the reactor can utilize only a part of natural sun light and cannot utilize visible light, energy efficiency of the reactor will be less than 5% at most. Some of physical or chemical changes of titanium dioxide should be necessary to absorb and utilize visible light. Otherwise, photocatalytic TiO_2 can utilize visible light by mixing a small amount of other inorganic substances such as chromic oxide (Cr_2O_3, VI). However, in this case, reduced photocatalytic activity should be expected.

Limitation of light source may not always be a drawback of photocatalytic TiO_2. Since it produces hydroxyl radicals in aqueous solution and hydroxyl radical can decompose most of organic compounds, prolonged release of hydroxyl radical might be harmful in living organisms such as human. In case of antibacterial orthodontic wire described in section 3, it was coated with photocatalytic TiO_2 for its additional feature. The fact that releases of hydroxyl radicals from the photocatalytic TiO_2 for decomposition of bacterial cell wall compartments may imply a negative supposition. Hydroxyl radicals may also act on normal oral epithelial cells. In this case, the limitation of TiO_2 could, in turn, be a simple solution for the problem. The fact that relatively low intensity of UV light in normal day light is an advantage in this case. Since, photocatalytic activity of TiO_2 is usually activated by UV light, it can be regulated by manually controlling the illumination time and period in dental clinics.

7. Conclusion

When Fujishima and Honda reported the remarkable characteristics of titanium dioxide in 1972, few people have noticed the potentials of this white powder. Combined with the powerful effect of reactive oxygen species it became an almost almighty substance that can be used in environmental cleanup industries, personal hygiene products and even food industries. Not many substances have been interested in such diverse fields. However, there are still some drawbacks to overcome in the application of photocatalytic TiO_2. That means it is still worthy of challenge in the field of photocatalysis research.

8. References

Ashikaga, T., Wada, M., Kobayashi, H., Mori, M., Katsumura, Y., Fukui, H., Kato, S., Yamaguchi, M. & Takamatsu, T. (2000) Effect of the photocatalytic activity of TiO_2 on plasmid DNA. *Mutation research,* 466, 1-7.

Balenseifen, J. W. & Madonia, J. V. (1970) Study of dental plaque in orthodontic patients. *Journal of dental research,* 49, 320-324.

Cho, M., Chung, H., Choi, W. & Yoon, J. (2004) Linear correlation between inactivation of E. coli and OH radical concentration in TiO_2 photocatalytic disinfection. *Water research,* 38, 1069-1077.

Chun, M. J., Shim, E., Kho, E. H., Park, K. J., Jung, J., Kim, J. M., Kim, B., Lee, K. H., Cho, D. L., Bai, D. H., Lee, S. I., Hwang, H. S., and Ohk, S. H. (2007) Surface modification of orthodontic wires with photocatalytic titanium oxide for its antiadherent and antibacterial properties. *The Angle orthodontist,* 77, 483-488.

Daneshvar, N., Hejazi, M. J., Rangarangy, B. & Khataee, A. R. (2004) Photocatalytic degradation of an organophosphorus pesticide phosalone in aqueous suspensions of titanium dioxide. *Journal of environmental science and health Part B, Pesticides, food contaminants, and agricultural wastes,* 39, 285-296.

Dongare, M. K., Sonawane, R. S. & Hegde, S. G. (2003) Preparation of titanium(IV) oxide thin film photocatalyst by sol-gel dip coating. *Mater Chem Phys,* 77, 744-750.

Elsaka, S. E., Hamouda, I. M. & Swain, M. V. (2011) Titanium dioxide nanoparticles addition to a conventional glass-ionomer restorative: Influence on physical and antibacterial properties. *Journal of dentistry,* 39, 589-598.

Fujishima, A. & Honda, K. (1972) Electrochemical photolysis of water at a semiconductor electrode. *Nature,* 238, 37-38.

Gerrity, D., Ryu, H., Crittenden, J. & Abbaszadegan, M. (2008) Photocatalytic inactivation of viruses using titanium dioxide nanoparticles and low-pressure UV light. *Journal of environmental science and health Part A, Toxic/hazardous substances & environmental engineering,* 43, 1261-1270.

Giavaresi, G., Giardino, R., Ambrosio, L., Battiston, G., Gerbasi, R., Fini, M., Rimondini, L. & Torricelli, P. (2003) In vitro biocompatibility of titanium oxide for prosthetic devices nanostructured by low pressure metal-organic chemical vapor deposition. *The International journal of artificial organs,* 26, 774-780.

Gluszek, J., Masalski, J., Furman, P. & Nitsch, K. (1997) Structural and electrochemical examinations of PACVD TiO_2 films in Ringer solution. *Biomaterials,* 18, 789-794.

Gonzalez-Elipe, A. R., Gracia, F. & Holgado, J. P. (2004) Photoefficiency and optical, microstructural, and structural properties of TiO_2 thin films used as photoanodes. *Langmuir,* 20, 1688-1697.

Ireland, J. C. & Valinieks, J. (1992) Rapid measurement of aqueous hydroxyl radical concentrations in steady-state HO · flux systems. *Chemosphere,* 25, 383-396.

Ireland, J. C., Klostermann, P., Rice, E. W. & Clark, R. M. (1993) Inactivation of *Escherichia coli* by titanium dioxide photocatalytic oxidation. *Applied and environmental microbiology,* 59, 1668-1670.

Kuhn, K. P., Chaberny, I. F., Massholder, K., Stickler, M., Benz, V. W., Sonntag, H. G. & Erdinger, L. (2003) Disinfection of surfaces by photocatalytic oxidation with titanium dioxide and UVA light. *Chemosphere,* 53, 71-77.

Lee, J. M., Kim, M. S. & Kim, B. W. (2004) Photodegradation of bisphenol-A with TiO_2 immobilized on the glass tubes including the UV light lamps. *Water research,* 38, 3605-3613.

Liga, M. V., Bryant, E. L., Colvin, V. L. & Li, Q. (2011) Virus inactivation by silver doped titanium dioxide nanoparticles for drinking water treatment. *Water research,* 45, 535-544.

Makino, T., Matsumoto, K., Ebara, T., Mine, T., Ohtsuka, T. & Mizuguchi, J. (2007) Complete decomposition of benzene, toluene, and particulate matter contained in the exhaust of diesel engines by means of thermally excited holes in titanium dioxide at high temperatures. *Jpn J Appl Phys 1*, 46, 6037-6042.

Matsunaga, T., Tomoda, R., Nakajima, T. & Wakea, H. (1985) Photoelectrochemical sterilization of microbial cells by semiconductor powders. *FEMS Microbiology Letters*, 29, 211-214.

Mills, A., Lee, S. K., Lepre, A., Parkin, I. P. & O'Neill, S. A. (2002) Spectral and photocatalytic characteristics of TiO_2 CVD films on quartz. *Photochemical & photobiological sciences : Official journal of the European Photochemistry Association and the European Society for Photobiology*, 1, 865-868.

Muneer, M., Philip, R. & Das, S. (1997) Photocatalytic degradation of waste water pollutants. Titanium dioxide-mediated oxidation of a textile dye, acid blue 40. *Res Chem Intermediat*, 23, 233-246.

Muranyi, P., Schraml, C. & Wunderlich, J. (2010) Antimicrobial efficiency of titanium dioxide-coated surfaces. *Journal of applied microbiology*, 108, 1966-1973.

Ohdaira, T., Nagai, H., Kayano, S. & Kazuhito, H. (2007) Antifogging effects of a socket-type device with the superhydrophilic, titanium dioxide-coated glass for the laparoscope. *Surgical endoscopy*, 21, 333-338.

Paspaltsis, I., Kotta, K., Lagoudaki, R., Grigoriadis, N., Poulios, I. & Sklaviadis, T. (2006) Titanium dioxide photocatalytic inactivation of prions. *The Journal of general virology*, 87, 3125-3130.

Sakamaki, S. T. & Bahn, A. N. (1968) Effect of orthodontic banding on localized oral lactobacilli. *Journal of dental research*, 47, 275-279.

Salih, F. M. (2002) Enhancement of solar inactivation of *Escherichia coli* by titanium dioxide photocatalytic oxidation. *Journal of applied microbiology*, 92, 920-926.

Sang, X., Phan, T. G., Sugihara, S., Yagyu, F., Okitsu, S., Maneekarn, N., Muller, W. E. & Ushijima, H. (2007) Photocatalytic inactivation of diarrheal viruses by visible-light-catalytic titanium dioxide. *Clinical laboratory*, 53, 413-421.

Saquib, M. & Muneer, M. (2003) Photocatalytic degradation of two selected textile dye derivatives, eosine yellowish and p-rosaniline, in aqueous suspensions of titanium dioxide. *Journal of environmental science and health Part A, Toxic/hazardous substances & environmental engineering*, 38, 2581-2598.

Scheie, A. A., Arneberg, P. & Krogstad, O. (1984) Effect of orthodontic treatment on prevalence of *Streptococcus mutans* in plaque and saliva. *Scandinavian journal of dental research*, 92, 211-217.

Schupbach, P., Glauser, R., Rocci, A., Martignoni, M., Sennerby, L., Lundgren, A. & Gottlow, J. (2005) The human bone-oxidized titanium implant interface: A light microscopic, scanning electron microscopic, back-scatter scanning electron microscopic, and energy-dispersive x-ray study of clinically retrieved dental implants. *Clinical implant dentistry and related research*, 7 Suppl 1, S36-43.

Singh, H. K., Muneer, M. & Bahnemann, D. (2003) Photocatalysed degradation of a herbicide derivative, bromacil, in aqueous suspensions of titanium dioxide. *Photochemical & photobiological sciences : Official journal of the European Photochemistry Association and the European Society for Photobiology*, 2, 151-156.

Yoshinari, M., Oda, Y., Kato, T. & Okuda, K. (2001) Influence of surface modifications to titanium on antibacterial activity in vitro. *Biomaterials,* 22, 2043-2048.

Zainal, Z., Lee, C. Y., Hussein, M. Z., Kassim, A. & Yusof, N. A. (2005) Electrochemical-assisted photodegradation of dye on TiO_2 thin films: investigation on the effect of operational parameters. *Journal of hazardous materials,* 118, 197-203.

Part 2

Growth and Genetic

6

Genetic Factors Affecting Facial Growth

James K. Hartsfield Jr.[1], Lorri Ann Morford[1] and Liliana M. Otero[1,2]
[1]*University of Kentucky*
[2]*Pontificia Universidad Javeriana*
[1]*USA*
[2]*Colombia*

1. Introduction

Malocclusion is the manifestation of complex genetic and environmental interactions on the development of the oral-facial region. Historically, orthodontists have been interested in genetics as a means to better understand why a patient has a particular occlusion, and to determine the best course of treatment for the malocclusion. The application of genetic information in treatment, however, has been hampered by several factors including: 1) the presumption that heritability studies have some clinical relevance to the individual patient, which they do not (Harris, 2008); 2) the presumption that whatever genetic factors may have contributed to the occlusion will also affect how the patient responds to treatment, which they may not; and 3) a lack of understanding to the extent at which genetic factors may interact with environmental factors (such as those created during orthodontic and dentofacial orthopedic treatments) to influence single gene (Mendelian) traits versus "Complex" traits which are more frequently observed in the clinic. (Hartsfield, 2011)

While it is essential to consider genetic factors when diagnosing the underlying cause for virtually all oral-facial anomalies and developmental variations, the importance of how genetic factors will affect the outcome of treatment is often not appreciated. Understanding the etiology of a malocclusion is important, e.g., if the patient is a thumb sucker, then that habit must stop. But in terms of etiology, the factors that influenced a malocclusion to develop may not be the same ones that will influence how the patient responds to treatment of that malocclusion. In addition, the patient's developmental stage during treatment is typically a later stage then when the basis of the malocclusion first formed. Although an environmental modification may alter the development of the phenotype at a particular moment, gross structural morphology, already present, may not change readily unless the environmental modification is sufficient to alter preexisting structure.(Buschang & Hinton, 2005) As every orthodontist knows, the ability of the practitioner to affect a change is dependent both on the time of intervention (treatment) and the patient's stage of development.

Knowing whether the cause of the problem is genetic has been cited as a factor in eventual outcome; that is, if the problem is genetic, then orthodontists may be limited in what they can do (or change), because of an intrinsic "predestination." This is a misapplication of genetics to clinical practice since most malocclusions we treat appear to not be the result of a single dominant (Mendelian) gene.(Mossey, 1999b) There are inappropriate uses of heritability estimates in the literature as a proxy for evaluating whether a malocclusion or some anatomic morphology is "genetic." This however has no relevance to the question. Regardless of the heritability estimate, there is not a yes or no answer. Heritability estimates only apply to the group that was studied and the environmental factors that they were exposed to up to that time. They do not necessarily apply to an individual at the time of the study, and are not predictive for an individual or the group in the future.(Harris, 2008) How genetic factors will influence the response to environmental factors, including treatment, and the long-term stability of its outcome as determined by genetic linkage or association studies, should be the greatest concern for the clinician as they are the only way leading to a better understanding of the genetic background of the individual patient in terms of their malocclusion and response to treatment.(Hartsfield, 2008) It is of critical importance in clinical practice to understand how genetic factors and their interaction with environmental factors may affect facial growth. The aim of this chapter is to review what is known about the genetic factors that affect facial growth with an emphasis on human studies involving malocclusion.

2. Genome, genotype, phenotype, modes of inheritance and epigenetics

An individual's **genome** is defined as the genetic information inherited from both of their parents. The information encoded in a patient's genome can influence growth and development when the coded information is converted into the form of **protein** (and/or regulatory molecules such as microRNAs (miRNAs)). This information is encoded by ~3.2 billion nucleotide base pairs (bps), comprised of adenine (A), thymine (T) , cytosine (C) and guanine (G) residues, that are organized into sequences on 23 pairs of chromosomes. Each individual has 22 pairs of **autosomal chromosomes** (chromosomes that exhibit the same copy number in both males and females) and 1 pair of **sex chromosomes** (XX or XY). One chromosome of each pair is inherited from the individual's mother and the other pair from their father. Collectively this genetic information is often referred to as a person's DNA or genetic code. Amazingly, the genetic sequences of all humans appear to be ~99.9% identical, and hence it is a mere 0.1% of the sequence information which codes for our individual differences.

It is estimated that the human genome is comprised of 25,000 genes (accounting for only ~2% of the entire genome), with the average gene length being ~3,000 bps of information. A **gene** is a specific sequence of information that provides the instructions for making a unique protein or set of related proteins. The location or "address" for any gene within a genome is called its **locus** (plural loci: i.e., referring to the physical location of more than one gene). A determination of the actual DNA code (A, T, C or G) for a specific location within a person's genome describes their **genotype** for that location. Since there is natural variation in the sequence of DNA, a specific gene at a locus can still vary among individuals and homologous chromosomes in the same individual. These different forms of the "same" gene are called **alleles**. When the alleles on homologous chromosome pairs are the same, they are said to be **homozygous**. When the alleles on homologous chromosome pairs are different, they are said to be **heterozygous**. The **mode of inheritance** describes how the genetic information is passed down one generation to the next.

Within a single individual, the majority of cells in the body will contain a complete copy of the genome the individual inherited from their parents. Only a small number of specialized cell types (e.g. mature erythrocytes, mature T- and B-cells of the immune system, sperm, and egg cells) eliminate a portion of inherited DNA to facilitate the cell's ability to perform a specialized function. Aside from these specialized cell types, most cells within an individual's body become (or differentiate into) a particular kind of cell (e.g. a muscle, nerve, or skin cell, etc...) or become part of a larger tissue or organ based upon the pattern of genes that are turned "on" or "off" within each cell. The process of turning a gene "on" is referred to as "gene expression" and most forms of gene expression lead to the production a protein or set of related proteins. Hence, a well differentiated cell like an osteoblast, does not become an osteoblast due to the presence of unique DNA codes found only is osteoblast cells or due to the loss of non-osteoblast related genetic information. An osteoblast becomes an osteoblast due to the genes and related proteins (or regulatory molecules) being expressed within the cell combined with the influence of any environmental factors that can alter these expression pattern(s).

The visible or measurable characteristics of an individual is their **phenotype**. A phenotype is determined based on the combination of: (1) the inherited genetic information being expressed by cells within the individual (e.g., the individual's genotype); (2) the environment in which the proteins (or regulatory molecules) are being expressed; and (3) any genotype-environment interactions that could influence protein (or regulatory molecule) expression or function. In contrast, a **trait** is a particular aspect or characteristic of the overall phenotype. An **inherited trait** is one that has the ability to be transferred from one generation to the next generation. A **syndrome** is a combination of traits that occur together in non random pattern that is different from the usual pattern.(Hartsfield & Bixler, 2011)

When the information in a single gene locus is essentially responsible for the development of a trait or syndrome, this trait or syndrome is said to be *monogenic*. If the gene locus is located on one of 22 autosomal chromosome pairs (chromosomes other than the X or Y sex chromosomes), and only one copy of a specific gene allele on the autosomal pair is sufficient to lead to the production of the trait or syndrome, then the individual is typically heterozygous for that allele and the effect on the inheritance pattern of the trait or syndrome is **autosomal dominant**. If the production of the trait or syndrome does not occur when only one copy of a particular allele is present at the locus on a paired set of autosomes, but does occur when two copies of that particular allele are present at the locus of a paired set of autosomes, then the inheritance pattern of the trait or syndrome is **autosomal recessive**. In this situation the "recessive" alleles are said to be homozygous.(Mossey, 1999a) This may be the case by having a common ancestor (inbreeding) in which the alleles are presumed to be identical, or by the random combination of alleles that although may not be of identical DNA sequence, still are operationally recessive.

The following are characteristic for **autosomal dominant inheritance**: (1) the trait or syndrome occurs in successive generations; (2) when an individual has the gene allele that results in the trait or syndrome, each child of theirs has a 50% chance of inheriting that gene allele; (3) males and females are equally likely to have the trait or syndrome; and (4) parents who do not have the trait or syndrome have offspring who do not have the trait or syndrome (see figure 1). However, there are notable caveats to these characteristics. Just because an individual has the "dominant" gene allele that would usually lead to the development of some particular trait or syndrome, such as Class III malocclusion, Treacher

Collins syndrome or Crouzon syndrome (a common craniosynostosis condition), the appearance of the trait or syndrome may "skip a generation" in what is called **non-penetrance** in the individual, or incomplete penetrance in a group of individuals who have the genotype but don't manifest the trait or syndrome.(Cruz et al., 2008; Everett et al., 1999; Hennekam et al., 2010) In addition, traits and syndromes with autosomal dominant inheritance typically have **varying degrees of severity** in individuals who show any evidence of the condition, which is termed **variable expressivity** of the phenotype. Thus analyzing the genome/genotype of even traits or syndromes with autosomal dominant may not "precisely" predict the phenotype, but certainly can often indicate there will be a major effect on growth and development to some degree. Variable expressivity also may apply to the pleiotropic effect of a particular genotype: that is the expression of a gene resulting in seemingly disparate traits in an individual. Thus even dominant traits that are said to be due to a change in a single gene can be influenced by the proteins from other genes and environmental factors (see figure 2).

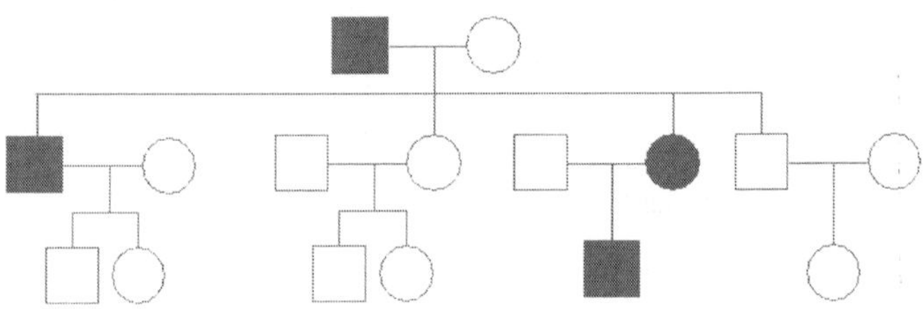

Fig. 1. Autosomal dominant Inheritance.

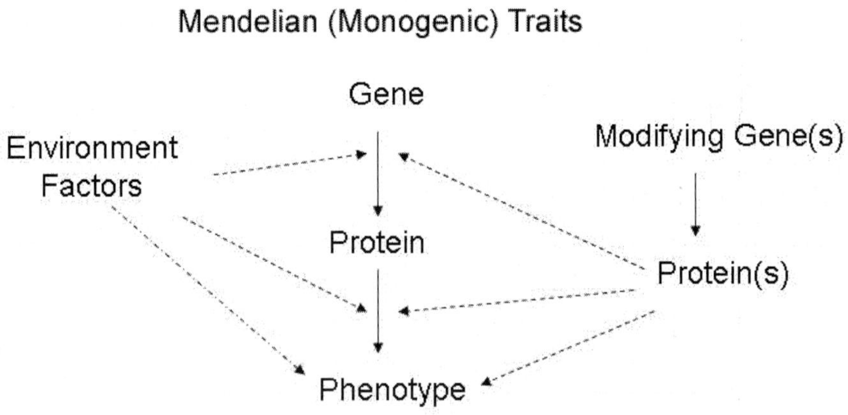

Fig. 2. Interaction of Genetic and Environmental Factors on an "Monogenic Dominant" Trait.

In **autosomal recessive inheritance** the transmission of the pedigree is typically horizontal (present only in siblings, see figure 3). Parents of a child with a trait or syndrome that has an autosomal recessive mode of inheritance are typically heterozygous ("carriers"). The heterozygous parents would then have a 25% of each child of theirs having the autosomal recessive trait or syndrome.

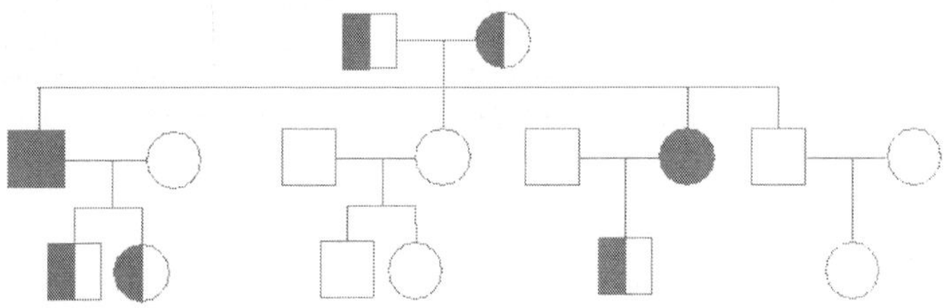

Fig. 3. Autosomal recessive inheritance.

For X linked traits, recessive genes on the one male X chromosome express themselves phenotypically as if they were dominant genes because a male usually only has one X chromosome (hemizygous). In this case the males with the genotype are affected in the pedigree, although in some cases the females can be affected as well. Females who are heterozygous for the gene associated with the X linked recessive phenotype may show some expression of the phenotype. This is because most of the genes on one of the X chromosomes in each cell of a female normally will be inactivated by a process called **lyonization (or X chromosome inactivation)**. Early in fetal development (at approximately the 16-cell morula stage), each cell of the developing female fetus inactivates almost all the genes on one of her two X chromosomes, and all cells that develop from that cell will show the inactivation of the same X chromosome. Depending on the ratio of cells with the X chromosome that has the recessive gene on it versus the X chromosome that does not have the recessive gene, the female may show some variable manifestation of the condition.

Most traits do not adhere to patterns of Mendelian inheritance. These traits are referred to as complex or common diseases and traits, and reflect their complex interaction between genes from more than one locus and environmental factors. Polygenic traits infer the effect of multiple genes on the phenotype, but can be affected by environmental factors also (see figure 4). The distinction between polygenic traits and multifactorial traits (both are traits influenced by environmental and multiple genetic factors) has been made for some multifactorial traits that are discrete (dichotomous) and that occur in an individual once a developmental threshold of genetic and environmental factors to produce the phenotype has been reached.

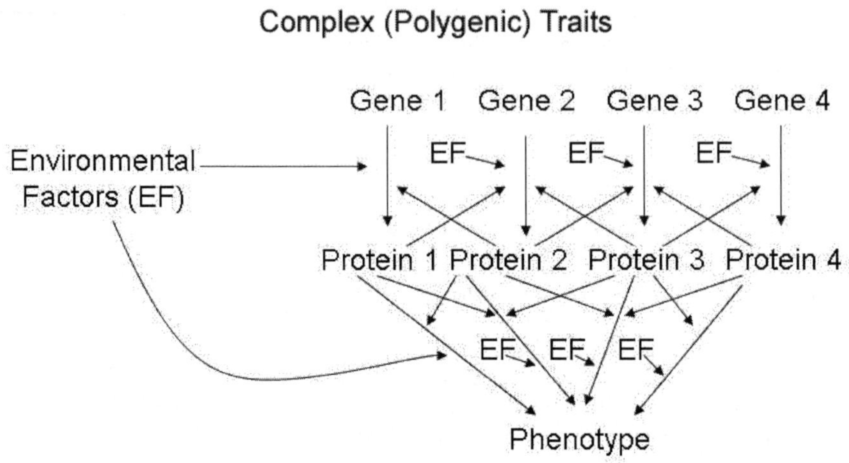

Fig. 4. Interaction of Genetic and Environmental Factors on a Complex Trait.

Epigenetics is the study of acquired and heritable changes in gene function that occur without a change in the DNA sequence. Environmental factors can influence epigenetic mechanisms such as DNA modification (i.e., methylation), histone modification (e.g., lysine and arginine methylation, acetylation, ubiquitination, phosphorylation, sumoylation, ADP ribosylation, deamination and proline isomerization)), and post-transcriptional silencing by RNA interference (microRNA, miRNA). All of these processes can result in gene activation and inactivation.(Lambert & Herceg, 2011) Epigenetic mechanisms can mediate the effect of the environment (e.g., dietary, hormonal and respiratory factors) on the human genome by controlling the transcriptional activity of specific genes, at specific points in time in specific organs.(Gabory et al., 2009; Schwartz, 2010) Malocclusion is a trait than can be greatly influenced by environmental factors. Corrucini suggested that the rapid increase in malocclusion in indigenous Australian people was produced by dietary factors concurrent with industrialization, and emphasized the importance of environmental influences on occlusal variation and the variability of apparent genetic determinants with respect to the environment or population in which they are measured.(Corruccini, 1984, 1990; Corruccini et al., 1990) Likewise Kawala et al. after studying the concordance of malocclusion in twins showed the distribution of within-pair malocclusions depended upon the gender of the individuals, and supported the impact of environmental factors.(Kawala et al., 2007)

In the consideration of environmental effects upon the development of malocclusion, it should not be forgotten that one's genome may influence the response to environmental factors. This is supported by the differences in shape of the mandibular condyles being "slightly greater" among four different inbred strains of mice on a hard diet than on a soft diet for six weeks. When the environment changed sufficiently, the response was different among animals with different genotypes that were not different before the environmental change.(Lavelle, 1983) Siblings may often have similar malocclusions not just because of common genetic or environmental factors, but also because of their shared genetic factors affecting how they respond to the shared environmental factors.(King et al., 1993) However, none of these studies on the effect of environmental factors were focused on epigenetic modifications as a result of environmental factors influencing malocclusion. As the exploration of epigenetics continues throughout biology and medicine, it may also be an interesting area to explore in facial growth.

3. Heritability and malocclusion

Most problems in orthodontics (or any outcome of growth), unless acquired by trauma, are not strictly the result of only genetic or only environmental factors. The ideal occlusion condition shows a proportional growth between the cranial base, the maxilla and the mandible; and involves the harmonious relation between skeletal bases and soft tissues (perioral musculature, lips and tongue).(Mossey, 1999b) The general morphology of craniofacial bones and teeth are largely genetically determined, although clearly variation is partly attributable to environmental factors.(Corruccini et al., 1990; Harris, 2008; Klingenberg et al., 2004; Kraus & Lufkin, 2006; Thesleff, 2006; Townsend et al., 2003) Genetic mechanisms predominate during embryonic craniofacial morphogenesis and in the etiology of many craniofacial abnormalities, therefore genetic factors must be considered in the etiology of malocclusion. However environment is also thought to influence dentofacial morphology postnatally, particularly during facial growth. In response to the presumption of the genome being the predetermining force for facial development and by inference skeletal malocclusion, the Functional Matrix Hypothesis by Moss theorized the primary role of function in craniofacial growth and development. Still, Moss did conclude that both genomic and environmental/epigenetic factors are necessary causes, that neither alone is a sufficient cause and that only the two interacting together furnish both the necessary and sufficient cause(s) of growth and development.(Moss, 1997b, 1997a)

One method employed to estimate this relative contribution of genetic and environmental factors is by calculating the heritability of a trait. Heritability in the broad since (H^2) includes all additive, interactive and other types of genetic and environmental influences. This is impossible to derive, since all the factors and how they interact is not known. Therefore heritability estimates in the literature are in the narrow sense (h^2), and represent the proportion of the total phenotypic variance in a sample that is contributed by additive genetic variance. However, the estimated ratio of genetic variation does not take into account gene-gene or gene-environment interaction.(Hartsfield, 2011) Numerous studies have examined how genetic variation contributes to either or both occlusal and skeletal variation among family members. It is difficult to estimate the influence of environmental (treatment) factors in craniofacial growth because the heritability studies of occlusion are typically based on twins and siblings who did not receive orthodontic treatment. Twin pairs and other groups of siblings containing one or more treated patients (with moderate to severe malocclusion) may have been excluded from most studies. Moreover the twin studies have not included extensive analysis of the parents, nor familial, and nutritional habits; and usually have not compared the twin group with a control group to ascertain environmental covariance (similarity due to twins and other siblings being in a common environment). Therefore, estimates of genetic and environmental contributions may have been affected by lack of accounting for a common environmental effect(Corruccini & Potter, 1980) and ascertainment bias.(King et al., 1993)

The cause of most skeletal- and dentoalveolar based malocclusions is essentially multifactorial in the sense that many diverse causes converge to produce the observed outcome.(King et al., 1993) Numerous studies have examined how genetic variation contributes to either or both occlusal and skeletal variation among family members.(Arya et al., 1973; Boraas et al., 1988; Byard et al., 1985; Cassidy et al., 1998; Chung & Niswander, 1975; Corruccini et al., 1986; Devor, 1987; Fernex et al., 1967; Gass et al., 2003; Harris et al., 1973; Harris et al., 1975; Harris & Smith, 1980; Harris & Johnson, 1991; Hauspie et al., 1985; Horowitz et al., 1960; Hunter et al., 1970; Johannsdottir et al., 2005; King et al., 1993; Kraus et al., 1959; Litton et al., 1970; Lobb, 1987; Lundstrom & McWilliam, 1987; Manfredi et al., 1997; Nakata et al., 1973; Nikolova, 1996; Proffit, 1986; Saunders et al., 1980; Susanne & Sharma, 1978; Watnick, 1972) In most studies (particularly those that try to account for bias from the effect of shared environmental factors, unequal means, and unequal variances in monozygotic and dizygotic twin samples),(Harris & Potter, 1997) variations in cephalometric skeletal dimensions are associated in general with a moderate to high degree of genetic variation, whereas in general, variation of occlusal relationships has little or no association with genetic variation.(Harris, 2008)

Although the heritability estimates are low, most of the studies that looked at occlusal traits found that genetic variation is positively correlated with phenotypic variation for arch width and arch length more than for overjet, overbite, and molar relationship. Still, arch size and shape are associated more with environmental variation than with genetic variation.(Cassidy et al., 1998) Because many occlusal variables reflect the combined variations of tooth position and basal and alveolar bone development, these variables (e.g., overjet, overbite, and molar relationship) cannot be less variable than the supporting structures. They will vary because of their own variation in position and those of the basilar structures.(Harris & Johnson, 1991) Heritability studies must be supplemented and to some degree superseded by studies linking or associating specific traits with variation in genetic markers such as single nucleotide polymorphisms (SNPs), variable number of tandem repeats, or other types of specific DNA variation.

For example, SNPs in the *EDA* gene and the gene for its receptor *XEDAR*, were found to be associated with dental crowding greater than 5 mm in a Hong Kong Chinese Class I malocclusion sample. It was thought that this may at least be due in part to variation in tooth size as the gene product of EDA is involved in tooth development, and mutations in EDA cause X-linked Hypohydrotic Ectodermal Dysplasia.(Ting et al., 2011) A possible affect on tooth size is consistent with the findings that in skeletal Class I crowding cases tooth size variation may more often play a role than skeletal growth.(Bernabe & Flores-Mir, 2006; Hashim & Al-Ghamdi, 2005; Poosti & Jalali, 2007; Ting et al., 2011) Although these genes are located on the X chromosome, the associations remained after adjustment for sex. This type of investigation is thought to help get around the problem of confounding environmental factors, although an increased analysis of epigenetic markers may show this is not that simple. Still these studies are the only way in which possible predictive data will be collected and tested.

4. Use of family data to predict growth

Siblings have been noted as often showing similar types of malocclusion. Examination of parents and older siblings has been suggested as a way to gain information regarding the treatment need for a child, including early treatment of malocclusion.(Harris & Kowalski, 1976; Litton et al., 1970; Niswander, 1975; Saunders et al., 1980) Niswander noted that the frequency of malocclusion is decreased among siblings of index cases with normal occlusion, whereas the siblings of index cases with malocclusion tend to have the same type of malocclusion more often. (Niswander, 1975) There are high correlation coefficient values between parents and their offspring for Class II and Class III malocclusions.(Nakasima et al., 1982) It has been shown that the craniofacial skeletal patterns of children with Class II (division 1) malocclusions are familial (i.e., occur more often in multiple members of some families), and that a high resemblance to the skeletal patterns occurs in their siblings with normal occlusion.(Harris et al., 1975) Although this was ascribed to the Class II (division 1) being "heritable," common environmental factors were not taken into account. From this it was concluded that the genetic basis for this resemblance is probably polygenic, and family skeletal patterns were used as predictors for the treatment prognosis of the child with a Class II malocclusion, although it was acknowledged that the current morphology of the patient is the primary source of information about future growth.(Harris & Kowalski, 1976)

Each child receives half of his or her genes from each parent, but not likely the same combination of genes as a sibling unless the children are monozygotic twins. When looking at parents with a differing skeletal morphology, knowing which of the genes in what combination from each parent is present in the child is difficult until the child's phenotype matures under the continuing influence of environmental factors. When considering polygenic traits, the highest phenotypic correlation that can be expected based on genes in common by inheritance from one parent to a child, or between siblings, is 0.5. Because the child's phenotype is likely to be influenced by the interaction of genes from both parents, the "mid-parent" value may increase the correlation with their children to 0.7 because of the regression to the mean of parental dimensions in their children. Squaring the correlation between the two variables derives the amount of variation predicted for one variable in correlation with another variable. Therefore, at best, using mid parent values, only 49% of the variability of any facial dimension in a child can be predicted by consideration of the average of the same dimension in the parents. Only 25% of the variability of any facial dimension in a child can be predicted, at best, by considering the same dimension in a sibling or one parent. Because varying effects of environmental factors interact with the multiple genetic factors, the usual correlation for facial dimensions between parents and their children is about 30%, yielding even less predictive power.(Hunter, 1990)

In most patients, the mode of inheritance for the craniofacial skeleton is polygenic (complex). However, in some families (e.g., with a relatively prognathic mandible compared with the maxilla), the mode of inheritance is not polygenic. Future research may investigate the genetic factors that do not fit a polygenic mode that may be present in some families. Identification of those factors will increase the ability to predict the likelihood of a particular resulting morphology. Unfortunately, orthodontists do not have sufficient information to make accurate predictions about the development of occlusion simply by studying the frequency of its occurrence in parents or even siblings. Admittedly, family patterns of resemblance are frequently obvious, and observed family tendencies should not be ignored.

Nonetheless, predictions must be made cautiously because genetic and environmental factors and their interaction are unknown and difficult to evaluate and predict with precision.(Hartsfield, 2011)

5. Genetic markers associated with variations in growth of complex etiology

5.1 Growth hormone receptor

Growth hormone is an important factor in craniofacial and skeletal growth. A variant in the growth hormone receptor and its gene (*GHR*), when there is a proline amino acid instead of threonine at the 561st residue in the protein, is referred to as the *GHR* P56IT allele. Of a normal Japanese sample of 50 men and 50 women, those who did not have the *GHR* P56IT allele had a significantly greater mandibular ramus length (condylion-gonion) than did those with the *GHR* P56IT allele. The average mandibular ramus height in those with the *GHR* P56IT allele was 4.65 mm shorter than the average for those without the *GHR* P56IT allele. This significant correlation between the *GHR* P56IT allele and shorter mandibular ramus height was confirmed in an additional 80 women.(Yamaguchi et al., 2001) Interestingly, the association was with the mandibular ramus height but not mandibular body length, maxillary length, or anterior cranial base length. This suggests a site-, area-, or region-specific effect. The study concluded that the *GHR* P56IT allele may be associated with mandibular height growth and can be a genetic marker for it. Still, whether the effect is directly on the mandible or some other nearby tissue or on another matrix is not clear. It has been suggested that *GHR* variants P561T and C422F are associated with mandibular ramus height in Japanese population and that the SNPs of the *GHR* gene associated with differences in mandibular ramus height in the Japanese are likely to be different in other ethnic groups. (Tomoyasu et al., 2009)

This is supported by the finding that although there is a possible association between the *GHR* polymorphisms P561T, C422F and "haplotype 4" in a Korean population, there was not significant association between these markers and mandibular height in African-Americans, European-Americans, and Hispanics.(Kang et al., 2009) This group suggested that this finding might partly explain the differing craniofacial morphology among different ethnicities. Analysis of the possible association between the P561T variant in the *GHR* gene and mandibular growth during early childhood did not find a difference between mandibular protrusion and normal occlusion. (Sasaki et al., 2009) To see what effect different diets would have on individuals with and without the *GHR* P56IT allele would be interesting as a means of looking at genetic and environmental factor interaction. Undoubtedly many other genes that may influence craniofacial structure, including ramus height, could be identified, and their variation could be studied along with different environmental factors (e.g., orthodontic treatment) and the resulting phenotype.

5.2 Growth differences during puberty

Increased accuracy in the estimation of pubertal facial growth would be of great benefit prior to the utilization of different therapeutic modalities including orthodontics, orthopedic growth modification and surgery. Research and discussion about facial growth and treatment in the literature have focused either on the timing of the greatest amount of facial growth, particularly for the mandible(Gu & McNamara, 2007; Hunter et al., 2007; Verma et al., 2009); or the estimated extent of facial growth to be attained.(Chvatal et al., 2005; Turchetta et al., 2007) As useful as average facial growth predictions based upon expected growth curves may be, more valid prediction must incorporate and account for the variation associated with individual genetic factors, particularly those that are highly pertinent to the pubertal growth spurt. The pubertal growth spurt response is mediated by the combination of sex steroids, growth hormone, insulin-like growth factor (IGF-I) and other endocrine, paracrine and autocrine factors. Testosterone and estradiol in mice have a direct, sex-specific stimulatory activity on male and female derived chondroprogenitor cell proliferation. Testosterone stimulated growth and local production of IGF-I and IGF-I-R in chondrocyte cell layers of an isolated organ culture of mice mandibular condyle.(Maor et al., 1999) Investigation into the effects of neonatal surgical castration and prepubertal chemical castration on craniofacial growth in rats showed that craniofacial growth was related to testosterone concentration. Administration of low doses of testosterone in boys with delayed puberty not only accelerates their statural growth rate, but their craniofacial growth rate as well.(Verdonck et al., 1998; Verdonck et al., 1999)

Ovariectomized and orchiectomized mice that sex hormone levels influenced condylar morphogenesis changed the internal structure of the mandibular condyle.(Fujita et al., 2001) It has been suggested that the suppression of sex hormone secretion in the growth phase might inhibit craniofacial growth and result in poor craniofacial development, particularly nasomaxillary bone and mandible, in new born and pubertal rats.(Fujita et al., 2004; Fujita et al., 2006) It has been demonstrated using administration of sex hormone specific receptor antagonists that growth of the mandible and femur is induced in response to the stimulation of the estrogen receptor beta (ERβ) in chondrocytes before and during early puberty in mice. In late and after puberty, the growth is induced by the stimulation of estrogen receptor alpha (ERα) in male and female mice. From this it was proposed that a screen of sex hormones could be used as an indicator of bone maturity to accurately predict the beginning and end of growth in orthodontic treatment.

CYP19A1 is the gene that encodes aromatase. This enzyme catalyzes the rate limiting step in estrogen biosynthesis by converting androgens. In order to best diagnose and treat the child or adolescent patient, the orthodontist needs to know as much as possible about the patient's growth potential. As useful as predictions based upon expected growth models starting from early in the patient's life may be, prediction must incorporate and account for the variation associated with individual genetic factors, especially those that are highly pertinent to the pubertal growth spurt.

Estrogens are a group of hormones involved in growth and development.(Honjo et al., 1992) Estrogen stimulates chondrogenesis, promotes the progressive closure of the epiphyseal growth plate, has an anabolic effect on the osteoblast and an apoptotic effect on the osteoclast, and increases bone mineral acquisition in axial and appendicular bone during adolescence and into the third decade.(Grumbach, 2000) Aromatase (also known as estrogen synthetase) is a key cytochrome P450 enzyme involved in estrogen biosynthesis.(Bulun et al., 2003) This steroidogenic enzyme catalyzes the final step of estrogen biosynthesis by converting testosterone and androstenedione to estradiol and estrone, respectively.(Guo et al., 2006) Regulation of this gene's transcription is critical for the testosterone/estrogen (T/E) ratio in the body since aromatase plays an important role in the conversion of androgens to estrogens. Some studies have shown that the T/E ratio is critical in the development of sex-indexed facial characteristics such as the growth of cheekbones, the mandible and chin, the prominence of eyebrow ridges and the lengthening of the lower face. (Schaefer et al., 2005; Schaefer et al., 2006)

The difference in the average sagittal jaw growth between the two groups of Caucasian males with different *CYP19A1* alleles with the greatest differences in growth per year was just over 1.5 mm per year during treatment for the maxilla, and 2.5 mm per year for the mandible. (Hartsfield Jr. et al., 2010) There was no statistical difference for the particular *CYP19A1* alleles in females. This is particularly impressive since at the beginning of treatment there was no significant difference among the males based upon the *CYP19A1* genotype. The significant difference only expressed itself over the time of treatment during the cervical vertebral stage associated with increased growth velocity.(Hartsfield et al., 2010) Interestingly the same result was found in a group of Chinese males and females, strongly suggesting that this variation in the *CYP19A1* gene may be a multi-ethnic marker for sagittal facial growth. (He et al., 2011) Although the difference in average annual sagittal mandibular and maxillary growth based upon this *CYP19A1* genotype were significant, as one factor in a complex trait (sagittal jaw growth), they account for only part of the variation seen, and therefore by itself has little predictive power. Further investigation of this and other genetic factors, their interactions with each other and with environmental factors will help to explain what has up to now been an unknown component of individual variations in facial growth.

5.3 Class II division 2 (Class II/2) malocclusion

There is evidence that Class II division 2, and particularly Class III malocclusions, can have a strong genetic component. The Class II division 2 (II/2) malocclusion is a relatively rare type of malocclusion, representing between 2.3% and 5% of all malocclusions in the western white population.(Ast et al., 1965; Mills, 1966) In one study 100% of 20 monozygotic (MZ) twin pairs were concordant for II/2 malocclusion, while only 10.7% of 28 dizygotic (DZ) twin pairs demonstrated concordance for the Class II/2 malocclusion. (Markovic, 1992) These findings suggest the effect of common genetic or environmental factors; however, the much lower concordance for DZ twins would suggest that multiple genetic factors rather than a single gene contribute to the risk for Class II/2. This was reinforced by Ruf et al. concluding that the etiology of Class II/2 malocclusion was unclear, with neither form nor function the sole controlling factor.(Ruf & Pancherz, 1999)

From a developmental viewpoint it is interesting that there is a strong association of Class II/2 malocclusion with dental developmental anomalies, more so than for other Angle malocclusion classes.(Basdra et al., 2001) Excluding 3rd molars, agenesis of other teeth was at least three times more common in Class II/2 subjects than in the general population. In addition, there were a significantly greater number of dental developmental anomalies present in Class II/2 subjects as compared to the general population. They found 56.6% of Class II/2 patients exhibited developmental tooth anomalies including hypodontia as compared to as many as 35% of the general population having agenesis of one or more third molar.(Basdra et al., 2000) In addition Peck et al. showed a statistically significant reduction in permanent maxillary incisor mesial-distal width associated with Class II/2.(Peck et al., 1998)

Further evidence for a polygenic complex etiology for Class II/2 was found in a study of 68 subjects (67 self reported as white and 1 white/African-American who was a child of one of the 18 probands). (Morrison, 2008) A proband is the affected individual through whom a family is first seen or studied for a genetic trait, syndrome or disorder. In this study, researchers included 50 reported first-degree relatives of each proband, with a minimum of 2 first-degree relatives of each proband. The findings showed a marked increase in the number of females affected with Class II/2 in both the probands and their first-degree relatives than affected males. Of the 36 first-degree relatives whose occlusion was analyzed, 6 (16.7%) were found to be Class II/2. The relative risk (RR) of first-degree relatives to have a Class II/2 was found to be 3.3 - 7.3. The confidence interval (CI) was 1.1-10.3 if the RR was 3.3 and 1.7-31.6 if the RR was 7.3.

Agenesis of one or more permanent teeth (excluding 3rd molars) was found in 2 (11.1%) of the 18 probands and 7 (14.0%) of the 50 first-degree relatives. Agenesis of one or more 3rd molars was found in 4 (22.2%) of the 18 probands and 12 (24.0%) of the 50 first-degree relatives. Agenesis of one or both permanent maxillary incisors was found in none of the 18 probands and 2 (4.0%) of the 50 first-degree relatives. One or more small teeth (excluding 3rd molars) were found in 4 (22.2%) of the 18 probands and 15 (30.0%) of the 50 first-degree relatives. Small maxillary permanent incisors were found in none of the 18 probands and 4 (8.0%) of the 50 first-degree relatives. Agenesis of one or more permanent teeth in combination with the presence of one or more small permanent teeth was found in 2 (11.1%) of the 18 probands and 7 (14.0%) of the 50 first-degree relatives. Of the 36 first-degree relatives evaluated for malocclusion, 6 (16.67%) were found to be Class II/2. The RR for first-degree relatives of the probands to have a Class II/2 malocclusion was 3.3 - 7.35.(Morrison, 2008)

These results indicate that first-degree relatives of Class II/2 probands have a significantly increased risk of having a Class II/2 malocclusion as compared with individuals from the general population. Were Class II/2 malocclusion to be the result of variation in a single gene, acting in either a dominant or recessive fashion, the relative risk would be expected to be much higher. Rather, the modest, albeit significant increase in risk appears consistent with results from previous studies, which suggest a multifactorial etiology for Class II/2 malocclusion.

The question could be raised as to whether or not anomalous maxillary lateral incisors are associated with the Class II/2 malocclusion phenotype, and therefore share common etiological factors. Basdra et al. showed that 13.9% of Class II/2 subjects had agenesis of maxillary lateral incisors and 7.5% had peg-shaped or small maxillary lateral incisors. In contrast, Morrison found none of the probands had agenesis of or small maxillary lateral incisors, although first-degree relatives of the Class II/2 probands showed similar frequencies of hypodontia and microdontia of other teeth as the II/2 probands. However, the frequencies of these dental anomalies in the probands and first degree relatives were not significantly greater than those in the general population.(Morrison, 2008) Thus it is unclear if Class II/2 probands and their first-degree relatives are at an increased risk of developing hypodontia and/or microdontia. Investigations of a larger sample of Class II/2 subjects and relatives to address that question and possible common etiological factors, including genes associated with tooth development and hypodontia, are needed.

A start on this was made when DNA markers (single nucleotide polymorphisms, also referred to as SNPs) in two genes associated with dental development and or hypodontia, *MSX1, PAX9, AXIN2. RUNX2* and *RUNX3* were investigated in 94 Class II/2 Caucasian subjects (31 with hypodontia) compared to 89 non-Class II/2 Caucasian subjects without hypodontia. (Morford et al., 2010b; Morford et al., 2010a) A borderline-association of all Class II/2 subjects with the *PAX9* SNP (rs8004560) was identified (p=0.06). A borderline-association of the same rs8004560 *PAX9* SNP was also identified for subjects with Class II/2 with hypodontia of any permanent tooth, excluding third-molars, when compared to non-Class II/2 without hypodontia (p=0.08) but not when compared to Class II/2 without hypodontia (p=0.46). No associations of Class II/2 with the *PAX9* rs1955734, *MSX1* rs3821949, *RUNX2* (rs1406846), *RUNX3* (rs6672420), or *AXIN2* (rs7591, rs2240308) genotypes were identified. There was a significant association (p=0.0286) for Class II/2 subjects (with or without hypodontia) and the *RUNX2* rs6930053 SNP. However, there was no association of *RUNX2* rs6930053 for subjects with Class II/2 that had hypodontia of any permanent tooth, including third-molars, when compared to Class II/2 subjects without hypodontia (p=0.3858). This suggests a mild impact of *PAX9* (or a locus in linkage-disequilibrium with it) on the development of Class II/2 with hypodontia, and that *RUNX2* (or genetic loci in linkage-disequilibrium with *RUNX2*) plays a role in Class II/2 development but not in the occasionally-associated hypodontia. These findings and other DNA markers should be investigated in a larger Caucasian and other ethnic groups.(Malinowski, 1983; Strohmayer, 1937; Suzuki, 1961)

5.4 Class III malocclusion

Although all Angle occlusion types a Class III malocclusion were initially only based on the sagittal relationship of the permanent first molars, it has generally been recognized that this dental relationship is often observed with a corresponding skeletal relationship as well. Thus, the Class III malocclusion is a complex disorder characterized by a combination of dental and skeletal features that characteristically result in the appearance of a prominent lower jaw. Often referred to as mandibular prognathism (taken from the Greek pro =forward and gnathos =jaw), skeletal aspects of this disorder can be a result of pure mandibular prognathism, maxillary hypoplasia/retrognathism, or a combination of the two. These phenotypic variations create a significant heterogeneity among Class III subjects that can vary according to sex and ethnicity, and account for some of the difficulty encountered when investigating the condition.(Singh, 1999) The familial nature of mandibular prognathism was first reported by Strohmayer (1937) as noted by Wolff et al (1993) in their analysis of the pedigree of the Hapsburg family.(Wolff et al., 1993)

The highest prevalence of Class III malocclusion is observed in East Asian populations such as Korean, Chinese, and Japanese (8%-40%).(Allwright, 1964; Ishii et al., 2002) By comparison, African populations exhibit a reduced prevalence rate (3-8%) compared to Asian samples(Emrich et al., 1965; Garner & Butt, 1985), as do individuals of European or European-American (Caucasian) decent (reports varying between 0.48%-9.5%, with most in the 3-5% range)(Davidov et al., 1961; Emrich et al., 1965; Goose et al., 1957; Helm, 1968; Horowitz, 1970; Ingervall, 1974; Laine & Hausen, 1983; Luffingham & Campbell, 1974; Massler & Frankel, 1951; Solow & Helm, 1968; Tipton & Rinchuse, 1991) While the prevalence in a sample of Native American Chippewa Indian children is relatively low (2.6-3.1%),(Grewe et al., 1968) North American Eskimos in Labrador, Canada have a class III prevalence of approximately 16%.(Zammit et al., 1995) (Zammit, Hans, et al. 1995)

Populations in South America are often a mixture of Caucasian/European, African and Amerindian decent. While the percentage of children in Bogotá, Colombia with Class III has been reported as 3.7%, Brazilian children exhibited a frequency between 4 -10%.(Grando et al., 2008; Martins Mda & Lima, 2009; Thilander et al., 2001) In areas of the Middle East, the prevalence of class III also displays variation with the highest prevalence in Egypt at 10.6%,(El-Mangoury & Mostafa, 1990) followed by 7.8% in Iran,(Borzabadi-Farahani et al., 2009) and 5.1% in Lebanon.(Saleh, 1999)

Several studies have suggested the existence of multiple patterns or sub-phenotypes of the Class III malocclusion based on anatomical appearance. For example, Ellis and McNamara reported considerable variation among class III patients. The most common combination of variables was a retrusive maxilla, protrusive maxillary incisors, retrusive mandibular incisors, a protrusive mandible, and a long lower facial height.(Ellis & McNamara, 1984) Although they did not find significant sex differences, Baccetti et al. showed a significant degree of sexual dimorphism in craniofacial features in subjects with class III malocclusion.(Baccetti et al., 2005) The female Class III subjects presented smaller linear dimensions in the maxilla, mandible, and anterior facial heights when compared with male subjects. The increase in mandibular growth was three times greater in males with class III than in subjects with normal occlusion.(Baccetti et al., 2007) Martone and colleagues suggested that craniofacial growth generates several head form types resulting in anatomic sub-groupings of Classes III.(Martone et al., 1992) Mackay et al (1992) identified five Class III subgroups, all of which exhibited mandibular prognathism.(Mackay et al., 1992) English children with Class III malocclusions divided into groups (normal anteroposterior positioned mandibles and protruded mandibles) according to their SNB angle were found to have significant differences in both groups relating to sagittal position of the maxilla and mandibular rotation.(Hashim & Sarhan, 1993)

Bui et al (2006) found five clusters representing distinct subphenotypes of class III malocclusion. The groupings of variables reflected anteroposterior and vertical dimensions rather than specific craniofacial structures, suggesting that different genes are involved in controlling dimension versus structure. The five subgroupings or "Prototype Clusters" were described as follows: (1) prognathic mandible with long face, (2) maxillary deficiency with decreased vertical dimension (low angle), (3) maxillary deficiency with increased vertical dimension (high angle), (4) mild prognathic mandible with normal vertical dimension, and (5) a combination of prognathic mandible and maxillary deficiency with normal vertical dimension.(Bui et al., 2006) Further studies of the variation of the subtypes of the Class III phenotype within families should facilitate increased understanding of the genetic and non-genetic factors involved.

The genetic factors appear to be heterogeneous, with monogenic (usually autosomal dominant with incomplete penetrance and variable expressivity) influences in some families and multifactorial (polygenic complex) influences in others.(Cruz et al., 2008; Downs, 1927 ; El-Gheriani et al., 2003; Krauss et al., 1959; Litton et al., 1970; Niswander, 1975; Stiles & Luke, 1953; Strohmayer, 1937; Thompson & Winter, 1988; Wolff et al., 1993) This contributes to the variety of anatomical changes in the cranial base, maxilla, and mandible that may be associated with "mandibular prognathism" or a Class III malocclusion.(Bui et al., 2006; Singh, 1999) The prevalence of Class III malocclusion varies among races and can show different anatomic characteristics between races.(Ishii et al., 2002) Considering this heterogeneity, and possible epistasis (the interaction between or among gene products on their expression) and even epigenetics, it is not surprising that genetic linkage and candidate gene studies to date have indicated the possible location of genetic loci influencing this trait in several chromosomal locations (see figure 5).(Falcão-Alencar et al., 2010; Frazier-Bowers et al., 2009; Jang et al., 2010; Li et al., 2010; Li et al., 2011; Tassopoulou-Fishell et al., 2011; Xue et al., 2010; Yamaguchi et al., 2005)

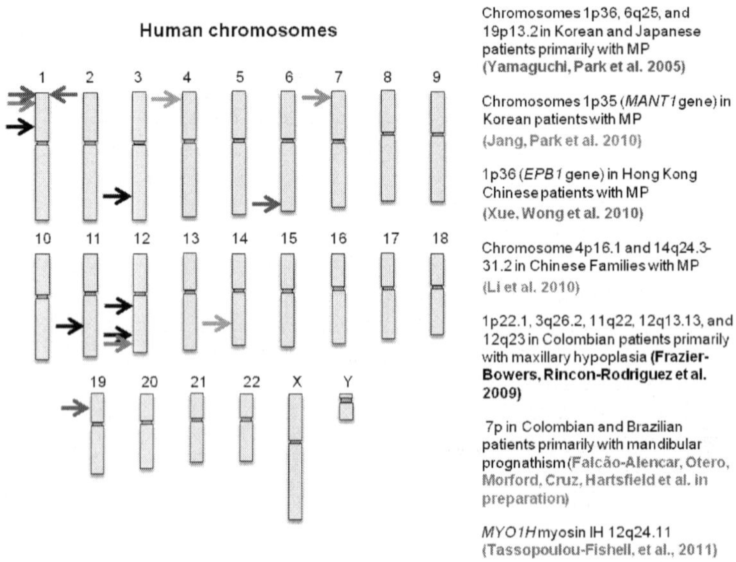

Fig. 5. Chromosome location of markers linked or associated with Class III malocclusion in humans.

6. Personalized orthdontics

In summary, "Personalized Medicine" is a new buzz phrase, based initially upon pharmacogenetics and now exploding as genome-wide association and pathway studies are undertaken. The understanding of the combination and interaction of genetic and environmental (including treatment) factors (nature and nurture together) that influence the growth treatment response of our patients is fundamental to the evidence based practice of orthodontics. Conclusions from retrospective studies must be evaluated by prospective testing to truly evaluate their value in practice. Genome-wide association studies, metabolic pathway analysis and candidate gene studies are necessary to further the evidence base for the practice of orthodontics to determine what the best treatment plan is for each patient in the era of truly personalized orthodontics.(Hartsfield, 2008)

7. References

Allwright, W.C. (1964). A survey of handicapping dentofacial anomalies among Chinese in Hong Kong. *Int Dent J*, Vol. 14, No. 1964), pp. 505-519,

Arya, B.S., Savara, B.S., Clarkson, Q.D. & Thomas, D.R. (1973). Genetic variability of craniofacial dimensions. *The Angle orthodontist,* Vol. 43, No. 2, (Apr 1973), pp. 207-215, 0003-3219 (Print)

Ast, D.B., Carlos, J.P. & Cons, N.C. (1965). The Prevalence and Characteristics of Malocclusion among Senior High School Students in Upstate New York. *American journal of orthodontics,* Vol. 51, No. (Jun 1965), pp. 437-445, 0002-9416

Baccetti, T., Reyes, B.C. & McNamara, J.A., Jr. (2005). Gender differences in Class III malocclusion. *The Angle orthodontist,* Vol. 75, No. 4, (Jul 2005), pp. 510-520, 0003-3219 (Print) 0003-3219 (Linking)

Baccetti, T., Reyes, B.C. & McNamara, J.A., Jr. (2007). Craniofacial changes in Class III malocclusion as related to skeletal and dental maturation. *American journal of orthodontics and dentofacial orthopedics : official publication of the American Association of Orthodontists, its constituent societies, and the American Board of Orthodontics,* Vol. 132, No. 2, (Aug 2007), pp. 171 e171-171 e112, 1097-6752 (Electronic) 0889-5406 (Linking)

Basdra, E.K., Kiokpasoglou, M. & Stellzig, A. (2000). The Class II Division 2 craniofacial type is associated with numerous congenital tooth anomalies. *European journal of orthodontics,* Vol. 22, No. 5, (Oct 2000), pp. 529-535, 0141-5387

Basdra, E.K., Kiokpasoglou, M.N. & Komposch, G. (2001). Congenital tooth anomalies and malocclusions: a genetic link? *European journal of orthodontics,* Vol. 23, No. 2, (Apr 2001), pp. 145-151, 0141-5387

Bernabe, E. & Flores-Mir, C. (2006). Dental morphology and crowding. A multivariate approach. *The Angle orthodontist,* Vol. 76, No. 1, (Jan 2006), pp. 20-25, 0003-3219 (Print) 0003-3219 (Linking)

Boraas, J.C., Messer, L.B. & Till, M.J. (1988). A genetic contribution to dental caries, occlusion, and morphology as demonstrated by twins reared apart. *Journal of dental research,* Vol. 67, No. 9, (Sep 1988), pp. 1150-1155, 0022-0345 (Print)

Borzabadi-Farahani, A., Borzabadi-Farahani, A. & Eslamipour, F. (2009). Malocclusion and occlusal traits in an urban Iranian population. An epidemiological study of 11- to 14-year-old children. *European journal of orthodontics,* Vol. 31, No. 5, (Oct 2009), pp. 477-484, 1460-2210 (Electronic) 0141-5387 (Linking)

Bui, C., King, T., Proffit, W. & Frazier-Bowers, S. (2006). Phenotypic characterization of Class III patients. *The Angle orthodontist,* Vol. 76, No. 4, (Jul 2006), pp. 564-569, 0003-3219 (Print) 0003-3219 (Linking)

Bulun, S.E., Sebastian, S., Takayama, K., Suzuki, T., Sasano, H. & Shozu, M. (2003). The human CYP19 (aromatase P450) gene: update on physiologic roles and genomic organization of promoters. *J Steroid Biochem Mol Biol,* Vol. 86, No. 3-5, (Sep 2003), pp. 219-224, 0960-0760 (Print)

Buschang, P.H. & Hinton, R.J. (2005). A Gradient of Potential for Modifying Craniofacial Growth. *Semin Orthod,* Vol. 11, No. 2005), pp. 219-226,

Byard, P.J., Poosha, D.V., Satyanarayana, M. & Rao, D.C. (1985). Family resemblance for components of craniofacial size and shape. *Journal of craniofacial genetics and developmental biology,* Vol. 5, No. 3, 1985), pp. 229-238, 0270-4145 (Print) 0270-4145 (Linking)

Cassidy, K.M., Harris, E.F., Tolley, E.A. & Keim, R.G. (1998). Genetic influence on dental arch form in orthodontic patients. *The Angle orthodontist,* Vol. 68, No. 5, (Oct 1998), pp. 445-454, 0003-3219 (Print)

Chung, C.S. & Niswander, J.D. (1975). Genetic and epidemiologic studies of oral characteristics in Hawaii's schoolchildren: V. Sibling correlations in occlusion traits. *Journal of dental research,* Vol. 54, No. 2, (Mar-Apr 1975), pp. 324-329, 0022-0345 (Print)

Chvatal, B.A., Behrents, R.G., Ceen, R.F. & Buschang, P.H. (2005). Development and testing of multilevel models for longitudinal craniofacial growth prediction. *American journal of orthodontics and dentofacial orthopedics : official publication of the American Association of Orthodontists, its constituent societies, and the American Board of Orthodontics,* Vol. 128, No. 1, (Jul 2005), pp. 45-56, 0889-5406 (Print)

Corruccini, R.S. & Potter, R.H. (1980). Genetic analysis of occlusal variation in twins. *American journal of orthodontics,* Vol. 78, No. 2, (Aug 1980), pp. 140-154, 0002-9416 (Print)

Corruccini, R.S. (1984). An epidemiologic transition in dental occlusion in world populations. *American journal of orthodontics,* Vol. 86, No. 5, (Nov 1984), pp. 419-426, 0002-9416 (Print)

Corruccini, R.S., Sharma, K. & Potter, R.H. (1986). Comparative genetic variance and heritability of dental occlusal variables in U.S. and Northwest Indian twins. *American journal of physical anthropology,* Vol. 70, No. 3, (Jul 1986), pp. 293-299, 0002-9483 (Print)

Corruccini, R.S. (1990). Australian aboriginal tooth succession, interproximal attrition, and Begg's theory. *American journal of orthodontics and dentofacial orthopedics : official publication of the American Association of Orthodontists, its constituent societies, and the American Board of Orthodontics,* Vol. 97, No. 4, (Apr 1990), pp. 349-357, 0889-5406 (Print) 0889-5406 (Linking)

Corruccini, R.S., Townsend, G.C., Richards, L.C. & Brown, T. (1990). Genetic and environmental determinants of dental occlusal variation in twins of different nationalities. *Hum Biol,* Vol. 62, No. 3, 1990), pp. 353-367.,

Cruz, R.M., Krieger, H., Ferreira, R., Mah, J., Hartsfield, J., Jr. & Oliveira, S. (2008). Major gene and multifactorial inheritance of mandibular prognathism. *American journal of medical genetics. Part A,* Vol. 146A, No. 1, (Jan 1 2008), pp. 71-77, 1552-4833 (Electronic) 1552-4825 (Linking)

Davidov, S., Geseva, N., Donveca, T. & Dehova, L. (1961). Incidence of prognathism in Bulgaria. *Dental Abstracts,* Vol. 6, No. 1961), pp. 240,

Devor, E.J. (1987). Transmission of human craniofacial dimensions. *Journal of craniofacial genetics and developmental biology,* Vol. 7, No. 2, 1987), pp. 95-106, 0270-4145 (Print)

Downs, W.G. (1927). Studies in the Causes of Dental Anomalies. . *Genetics* Vol. 12, No. 6, (Nov 1927 1927), pp. 570-580, 0016-6731 (Print) 0016-6731 (Linking)

El-Gheriani, A.A., Maher, B.S., El-Gheriani, A.S., Sciote, J.J., Abu-Shahba, F.A., Al-Azemi, R. & Marazita, M.L. (2003). Segregation analysis of mandibular prognathism in Libya. *Journal of dental research,* Vol. 82, No. 7, (Jul 2003), pp. 523-527, 0022-0345 (Print) 0022-0345 (Linking)

El-Mangoury, N.H. & Mostafa, Y.A. (1990). Epidemiologic panorama of dental occlusion. *The Angle orthodontist,* Vol. 60, No. 3, (Fall 1990), pp. 207-214, 0003-3219 (Print) 0003-3219 (Linking)

Ellis, E., 3rd & McNamara, J.A., Jr. (1984). Components of adult Class III malocclusion. *J Oral Maxillofacial Surg,* Vol. 42, No. 5, (May 1984), pp. 295-305, 0278-2391 (Print) 0278-2391 (Linking)

Emrich, R.E., Brodie, A.G. & Blayney, J.R. (1965). Prevalence of Class 1, Class 2, and Class 3 malocclusions (Angle) in an urban population. An epidemiological study. *Journal of dental research,* Vol. 44, No. 5, (Sep-Oct 1965), pp. 947-953, 0022-0345 (Print) 0022-0345 (Linking)

Everett, E.T., Britto, D.A., Ward, R.E. & Hartsfield, J.K., Jr. (1999). A novel FGFR2 gene mutation in Crouzon syndrome associated with apparent nonpenetrance. *The Cleft palate-craniofacial journal : official publication of the American Cleft Palate-Craniofacial Association,* Vol. 36, No. 6, (Nov 1999), pp. 533-541, 1055-6656 (Print)

Falcão-Alencar, G., Ortero, L., Cruz, R.M., Foroud, T.M., Dongbing, L., Koller, D., Morford, L.A., Ferrari, I., Oliveira, S.F. & Hartsfield, J.K. (2010). *Evidence for Genetic Linkage of the Class III Craniofacial Phenotype With Human Chromosome 7 in 36 South American Families,* (abstract/program #975). Presented at the 60th Annual Meeting of The American Society of Human Genetics, November 3, 2010, Washington, DC).

Fernex, E., Hauenstein, P. & Roche, M. (1967). [Heredity and craniofacial morphology]. *Report of the congress. European Orthodontic Society,* Vol. No. 1967), pp. 239-257,

Frazier-Bowers, S., Rincon-Rodriguez, R., Zhou, J., Alexander, K. & Lange, E. (2009). Evidence of linkage in a Hispanic cohort with a Class III dentofacial phenotype. *Journal of dental research,* Vol. 88, No. 1, (Jan 2009), pp. 56-60, 1544-0591 (Electronic) 0022-0345 (Linking)

Fujita, T., Kawata, T., Tokimasa, C., Kohno, S., Kaku, M. & Tanne, K. (2001). Breadth of the mandibular condyle affected by disturbances of the sex hormones in ovariectomized and orchiectomized mice. *Clinical orthodontics and research,* Vol. 4, No. 3, (Aug 2001), pp. 172-176, 1397-5927 (Print) 1397-5927 (Linking)

Fujita, T., Ohtani, J., Shigekawa, M., Kawata, T., Kaku, M., Kohno, S., Tsutsui, K., Tenjo, K., Motokawa, M., Tohma, Y. & Tanne, K. (2004). Effects of sex hormone disturbances on craniofacial growth in newborn mice. *Journal of dental research,* Vol. 83, No. 3, (Mar 2004), pp. 250-254, 0022-0345 (Print) 0022-0345 (Linking)

Fujita, T., Ohtani, J., Shigekawa, M., Kawata, T., Kaku, M., Kohno, S., Motokawa, M., Tohma, Y. & Tanne, K. (2006). Influence of sex hormone disturbances on the internal structure of the mandible in newborn mice. *European journal of orthodontics,* Vol. 28, No. 2, (Apr 2006), pp. 190-194, 0141-5387 (Print) 0141-5387 (Linking)

Gabory, A., Attig, L. & Junien, C. (2009). Sexual dimorphism in environmental epigenetic programming. *Molecular and cellular endocrinology,* Vol. 304, No. 1-2, (May 25 2009), pp. 8-18, 1872-8057 (Electronic) 0303-7207 (Linking)

Garner, L.D. & Butt, M.H. (1985). Malocclusion in black Americans and Nyeri Kenyans. An epidemiologic study. *The Angle orthodontist,* Vol. 55, No. 2, (Apr 1985), pp. 139-146, 0003-3219 (Print) 0003-3219 (Linking)

Gass, J.R., Valiathan, M., Tiwari, H.K., Hans, M.G. & Elston, R.C. (2003). Familial correlations and heritability of maxillary midline diastema. *American journal of orthodontics and dentofacial orthopedics : official publication of the American Association of Orthodontists, its constituent societies, and the American Board of Orthodontics,* Vol. 123, No. 1, (Jan 2003), pp. 35-39, 0889-5406 (Print)

Goose, D.H., Thomson, D.G. & Winter, F.C. (1957). Malocclusion in schoolchildren of the west Midlands. *British Dental Journal,* Vol. 102, No. 1957), pp. 174-178,

Grando, G., Young, A.A., Vedovello Filho, M., Vedovello, S.A. & Ramirez-Yanez, G.O. (2008). Prevalence of malocclusions in a young Brazilian population. *International journal of orthodontics,* Vol. 19, No. 2, (Summer 2008), pp. 13-16, 1539-1450 (Print) 1539-1450 (Linking)

Grewe, J.M., Cervenka, J., Shapiro, B.L. & Witkop, C.J., Jr. (1968). Prevalence o f malocclusion in Chippewa Indian children. *Journal of dental research,* Vol. 47, No. 2, (Mar-Apr 1968), pp. 302-305, 0022-0345 (Print) 0022-0345 (Linking)

Grumbach, M.M. (2000). Estrogen, bone, growth and sex: a sea change in conventional wisdom. *J Pediatr Endocrinol Metab,* Vol. 13 Suppl 6, No. 2000), pp. 1439-1455, 0334-018X (Print)

Gu, Y. & McNamara, J.A. (2007). Mandibular growth changes and cervical vertebral maturation. a cephalometric implant study. *The Angle orthodontist,* Vol. 77, No. 6, (Nov 2007), pp. 947-953, 0003-3219 (Print)

Guo, Y., Xiong, D.H., Yang, T.L., Guo, Y.F., Recker, R.R. & Deng, H.W. (2006). Polymorphisms of estrogen-biosynthesis genes CYP17 and CYP19 may influence age at menarche: a genetic association study in Caucasian females. *Human molecular genetics,* Vol. 15, No. 16, (Aug 15 2006), pp. 2401-2408, 0964-6906 (Print)

Harris, E.F. & Smith, R.J. (1980). A study of occlusion and arch widths in families. *American journal of orthodontics,* Vol. 78, No. 2, (Aug 1980), pp. 155-163, 0002-9416 (Print)

Harris, E.F. & Johnson, M.G. (1991). Heritability of craniometric and occlusal variables: a longitudinal sib analysis. *American journal of orthodontics and dentofacial orthopedics : official publication of the American Association of Orthodontists, its constituent societies, and the American Board of Orthodontics,* Vol. 99, No. 3, (Mar 1991), pp. 258-268, 0889-5406 (Print)

Harris, E.F. & Potter, R.H. (1997). Sources of bias in heritability studies. *American journal of orthodontics and dentofacial orthopedics : official publication of the American Association of Orthodontists, its constituent societies, and the American Board of Orthodontics,* Vol. 112, No. 3, (Sep 1997), pp. 17A-21A, 0889-5406 (Print)

Harris, E.F. (2008). Interpreting Heritability Estimates in the Orthodontic Literature. *Semin Orthod,* Vol. 14, No. 2008), pp. 125-134,

Harris, J.E., Kowalski, C.J. & Watnick, S.S. (1973). Genetic factors in the shape of the craniofacial complex. *The Angle orthodontist,* Vol. 43, No. 1, (Jan 1973), pp. 107-111, 0003-3219 (Print)

Harris, J.E., Kowalski, C.J. & Walker, S.J. (1975). Intrafamilial dentofacial associations for Class II, Division 1 probands. *American journal of orthodontics,* Vol. 67, No. 5, (May 1975), pp. 563-570, 0002-9416 (Print)

Harris, J.E. & Kowalski, C.J. (1976). All in the family: use of familial information in orthodontic diagnosis, case assessment, and treatment planning. *American journal of orthodontics,* Vol. 69, No. 5, (May 1976), pp. 493-510, 0002-9416 (Print)

Hartsfield, J.K., Jr. (2008). Personalized Orthodontics, The Future of Genetics in Practice. *Semin Orthod,* Vol. 14, No. 2008), pp. 166-171,

Hartsfield, J.K., Jr., Zhou, J. & Chen, S. (2010).In: *Surgical Enhancement of Orthodontic Treatment, Craniofacial Growth Series, Department of Orthodontics and Pediatric Dentistry and Center for Human Growth and Development,* J.A. McNamara & S.D. Kapila, pp. 267-281, The University of Michigan,Ann Arbor

Hartsfield, J.K., Jr. (2011).5, In: *Orthodontics : current principles and techniques,* L.W. Graber, R.L. Vanarsdall & K.W.L. Vig, pp. 139-156, Elsevier Mosby,0323066410 St Louis

Hartsfield, J.K., Jr. & Bixler, D. (2011).6, In: *McDonald's and Avery's dentistry for the child and adolescent,* J.A. Dean, D.R. Avery & R.E. McDonald, pp. 64-84, Mosby/Elsevier,9780323057240, St. Louis, Mo.

Hartsfield Jr., J.K., Zhou, J. & Chen, S. (2010). Genetic Variation in the CYP19A1/Aromatase Gene and Facial Growth. *Journal of dental research,* Vol. 89, No. Special Issue A, 2010), pp. Abstract 63, (www.dentalresearch.org).

Hashim, H.A. & Sarhan, O.A. (1993). Dento-skeletal components of class III malocclusions for children with normal and protruded mandibles. *The Journal of clinical pediatric dentistry,* Vol. 18, No. 1, (Fall 1993), pp. 12-16, 1053-4628 (Print) 1053-4628 (Linking)

Hashim, H.A. & Al-Ghamdi, S. (2005). Tooth width and arch dimensions in normal and malocclusion samples: an odontometric study. *J Contemp Dent Pract,* Vol. 6, No. 2, (May 15 2005), pp. 36-51, 1526-3711 (Electronic) 1526-3711 (Linking)

Hauspie, R.C., Susanne, C. & Defrise-Gussenhoven, E. (1985). Testing for the presence of genetic variance in factors of face measurements of Belgian twins. *Annals of human biology,* Vol. 12, No. 5, (Sep-Oct 1985), pp. 429-440, 0301-4460 (Print)

He, S., Hartsfield, J., Guo, Y., Cao, Y., Wang, S. & Chen, S. (2011). *Association between CYP19A1 SNPs and haplotypes and pubertal sagittal jaw growth,* Submitted to the Journal of Dental Research.

Helm, S. (1968). Malocclusion in Danish children with adolescent dentition: an epidemiologic study. *American journal of orthodontics,* Vol. 54, No. 5, (May 1968), pp. 352-366, 0002-9416 (Print) 0002-9416 (Linking)

Hennekam, R.C.M., Allanson, J.E., Krantz, I.D. & Gorlin, R.J. (2010). *Gorlin's syndromes of the head and neck* (edition), Oxford University Press, 9780195307900 (alk. paper), Oxford; New York

Honjo, H., Tamura, T., Matsumoto, Y., Kawata, M., Ogino, Y., Tanaka, K., Yamamoto, T., Ueda, S. & Okada, H. (1992). Estrogen as a growth factor to central nervous cells. Estrogen treatment promotes development of acetylcholinesterase-positive basal forebrain neurons transplanted in the anterior eye chamber. *J Steroid Biochem Mol Biol,* Vol. 41, No. 3-8, (Mar 1992), pp. 633-635, 0960-0760 (Print)

Horowitz, H.S. (1970). A study of occlusal relations in 10 to 12 year old Caucasian and Negro children--summary report. *International dental journal,* Vol. 20, No. 4, (Dec 1970), pp. 593-605, 0020-6539 (Print) 0020-6539 (Linking)

Horowitz, S.L., Osborne, R.H. & DeGeorge, F.V. (1960). A Cephalometric Study Of Craniofacial Variation In Adult Twins. *The Angle orthodontist,* Vol. 30, No. 1, 1960), pp. 1-5,

Hunter, W.S., Balbach, D.R. & Lamphiear, D.E. (1970). The heritability of attained growth in the human face. *American journal of orthodontics,* Vol. 58, No. 2, (Aug 1970), pp. 128-134, 0002-9416 (Print) 0002-9416 (Linking)

Hunter, W.S. (1990). *Heredity in the craniofacial complex.* (edition), Saunders, Philadelphia

Hunter, W.S., Baumrind, S., Popovich, F. & Jorgensen, G. (2007). Forecasting the timing of peak mandibular growth in males by using skeletal age. *American journal of orthodontics and dentofacial orthopedics : official publication of the American Association of Orthodontists, its constituent societies, and the American Board of Orthodontics,* Vol. 131, No. 3, (Mar 2007), pp. 327-333, 1097-6752 (Electronic)

Ingervall, B. (1974). Prevalence of dental and occlusal anomalies in Swedish conscripts. *Acta odontologica Scandinavica,* Vol. 32, No. 2, 1974), pp. 83-92, 0001-6357 (Print) 0001-6357 (Linking)

Ishii, N., Deguchi, T. & Hunt, N.P. (2002). Craniofacial differences between Japanese and British Caucasian females with a skeletal Class III malocclusion. *European journal of orthodontics,* Vol. 24, No. 5, (Oct 2002), pp. 493-499, 0141-5387 (Print) 0141-5387 (Linking)

Jang, J.Y., Park, E.K., Ryoo, H.M., Shin, H.I., Kim, T.H., Jang, J.S., Park, H.S., Choi, J.Y. & Kwon, T.G. (2010). Polymorphisms in the Matrilin-1 gene and risk of mandibular prognathism in Koreans. *Journal of dental research,* Vol. 89, No. 11, (Nov 2010), pp. 1203-1207, 1544-0591 (Electronic) 0022-0345 (Linking)

Johannsdottir, B., Thorarinsson, F., Thordarson, A. & Magnusson, T.E. (2005). Heritability of craniofacial characteristics between parents and offspring estimated from lateral cephalograms. *American journal of orthodontics and dentofacial orthopedics : official publication of the American Association of Orthodontists, its constituent societies, and the American Board of Orthodontics,* Vol. 127, No. 2, (Feb 2005), pp. 200-207; quiz 260-201, 0889-5406 (Print) 0889-5406 (Linking)

Kang, E.H., Yamaguchi, T., Tajima, A., Nakajima, T., Tomoyasu, Y., Watanabe, M., Yamaguchi, M., Park, S.B., Maki, K. & Inoue, I. (2009). Association of the growth hormone receptor gene polymorphisms with mandibular height in a Korean population. *Archives of oral biology,* Vol. 54, No. 6, (Jun 2009), pp. 556-562, 1879-1506 (Electronic) 0003-9969 (Linking)

Kawala, B., Antoszewska, J. & Necka, A. (2007). Genetics or environment? A twin-method study of malocclusions. *World journal of orthodontics,* Vol. 8, No. 4, (Winter 2007), pp. 405-410, 1530-5678 (Print) 1530-5678 (Linking)

King, L., Harris, E.F. & Tolley, E.A. (1993). Heritability of cephalometric and occlusal variables as assessed from siblings with overt malocclusions. *American journal of orthodontics and dentofacial orthopedics : official publication of the American Association of*

Orthodontists, its constituent societies, and the American Board of Orthodontics, Vol. 104, No. 2, (Aug 1993), pp. 121-131, 0889-5406 (Print)

Klingenberg, C.P., Leamy, L.J. & Cheverud, J.M. (2004). Integration and modularity of quantitative trait locus effects on geometric shape in the mouse mandible. *Genetics,* Vol. 166, No. 4, (Apr 2004), pp. 1909-1921, 0016-6731 (Print) 0016-6731 (Linking)

Kraus, B.S., Wise, W.J. & Frei, R.H. (1959). Heredity and the craniofacial complex. *American journal of orthodontics,* Vol. 45, No. 1959), pp. 172,

Kraus, P. & Lufkin, T. (2006). Dlx homeobox gene control of mammalian limb and craniofacial development. *American journal of medical genetics. Part A,* Vol. 140, No. 13, (Jul 1 2006), pp. 1366-1374, 1552-4825 (Print) 1552-4825 (Linking)

Krauss, B., Wise, W. & Frei, R. (1959). Heredity and the craniofacial complex. *American journal of orthodontics,* Vol. 45, No. 1959), pp. 172-217,

Laine, T. & Hausen, H. (1983). Occlusal anomalies in Finnish students related to age, sex, absent permanent teeth and orthodontic treatment. *European journal of orthodontics,* Vol. 5, No. 2, (May 1983), pp. 125-131, 0141-5387 (Print) 0141-5387 (Linking)

Lambert, M.-P. & Herceg, Z. (2011). *Mechanisms of Epigenetic Gene Silencing,* Epigenetic Aspects of Chronic Diseases. H.I. Roach, F. Bronner & R.O.C. Oreffo. Springer, London. 41-53

Lavelle, C.L. (1983). Study of mandibular shape in the mouse. *Acta Anat (Basel),* Vol. 117, No. 4, 1983), pp. 314-320, 0001-5180 (Print)

Li, Q., Zhang, F., Li, X. & Chen, F. (2010). Genome scan for locus involved in mandibular prognathism in pedigrees from China. *PLoS One,* Vol. 5, No. 9, 2010), pp. 1932-6203 (Electronic) 1932-6203 (Linking)

Li, Q., Li, X., Zhang, F. & Chen, F. (2011). The identification of a novel locus for mandibular prognathism in the Han Chinese population. *Journal of dental research,* Vol. 90, No. 1, (Jan 2011), pp. 53-57, 1544-0591 (Electronic) 0022-0345 (Linking)

Litton, S.F., Ackermann, L.V., Isaacson, R.J. & Shapiro, B.L. (1970). A genetic study of Class 3 malocclusion. *American journal of orthodontics,* Vol. 58, No. 6, (Dec 1970), pp. 565-577, 0002-9416 (Print) 0002-9416 (Linking)

Lobb, W.K. (1987). Craniofacial morphology and occlusal variation in monozygous and dizygous twins. *The Angle orthodontist,* Vol. 57, No. 3, (Jul 1987), pp. 219-233, 0003-3219 (Print) 0003-3219 (Linking)

Luffingham, J.K. & Campbell, H.M. (1974). The need for orthodontic treatment. A pilot survey of 14 year old school children in Paisley, Scotland. *Transactions. European Orthodontic Society,* Vol. No. 1974), pp. 259-267,

Lundstrom, A. & McWilliam, J.S. (1987). A comparison of vertical and horizontal cephalometric variables with regard to heritability. *European journal of orthodontics,* Vol. 9, No. 2, (May 1987), pp. 104-108, 0141-5387 (Print)

Mackay, F., Jones, J.A., Thompson, R. & Simpson, W. (1992). Craniofacial form in class III cases. *British journal of orthodontics,* Vol. 19, No. 1, (Feb 1992), pp. 15-20, 0301-228X (Print) 0301-228X (Linking)

Malinowski, A. (1983). Changes in dimensions and proportions of the human mandible during fetal period. *Collegium antropologicum,* Vol. 7, No. 1983), pp. 65-70,

Manfredi, C., Martina, R., Grossi, G.B. & Giuliani, M. (1997). Heritability of 39 orthodontic cephalometric parameters on MZ, DZ twins and MN-paired singletons. *American journal of orthodontics and dentofacial orthopedics : official publication of the American Association of Orthodontists, its constituent societies, and the American Board of Orthodontics,* Vol. 111, No. 1, (Jan 1997), pp. 44-51, 0889-5406 (Print) 0889-5406 (Linking)

Maor, G., Segev, Y. & Phillip, M. (1999). Testosterone stimulates insulin-like growth factor-I and insulin-like growth factor-I-receptor gene expression in the mandibular condyle--a model of endochondral ossification. *Endocrinology,* Vol. 140, No. 4, (Apr 1999), pp. 1901-1910, 0013-7227 (Print) 0013-7227 (Linking)

Markovic, M.D. (1992). At the crossroads of oral facial genetics. *European journal of orthodontics,* Vol. 14, No. 6, (Dec 1992), pp. 469-481, 0141-5387 (Print) 0141-5387 (Linking)

Martins Mda, G. & Lima, K.C. (2009). Prevalence of malocclusions in 10- to 12-year-old schoolchildren in Ceara, Brazil. *Oral health & preventive dentistry,* Vol. 7, No. 3, 2009), pp. 217-223, 1602-1622 (Print) 1602-1622 (Linking)

Martone, V.D., Enlow, D.H., Hans, M.G., Broadbent, B.H., Jr. & Oyen, O. (1992). Class I and Class III malocclusion sub-groupings related to headform type. *The Angle orthodontist,* Vol. 62, No. 1, (Spring 1992), pp. 35-42; discussion 43-34, 0003-3219 (Print) 0003-3219 (Linking)

Massler, M. & Frankel, J.M. (1951). Prevalence of malocclusion in children aged 14 to 18 years. *American journal of orthodontics,* Vol. 37, No. 10, (Oct 1951), pp. 751-768, 0002-9416 (Print) 0002-9416 (Linking)

Mills, L.F. (1966). Epidemiologic studies of occlusion. IV. The prevalence of malocclusion in a population of 1,455 school children. *Journal of dental research,* Vol. 45, No. 2, (Mar-Apr 1966), pp. 332-336, 0022-0345

Morford, L.A., Coles, T.J., Fardo, D.W., Wall, M.D., Morrison, M.W., Kula, K.S. & Hartsfield, J.K., Jr. (2010a). *Assocaiton analysis of Class II division 2 (CII/D2) with RUNX2 and RUNX3* Journal of dental research. 89 (Special Iss B) abstract #1948:

Morford, L.A., Wall, M.D., Morrison, M.W., Kula, K.S. & Hartsfield, J.K., Jr. (2010b). *Association Analysis of Class-II Division-2 (CII/D2) with PAX9 and MSX1,* Journal of dental research. 89 (Special Iss A) abstract #633:

Morrison, M.W. (2008). *Relative Risk of Class II division 2 Malocclusion in First-Degree Relatives of Probands with Class II division 2 Malocclusion,* Department of Orthodontics and Oral Facial Genetics. Indiana University School of Dentistry, Master of Science in Dentistry degree:

Moss, M.L. (1997a). The functional matrix hypothesis revisited. 4. The epigenetic antithesis and the resolving synthesis. *American journal of orthodontics and dentofacial orthopedics : official publication of the American Association of Orthodontists, its constituent societies, and the American Board of Orthodontics,* Vol. 112, No. 4, 1997a), pp. 410-417.,

Moss, M.L. (1997b). The functional matrix hypothesis revisited. 3. The genomic thesis. *American journal of orthodontics and dentofacial orthopedics : official publication of the*

American Association of Orthodontists, its constituent societies, and the American Board of Orthodontics, Vol. 112, No. 3, 1997b), pp. 338-342.,

Mossey, P.A. (1999a). The heritability of malocclusion: Part 1--Genetics, principles and terminology. *British journal of orthodontics,* Vol. 26, No. 2, (Jun 1999a), pp. 103-113, 0301-228X (Print)

Mossey, P.A. (1999b). The heritability of malocclusion: part 2. The influence of genetics in malocclusion. *British journal of orthodontics,* Vol. 26, No. 3, (Sep 1999b), pp. 195-203, 0301-228X (Print) 0301-228X (Linking)

Nakasima, A., Ichinose, M., Nakata, S. & Takahama, Y. (1982). Hereditary factors in the craniofacial morphology of Angle's Class II and Class III malocclusions. *American journal of orthodontics,* Vol. 82, No. 2, (Aug 1982), pp. 150-156, 0002-9416 (Print) 0002-9416 (Linking)

Nakata, N., Yu, P.I., Davis, B. & Nance, W.E. (1973). The use of genetic data in the prediction of craniofacial dimensions. *American journal of orthodontics,* Vol. 63, No. 5, (May 1973), pp. 471-480, 0002-9416 (Print) 0002-9416 (Linking)

Nikolova, M. (1996). Similarities in anthropometrical traits of children and their parents in a Bulgarian population. *Annals of human genetics,* Vol. 60, No. Pt 6, (Nov 1996), pp. 517-525, 0003-4800 (Print) 0003-4800 (Linking)

Niswander, J.D. (1975). Genetics of common dental disorders. *Dent Clin North Am,* Vol. 19, No. 1, (Jan 1975), pp. 197-206, 0011-8532 (Print)

Peck, S., Peck, L. & Kataja, M. (1998). Class II Division 2 malocclusion: a heritable pattern of small teeth in well-developed jaws. *The Angle orthodontist,* Vol. 68, No. 1, (Feb 1998), pp. 9-20, 0003-3219

Poosti, M. & Jalali, T. (2007). Tooth size and arch dimension in uncrowded versus crowded Class I malocclusions. *J Contemp Dent Pract,* Vol. 8, No. 3, 2007), pp. 45-52, 1526-3711 (Electronic) 1526-3711 (Linking)

Proffit, W.R. (1986). On the aetiology of malocclusion. The Northcroft lecture, 1985 presented to the British Society for the Study of Orthodontics, Oxford, April 18, 1985. *British journal of orthodontics,* Vol. 13, No. 1, (Jan 1986), pp. 1-11, 0301-228X (Print)

Ruf, S. & Pancherz, H. (1999). Class II Division 2 malocclusion: genetics or environment? A case report of monozygotic twins. *The Angle orthodontist,* Vol. 69, No. 4, (Aug 1999), pp. 321-324, 0003-3219

Saleh, F.K. (1999). Prevalence of malocclusion in a sample of Lebanese schoolchildren: an epidemiological study. *Eastern Mediterranean health journal = La revue de sante de la Mediterranee orientale = al-Majallah al-sihhiyah li-sharq al-mutawassit,* Vol. 5, No. 2, (Mar 1999), pp. 337-343, 1020-3397 (Print) 1020-3397 (Linking)

Sasaki, Y., Satoh, K., Hayasaki, H., Fukumoto, S., Fujiwara, T. & Nonaka, K. (2009). The P561T polymorphism of the growth hormone receptor gene has an inhibitory effect on mandibular growth in young children. *European journal of orthodontics,* Vol. 31, No. 5, (Oct 2009), pp. 536-541, 1460-2210 (Electronic) 0141-5387 (Linking)

Saunders, S.R., Popovich, F. & Thompson, G.W. (1980). A family study of craniofacial dimensions in the Burlington Growth Centre sample. *American journal of orthodontics,* Vol. 78, No. 4, (Oct 1980), pp. 394-403, 0002-9416 (Print) 0002-9416 (Linking)

Schaefer, K., Fink, B., Mitteroecker, P., Neave, N. & Bookstein, F.L. (2005). Visualizing facial shape regression upon 2nd to 4th digit ratio and testosterone. *Collegium antropologicum,* Vol. 29, No. 2, (Dec 2005), pp. 415-419, 0350-6134 (Print) 0350-6134 (Linking)

Schaefer, K., Fink, B., Grammer, K., Mitteroecker, P., Gunz, P. & Bookstein, F.L. (2006). Female appearance: facial and bodily attractiveness as shape. *Psych Sci,* Vol. 48, No. 2006), pp. 187-204,

Schwartz, D.A. (2010). Epigenetics and environmental lung disease. *Proceedings of the American Thoracic Society,* Vol. 7, No. 2, (May 2010), pp. 123-125, 1943-5665 (Electronic) 1546-3222 (Linking)

Singh, G.D. (1999). Morphologic determinants in the etiology of class III malocclusions: a review. *Clinical anatomy,* Vol. 12, No. 5, 1999), pp. 382-405, 0897-3806 (Print) 0897-3806 (Linking)

Solow, B. & Helm, S. (1968). A method for tabulation and statistical evaluation of epidemiological malocclusion data. *Acta odontologica Scandinavica,* Vol. 26, No. 1, (May 1968), pp. 63-88, 0001-6357 (Print) 0001-6357 (Linking)

Stiles, K. & Luke, J. (1953). The inheritance of malocclusion due to mandibular prognathism. *J of Hereditary,* Vol. 44, No. 1953), pp. 241-245,

Strohmayer, W. (1937). Die Vereburg des Hapsburger Familientypus. *Nova Acta Leopoldina,* Vol. 5, No. 1937), pp. 219-296,

Susanne, C. & Sharma, P.D. (1978). Multivariate analysis of head measurements in Punjabi families. *Annals of human biology,* Vol. 5, No. 2, (Mar 1978), pp. 179-183, 0301-4460 (Print)

Suzuki, S. (1961). Studies on the so-called reverse occlusion. *The Journal of Nihon University School of Dentistry,* Vol. 3, No. 1961), pp. 51-58,

Tassopoulou-Fishell, M., Deeley, K., Harvey, E., Sciote, J. & Viera, A. (2011). MYO1H contributes to Class III malocclusion. *Journal of dental research,* Vol. 90 (Special Iss A) abstract #248, No. 2011), pp.

Thesleff, I. (2006). The genetic basis of tooth development and dental defects. *American journal of medical genetics. Part A,* Vol. 140, No. 23, (Dec 1 2006), pp. 2530-2535, 1552-4825 (Print) 1552-4825 (Linking)

Thilander, B., Pena, L., Infante, C., Parada, S.S. & de Mayorga, C. (2001). Prevalence of malocclusion and orthodontic treatment need in children and adolescents in Bogota, Colombia. An epidemiological study related to different stages of dental development. *European journal of orthodontics,* Vol. 23, No. 2, (Apr 2001), pp. 153-167, 0141-5387 (Print) 0141-5387 (Linking)

Thompson, E.M. & Winter, R.M. (1988). Another family with the 'Habsburg jaw'. *Journal of medical genetics,* Vol. 25, No. 12, (Dec 1988), pp. 838-842, 0022-2593 (Print) 0022-2593 (Linking)

Ting, T.Y., Wong, R.W. & Rabie, A.B. (2011). Analysis of genetic polymorphisms in skeletal Class I crowding. *American journal of orthodontics and dentofacial orthopedics : official publication of the American Association of Orthodontists, its constituent societies, and the*

American Board of Orthodontics, Vol. 140, No. 1, (Jul 2011), pp. e9-15, 1097-6752 (Electronic) 0889-5406 (Linking)

Tipton, R.T. & Rinchuse, D.J. (1991). The relationship between static occlusion and functional occlusion in a dental school population. *The Angle orthodontist,* Vol. 61, No. 1, (Spring 1991), pp. 57-66, 0003-3219 (Print) 0003-3219 (Linking)

Tomoyasu, Y., Yamaguchi, T., Tajima, A., Nakajima, T., Inoue, I. & Maki, K. (2009). Further evidence for an association between mandibular height and the growth hormone receptor gene in a Japanese population. *American journal of orthodontics and dentofacial orthopedics : official publication of the American Association of Orthodontists, its constituent societies, and the American Board of Orthodontics,* Vol. 136, No. 4, (Oct 2009), pp. 536-541, 1097-6752 (Electronic) 0889-5406 (Linking)

Townsend, G., Richards, L. & Hughes, T. (2003). Molar intercuspal dimensions: genetic input to phenotypic variation. *Journal of dental research,* Vol. 82, No. 5, (May 2003), pp. 350-355, 0022-0345 (Print)

Turchetta, B.J., Fishman, L.S. & Subtelny, J.D. (2007). Facial growth prediction: a comparison of methodologies. *American journal of orthodontics and dentofacial orthopedics : official publication of the American Association of Orthodontists, its constituent societies, and the American Board of Orthodontics,* Vol. 132, No. 4, (Oct 2007), pp. 439-449, 1097-6752 (Electronic)

Verdonck, A., De Ridder, L., Verbeke, G., Bourguignon, J.P., Carels, C., Kuhn, E.R., Darras, V. & de Zegher, F. (1998). Comparative effects of neonatal and prepubertal castration on craniofacial growth in rats. *Archives of oral biology,* Vol. 43, No. 11, (Nov 1998), pp. 861-871, 0003-9969 (Print) 0003-9969 (Linking)

Verdonck, A., Gaethofs, M., Carels, C. & de Zegher, F. (1999). Effect of low-dose testosterone treatment on craniofacial growth in boys with delayed puberty. *European journal of orthodontics,* Vol. 21, No. 2, (Apr 1999), pp. 137-143, 0141-5387 (Print) 0141-5387 (Linking)

Verma, D., Peltomaki, T. & Jager, A. (2009). Reliability of growth prediction with hand-wrist radiographs. *European journal of orthodontics,* Vol. 31, No. 4, (Aug 2009), pp. 438-442, 1460-2210 (Electronic)

Watnick, S.S. (1972). Inheritance of craniofacial morphology. *The Angle orthodontist,* Vol. 42, No. 4, (Oct 1972), pp. 339-351, 0003-3219 (Print) 0003-3219 (Linking)

Wolff, G., Wienker, T.F. & Sander, H. (1993). On the genetics of mandibular prognathism: analysis of large European noble families. *Journal of medical genetics,* Vol. 30, No. 2, (Feb 1993), pp. 112-116, 0022-2593 (Print) 0022-2593 (Linking)

Xue, F., Wong, R.W. & Rabie, A.B. (2010). Genes, genetics, and Class III malocclusion. *Orthodontics & craniofacial research,* Vol. 13, No. 2, (May 2010), pp. 69-74, 1601-6343 (Electronic) 1601-6335 (Linking)

Yamaguchi, T., Maki, K. & Shibasaki, Y. (2001). Growth hormone receptor gene variant and mandibular height in the normal Japanese population. *American journal of orthodontics and dentofacial orthopedics : official publication of the American Association of Orthodontists, its constituent societies, and the American Board of Orthodontics,* Vol. 119, No. 6, (Jun 2001), pp. 650-653, 0889-5406 (Print)

Yamaguchi, T., Park, S.B., Narita, A., Maki, K. & Inoue, I. (2005). Genome-wide linkage analysis of mandibular prognathism in Korean and Japanese patients. *Journal of dental research,* Vol. 84, No. 3, (Mar 2005), pp. 255-259, 0022-0345 (Print) 0022-0345 (Linking)

Zammit, M.P., Hans, M.G., Broadbent, B.H., Johnsen, D.C., Latimer, B.M. & Nelson, S. (1995). Malocclusion in Labrador Inuit youth: a psychosocial, dental and cephalometric evaluation. *Arctic medical research,* Vol. 54, No. 1, (Jan 1995), pp. 32-44, 0782-226X (Print) 0782-226X (Linking)

A Simplified Method to Determine the Potential Growth in Orthodontics Patients

Gladia Toledo Mayarí
School of Dentistry/ Havana Medical University
Cuba

1. Introduction

The current Orthodontics worries is about the early correction of malocclusion, giving importance to the harmonization of the bone bases in connection with the discrepancy and positioning of the teeth, that can be corrected in any time of life, for what is of great importance is to know the biggest peak of growth (Peluffo, 2001; Quirós 2000).

The maturation stages can have a considerable influence in the diagnosis, the goals of the treatment, the planning and the eventual result of the orthodontic treatment (Madhu et al., 2003; Toledo 2004).

The clinical decisions with regards to the use of the extraoral force, functional appliances, the treatment without extractions and the orthognatic surgeon is based on the considerations of the growth, for this reason, the prediction of the quantity of active growth, mainly in the craniofacial complex, are useful to the orthodontists (Toledo, 2004).

The orthodontic diagnosis has a group of stages in those that have multiple evaluation factors which are used in the study of the malocclusions. In general evaluation of a patient, it is important to consider the general physical development and the potential growth (Quirós 2000).

The pubertal growth spurt of is an advantageous period in the orthodontic treatment and it should be kept in mind in connection with the planning of the treatment. One of the objectives of the orthodontic treatment during the adolescence, in the cases with skeletal discrepancies is to take advantage of the changes of growth of the patient. (Fiani, 1998; Padrós & Creus, 2002).

In the adolescent, the phase of somatic maturity can influence in the selection of the appliances, the course of the treatment and the retention after the therapy (Geran et al. 2006). Because of this the study and the knowledge of the maturation stage and the phase of growth of the patient, is very important for making more efficient therapy. Authors like Nanda (Nanda, 1955), Björk and Helm (Björk & Helm, 1967), and Hägg and Taranger (Hägg & Taranger, 1980a, 1980b, 1982) established that the pattern of growth and facial development is similar to that of the general skeletal growth, and that the maximum peak of pubertal growth of the craniofacial structures occurs between 6 and 8 months after the maximum peak of pubertal growth in the stature.

Due to the wide individual variation, the chronological age cannot be used in the evaluation of the pubertal growth (Fiani, 1998), for that reason is appealed to determine the biological age. It is calculated starting from the bone, dental, morphological and sexual ages (Ceglia, 2005).

The study of the bone maturation is the surest and reliable method to evaluate the biological age of the individuals and to fix the physiologic maturity (Gutiérrez Muñiz et al. 2006).

In spite of the difficulties that outline the different existent methods (quality of the X-ray, minimum modifications of the projection, variability intra and inter observant, errors in the reading of the online systems, population in which the method is based, etc.) the evaluation of the bone maturation is indispensable in the clinical practice, since it is a parameter of great importance in the study of the alterations of the growth (Paesano et al, 1998).

The hand, the wrist and the distal epiphysis of the radius and the ulna present a great number of secondary centers of ossification on the whole, and they can reproduce in a single X-ray. For this reason, they are often chosen as study centers when it is sought to determine the state of skeletal maturation, although other centers of ossification of secondary epiphysis can be used, such as, the elbow and the tarsal bones (Cha, 2003).

Todd, in 1937, was the first author that mentioned the term "determinant of the maturity", when referring to the gradual changes that occur on the growth of the cartilage during the trial of coalition of the epiphysis with the diaphysis and that they can be determined by studying radiographic plaques (Quirós Álvarez, 2006). Years later Greulich and Pyle called them indicators of maturity and in 1959 they established the norms of skeletal age to value the bone maturation of the complete hand (Greulich & Pyle, 1959). As the different epiphyses don't often mature at the same time, discrepancies that are resolved with subjective trials which subtract precision to the method arise (Tanner et al. 1983).

Tanner and Whitehouse (Tanner et al. 1983), develop the method Tanner - Whitehouse 2 (TW2) to evaluate the bone development, through X-rays of the lefts hand and wrist, which has had great acceptance for their precision, being used at the present time in numerous countries (Izaguirre de Espinoza et al. 2003; Jiménez Hernández et al., 1986; Ortega et al., 2006).

In 1979, the professor Jordan (Jordan, 1979) publishes the results of the Study of Physical Growth in Cuba, where it uses the method TW2 in the determination of the bone maturation. Later on, in 1987 a group of investigators of the Department of Growth and Human Development determine the patterns of the Cuban population's bone maturation for sex and race through the method TW2 (Jiménez JM et al., 1987). This method is one of those that is used in Cuba in the evaluation of the bone maturation (Abreu Suárez et al., 1995).

Some authors have looked in the X-rays of the hand specific indicators of the spurt of pubertal growth (Fishman, 1982). Björk and Helm (Björk & Helm, 1967) and Gupta (Gupta, 1995) point out as a reliable indicator of the installation of the puberty, the beginning of the ossification of the sesamoid bone. Toledo (Toledo, 2004) and Rakosi and Jonas (Rakosi & Jonas, 1992) affirm that the appearance of the hook of the hamate bone is also a good indicator of the installation of the puberty.

In Maxillary Orthopedics one of the most utilized methods in the evaluation of the growth potential has been the one of Grave and Brown (Rakosi & Jonas, 1992; Tedaldi et al., 2007) that it divides the process of maturation of the bones of the hand in nine stages, between the 9th and the 17th year of age. The ossification characteristics are detected to the level of the phalanges, bones of the carpus and radius, and the stages of growth of the fingers are valued according to the relationship between the epiphysis and the diaphysis (Fiani, 1998). The evaluation of the Grave and Brown's method is recommended by Ortiz et al. (Ortiz et al., 2007), Spinelli Casanova et al. (Spinelli Casanova et al, 2006) and Pancherz and Hägg (Pancherz & Hägg, 1985) before the therapeutic interceptive in Orthodontics patients, to choose the ideal treatment according to the stages of bone maturation that the patient presents, diminishing this way the time in the use of the appliances and making them more effective. Previous to the realization of this investigation (Toledo Mayarí & Otaño Lugo, 2010a, 2010b, 2010c), was not reported in Cuba the use of Grave and Brown's method.

The inconvenience that presents the evaluation of the bone maturation through the hand in orthodontics patients , is the use of an additional X-ray for the patient, besides that this is not carried out with the dental X-ray machine, being necessary to remit the patient to a radiology service.

The current tendency in Orthodontics is to reduce the number of X-rays to the strictly necessary ones (Bujaldón Daza et al., 1998), for that indexes of skeletal maturation have been developed with the profiles of the bodies of the cervical vertebras that generally appear in the lateral teleradiography of skull used for the orthodontist diagnostic (Ortiz et al., 2007), being discharges correlations in the evaluations of the bone age between the cervical vertebras and the bones of the hand (Edilmar et al., 2005; Gandini et al., 2006; Hassel & Farman, 1995; San Roman et al., 2002; Uysal et al., 2006).

Also with the objective of substituting the X-ray of the hand that constitutes an additional exhibition to radiations in the patients of Orthodontics, Leite et al. (Leite et al., 1987), analyze the first three fingers, which include in the lateral teleradiography of skull and they don't find significant differences between the analysis of the bone maturation of the total hand and that of the three fingers. Shigemi Goto et al. (Shigemi Goto et al., 1996) and Rossi et al. (Rossi et al., 1999), analyze the changes at level of the first finger, in the distal phalanx and in the proximal respectively, finding that the evaluations at level of the phalanges constitute a quick and useful clinical method, to evaluate the growth potential in patient of Orthodontics. Madhu et al. (Madhu et al., 2003) and Ozer et al.((Ozer et al., 2006) use the stages of maturation of the middle phalange of the third finger, visualized in an X-ray of 41x31mm., taken with a machine of dental X rays conventional, where they find out that the evaluation of the stages of maturation of the middle phalanx of the third finger, constitutes an alternative method that can be used to determine the bone maturation, of the children in growth. Previous to the realization of this investigation, was not reports that in Cuba the patient's growth potential was evaluated through the middle phalange of the third finger, that which motivated us to determine the stages of maturation of that phalange and to identify the concordance between these and the stages of skeletal maturation, whereas clause that of existing concordance among the same ones, we will have a simplified method, for the determination of the growth potential, without the necessity of using an X-ray of the hand and an additional X-rays machine.

Problem of Investigation:

Whereas clause that in Orthodontics the evaluation of the growth potential has influence in the diagnosis, the treatment plan, the results and the prognostic of the treatment, and that the evaluation of the bone maturation through the X-ray of the hand, that is the anatomical area that is used in the evaluation of the bone maturation in Cuba, constitutes an additional X-ray for the tributary patients of orthodontist treatment, it would be necessary to respond:

What is the bone age of our patients?

What stages of skeletal maturation and of maturation of the middle phalange of the third finger they do present the same ones?

What is the relationship between the bone age and the chronological age, the stages of skeletal maturation and the stages of maturation of the middle phalange of the third finger in our patients?

What concordance does it exist among the methods to determine the growth potential in patient of Orthodontics?

The formulation of these questions forms the bases of a hypothesis that can be defined as it continues:

Considering that the growth potential constitutes the grade of growth becomes for the individual between the state in the moment of the exam and the definitive ceasing of this. In the determination of this potential, inside the diagnosis in Orthodontics, you can substitute the radiographic of the hand, being clinically useful the analysis of the bone maturation through the middle phalange of the third finger.

To give answers to the questions and the hypothesis, the following objectives were formulated:

General objective: To propose a simplified method to determine the growth potential in Orthodontics patient.

Specific objectives:

1. To determine according to sex and chronological age: the bone age, the stages of skeletal maturation and the stages of maturation of the middle phalange of the third finger.
2. To identify the relationship between the bone age and: the chronological age, the stages of skeletal maturation and the stages of maturation of the middle phalange of the third finger.
3. To identify the concordance between the studied methods.

2. Background

In this epigraph are approached theoretical aspects of great importance in the specialty of Orthodontics that were considered in this investigation, due to the great majority of the children that go to the clinic and they are tributary of orthodontic treatment, they are in periods of growth and development, reason why when ignoring their biological age, we could incur in errors when outlining a diagnosis, prognostic and treatment plan.

The terms of growth and development are used to indicate the series of changes of volume, forms and weight that suffers the organism from the fecundation until the mature age (Cannut Brusola, 1988; J. Mayoral & G. Mayoral, 1990).

The growth in an individual's active development, is a continuous phenomenon that begins in the moment of the conception and it culminates at the end of the puberty, period during which reaches the maturity in their physical, psycho-social and reproductive aspects. Both processes have characteristic communes to all the individuals of the same species, what makes them predictable, however, they present wide differences between the subjects, given by the pattern's of growth individual character and development. This typical pattern emerges on one hand of the interaction of genetic and environmental factors that establish the growth potential and for other, the magnitude that this potential is expressed (Proffit, 1994).

The chronological age, that constitutes the time lapsed from the birth until the moment of the exam (Proffit, 1994), it doesn't always allow to value the development and the patient's somatic maturation, for that is appear to determine the biological maturity (Fiani, 1998).

According to Gutiérrez Muñiz et al. (Gutiérrez Muñiz et al., 2006) "the concept of biological maturity is defined as the successive transformations through the time, from the conception until the adulthood, existing two applicable fundamental methods at the present time for its evaluation: the bone age and the dental age".

The bone age is established determining radiograph of the number and size of the centers of ossification epiphysis, which should be compared with the existent norms for each age and sex (Recalde Cortes et al. 1997; Tanner et al., 1983). Each bone begins with a primary center of ossification that will grow progressively at the same time that is remodeled being able to acquire an or more epiphysis and finally it will acquire the mature form with the coalition from the epiphysis to the body of the bone. The sequence for each bone is the same as for the events that will happen in it, taking place independently late to the grade or advance with regard to the chronological age (Cattani, 2003; Fiani, 1998; Proffit, 1994).

The potential growth constitutes the grade of growth becomes for the individual between the state in the moment of the exam and the definitive ceasing of this (Proffit, 1994). It is given by the existent relationship between the bone age and the chronological age: to smaller bone age for a certain chronological age the individual's growth potential will be bigger, that is to say, the grade late of the bone age in connection with the chronological age reflects theoretically the years of growth residual extra or, that is the same thing, the years of growth that he has left before the closing of the epiphysis (Cattani, 2003; Proffit, 1994).

Theoretically, any part of the body can be used to determine the bone age, but in practice the hand and the wrist, are the most used, because they possess a great number of bones and epiphyses in development what allows the pursuit of the changes that happen through the years of the growth (Freitas et al. 2004; Jordan, 1979). They are also the most convenient areas to value the bone maturation, to be far from the gonads and to need less radiation (Jordán et al. 1987; Recalde Cortes et al. 1997).

The methods that are used to evaluate the growth potential of the left hand are: the TW2 that determines the bone age according to the maturation stages of each one of the bones; and the Grave and Brown that divides the process of maturation of the bones in nine stages of skeletal maturation. These two methods have disadvantage for the Orthodontics patients because the use of an additional X-ray, which is not carried out in the dental X rays machine, being necessary the patient's remission.

The current tendency in Orthodontics in the evaluation of the bone maturation is to reduce the number of X-rays to the strictly necessary ones (Bujaldón Daza et al., 1998), for that investigators exist as: Hassel and Farman (Hassel & Farman, 1995) that they try to develop some indexes of skeletal maturation with the profiles of the bodies of the cervical vertebras that appear in the lateral teleradiography of skull used for the orthodontist diagnostic. The advantages of using the cervical vertebras, it is centered in the reduction of radiographies to those that are subjected to the patients and for the easiness of consenting to the same ones (Ortiz et al., 2007).

Also in patient of Orthodontics with the objective of doing without of the X-ray of the hand that constitutes an additional exhibition to radiations, and it implies the use of a machine of rays X that is not used in a conventional way in Dentistry; the evaluation of the bone maturation has been used and of the growth potential through the development of the phalanges, that also has the purpose of simplifying the estimate, since alone the changes are analyzed at level of some phalanges, according to the relationship between the epiphysis and the diaphysis (Madhu et al., 2003).

Inside the diagnosis in Orthodontics, it is very important the evaluation of the growth potential, since most of the patients that require orthodontist treatment, are in a period of active growth, and with the treatment it can modify the facial growth, well be braking it, accelerating it or forward a normal vector (Tedaldi et al, 2007). According to Proffit (Proffit, 1994) it is not possible to modify a growth that is not taking place, and if a functional apparatus is placed on a patient that is not growing, the obtained result will be almost totally a dental mobilization.

The children with maxillary discrepancies usually benefit from the application of techniques to modify the growth. Since the bones of the face, and in particular the maxillary ones, suffer spontaneous changes during the different phases of growth, before establishing a treatment to correct skeletal malocclusions, it is necessary to know the opportune moment to begin the same one, according to the growth potential that the patient presents, to make more efficient our therapy (Tedaldi et al., 2007, Proffit, 1994).

The guiding principle is that growth can only be modified when it is occurring (Proffit, 1994), there is the importance of knowing the growth potential that the patient presents, when we carry out the diagnosis of the skeletal problems. Keeping in mind these aspects motivates ourselves to determine in the same sample three appraisal methods of the growth potential (Method TW2, Serious method and Brown, and determination of the stages of maturation of the half phalange of the third finger), with the objective of to propose a simplified method to determine the growth potential in patient of Orthodontics.

3. Methodological design

A cross-sectional technological innovation research was conducted in the period of January 2004 to April 2007, in the Clinic of Orthodontics of Havana School of Dentistry, in a sample of 150 patients between 8 and 16 years of age. A sampling was used by quotas according to sex and age, being divided in two groups, 75 for each sex. The patients were selected with previous condition to present good state of general health; to have measures of weight and height, that were between 10 and 90 percentile, of the Cuban Score of Weight for Height (Gutiérrez Muñiz et al., 2006); absence of chronic illnesses; absence of oligodontias; absences of congenital malformations; that they didn't have treatment corrective of the spinal column ; the need for the characteristics of their malocclusion, the realization of a lateral teleradiography of skull to complete their diagnosis; and to have signed the informed consent in writing.

3.1 Variables

Were studied the variables: chronological age, bone age (TW2), sex, stages of skeletal maturation and stages of maturation of the middle phalanx of the third finger.

Chronological age: Was considered the decimal age (Jordán, 1979): For the calculation, we subtracted the boy's date of birth and the date of the exam. The numeral was provided by the last two digits of the year and the decimal fraction was looked for in the table of decimal age.

Bone age (TW2): Was calculated in dependence of the sum of the punctuation of each stage for Radius, Ulna and Fingers, according to the patterns of the Cuban population's bone maturation, for the method TW2 (Jiménez et al., 1987).

Sex: Female and male.

Stages of skeletal maturation: Was classified according to Grave and Brown's method in stages of the 1 at 9.

Stages of maturation of the middle phalanx of the third finger: Was classified according to the relationship among the epiphysis and the diaphysis in one of the following stages (Toledo, 2004):

a. The epiphysis has smaller width than the diaphysis.
b. The epiphysis has the same width with the diaphysis.
c. The epiphysis surrounds the diaphysis by way of cap.
d. Begins the coalition between the epiphysis and the diaphysis.
e. Where the epiphysis becomes ossified with the diaphysis.

3.2 Ethical aspects

With all the patients that participated in the investigation and their parents, an interview was conducted before the beginning of that, where they were explained on what it consisted with the study, frequency, evaluation type and the radiological protection measures that would be taken for not damaging the patient's health. If they agreed, the patients and their parents should sign the informed consent, approving their holding in the study.

3.3 Technical and procedures of obtaining the information

3.3.1 For the determination of: The bone age and the stages of skeletal maturation

Firstly you proceeded to each observer's training in the appraisal methods of the studied maturation. The information was picked up and analyzed by two residents and two specialists of Orthodontics, each resident and each specialist determined in the same sample, one of the two methods of study of the maturation analyzed in this investigation (method TW2 and method of Grave and Brown).

To each patient was made the clinical history of Orthodontics and was realized an radiographic of the left hand (Fig. 1) where they were determined: the bone age for the method TW2 (Jiménez et al, 1987) and the stages of skeletal maturation for the method of Grave and Brown (Tedaldi et al. 2007).

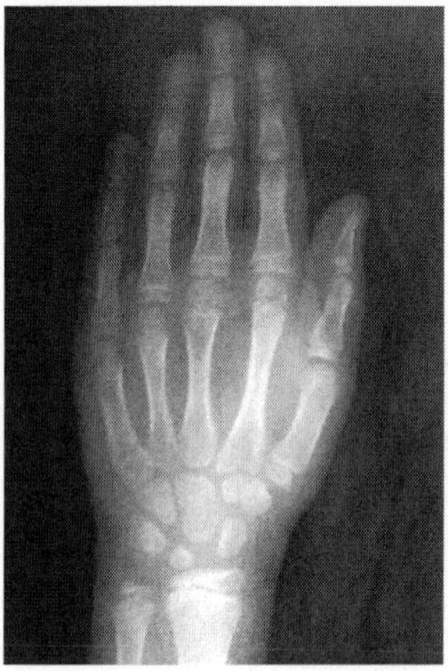

Fig. 1. Radiographic of the left hand.

The radiographic of the left hand was realized with the same regulations that the utilized ones in the National Study of Growth and Human Development in Cuba, carried out by Jordan (Jordán, 1979).

Each radiographic of the left hand was evaluated by the resident and the specialist in a first observation and in three weeks later in a second observation; that is to say a total of four times to calculate the variability inter and intra observant. The cases where discrepancy existed they were studied again to obtain the final results.

3.3.2 To determine the stages of skeletal maturation of the middle phalanx of the third finger of the left hand

In a paper of size Letter (21,59 cm. x 27,94 cm.), at a distance of 10 cm. of the superior margin and 10 cm. of the left margin, the contour of a film dental standard, Kodak marks, of 41x31 mm. was traced, and it was clipped by the traced area, being an opening in the paper with the dimensions of the dental film.

The paper was placed on the X-rays of the left hand of the 150 studied patients, it was made coincide the opening of the paper on the union between the middle phalanx and the proximal phalanx of the third finger and it was placed on a fixed negatoscope (Fig. 2).

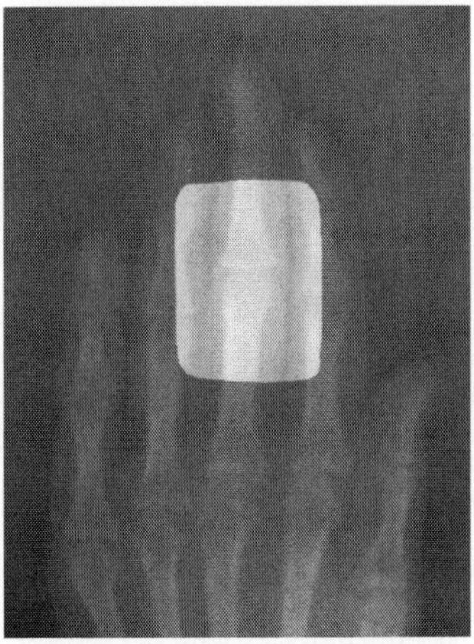

Fig. 2. Placement of the prepared paper on the union between the middle phalanx and the proximal phalanx of the third finger, in the radiographic of the left hand.

The analysis of the radiographic was carried out using a compass to measure the bone size in the middle phalanx and the maturation stage was classified with A to E, according to the classification proposed by Toledo (Toledo, 2004). With this procedure it was possible to locate each patient evaluated in a stage of maturation of the middle phalanx of the third finger, the same one was carried out by the main investigator and a specialist in Orthodontics, member of the investigation team, in two different opportunities to calculate the variability intra and inter observant.

3.4 Technical and procedures of elaboration and analysis

The information was stored in a data base automated in the system Excel, of the package Office 2003 on Windows XP professional and for the prosecution of the results the statistical packages SPSS version 11.5 and STATISTICA version 6.1 were used.

To calculate the variability intra and inter observant in the studied methods, the coefficient Kappa was applied (Begole, 2003).

The percentage was used for the qualitative variables and for the quantitative variables the arithmetic mean like measure summary and the standard deviation like variation measure (Bayarre et al. 2005).

You prove statistics employees: The association grade was calculated among the quantitative variables by means of the lineal correlation coefficient of Pearson (Begole, 2003) and the association grade among the variables in ordinal scales by means of the correlation coefficient of ranges of Spearman (Begole, 2003). To calculate the concordance among the results obtained in the studied methods, the coefficient Kappa was applied (Begole, 2003).

In all the used statistical tests, the used level of significance was of 0.05.

The results were presented in tables designed to the effect.

4. Results

In this epigraph the main results are presented, it contains the analysis of 6 tables.

The analysis of the variability intra and inter observant, their agreement was evaluated regarding the methods studied by means of an index Kappa. With relationship to the variability intra observant, that is to say, the level of discrepancy with regard to the valuations of oneself after three weeks, discrepancies didn't exist, in the three valued methods, being the agreement of 1,000 in the 150 cases, in each one of the methods. With relationship to the variability inter observant, that is to say, the level of discrepancy with regard to the valuations among the two observants, discrepancies didn't exist among these, being the agreement of 1,000 in the 150 cases, for these three methods.

4.1 Determination according to sex and chronological age of: The bone age, the stages of skeletal maturation and the stages of maturation of the middle phalanx of the third finger

4.2 Identification of the relationship among the bone age and: The chronological age, the stages of skeletal maturation and the stages of maturation of the middle phalanx of the third finger

Table 1 shows the arithmetic mean and the standard deviation of the chronological age and the bone age, calculated by the method TW2, according to groups of ages in the feminine sex, were found that in the groups of ages that were between the 8,00 and the 12,99 years and of 15.00 to 16.99 years, the bone age was bigger than the chronological one, being smaller in the remaining groups of ages. The coefficient of lineal correlation of Pearson among the bone age (TW2) and the chronological one presented a value of 0,977; that which signifies a very strong positive correlation, highly significant (p <0,010).

Group of Ages	Chronological age		Bone age (TW2)	
	X_1	DE_1	X_2	DE_2
8,00-8,99	8,38	0,33	8,72	1,22
9,00-9,99	9,87	0,17	10,55	0,47
10,00-10,99	10,53	0,33	10,58	0,98
11,00-11,99	11,58	0,24	12,36	0,47
12,00-12,99	12,75	0,20	13,32	0,89
13,00-13,99	13,42	0,28	12,57	0,73
14,00-14,99	14,86	0,01	14,78	0,46
15,00-16,99	15,19	0,14	15,20	0,70

r= 0,977 p = 0,000 n =75
r (lineal correlation coefficient of Pearson among bone age (TW2) and chronological age).

Table 1. Arithmetic mean (X) and standard deviation (DE) of chronological age and bone age (TW2) by groups of age in females.

Table 2 shows the arithmetic mean and the standard deviation of the chronological age and the bone age calculated by the method TW2 according to groups of ages in the masculine sex, it was found that in the groups of ages that were between 8,00 and 12,99 years, the bone age was smaller than the chronological one, being bigger starting from 13,00 years. The coefficient of lineal correlation of Pearson among the bone age (TW2) and the chronological one presented a value of 0,983; that which signifies a very strong positive correlation, highly significant (p <0,010).

Group of Ages	Chronological age		Bone age (TW2)	
	X_1	DE_1	X_2	DE_2
8,00-9,99	8,98	0,66	8,94	0,97
10,00-10,99	10,83	0,03	9,96	0,87
11,00-11,99	11,40	0,35	11,35	0,92
12,00-12,99	12,66	0,35	12,36	0,94
13,00-13,99	13,44	0,20	14,24	0,47
14,00-14,99	14,52	0,20	14,83	0,37
15,00-15,99	15,55	0,20	15,61	0,48
16,00-16,99	16,40	0,20	16,46	0,61

r = 0,983 p = 0,000 n =75
r (lineal correlation coefficient of Pearson among bone age (TW2) and chronological age).

Table 2. Arithmetic mean (X) and standard deviation (DE) of chronological age and bone age (TW2) by groups of age in males.

Table 3 shows the arithmetic mean and the standard deviation of the chronological age and the bone age (TW2) according to stages of skeletal maturation and sex, it was found that in each maturation stage, the averages of the chronological age were smaller in the feminine sex than in the masculine one. With relationship to the bone age calculated by the method TW2, in the feminine sex the averages of the same one went superior to those of the chronological age, in all the studied stages, however, in the masculine sex the bone age overcame the chronological one in the stages 4, 5, 6 and 8. The stages 4 and 5 are those of more clinical significance, belonged together with the chronological ages of 11,35 and 11,77 years in the feminine sex and 13,76 and 13,82 years in the masculine one and with the bone ages of 11,78 and 12,34 years in the feminine sex and of 14,20 and 14,57 years in the masculine one. It was observed that the females were earlier in their maturation stages than the males and that the stages advanced as it increased the chronological age and the bone age of the patients, in both sexes. The coefficient of correlation of ranges of Spearman among the bone age (TW2) and the stages of skeletal maturation presented a value of 0,855 in the feminine sex and 0,903 in the masculine one, both sexes showed a positive correlation, very significant (p <0,010). In the studied sample they were not patient in the stage 9.

Stages of skeletal maturation	Chronological age				Bone age (TW2)			
	Female		Male		Female		Male	
	X_1	DE_1	X_1	DE_1	X_2	DE_2	X_2	DE_2
1	8,59	0,66	11,38	1,34	8,97	1,25	10,66	1,11
2	10,06	0,54	11,61	0,87	10,25	0,71	10,50	1,20
3	11,63	1,35	11,71	0,65	11,82	0,84	10,50	0,89
4	11,35	1,71	13,76	0,80	11,78	1,18	14,20	0,14
5	11,77	1,18	13,82	1,13	12,34	0,99	14,57	0,72
6	13,34	0,97	14,96	0,97	13,77	0,79	15,46	0,54
7	15,31	0,17	16,35	0,48	15,45	0,07	16,08	0,62
8	14,24	0,98	16,25	0,23	14,45	1,03	16,56	0,28

Sex Female rho= 0,855 p = 0,000 n =75
Sex Male rho= 0,903 p = 0,000 n =75
rho (Correlation coefficient of Spearman among bone age (TW2) and stages of skeletal maturation.

Table 3. Arithmetic mean (X) and standard deviation (DE) of chronological age and bone age (TW2) by stages of skeletal maturation and sex.

Table 4 shows arithmetic mean and the standard deviation of the chronological age and the bone age (TW2) according to stages of maturation of the middle phalanx of the third finger and sex, it was found that in all the maturation stages the averages of the chronological age were smaller in the feminine sex than in the masculine one. In feminine sex the bone age overcame the chronological one in all the stages and in the masculine one in the stages B, C and E. The stage C (cap stage), it happened that 11,77 year-old chronological age and the bone one of 12,34 years, with a standard deviation of 1,18 and 0,99 years respectively in the females, while in the males, went to the 13,82 years and 14,57 years, with a standard deviation of 1,13 and 0,72 years respectively. It was observed that the females were earlier in their maturation stages than the males. The coefficient of correlation of ranges of Spearman among the bone age (TW2) and the stages of maturation of the middle phalanx of the third finger presented a value of 0,888 in the feminine sex and 0,921 in the masculine one, both sexes showed a positive correlation, very significant (p <0,010).

Stages of maturation of the middle phalanx of the third finger	Chronological age				Bone age (TW2)			
	Female		Male		Female		Male	
	X_1	DE_1	X_1	DE_1	X_2	DE_2	X_2	DE_2
A	8,59	0,66	11,38	1,34	8,97	1,25	10,66	1,11
B	11.55	1.4	13.06	0.71	11.52	0.92	13.25	0.92
C	11,77	1,18	13,82	1,13	12,34	0,99	14,57	0,72
D	13.83	1.23	15.93	0.86	13.59	1.17	15.7	0.63
E	14.24	0.98	16.25	0.23	14.45	1.03	16.56	0.28

Sex Female rho= 0,888 p = 0,000 n =75
Sex Male rho= 0,921 p = 0,000 n =75
rho (Correlation coefficient of Spearman among bone age (TW2) and stages of maturation of the middle phalanx of the third finger

Table 4. Arithmetic mean (X) and standard deviation (DE) of chronological age and bone age (TW2) by stages of maturation of the middle phalanx of the third finger and sex.

4.3 Identification of concordance between the studied methods

Table 5 shows the percentages of females according to the stages of skeletal maturation and stages of maturation of the middle phalanx of the third finger, it was found that in the stage of skeletal maturation 1, 100,00% was in the stage A of maturation of the middle phalanx of the third finger; in the stages 2, 3 and 4, 100% was in the stage B of the phalanx; in the stage 5, 100% was in the C; in the 6 and the 7, 100,00% was in the stage D and in the stage 8, 100,00% was in the stage E of the phalanx. The coefficient of concordance Kappa between the stages of skeletal maturation and the stages of maturation of the middle phalanx of the third finger, presented a value of 1,000 that which evidenced a perfect concordance, very significant (p <0.010).

Stages of skeletal maturation	Total	Stages of maturation of the middle phalanx of the third finger									
		A		B		C		D		E	
		#	%	#	%	#	%	#	%	#	%
1	12	12	100,00	-	-	-	-	-	-	-	-
2	8	-	-	8	100,00	-	-	-	-	-	-
3	10	-	-	10	100,00	-	-	-	-	-	-
4	4	-	-	4	100,00	-	-	-	-	-	-
5	15	-	-	-	-	15	100,00	-		-	-
6	6	-	-	-	-	-	-	6	100,00	-	-
7	2	-	-	-	-	-	-	2	100,00	-	-
8	18	-	-	-	-	-	-	-	-	18	100,00

Coefficient Kappa = 1,000 p=0,000 n=75

Table 5. Percentage of females according to stages of skeletal maturation and stages of maturation of the middle phalanx of the third finger.

Table 6 shows the percentages of males according to the stages of skeletal maturation and stages of maturation of the middle phalanx of the third finger, it was found that in the stage of skeletal maturation 1, 100,00% was in the stage A of maturation of the middle phalanx of the third finger; in the stages 2, 3 and 4, 100% was in the stage B of the phalanx; in the stage 5, 100% was in the C; in the 6 the biggest percent was in the D (75,00); in the 7, 100,00% was in the stage D and in the stage 8, 100,00% was in the stage E of the phalanx. The coefficient of concordance Kappa between the stages of skeletal maturation and the stages of maturation of the middle phalanx of the third finger, presented a value of 0,964; that which evidenced a high concordance, very significant (p <0.010).

Stages of skeletal maturation	Total	Stages of maturation of the middle phalanx of the third finger									
		A		B		C		D		E	
		#	%	#	%	#	%	#	%	#	%
1	15	15	100,00	-	-	-	-	-	-	-	-
2	11	-	-	11	100,00	-	-	-	-	-	-
3	12	-	-	12	100,00	-	-	-	-	-	-
4	2	-	-	2	100,00	-	-	-	-	-	-
5	20	-	-	-	-	20	100,00	-	-	-	-
6	8	-	-	-	-	2	25,00	6	75,00	-	-
7	5	-	-	-	-	-	-	5	100,00	-	-
8	2	-	-	-	-	-	-	-	-	2	100,00

Coefficient Kappa = 0,964 p=0,000 n=75

Table 6. Percentage of males according to stages of skeletal maturation and stages of maturation of the middle phalanx of the third finger.

5. Discussion

In this epigraph, one discussed the most important results and they were compared with the results of other investigations, with foundations starting from the revised bibliography.

With relationship to the variability intra and inter observant results were completely coincident in the three studied methods. The author considers that the results are due to the previous training of the investigators in each one of the studied evaluation methods.

With relationship to the variability intra observant and inter observant in the analysis of the stage of maturation of the middle phalanx of the third finger, coincidence existed among the four carried out observations. The author considers that the results are due to the simplification of this method, since in the same alone the changes are analyzed at level of a single phalanx.

In the studied sample, the bone age of the patients, calculated through the method TW2, didn't coincide with the chronological age. These results coincide with those of Malavé and Rojas (Malavé & Rojas, 2000) whom they outlined that, the chronological age is not a good indicator of the level of an individual's bone maturation.

In the three methods of study of the analyzed maturation, it was found that the females matured before the males of their same age. These results coincide with studies carried out for Grave and Townsend (Grave & Townsend, 2003), Demirjian et al. (Demirjian et al, 1985) and Liversidge and Speechly (Liversidge & Speechly, 2001), who they find that, the females mature more early than the males, that which is important to consider in the general evaluation of the orthodontist patient.

There were a positive, very significant correlation (p <0,010) among the bone age (TW2) and the stages of skeletal maturation in both sexes (rho = 0,855 for the females and rho = 0,903 for the males). These results coincide with other carried out studies (Moore et al., 1990; Uysal et al., 2006).

In the analysis of the stages of maturation of the half phalange of the third finger it was found that the females were earlier in their maturation stages than the males. These results belong together with those obtained in other methods analyzed in this investigation and they coincide with those of Hägg and Taranger (Hägg & Taranger, 1980a, 1980b, 1982) who they find that, the females mature early, that which is important to consider in the planning of the orthodontist treatment.

The coefficient of correlation of Spearman among the bone age (TW2) and the stages of maturation of the middle phalanx of the third finger showed positive, very significant correlations (p <0,010); in both sexes (0,888 in the feminine one and 0, 921 in the masculine one). These results coincide with other studies that analyze the bone maturation through the development of the phalanges: Leite et al. (Leite et al., 1987) they carry out a longitudinal study, through which value the age skeletal analyzing the first one, second and third fingers of the hand, in a sample of 19 males radiographies and 20 females whose radiographic of the annual hand-wrist had taken from the 10 to the 16 years for the girls and of 12 to 18 years for the males and they find that although differences exist between the analysis of the total hand and that of the three fingers, the method of the three fingers never strays of that of the hand-wrist for more than 2.89 months for the males with a minimum deviation of 0.32 months and for the females, the maximum deviation was of 4.45 months with a minimum of 1.55 months. They also find that the maximum deviations happen during the time of coalition of the epiphysis with the diaphysis when the growth is coming closer to their finalization and consequently they are not of clinical importance. These authors conclude that the advantage of the use of the method of the three fingers is that they can incorporate in the lateral teleradiography, eliminating this way the necessity of other radiographies.

Shigemi Goto et al. (Shigemi Goto & Yamada Miyazawa, 1996) carry out a study in which analyze the ossification of the distal phalanx of the first finger like an indicator of maturity for the initiation of the orthodontist treatment in 2 Japanese women with Class III malocclusion, where they conclude that the determination of the phases of maturation skeletal of the distal phalanx of the first finger, it can be a quick and useful clinical method, to evaluate the potential of residual growth in the cases of Class III.

Rossi et al. (Rossi et al., 1999) carry out a study in 72 feminine patients with ages understood between 8 and 13 years of age, where they analyze the proximal phalanx of the first finger and they find that in the patients that were in the epiphysis stage C, they were next to the peak of maximum speed of growth pubertal.

In relation of the concordance between the stages of skeletal maturation and the stages of maturation of the middle phalanx of the third finger, in the studied sample a high concordance existed, very significant (p <0,010) in both sexes, being perfect in the feminine sex (1,000). That which coincides with other carried out studies: Rajagopal and Sudhanshu (Rajagopal & Sudhanshu, 2002) carry out a study with the objective of determining the dependability of using radiographic of the middle phalanx of the third finger as an indicator of skeletal maturation, in a sample of 75 girls and 75 children, between the 9 and 17 years of age; where they compare the stages of maturation of the cervical vertebras, and the stages of maturation of the middle phalanx of the third finger and they conclude that the assessment of the growth puberal based on the observations of the middle phalanx of the third finger observed by means of standard X-rays, is an useful method and it has as advantages: the smallest exhibition to the X rays and that X rays supplementary machine is not needed.

Madhu et al. (Madhu et al., 2003) carry out a study with the objective of obtaining a unique and simple method to determine the skeletal maturation using the stages of development of the middle phalanx of the third finger that one observes in a radiographic, taken with a conventional X ray dental machine; in a sample of 67 patients, 35 males between 10 and 18 years of age and 32 females between 8 and 16 years. To the patients they carry out them lateral teleradiographies of skull and an X-ray of the area of the middle phalanx of the third finger, where they determine the stages of maturation of the cervical vertebras of the patients in previous stages to the peak puberal, patient that were in the peak of growth puberal and patient in those that it had already happened the peak of growth puberal and the stages of the middle phalanx of the third finger are classified in 3 stages: patient in the previous period to reach the peak pubertal of growth, patient that are in the period of growth pubertal and those patients that the period of growth pubertal had passed. These authors find agreement among the results obtained in the analysis of the cervical vertebras and of the middle phalanx of the third finger and they conclude that the analysis of the maturation of the middle phalanx of the third finger, is an alternative method that can be used to determine the skeletal maturation of the children in growth.

Ozer et al. (Ozer et al., 2006) carry out a study in 150 masculine patients, with ages understood among 9 and 19 years that were in orthodontist treatment, with the purpose of determining the correlation between the index of maturation of the cervical vertebras and the stages of maturation of the middle phalanx of the third finger, for that which they carry out lateral teleradiography of skull and X-rays of the middle phalanx of the third finger of the left hand, finding high correlation coefficients between the stages of vertebral maturation and those of the phalanges. They conclude that the middle phalanx of the third finger can be used in the evaluation of the skeletal maturation of the patients.

From the clinical point of view in the planning of an orthodontist treatment, we should consider if the patient has begun the spurt of pubertal growth, if this is happening in that moment or if it has concluded (Tedaldi, 2007). With the analysis of the stages of maturation of the middle phalanx of the third finger, visualized in an X-ray of 41 x 31 mm., is possible to determine: if the patient has not reached the spurt of pubertal growth (Stage A), if it is next or this event already began (B), if it is in its maximum peak (C) or if it is in the descending curve of growth pubertal (D and E) (Toledo Mayarí & Otaño Lugo, 2010).

Due to the high correlation coefficient found in this sample, between the stages of maturation of the middle phalanx of the third finger and the bone age in both sexes, as well as to the high concordance found in this study, among the evaluation of the maturation through the left hand and the analysis of the middle phalanx of the third finger, which was perfect in the feminine sex, and considering the current tendency in Orthodontics of reducing the number of radiations, we propose inside the diagnosis for the evaluation of the potential growth of the patients, the realization of an X-ray of 41 x 31 mm. of the middle phalanx of the third finger of the left hand (Fig. 3), with the following requirements:

An auxiliary table will be used, where the radiography of 41x31 mm. will be placed, with the vertical bigger axis coinciding with the same position of the phalanx and with the active face in front of the focus. The radiograph will be located on the union between the middle and proximal phalanx of the third finger of the left hand, with the coincident located reference point with the proximal phalanx. The focus will be centered in perpendicular sense to the table, with an angle of 90 °, at a distance focus film, using short cone, of 11 cm. with a time of exhibition of 0,5 second. The calibration of the machine will be of 110 volt / 10 MA / seg. They will take all the measures of protection radiological established (Ugarte et al., 2004) and a dental machine of X rays and dental films standard of 41x31mm., Kodak marks. The one revealed will be executed looking for soft revealed low contrasts.

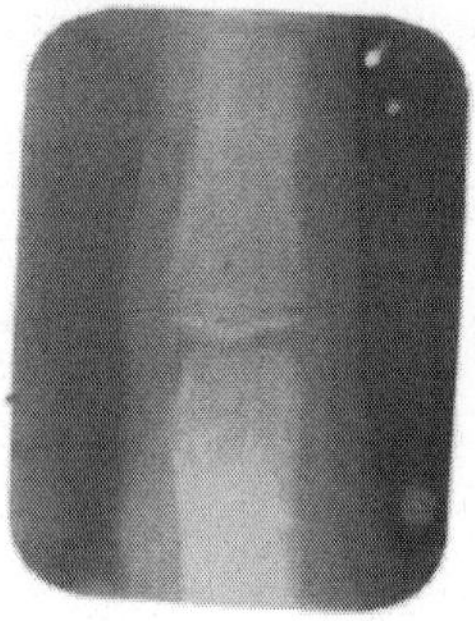

Fig. 3. Radiographic of middle phalanx of the third finger.

The author considers that, in the patients, it is not necessary to carry out a lateral teleradiography of skull, the evaluation of the potential of growth, inside the diagnosis in Orthodontics, one can make through the stages of maturation of the middle phalanx of the third finger of the left hand, which contributes the following benefits:

It constitutes a simplified method that can be applied in any service of Orthodontics and it allows planning for the treatment of orthodontics in dependence of the potential of growth which the patient presents that makes more efficient therapy.

It allows bigger efficiency and decrease of the costs and it can be carried out in the dental X rays machine, for what includes relative savings to the depreciation of the machine of X-rays and the energy consumption.

They diminish the quantity from radiations to those that are exposed to the patients and the auxiliary personnel (technicians in radiology), as well as, the radiations in the local where the radiographies were taken.

6. Conclusions

The evaluation of the potential of growth that the patients of Orthodontics present can be made by means of the realization of radiography of the middle phalanx of the third finger of the left hand.

In the three certain methods, it was found that the females mature before the males of their same age.

It existed a high correlation and concordance among the studied methods of determination of the potential growth.

The substitution of the radiography of the left hand, for the radiography of the middle phalanx of the third finger, allows the realization of that in the own service of Dentistry, with the benefits that it reports as for the patient's better attention.

The results of this study prove the hypothesis formulated and constituted part of the Thesis in option to PhD degree in Dentistry of the author.

7. Acknowledgment

This research project would not have been possible without the support of many people. The author wishes to express her gratitude to her mother Dr. Zoila Gúdula Mayarí Cano, who introduced her into Dentistry, her tutor, Prof. PhD. Rigoberto Otaño Lugo of blessed memory who was abundantly helpful and offered invaluable assistance, support and guidance. Deepest gratitude also goes to all the members of the investigation team, without whose knowledge and assistance this study would not have been successful.

8. References

Abreu Suárez, G., González Valdés, J A., Jordán Rodríguez, J. & Chiong Molina, D. (1995). Growth and bone maturation in asthmatic children. *Rev Cub Aliment Nutr*, Vol.9, No.2, pp. 106-12.

Bayarre, H. et al. (2005). *Descriptive Statistic and statistic of Health*, Editorial Medical Sciences, Havana City, Cuba

Begole, EA. (2003). Statistic for the orthodontist, In: *Orthodontics. General and Technical principles*, Graber TM, Vanarsdall (h) RL, 3a ed., Pan-American Medical editorial, Buenos Aires, Argentina.

Björk, A. & Helm, S. (1967). Prediction of age of maximum puberal growth in body height. *Angle Orthod*, Vol.37, No.2, pp. 134 - 43.

Bujaldón Daza, JM., Rodríguez Argáiz. R. & Bujaldón Daza, AL. (1998). Study preliminary about the validity of the index of maturation of the cervical vertebras as diagnostic tool in the orthodontist planning, *RCOE*, Vol.3, No.8, pp 751-760.

Cannut Brusola, JA. (1988). *Clinical orthodontics*, Scientific and Technical editions, S.A., Barcelona, España.

Cattani, A. (2003). *Studies Health and the adolescent's development. Module I: Lesson 1. Growth and development puberal during the adolescence*, [on-line article], 11.05.2005.Available from: http://escuela.med.puc.cl/paginas/OPS/Curso/Lecciones/Leccion01/M1L1Leccio n.html.

Ceglia, A. (2005). Indicative of maturation of the bone, dental and morphological age. *Revista Latinoamericana de Ortodoncia y Odontopediatría*. [online], 03.02.2007; Available from: http://www.ortodoncia.ws/publicaciones/2005/indicadores_maduracion_edad_o sea_dental_morfologica.asp .

Cha, KS. (2003). Skeletal changes of maxillary protraction in patients exhibiting skeletal class III malocclusion: a comparison of three skeletal maturation groups. *Angle Orthod*, Vol.73, No.1, pp. 2635.

Demirjian, A., Bushchang, PH., Tanguay, R. & Patterson, DK. (1985). Interrelationships of measure of somatic, skeletal dental and sexual maturity. *Am J Orthod Dentofac Orthop*, Vol.88, pp. 433- 8.

Edilmar, M., Tavano, O., & Carvalho, IM. (2005). Cervical vertebral like estimate do grow and development in patient with lip-palatal fissures. *Salusvita* Vol.24, No.1, pp. 11-28.

Fiani, E. (1998). Indicative of maturation skeletal, bone, dental and morphological age. *Rev Cub Ortod*, Vol.13, No.2, pp. 121 - 125.

Fishman, LS. (1982). Radiographic evaluation of skeletal maturation. A clinically oriented method based on hand-wrist films. *Angle Orthod*, Vol.52, pp. 88-111.

Freitas, D., Maia, J., Beunen, G., Lefevre, J., Claessens, A., Marques, A. et al. (2004). Skeletal maturity and socio-economic status in Portuguese children and youths: the Madeira growth study. *Ann Hum Biol*, Vol.31, No.4, pp. 408-20.

Gandini, P., Mancini, M. & Andreani, F.(2006). A comparison of hand-wrist bone and cervical vertebral analyses in measuring skeletal maturation. *Angle Orthod*, Vol.76, No.6, pp. 984-9.

Geran, RG., McNamara, JJr., Baccetti, T., Franchi, L. & Shapiro, L. (2006). A prospective long-term study on the effects of rapid maxillary expansion in the early mixed dentition. *Am J Orthod Dentofac Orthop*, Vol.129, No.5, pp. 454-62.

Grave, K. & Townsend, G. (2003). Cervical vertebral maturation as a predictor of the adolescent growth spurt. *Aust Orthod J*, Vol.19, No.2, pp. 44-47.

Greulich, WW. & Pyle, SI. (1959). *Radiographic Atlas of Skeletal Development of the Hand and Wrist*. 2nd ed., Oxford University Press, London, England.

Gupta, S. (1995). Assessment of puberty growth spurt in boys and girls: a dental radiographic method. *J Indian Soc Pedod Prev Dent*, Vol.13, No.1, pp.4 - 9.

Gutiérrez Muñiz, JA., Berdasco Gómez, A., Esquivel Lauzurique, M., Jiménez Hernández, JM., Posada Lima, E., Romero del Sol, JM. et al. (2006). Growth and Development. In: *Pediatrics*, Collective of Authors, T1. [online]. 14.02.2007. Editorial Medical Sciences; Havana, Cuba. Available from:
http://www.bvs.sld.cu/libros_texto/pediatria_tomoi/parteii_cap06.pdf.

Hägg, U. & Taranger, J. (1982). Maturation indicators and the pubertal growth spurt. *Am J Orthod Dentofac Orthop*, Vol.82, No.4, pp. 299 - 309.

Hägg, U. & Taranger, J. (1980). Menarche and voice change as indicators of the pubertal growth spurt. *Acta Odontol Scand*, Vol.38, pp. 170 - 86.

Hägg, U. & Taranger, J. (1980). Skeletal stages of the hand and wrist as indicators of the pubertal growth spurt. *Acta Odontol Scand*, Vol.38, pp. 187 - 200.

Hassel, B. & Farman, AG. (1995). Skeletal maturation evaluation using cervical vertebrae. *Am J Orthod Dentofac Orthop*, Vol.107, pp. 58-66.

Izaguirre de Espinoza, I., Macías de Tomei, C., Castañeda de Gómez, M. &, Méndez Castellano H. (2003). Atlas Venezuelan bone maturation. *An Venez Nutr*, Vol.16, No.1, pp. 23-30.

Jiménez Hernández, JM., Romero del Sol, JM., Rubén Quesada, M., Barrera Yanes, R, Berdasco Gómez, A. &, Jordán Rodríguez, J. (1986). Study of bone maturation by sex and race. *Rev Cub Ped*, Vol.58, No.5, pp. 533-45.

Jiménez, JM., Romero, JM., Barrera, R., Rúben, M., Berdasco, A. & Jordán, J. (1987). *Patron of Cuban population's bone maturation*. ISCMH, Havana City, Cuba.

Jordán, RJ. (1979). *Human Development*, Editorial Scientific-technique, Havana, Cuba.

Jordán J., Berdasco, A., & J iménez, JM. (1987). *Bone maturation. Method TW2*, ISCMH, Havana City, Cuba

Leite, HR., O'Reilly, MT. & Close, J. (1987). Skeletal age assessment with first, second and third fingers. *Am J Orthod Dentofac Orthop*; Vol.92, pp 492-8.

Liversidge, HM. & Speechly, T. (2001). Growth of permanent mandibular teeth of British children aged 4 to 9 years. *Ann Hum Biol*, Vol.28, No.3, pp. 256-62.

Madhu, S., Hedge, AM. & Munshi, AK. (2003). The developmental stages of the middle phalanx of the third finger (MP3): a sole indicator in assessing the skeletal maturity? *J Clin Pediatr Dent*, Vol.27, No.2, pp.149-56.

Malavé, Y. & Rojas, I. (2000). Análisis Carpal como Indicador de Maduración Ósea. *Acta Odontol Venez* [online] 2000, Vol.38, No.3, pp.4-9. Available from http://www2.scielo.org.ve/scielo.php?script=sci_arttext&pid=S0001-63652000000300002&lng=en&nrm=iso .

Mayoral, J. & Mayoral, G. (1990). *Orthodontics: Fundamental principles and practice*. 6a ed., Labor S.A., Barcelona, Spain.

Moore, RN., Moyer, BA. & DuBois, LM. (1990). Skeletal maturation and craniofacial growth. *Am J Orthod Dentofac Orthop*, Vol.98, pp.33-40.

Nanda, R. (1955). The rate of growth of several facial components measured from serial cefalometric roentgenograms. *Am J Orthod Dentofac Orthop*, Vol.41, pp.129-141.

Ortega, AI., Haiter-Neto, F., Bovi Ambrosano, GM., Bóscolo, FN., Almeida, SM. &, Spinelli Casanova, M. (2006). Comparison of TW2 and TW3 skeletal age differences in a Brazilian population. *J Appl Oral Sci.* [online]. 27.09.2007. Vol.14, No.2, Available from:
http://www.scielo.br/scielo.php?script=sci_arttext&pid=S1678-77572006000200014 .

Ortiz, M., Godoy, S., Fuenmayor, D., Farias, M., Quirós, O., Rondón, S. & Harry, L. (2007). Method of bone maturation of the cervical vertebras, in patient of the Graduate of Orthodontics Interceptiva, UGMA-2006. *Revista Latinoamericana de Ortodoncia y Odontopediatría* [online]. 29.06.2007. Available from:
http://www.ortodoncia.ws/publicaciones/2007/maduracion_osea_vertebras_cervicales.asp .

Ozer, T., Kama, JD. &, Ozer, SY. (2006). A practical method for determining pubertal growth spurt. *Am J Orthod Dentofac Orthop*, Vol.130, No. 2, pp. 131-6.

Padrós, E. & Creus, M. (2002). Revision of the methods to study the growth craniofacial in orthodontics. *Ortod Clínic*, Vol.5, No. 2, pp. 100-116.

Paesano, PL., Vigone, MC., Siragusa, V., Chiumello, G., DelMaschio, A. & Mora, S (1998). Assessment of skeletal maturation in infants: comparison between two methods in hypothyroid patients. *Pediatr Radiol*, Vol.28, pp. 622-26.

Pancherz H. & Hägg V. (1985). Dentofacial orthopedic in relation to somatic maturation: An analysis of 7 consecutive cases treated with the Herbst appliance. *Am J Orthod Dentofac Orthop*, Vol.88, pp. 273 – 87.

Peluffo, PL. (2001). Indicators of maturation. Bone age and cervical vertebrae. *Rev Odont Interdis*, Vol.11, No. 3, pp. 9-15.

Proffit, WR. (1994). *Orthodontics: Theory and practice*. 2a ed., Mosby- Doyma Libros, S. A., Madrid, Spain.

Quirós Álvarez, OJ. (2006). *Base Bio mechans and Clinical Applications on Interceptive Orthodontics.* Actualidades Médico Odontológicas Latinoamericanas, Caracas, Venezuela.

Quirós Álvarez, OJ. (2000). *Manual of Maxillary Functional Orthopedics and Interceptive Orthodontics.* Actualidades Médico Odontológicas Latinoamericanas, Caracas, Venezuela.

Rajagopal, R. & Sudhanshu, K. A. (2002). Comparison of modified MP3 stages and the cervical vertebrae as growth indicators. *J Clin Orthod,* Vol.7, pp. 398-406.

Rakosi, T. & Jonas, I. (1992). *Atlas of Maxillary Orthopedics. Diagnostic.* Scientific and Technical editions, S. A., Barcelona, Spain.

Recalde Cortes, C., López Santomauro, D. & Palleiro, AM. (1997). Hand radiography, their clinical value. CEDDU, Vol. VIII, No.1, pp. 51-67.

Rossi Rowdley, R., Sandro Gomes, A. & Pacheco Thomé, MC. (1999). Correlation among dental stages mineralization and estimative of skeletal maturation. *Ortodontia,* Vol. 32, No. 3, pp. 48-58.

San Roman, P., Palma, JC., Oteo, MD. & Nevado, E. (2002). Squeletal maturation determined by cervical vertebrae development. *Eur J Orthod,* Vol.24, pp. 303-11.

Shigemi Goto, A. & Yamada Miyazawa, N. (1996) Ossification of the distal phalanx of the first digit as a maturity indicator for initiation of orthodontic treatment of Class III malocclusion in Japanese women. *Am J Orthod Dentofac Orthop,* Vol.110, pp. 490-501.

Spinelli Casanova, M., Ortega, AI., Haiter-Neto, F. & de Almeida, SM. (2006). Comparative Analyze bone maturation by Grave-Brown's method among conventional images and digitized. *Dental J Press Orthodon Facial Orthop* [online]. 22.06.2007, Vol. 11, No. 5, pp. 104-109. Available from:
http://www.scielo.br/pdf/dpress/v11n5/a11v11n5.pdf .

Tanner, JM., Whitehouse, RH., Cameron, N., Marshall, WA., Healy, MJR., & Goldstein, H. (1983). *Assessment of skeletal maturity and prediction of adult height (TW2 method).* 2nd ed.. Academic Press, London, England.

Tedaldi, J., Calderón, R., Mayora, L., Quirós, O., Farias, M., Rondón, S., et al. (2007). Maloclussions treatment according to the stage of maturation carpal. Bibliographical revision. *Revista Latinoamericana de Ortodoncia y Odontopediatría.* [online], 29.06.2007; Available from:
http://www.ortodoncia.ws/publicaciones/2007/tratamiento_maloclusiones.asp.

Toledo Mayarí, G. & Otaño Lugo, R. (2010). A simplified method to determine the potential growth in Orthodontics patients. *Rev Cubana Estomatol,* Vol.47, No.2, pp. 134-142.[online]. 23.09.2011. Available from:
http://scielo.sld.cu/pdf/est/v47n2/est02210.pdf .

Toledo Mayarí, G. & Otaño Lugo, R. (2010). Concordance among skeletal maturation stages and dental calcification stages. *Rev Cubana Estomatol,* Vol.47, No.2, pp. 207-214. [online]. 23.09.2011. Available from:
http://scielo.sld.cu/pdf/est/v47n2/est09210.pdf

Toledo Mayarí, G. & Otaño Lugo, R. (2010). Assessment of bone maturation in cervical vertebrae in Orthodontics patients. *Rev Cubana Estomatol,* Vol.47, No.3, pp. 326-335. [online]. 23.09.2011. Available from:
http://scielo.sld.cu/pdf/est/v47n3/est06310.pdf

Toledo, V. (2004). *Orthognatic Surgeon Simplification of the treatment Surgical Orthodontic in Adults.*, Amorca Caracas, Venezuela.

Ugarte Suárez, JC., Banasco Domínguez, J. & Ugarte Moreno, D. (2004). *Manual of Imagenology*. 2a ed., Editorial Medical Sciences, Havana City, Cuba.

Uysal, T., Ramoglu, IF., Basciftci, FA. & Sari, ZA. (2006). Chronologic age and skeletal maturation of the cervical vertebrae and hand-wrist: is there a relationship? *J Orthod Dentofac Orthop*, Vol.130, No.5, pp. 622-8.

Part 3

Orthodontic Therapy

8

Three-Dimensional Imaging and Software Advances in Orthodontics

Ahmed Ghoneima[1,2], Eman Allam[1], Katherine Kula[1] and L. Jack Windsor[1]
[1]*Indiana University School of Dentistry, Indianapolis,*
[2]*Faculty of Dental Medicine, Al-Azhar University, Cairo*
[1]*USA*
[2]*Egypt*

1. Introduction

The technological advances and innovations of imaging systems for orthodontic practice require a continuous update of their applications and assessments of their strength and weakness, as well as guidelines for utilization. Orthodontists are challenged by the increasing number and complexity of these systems and softwares. Accurate diagnostic imaging is an essential requirement for the optimal diagnosis and treatment planning of orthodontic patients. In addition, it is a critical tool that allows the clinician to monitor and document the treatment progress and outcome. The purpose of this chapter is to update orthodontists about the current options and applications of the latest imaging techniques in orthodontic practice and to review the existing software advances.

2. Cone beam technology in orthodontics

The cone-beam computed tomography (CBCT) scanners were introduced in the late 1990s. Shortly after, the US Food and Drug Administration (FDA) approved the first CBCT unit in 2001. Since then, there has been an enormous interest in this new technology for its clinical and research applications. The CBCT is an imaging acquisition technique that utilizes a volumetric scanning machine. This technology is based on a cone-shaped X-ray beam directed at a flat two-dimensional (2D) detector. As both rotate around the patient's head, a series of 2D images are generated. The software then reconstructs the images into three-dimensional (3D) data set using a specialized algorithm (De Vos et al., 2009; Molen, 2011).

Currently, there are more than 43 CBCT systems from 20 different companies available commercially. The most commonly used of these CBCT imaging aquistion systems are the 3D Accuitomo (J. Morita, Kyoto, Japan), CB MercuRay (Hitachi Medical Corporation, Osaka, Japan), iCAT (Imaging Sciences International, Hatfield, PA), Galileos (Sirona Dental Systems LLC, Charlotte, NC), New-Tom 3G (QR srl, Verona, Italy), Scanora 3D (SOREDEX, Milwaukee, WI), and Kodak 9500 (Kodak Dental Systems, Rochester, NY). There are big variations in the quality and characteristics of the images or the reconstructed volumes and the radiation doses between most of these CBCT systems. Machines with reduced radiation doses and less powerful tubes are often associated with poor image quality, low contrast resolution and increased noise. The exposure parameters, the source-detector distance, the field of view (FOV), the data reconstruction algorithm, and the software used are among the major factors responsible for those variations. The currently available CBCT units utilize radiation doses ranging from 87 to 206 μSv for a full craniofacial scan. These radiation doses are slightly higher than the conventional radiographic techniques such as the lateral cephalograms or the panoramic radiographs and markedly lower than that of multi-slice CT. The scan time varies between 10 to 75 seconds, depending on the FOV and the CBCT unit used (Molen, 2011; Kapila et al., 2011).

Craniofacial imaging is a crucial component of an orthodontic patient's record. The gold standard for orthodontic records is the attempt to achieve an accurate replication of the real anatomical structures or the "anatomic truth". Although the use of the traditional imaging views in orthodontics has been adequate, the achievement of the ideal imaging goal of replicating the anatomic truth has been limited by the available technology such as the 2D frontal and lateral cephalograms, panoramic radiographs, and intraoral/extraoral photographs. Recently, more emphasis has been placed on the CBCT technology, the 3D images, and virtual models. The main advantage for the use of CBCT is that the clinician can get more accurate data from one scan than from the many 2D radiographs traditionally used with less radiation exposure (Mah & Hatcher, 2005) (Figure 1).

The 3D CBCT data can greatly expand the orthodontist's diagnostic capabilities. It offers a comprehensive evaluation of the dentition and is very useful for identifying abnormalities such as missing teeth, supernumerary teeth, eruption disturbances, teeth malpositions, and/or root irregularities that could delay or prevent tooth movement. CBCT can be considered the technique of choice for examining and localizing impacted teeth. The exact position of impacted tooth and its relations to the adjacent roots or important anatomical structures such as the maxillary sinus or the mandibular canal when planning surgical exposure and subsequently orthodontic management can be precisely assessed by 3D CBCT (Mah et al., 2011) (Figures 2 and 3).

Using CBCT scans, alveolar bone can be assessed from all aspects not only on the mesial and distal surfaces of the tooth. This allows for the assessment of the width of available bone for buccolingual movement of teeth during orthodontic management especially in cases requiring arch expansion or labial movement of incisors. Fenestrations, dehiscence, and/or external apical root resorption can be precisely visualized on the 3D images. Evaluation of alveolar bone volume, which is especially important in periodontally compromised adult orthodontic patients, is one of the beneficial uses of CBCT in orthodontics. The width of alveolar ridges for placement of implants is another variable that can be investigated (Halazonetis, 2005; Valiathan et al., 2008).

Preoperative implant site assessment is probably one of the most useful applications of CBCT in orthodontics. In the orthodontic field, osseo-integrated implants are either used for anchorage or as a prosthetic replacement of missing teeth. The accurate determination of root angulations and the available space are essential for successful placement of the implant. CBCT can be used to accurately assess the space availability and root angulation, as well as the 3D quantification of the alveolar bone at the implant site (Mah & Hatcher, 2005) (Figure 4).

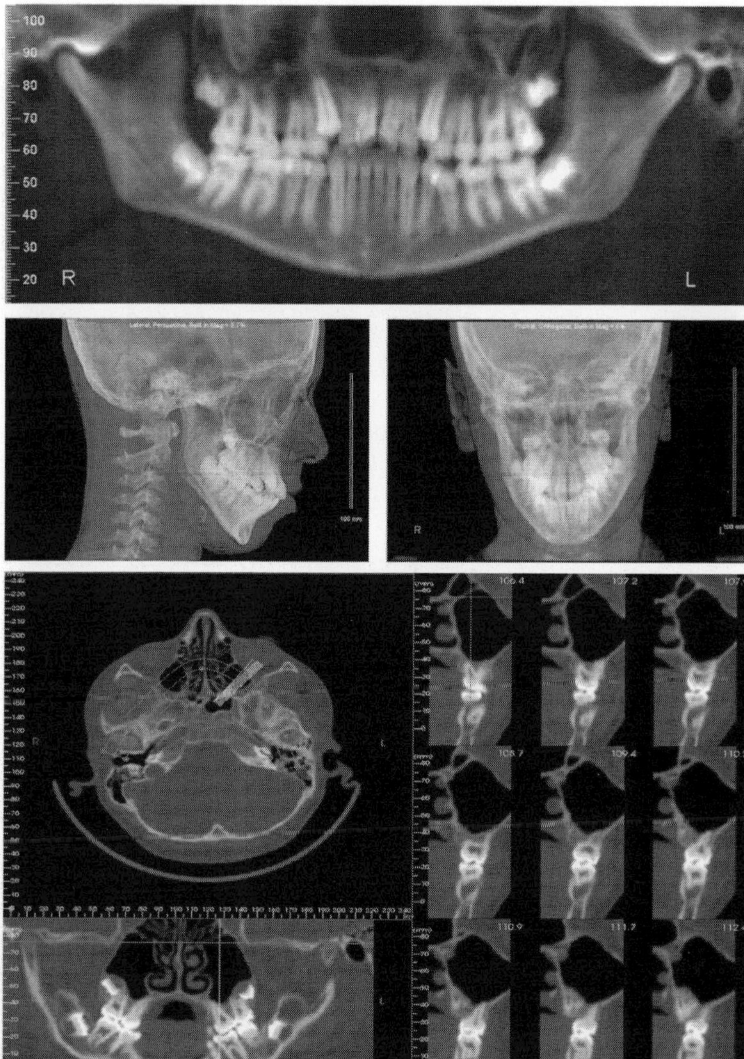

Fig. 1. CBCT data can be easily reconstructed into traditional panoramic, lateral, or postero-anterior cephalometric images, as well as cross section views. In this way, the clinician can get more information from the scan than from multiple 2D radiographs with less radiation exposure. Images created by the Dolphin and InVivoDental softwares from a single CBCT scan.

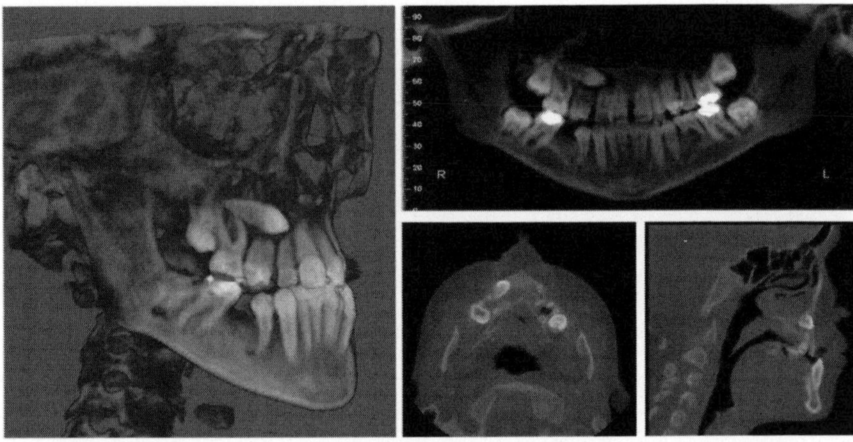

Fig. 2. A 15 years old female with impacted canine that was initially diagnosed on the panoramic radiograph, but could not be precisely located in relationship to the present teeth. Using the axial and sagittal sections of the CBCT data, the labial location could be confirmed. In addition, the 3D volume allowed for viewing the impacted canine from any angle.

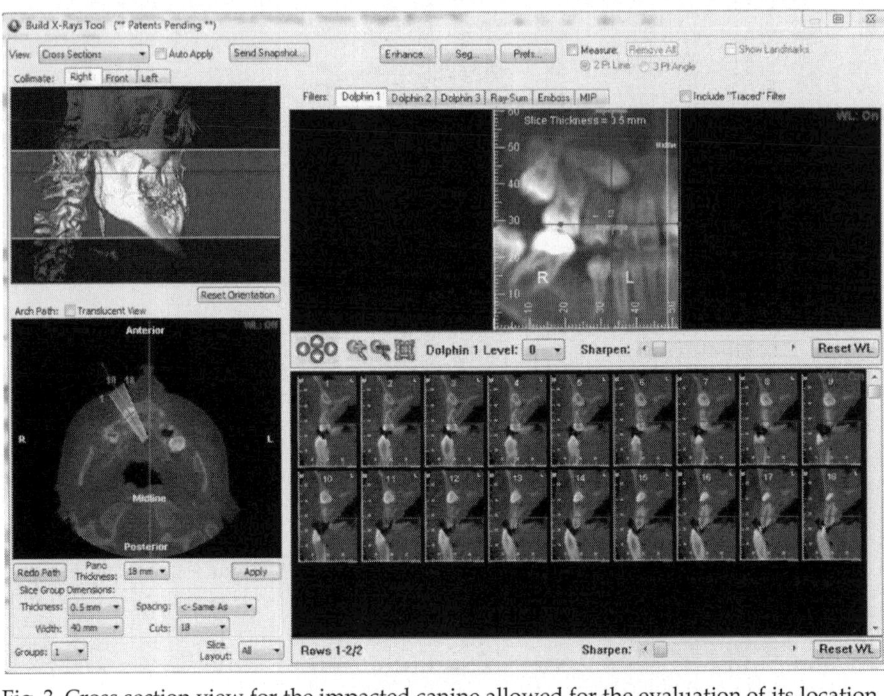

Fig. 3. Cross section view for the impacted canine allowed for the evaluation of its location and relationship to other structures slice by slice in 1 view (slice thickness 0.5 mm).

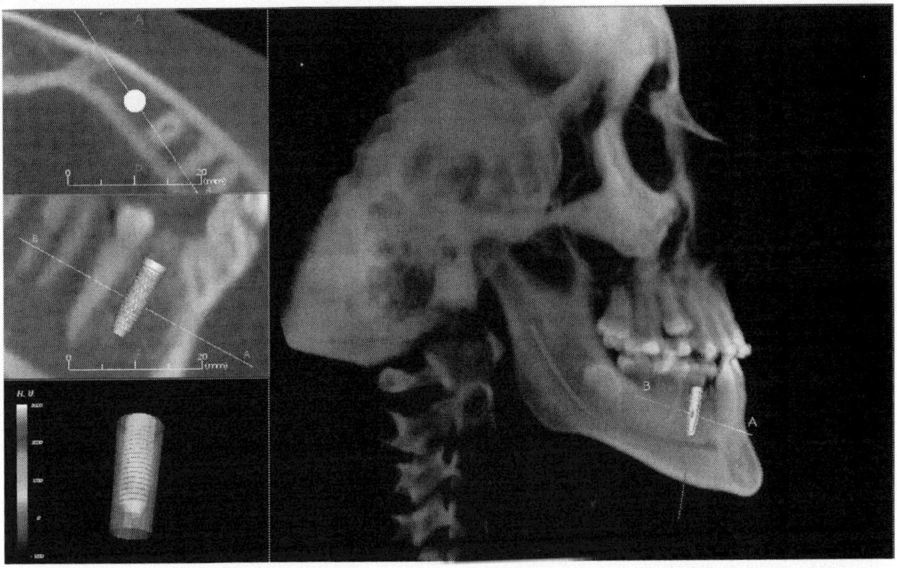

Fig. 4. Axial and sagittal sections showing the buccal and lingual bone thickness, as well as the relationship between the implant and the inferior alveolar nerve (labeled in red color). The 3D view is important in the evaluation of space availability.

Orthodontic patients with temporomandibular joint (TMJ) disorders are common. When these disorders occur during development, they may alter the facial growth pattern and may also affect the growth of the ipsilateral part of the mandible with compensations in the maxilla, tooth position, occlusion, and cranial base. CBCT allows the clinicians to assess and quantify these changes associated with TMJ disorders more accurately than the 2D images as these changes occur in the vertical, horizontal, and transverse directions. CBCT is especially indicated when more information about the morphology and internal structure of the osseous components of the TMJ is required. Studies have shown that CBCT images provide higher reliability and accuracy than CT and panoramic radiographs in the detection of condylar cortical erosion. CBCT images also allow for the visualization of the TMJs from different views and efficient evaluation of its relationship to the dentition and occlusion (Huang, et al., 2005; Hilgers et al., 2005; Honey et al., 2007) (Figure 5).

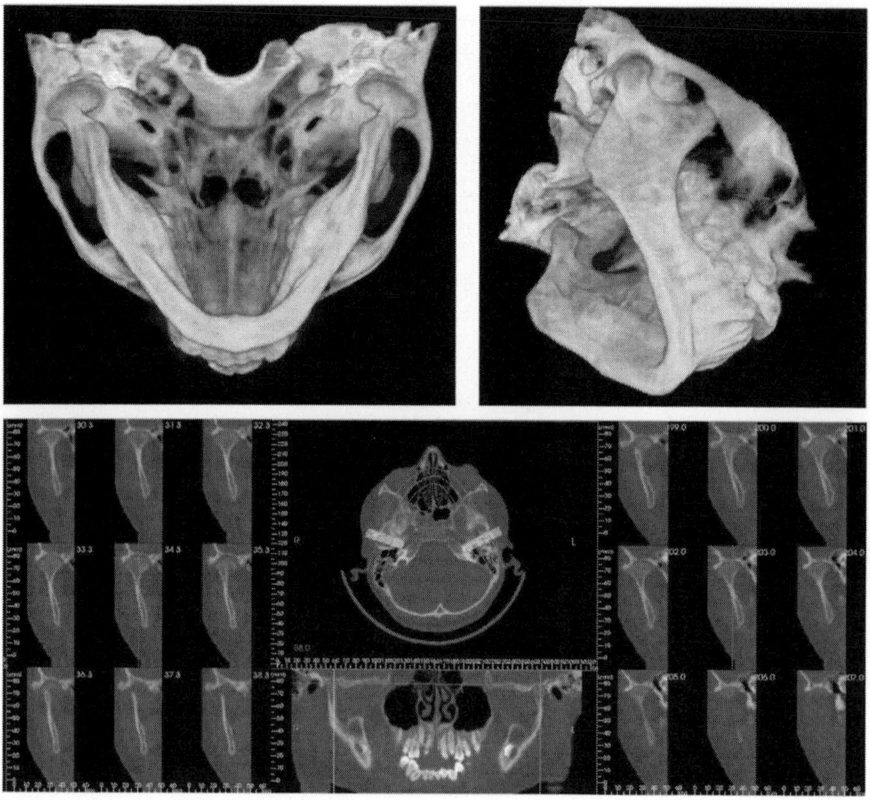

Fig. 5. 3D CBCT volume allows for better visualization and provides more details about the morphology and position of the TMJ and the condyles from different views. In addition, the TMJ cross-section view permits complete and thorough examination of the joint through a group of cross section slices.

Digital study models have been introduced as the digital alternative to the traditional stone cast record. A gradual transition from the plaster models decade to the digital models is expected to occur in the near future. The rapid growth and acceptance of these digital models among the orthodontists has been driven by many factors. They are easier and faster to obtain, to store, transfer, and retrieve. Patients benefit from shorter appointment time when impressions are not needed, and the clinicians benefit from the superior diagnosis and treatment simulation provided by better presentation of the dentition and manipulation of the images (Enciso et al., 2003).

The digital models allow the clinician to obtain additional diagnostic information that are not available with the use of the plaster models such as root shape, position, and angulations. The relationship of the roots to anatomic structures such as the mandibular nerve, as well as quantitative bone density information, can also be evaluated. Crown to root ratios can be estimated and other different dental measurements can be performed easily. Several studies have proved that the digital models created from CBCT scans or obtained from laser scanning of a dental impression or study model are as accurate and as reliable as plasters models (Dalstra & Melsen, 2009; Hernandez-Soler et al., 2011). Perhaps a major advantage of the digital models is the virtual setup capability with complete 3D anatomy by including the roots and the alveolar bone. The virtual setup provides superior case presentation, treatment simulation, aesthetic predictions, and results visualization. It also allows for including the torque and labiolingual inclination calculations in the dental setup (Hernandez-Soler et al., 2011) (Figures 6 and 7).

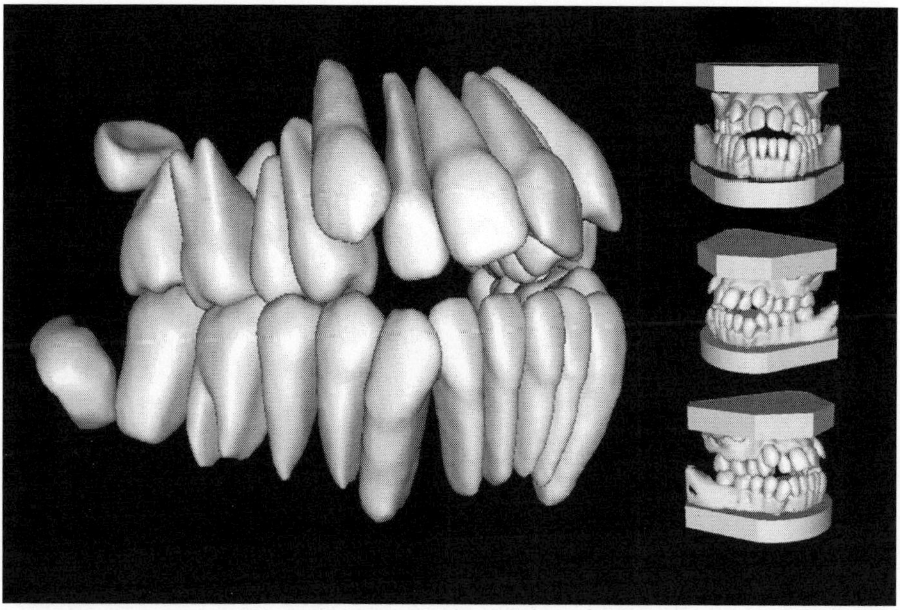

Fig. 6. Computer-generated models reconstructed from the digital imaging and communications in medicine (DICOM) data using the InVivoDental software showing not only the crowns of the teeth but also the roots.

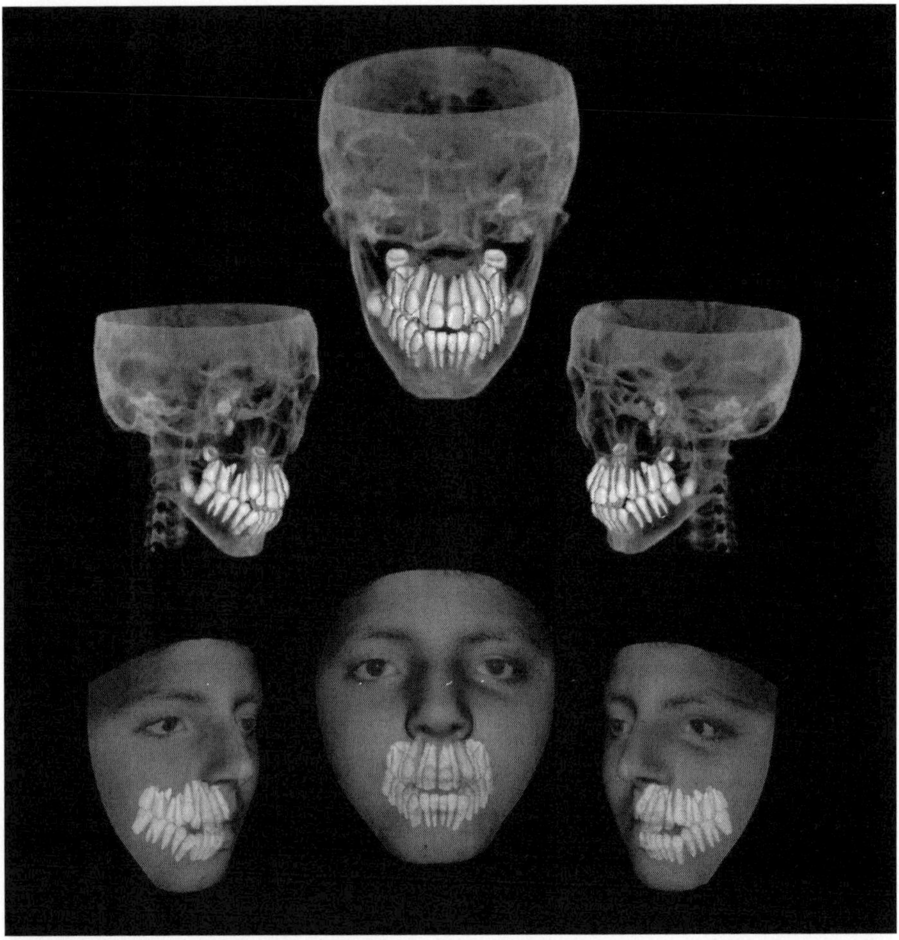

Fig. 7. Dual volume superimposition: the digital model superimposed on a 3D skull volume and a 3D facial photograph provides an excellent tool for treatment simulation and for the evaluation of the anatomical relationships between the teeth, the skeletal, and the soft tissues.

3. Cone beam computed tomography and airway analysis

Airway disorders are a common cause of malocclusions and might result in the classical appearance of adenoid facies. The results of a retrospective review of 500 orthodontic patients showed that 18.2 percent of the patients had airway-related problems. Variations in airway morphology and dimensions are commonly related to hereditary or functional disorders. Despite the cause or the effect, any airway problem has to be properly diagnosed and treated as soon as it is identified. Methods that are traditionally used to assess the airway include cephalometry, rhinoendoscopy, and tomography (Subtenley & Baker, 1965; Fujiki & Rossato, 1999; Filho et al., 2001; Abramson et al., 2010).

Mandibular advancement device, tongue retraining device, and a continous positive airflow pressure appliance are the most common orthodontic therapeutic options for patients with breathing disorders. The assessment of the patient's airway plays a primary role in planning the management strategy, especially in patients suffering from mouth breathing, adenoid hypertrophy, or sleep apnea. The 2D lateral cephalograms offer limited information due to the difficulty in identifying the soft tissue contour in the third dimension thus restricting evaluation of areas and volumes. Currently, there appears to be no better way to assess the airway than by using CBCT imaging (Halazonetis, 2005; Aboudara et al., 2009).

3D CBCT images offer accurate representation of the airway. The CBCT data with the use of different software systems allows better visualization, volumetric measurements, and patency assessment of the airway, as well as the precise distinction between the soft tissues and the airway space. Several studies questioned the reliability of the 3D methods and indicated high reliability and accuracy of area and volume measurements using this technique. Clinicians can more easily perform the volumetric measurements and also calculate the cross-sectional areas of the airway in 3 planes of space: coronal, sagittal, and axial. In addition, the option provided by some softwares for detecting and measuring the most constricted area in the airway provides essential diagnostic clinical information especially in obstructive sleep apnea patients (Ogawa et al., 2007; Aboudara et al., 2009; Abramson et al., 2010) (Figures 8 and 9).

4. 3D cephalometry

Cephalometric analysis in orthodontics is an important diagnostic tool for the assessment of craniofacial morphology. The lateral cephalograms enable orthodontists to determine the size and shape of the jaws, their position in sagittal and vertical relation to the anterior base of the skull, and their position in relation to each other. An analytical method is used to identify and analyze the necessary parameters. It involves determining hard tissue and soft tissue landmarks, and making angular and linear measurements. The information provided by the lateral cephalogram about the vertical and sagittal structure of the facial skull cannot be obtained by any other diagnostic measure. However, cephalometric measurements on the 2D images suffer from several limitations such as the difficulty in locating some reference points and landmarks, image distortion, differences in magnifications, superimposition of the bilateral craniofacial structures, and measurement errors. Another important drawback of lateral and frontal cephalograms is the lack of information about cross-sectional area and volume (Adams et al., 2004; Lenza et al., 2010).

CBCT provide a 3D method for cephalometric analysis (Figure 10). Compared with the traditional cephalometric radiographs, the CBCT produces images that are anatomically true (real-size 1:1 scale) with accurate volumetric 3D depiction of hard and soft tissues of the skull and lack of superimposition of the anatomical structures. Other advantages of this method over the 2D cephalometric analysis include the reduced radiation exposure (as the 3D visualization software generates a 2D lateral image from the 3D data set) and the high precision of the linear and angular measurements obtained. Reliability studies demonstrated that cephalograms reconstructed from CBCT data have no statistically significant differences in linear and angular measurements relative to traditional cephalograms, whereas measurement error from CBCT images are lower than those from cephalograms (Kumar et al., 2007; Moshiri et al., 2007; Kumar et al., 2008).

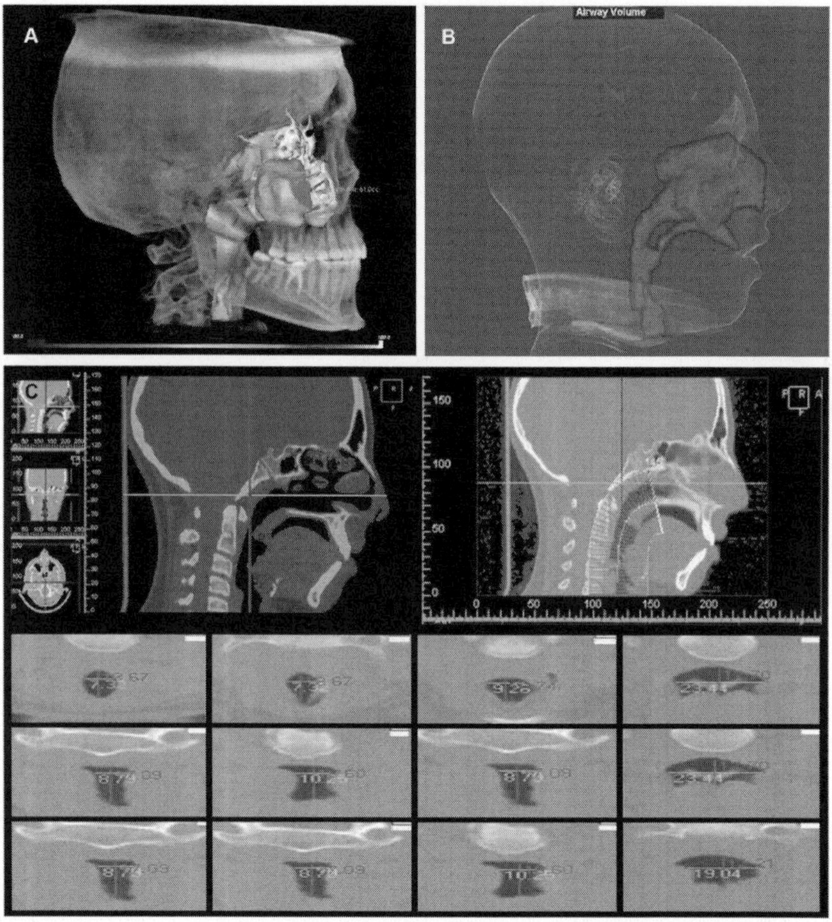

Fig. 8. Volumetric measurements of the airway can be done using different softwares each with a different way of performing the calculations. A) using the InVivoDental software (Anatomage Inc, San Jose, CA), the operator first manually trace the airway passage and then the software will calculate it selectively, B) total airway volume can be calculated by filling in the airway space automatically using the Dolphin software (Dolphin Imaging & Management solutions, Chatsworth, CA), and C) using 3dMD software (3dMD LLC, Atlanta, GA), segmentation for the airway is done first and then the selected areas to be measured will be automatically turned up to a multiple axial slices and the software will calculate the height and width of each slice and give the total airway volume.

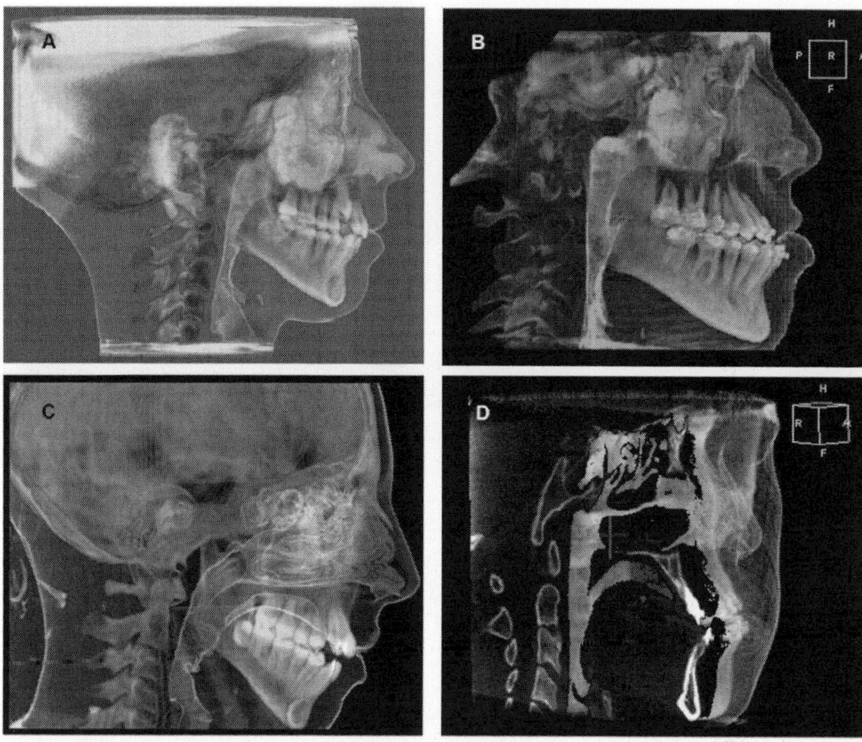

Fig. 9. Volume-rendered CBCT images for the airway in either color enhanced form (A, B, and C) or shaded form (D) where the colors or the shadow are used to aid better visualization and assessment of the airway, as well as correlations with the surrounding head and neck structures. Images generated using the Dolphin software (A), 3dMD (B and D), and InVivoDental (C).

For 3D cephalometry, the anatomical landmarks are identified on 3D surface-rendered volumes or models obtained from CBCT data. In the tracing step, cephalometric planes are defined using either three or four landmarks instead of the two landmarks traditionally used in 2D cephalometry. Beside the elimination of the superimposition of bilateral structures and unequal enlargement artifacts, this also allows for the evaluation of the right and the left sides of the skull independently. The quality and the visibility of the 3D cephalometric landmarks and parameters vary among the different scanners and depend mainly on the scan field of view (FOV) selection, the 3D model segmentation threshold, and image artifacts (Swennen & Schutyser, 2006; Halazonetis, 2005).

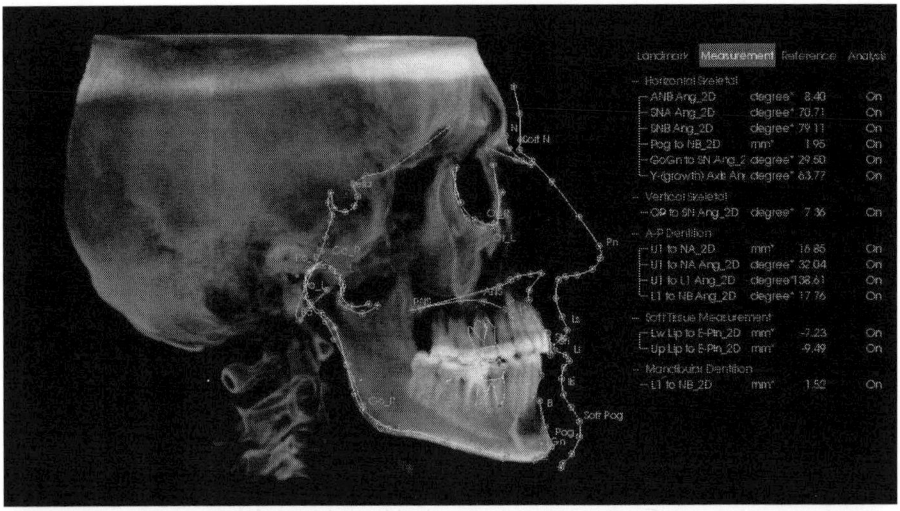

Fig. 10. Linear and angular parameters used for 3D cephalometric analysis (InVivoDental software).

5. 3D superimposition

One of the main advantages of the CBCT is that it allows superimposition of serial images to evaluate the growth and treatment changes. This is an efficient way for showing areas of bone displacement and remodeling, as well as demonstrating the changes in size, shape, and shift in positions of skeletal and soft tissues as a result of either orthodontic or surgical treatments. The 2D cepahalograms have been traditionally used to evaluate these growth or treatment changes based on stable reference structures or anatomical landmarks. The traditional approach to lateral cephalometric superimposition is based on using the most stable anatomical landmarks. For example, the sella turcica for the cranial base registration, the lingual curvature of the palate for the maxillary bony structures, the internal cortical outline of the symphysis, and the mandibular canal for the mandible. However, a major limitation of the 2D representation of a 3D structure with the difficulty in identification of the landmarks is due to the superimposition of multiple structures. In contrast, 3D images provided easier and more accurate anatomical landmark registration (Cevidanes et al., 2005; Lagravere et al., 2006).

The available software tools and options allow optimal alignment of the 3D CBCT datasets at different time points with high precision and accuracy after identification of specific anatomical landmarks and structures. The computed registration is then applied to the segmented structures to measure changes due to orthodontic treatment or surgery. Surface distance calculations are then used for the purpose of accurate quantification of the changes or displacement due to either growth or treatment. Color mapping can show surface area distance differences between two 3D objects or 3D facial photographs (Cevidanes et al., 2005) (Figures 11, 12, and 13).

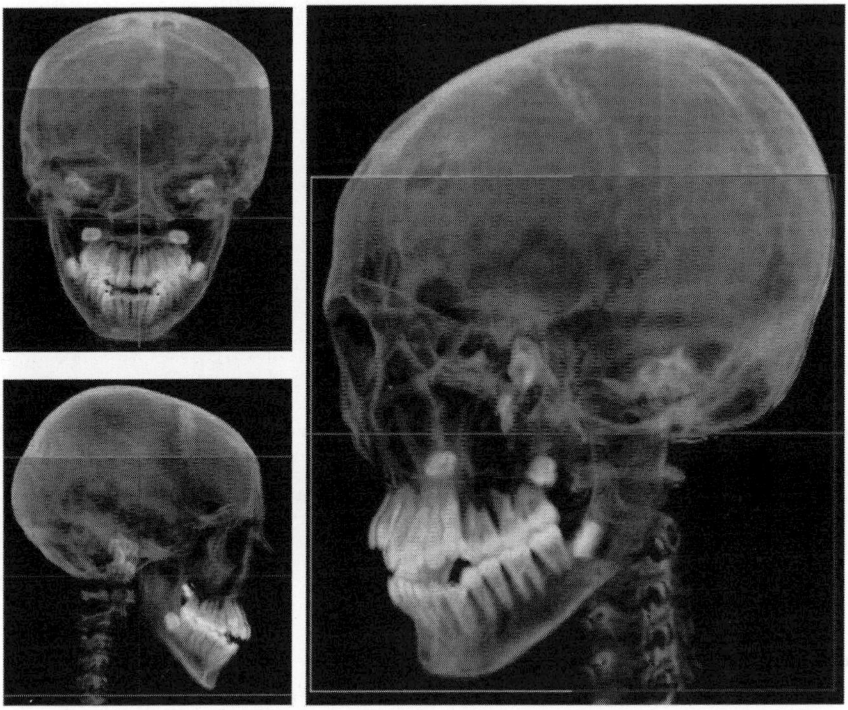

Fig. 11. Demonstration of superimposition of the pre- (brown) and post- (blue) treatment skull models of a 12 years old patient treated with rapid maxillary expansion for a constricted maxillary arch. The use of different colors highlights the changes between the two scans.

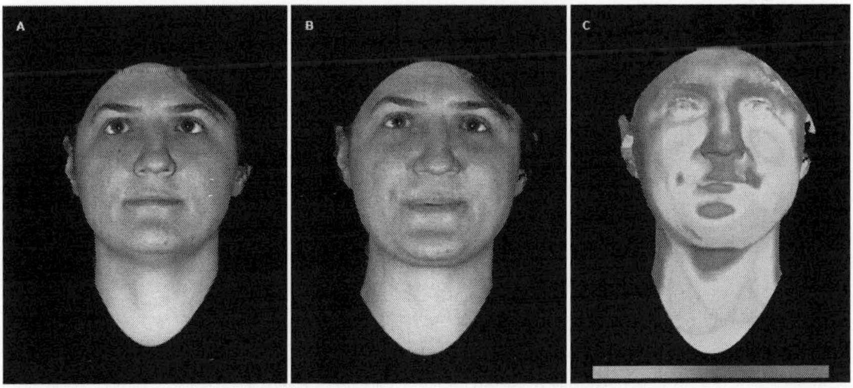

Fig. 12. Three-dimensional facial photograph of a trumpet player: in the rest position (A), during blowing (B), and color mapping (C) used to demonstrate the differences between the two positions.

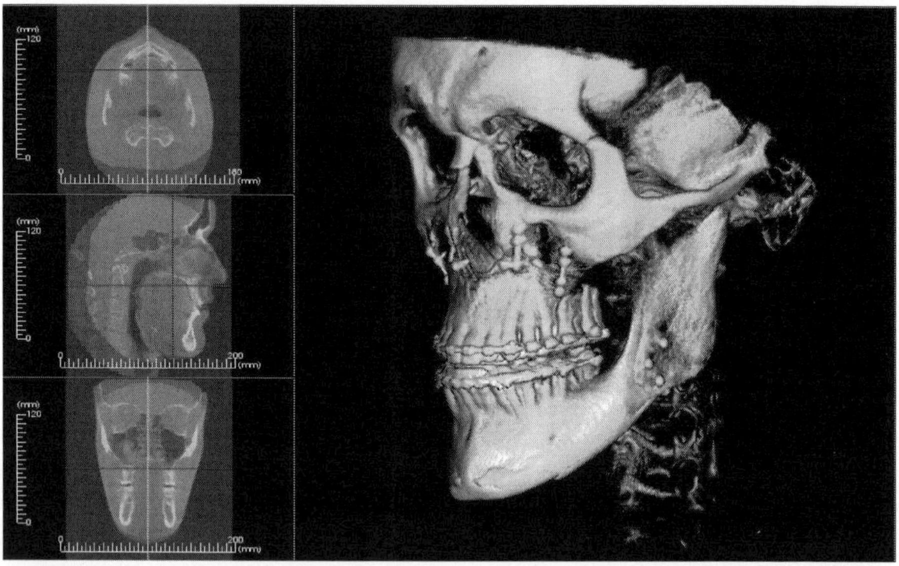

Fig. 13. The changes and shift in position of skeletal structures resulting from orthognathic surgery for correction of mandibular prognathism in 23 years old female patient demonstrated by superimposition of serial 3D images of skull volumes using 2 different color codes.

6. 3D facial photographs

With the introduction of a new system and software, the applicability of 3D photographs in daily orthodontic practice became possible. Photographic soft tissue profile analysis, evaluation of the craniofacial growth and development, orthodontic diagnosis, and measurements of the aesthetic facial parameters can all be professionally performed on these photographs.

One of the gold standard diagnostic tools in orthognathic surgery and preoperative orthodontic treatment is the 2-D facial photographs that consequently reveal limitations in describing the 3D structures of a patient's face. CBCT and the newly introduced imaging techniques such as the 3D stereophotogrammetry (3D photographs) allows exploring the human face 3-dimensionally with multiple useful applications that ranges from using the facial scans to measure all the aesthetic facial parameters to orthodontic diagnosis and evaluation of the craniofacial growth and development (Lane & Harrell, 2008).

Stereophotogrammetry is a method of obtaining an image by means of one or more stereo pairs of photographs being taken simultaneously. The 3D photo camera is used to capture the soft tissue surface of the face with correct geometry and texture information. The technique is based on the triangulation and fringe projection method. Image fusion (i.e., registration of a 3D photograph upon a CBCT) results in an accurate and photorealistic digital 3D data set of a patient's face (Maal et al., 2008).

The registration of pre- and post-operative 3D photographs has many important applications, which mainly include the evaluation of treatment outcomes in orthognathic surgery or orthodontic treatment. After registration or matching of the 3D photographs, the differences between the pre- and post-photographs can be visualized by a color scale or map. In this way, results of the treatment can be evaluated quantitatively and objectively. Other useful applications of comparing different 3D photographs are the evaluation of pathological lesions or swelling such as abscess or tumors over time, cross-sectional growth changes, and the establishment of databases for normative populations. For clinical use, the registration process of pre- and post-treatment 3D photographs has to be very accurate (Metzger et al., 2007; Maal et al., 2010).

One of the recently introduced software features allow the facial photograph to be morphed onto a digital imaging and communications in medicine (DICOM) dataset where the 3D volume can generate a simulated 3D projection of the face in any frontal, lateral, or user-defined view of the face. By changing the translucency of the image, the correlation between the facial soft tissues to the skeleton can be determined. This has great implications in planning orthognathic surgery, orthodontic treatment, or other craniofacial therapies that could affect the facial appearance (Harrell, 2009; Schendel & Lane, 2009) (Figure 14).

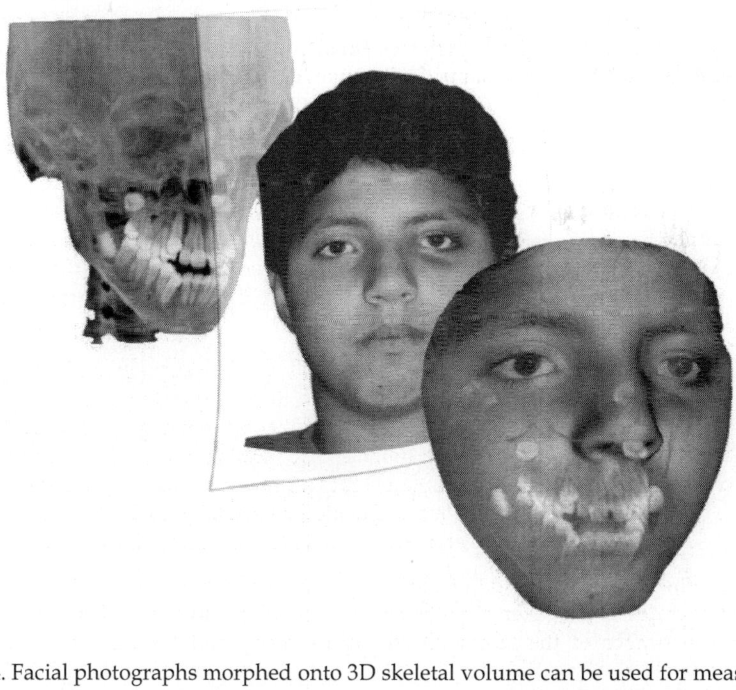

Fig. 14. Facial photographs morphed onto 3D skeletal volume can be used for measurements of the aesthetic facial parameters and soft tissue profile analysis, as well as treatment simulation.

7. Conclusion

CBCT has become widely available and acceptable by the orthodontic community especially as the radiation exposure and cost decreases. The continuous advancements in the imaging machines, techniques, and softwares have added valuable improvement in its diagnostic capabilities. In addition, the ease of image manipulation and its relevancy to the clinical setting offers orthodontists and clinicians the chance for improved diagnosis. Craniofacial imaging is expected to become totally digital in the near future. The orthodontic community needs to increase their knowledge, and evaluate its clinical relevancy and reliability, as well as consider its other applications.

8. References

Aboudara, C., Nielsen, I. & Huang, J. (2009). Comparison of human airway space using conventional lateral headfilms and three-dimensional reconstruction from cone-beam computed tomography. Am J Orthod Dentofac Orthop 135:468-479.

Abramson, Z., Susarla, S., August, M., Troulis, M. & Kaban, L. (2010). Three-dimensional computed tomographic analysis of airway anatomy in patients with obstructive sleep apnea. J Oral Maxillofac Surg 68:354-362.

Adams, G., Gansky, S., Miller, A., Harell, W. & Hatcher D. (2004). Comparison between traditional 2-dimensional cephalometry and a 3-dimensional approach on human dry skull. Am J Orthod Dentofac Orthop 126:397-409.

Cevidanes, L., Bailey, L. & Tucker, GR.(2005). Superimpositon of 3D cone-beam CT models of orthognathic surgery patients. Dentomaxillofac Radiol 34:369-375.

Cevidanes, L., Oliveira, A., Grauer, D., Styner, M. & Proffit, W. (2011). Clinical application of 3D imaging for assessment of treatment outcomes. Semin Orthod 17:72-80.

Dalstra, M. & Melsen, B. (2009). From alginate impressions to virtual digital models. J Orthod 36:36-41.

De Vos, W., Casselman, J. & Swennen, G. (2009). Cone-beam computerized tomography (CBCT) imaging of the oral and maxillofacial region: A systemic review of the literature. Int J Oral Maxillofac Surg 38(6):609-25.

Enciso, R., Memon, A. & Fidaleo, D. (2003). The virtual craniofacial patient: 3D jaw modeling and animation. Stud Health Technol Inform 94:65-71.

Filho, D., Raveli, D., Raveli, R., De Castro, L. & Gandin, L. (2001). A comparison of nasopharyngeal endoscopy and lateral cephalometric radiography in the diagnosis of nasopharyngeal airway obstruction. Am J Orthod Dentofac Orthop 120:348-352.

Fujiki, P. & Rossato, C. (1999). Influencia da hipertrofa adenoideana no crescimento e desenvolvimento craniodentofacial. Ortodontia 32:70-79.

Halazonetis, D. (2005). From 2-dimensional cephalograms to 3-dimensional computed tomography scans. Am J Orthod Dentofac Orthop 127: 627–637

Harrell, W. (2009). 3D diagnosis and treatment planning in orthodontics. Semin Orthod 15:35-41.

Hernandez-Soler, V., Enciso, R. & Cisneros, G. (2011). The virtual patient specific-model and the virtual dental model. Semin Orthod 17:46-48.

Hilgers, M., Scarfe, S. & Scheetz, J. (2005). Accuracy of linear temporomandibular joint measurements with cone beam computed tomography and digital cephalometric radiography. Am J Orthod Dentofacial Orthop 128:803-811.

Honey, O., Scarfe, W. & Hilgers, M. (2007). Accuracy of cone-beam computed tomography imaging of the temporomandibular joint: Comparisons with panoramic radiology and linear tomography. Am J Orthod Dentofacial Orthop 132:429-438.

Huang, J., Bumann, A. & Mah, J. (2005). Three dimensional radiographic analysis in orthodontics. JCO 7:421-428.

Kapila, S., Conley RS. & Harrell, Jr. (2011). The current status of cone beam computed tomography imaging in orthodontics. Dentomaxillofacial Radiology 40:24-34.

Kumar, V., Ludlow, J., Mol, A. & Cevidanes, L. (2007). Comparison of conventional and cone beam CT synthesized cephalograms. Dentomaxillofacial Radiology 36: 263–269

Kumar, V., Ludlow, J., Cevidanes, L. & Mol, A. (2008). In vivo comparison of conventional and cone beam CT synthesized cephalograms. Angle Orthodontist 78: 873–879

Lagravere, M., Hansen, L., Harzer, W. & Major, P. (2006). Plane orientation for standardization in 3-dimensional cephalometric analysis with computerized tomography imaging. Am J Orthod Dentofac Orthop 129:601-4.

Lane, C. & Harrell, W. (2008). Completing the 3-dimensional picture. Am J Orthod Dentofac Orthop 133:612-20.

Lenza, M., Lenza, MM., Dalstra, M., Melsen, B. & Cattaneo, PM. (2010). An analysis of different approaches to the assessment of upper airway morphology: a CBCT study. Orthod Craniofac Res 13:96-105.

Maal, T., Plooij, J., Rangel, F., Mollemans, W., Schutyser, F. & Berge, S. (2008). The accuracy of matching three-dimensional photographs with skin surfaces derived from cone-beam computed tomography. J Oral Maxillofac Surg 37:641-646.

Maal, T., Loon, B., Plooij, J., Rangel, F., Ettema, A., Borstlap, W. & Berge, S. (2010). Registration of 3-dimensional facial photographs for clinical use. J Oral Maxillofac Surg 68:2391-2401.

Mah, J.& Hatcher, D. (2005) Craniofacial imaging in orthodontics. In: Graber, TM., Vanarsdall, RL. & Vig, KWL., editors. Orthodontics, current principles and techniques. 4th ed. St Louis: Mosby.

Mah, J., Yi, L., Huang, R. & Choo, H. (2011). Advanced applications of cone beam computed tomography in orthodontics. Semin Orthod 17:57-71.

Metzger, MC., Hohlweg-Majert, B. & Schon, R. (2007). Verification of clinical precision after computer-aided reconstruction in craniomaxillofacial surgery. Oral Surg Oral Med Oral Pathol Oral Radiol Endod 104:e1.

Molen, A. (2011). Comparing cone beam computed tomography systems from an orthodontic perspective. Semin Orthod 17:34-38.

Moshiri, M., Scarfe, W., Hilgers, M., Scheetz, J., Silveira, A. & Farman, A. (2007). Accuracy of linear measurements from imaging plate and lateral cephalometric images derived from cone-beam computed tomography. Am J Orthod Dentofac Orthop 132: 550–560

Ogawa, T., Enciso, R., Shintaku, W. & Clark, G. (2007). Evaluation of cross-section airway configuration of obstructive sleep apnea. Oral Surg Oral Med Oral Pathol Oral Radiol Endod 103:102-8.

Schendel, S. & Lane, C. (2009). 3D orthognathic surgery simulation using image fusion. Semin Orthod 15:48-56.

Subtelney, J. & Baker, H. (1956). The significance of adenoid tissue in velopharyngeal function. Plastic and Reconstructive Surgery 17:235-250.

Swennen, G. & Schutyser, F. (2006). Three-dimensional cephalometry: spiral multi-slice vs cone-beam computed tomography. Am J Orthod Dentofac Orthop 130: 410–416

Valiathan, A., Dhar, S. & Verma, N. (2008). 3D CT imaging in orthodontics: Adding a new dimension to diagnosis and treatment planning. Trends Biomater Artif Organs 21(2):116-120.

9

The Use of Mini-Implants (Temporary Anchorage Devices) in Resolving Orthodontic Problems

P. Salehi, S. Torkan, S.M.M. Roeinpeikar
Orthodontic Research Center, Shiraz University of Medical Sciences, Shiraz Iran

1. Introduction

In orthodontic treatment, the final goal is to achieve the desired tooth movement and to reduce the number of unwanted side effects and eventually to improve patient's esthetics.[1] Therefore, different methods for anchorage control has been suggested, such as using the opposing arch, extraoral anchorage, increasing the number of teeth in the anchorage unit or circum-oral musculature.

Nowadays, with the advent of mini-implants, maximum anchorage has become possible and unwanted side effects have been reduced to a minimum. Mini-implants which are also known as Temporary Anchorage Devices (TADs) are small titanium bone screw or stainless steel bone screws which are placed either in buccal alveolar bone or the palatal side. These bone screws can be placed on the paramedian areas of the palate in growing children. [2, 3] The use of TADs can ensure a rigid intra-oral anchorage through which different tooth movements in all three planes of space can be provided. This might as well serve as an alternative to orthognathic surgery, especially in those instances where changes in the vertical dimension are required.[4] They can vary in size form 5-12 mm in length and from 1.2-20 mm in diameter. [5]

Among the pioneers in this field, Linkow was one of the first to use blade implants as an anchorage method for cl II elastics, [6] Later, in 1983, Creekmore and Eklund used vitallium screws placed in the anterior nasal spine region to intrude maxillary incisors as much as 6 mm. [7] it was until later in 1997, that Kanomi described the intrusion of mandibular anterior teeth using mini-implants. [8] Gelgor et al. reported as much as 88% success in molar distalization when the first and second molars were present following immediate loading. [9]

It has been reported that mini-implants can be further divided into two group: 1) those that provide mechanical retention and 2) those that osseointegrate. [10] The process of osseointegration is a histological phenomenon through which the bony tissue is formed around the implant without the presence of fibrous tissue at the interface of implant-bone, [11-13] however, in mechanical retention, those areas which are in direct contact with the bone are in charge of providing the primary stability; while there might be gaps in other areas between the mini-implant and the bone. [10] Osseointegrated devices need a healing period during which they should not be loaded. Anyhow, it has been reported that immediate loading up to 5 N does not affect the stability of miniscrew or loss of anchorage. [14, 15]

The decision making based on which the site for mini-implant placement is determined depends on the quality and quantity of bone in a particular region as well as interdental root space and the type of malocclusion. [5] The recommended anatomic sites for placement of mini-implant in maxilla include the interdental alveolar process , maxillary tuberosity, palate or anterior nasal spine.[16] As for mandible, the proper anatomic places are symphysis and parasymphysial area, interdental alveolar process and retromolar area. [16]

Correction of vertical problems has become easier with the advent of mini-implants. The envelope of orthodontic tooth movement has well increased and less emphasis needs to be placed upon patient's compliance. Treatment of different patients addressing their orthodontic problems (specially vertical problems) are presented in this chapter.

2. Patients and methods

2.1 Case 1: T.P.

The patient is a 15 year old male who was suffering from crowding both in the upper and lower arches. In order to alleviate the crowding, the patient had extracted the four first premolars based on an old myth that this will resolve the crowding. The spaces did not obviously close following extraction and the patient was referred to the orthodontist due to deep bite and the presence of spacing both in the upper and lower arches. (Figure 1-a to 1-c and 2-a to 2-f) The patient's chief complaint was the presence of spaces in both the maxillary and mandibular arches.

Clinical examination of patient show a slightly retrusive mandible and a nice posed smile. The intraoral photographs exhibit increased overbite, mild maxillary anterior crowding and a class II canine and molar relationship on both sides.

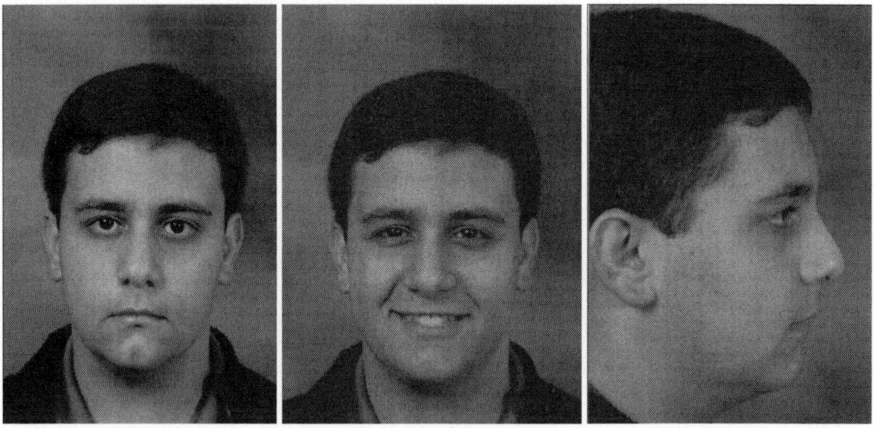

Fig. 1. Figure 1-a to 1-c, patient T.P, pretreatment facial photographs. The patient exhibits a nice social or posed smile, but a convex profile. An analysis of the E-line and S-line of the patient shows that the lips are retruded and therefore, the teeth cannot be further retracted.

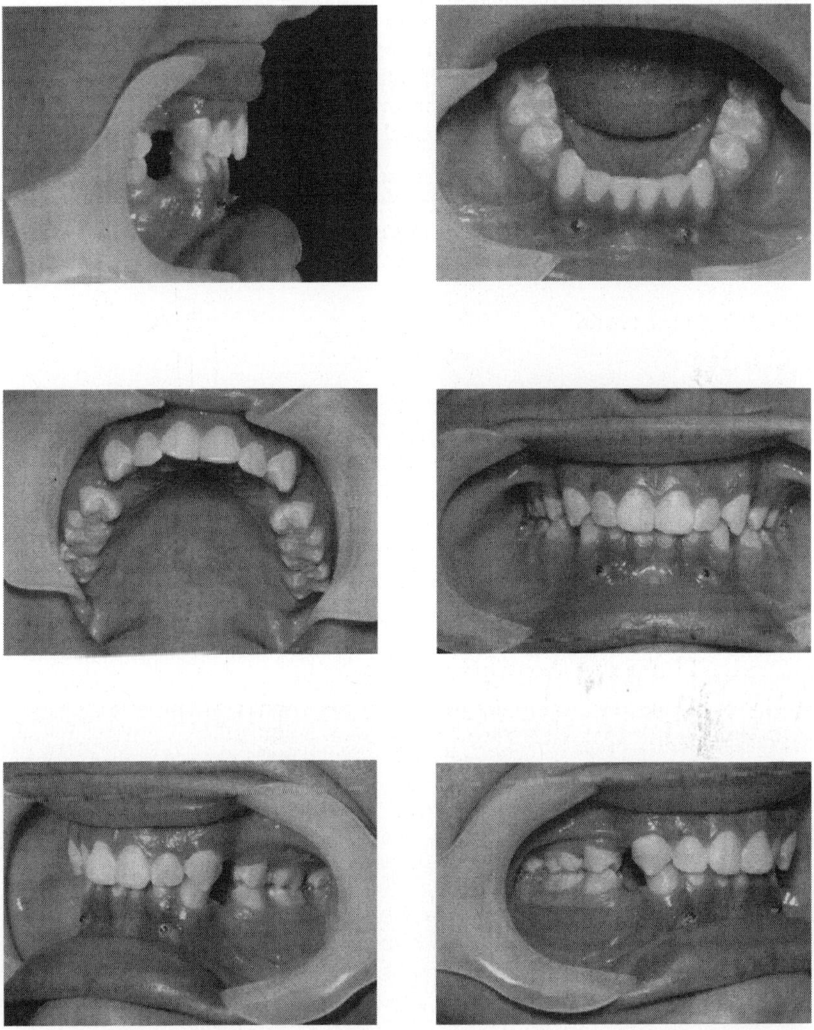

Fig. 2. Figs 2-a to 2-f, the patient had already extracted his four first premolars hoping that this would alleviate the mild crowding present. This had only led to a deep bite and four extraction spaces which looked unaesthetic.

x

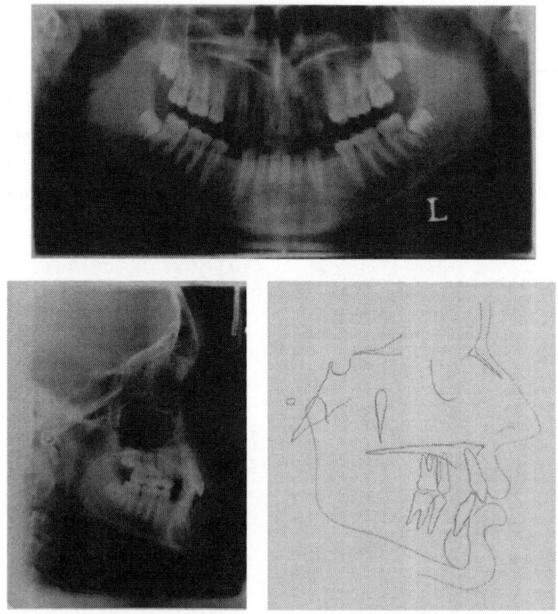

Fig. 3. Figs 3-a to 3-c, pretreatment lateral cephalograms, cephalometric tracing and panoramic radiograph.

Correction of deep bite can be achieved through different methods: extrusion of posterior teeth, upper incisors flaring, upper or lower incisors intrusion. Factors such as lower face height and upper incisor display dictate the technique through which deep bite can be addressed.[17]

Intrusion of anterior teeth has always been challenging and more difficult to attain than extrusion. [18] For intrusion to be successful and efficient, light, continuous forces are desired. [17, 19] This method can be successfully carried out in patients with an increased interlabial gap, increased vertical dimension and excessive gingival display.[20]

Case T.P exhibits acceptable posed smile at rest and upon smiling, therefore, intrusion of the upper incisors would not be a wise choice. Extrusion of posterior teeth, even though easier to achieve has a higher tendency for relapse but it tends to rotate the mandible backward and downward and thus aggravate the convex profile.[21] Based on the aforementioned factors, intrusion of lower incisors is the logical treatment approach.

Lower and upper arch were set up with 0.018-in slot standard edgewise braces. In the lower arch, segmented technique was used to intrude anterior teeth. Two mini-implants, 1.6 mm in diameter and 8.0 mm in length were placed between the roots of mandibular lateral incisors and canines for en masse intrusion of lower incisors by chain elastics. In the rest of treatment the lower anterior teeth were tied to the miniscrews in order to prevent them from relapse after their intrusion and to prepare anchorage for upper and lower posterior teeth to protract.

After intrusion the lower arch was replaced by a continuous arch wire. The mini-implants were used in this stage of treatment for upper and lower posterior segment protraction. Lower posterior teeth were protracted one by one. Protraction of upper posterior teeth was done by class III elastics. So, the miniscrews were used as an indirect anchorage to close the spaces in the upper arch. In addition, As the upper anterior teeth were not retracted and the canine relationship was class II it was necessary for the lower anterior teeth to be protracted by increased lower arch wire and use of miniscrews. (Figures 4-a to 4-c)

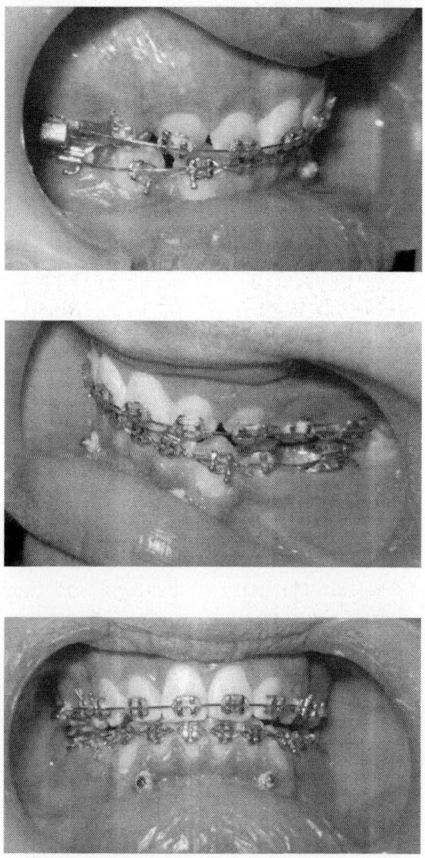

Fig. 4. Figs 4-a to4-c, progress intraoral photographs, Protrusion of upper and lower anterior teeth along with intrusion of lower incisors was needed to achieve the optimal overbite.

At 12 months, treatment was completed (figure 5-a to 5-h and figures 6-a to 6-c). Fixed retainers extending from premolar to premolar were bonded in maxilla and mandible.

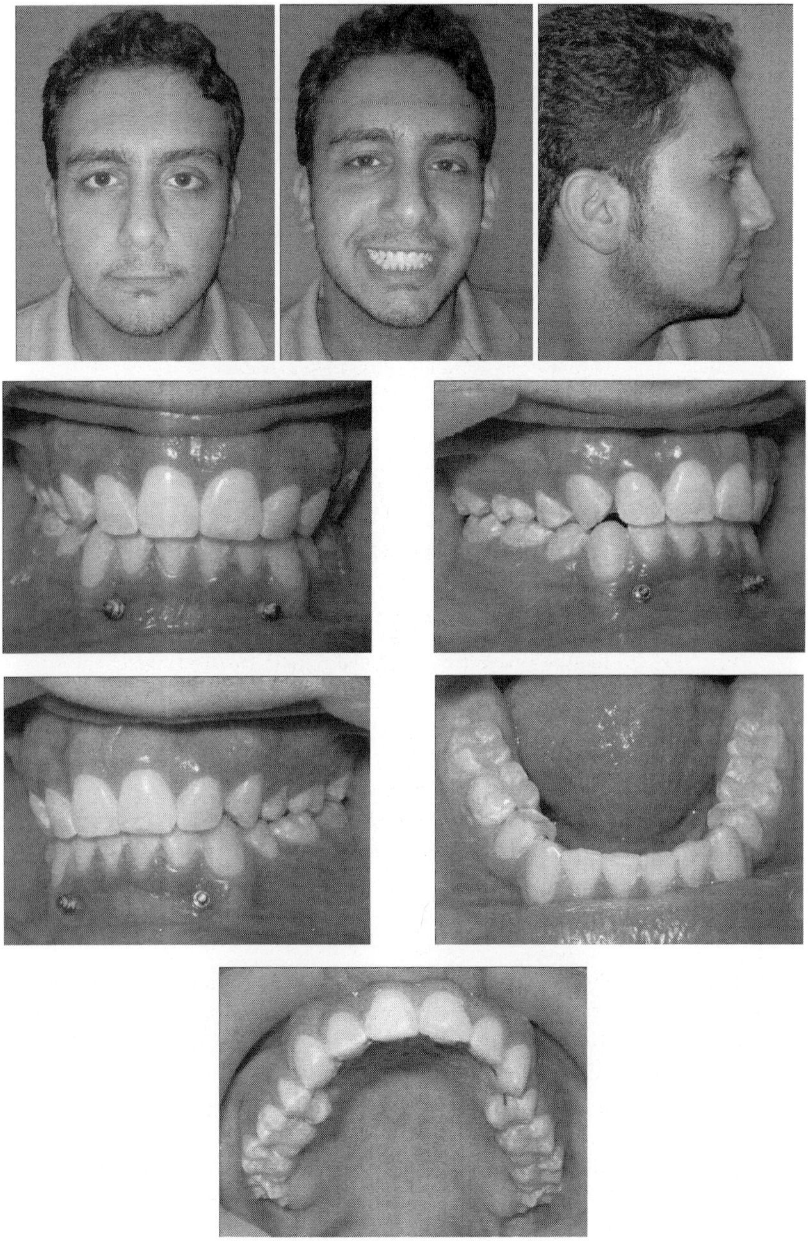

Fig. 5. Figs 5-a to 5-h at 11 months, treatment is completed. Notice the marked improvement in the facial profile and overbite.

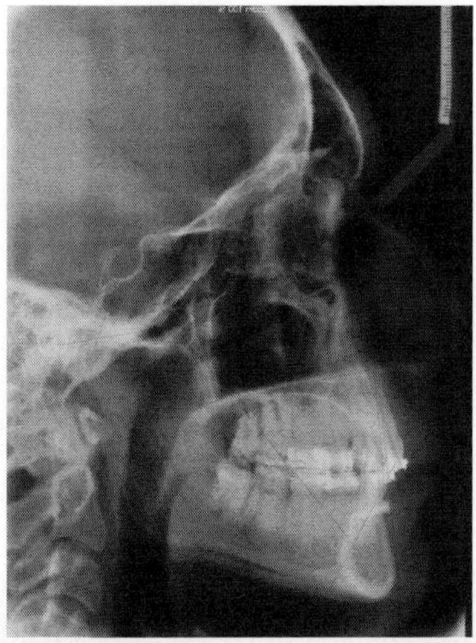

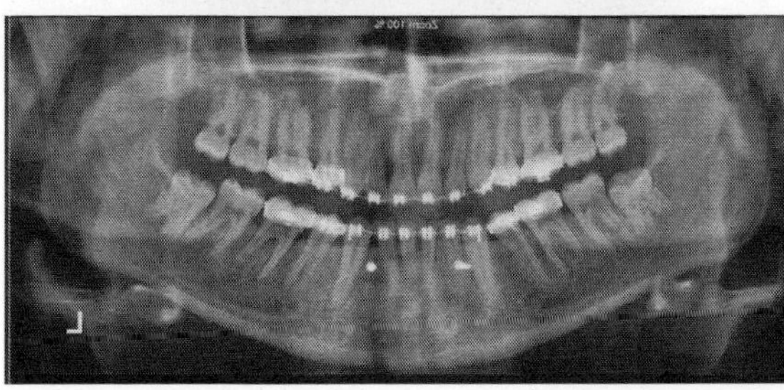

Fig. 6. Figs 6-a to 6-c, posttreatment cephalogram and panoramic radiograph.

2.2 Case 2: J.V.

The patient is a 16-year-old girl with a class II canine relationship on both sides and a very deep overbite. Her chief complaint was irregular teeth.

The pretreatment facial photographs show a retrsuive mandible and moderate crowding of the maxillary anterior teeth. The pretreatment intraoral photographs exhibited full class II molar and canine relationship on both sides, severe deep bite along with retroinclination of maxillary central incisors (fig 7-a to 7-I)

Cephalometric analysis showed a class II skeletal relationship due to mandibular deficiency (SNB angle, 71°), A-point was also retruded (SNA angle, 75°). The FMA was within the normal range (26°). Maxillary incisor to SN plane was 87° which is much smaller than the normal range. IMPA was 94° which is within the normal range. In other words, the maxillary incisors were linguoversion and mandible is slightly retruded.

The ideal treatment was to create a normal overbite and overjet relationship, reduce the anteroposterior skeletal discrepancy and obtain a class I canine and molar relationship.

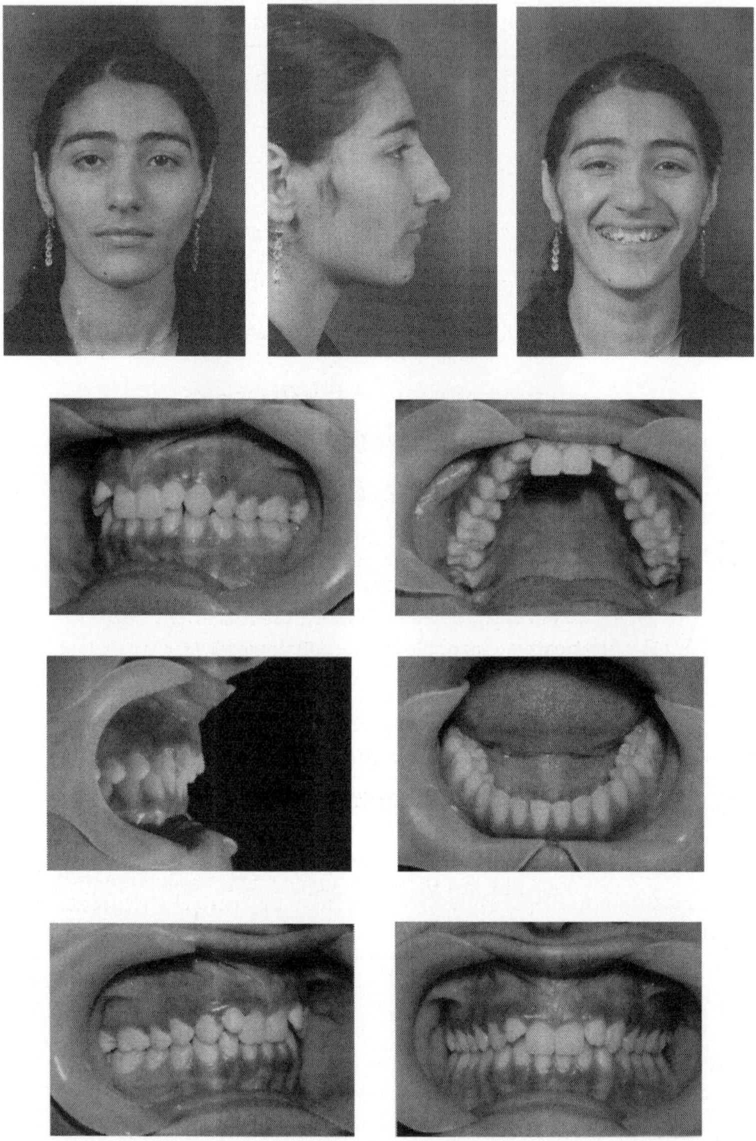

Fig. 7. Fig 7-a to 7-i, pretreatment facial and intraoral photographs. Notice the retruded mandible and marked retroinclination of maxillary central incisors.

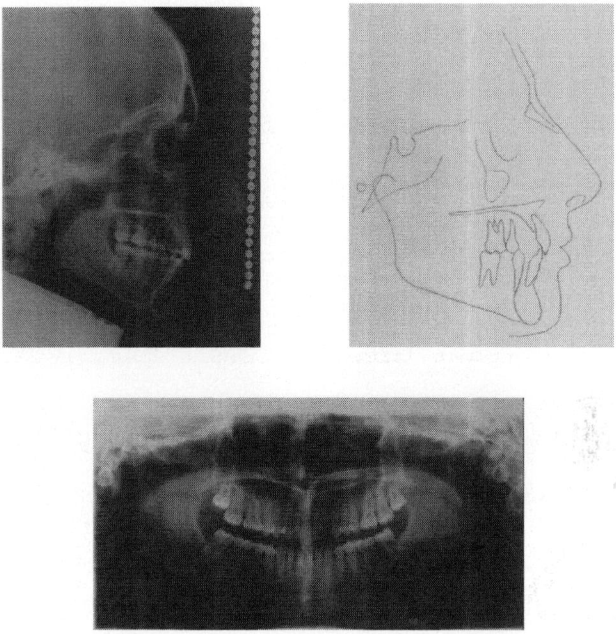

Fig. 8. Figs 8-a to 8-c, pretreatment cephalogram, cephalometric tracing and panoramic radiograph.

The ideal treatment approach would be orthognathic surgery during which maxillary anterior teeth are proclined forward to obtain some overjet and move the mandible forward. However, the patient is past the age of growth modification and is not willing to undertake surgery as well. The treatment alternative would be distalization of maxillary dentition to provide space for leveling and aligning of maxillary incisors. However, distalizing the teeth tends to extrude them which makes the mandible to rotate backward and downward and thus worsen the facial profile. Therefore, it is essential that distalization of maxillary molars be carried out without extrusion.

Missing of mandibular third molars permitted the second upper molars to be extracted. Therefore, Initially maxillary second molars were extracted and it was decided that the maxillary third molars would eventually replace the extracted teeth . Then, a segmented arch technique (o.o18-in slot) was fabricated in the maxillary arch to prevent protrusion of the maxillary incisors while distalization of maxillary molars was being carried out. Two mini-implants 2mm in diameter and 10 mm in length were placed in paramedian midsagittal raphe. A transpalatal bar (0.38-in) was fabricated which was soldered to the bands cemented on maxillary molars. Anchorage was provided from the mini-implants to distalize the maxillary molars and at the same time prevent extrusion of maxillary molars. (figure 9-a to 9-f)

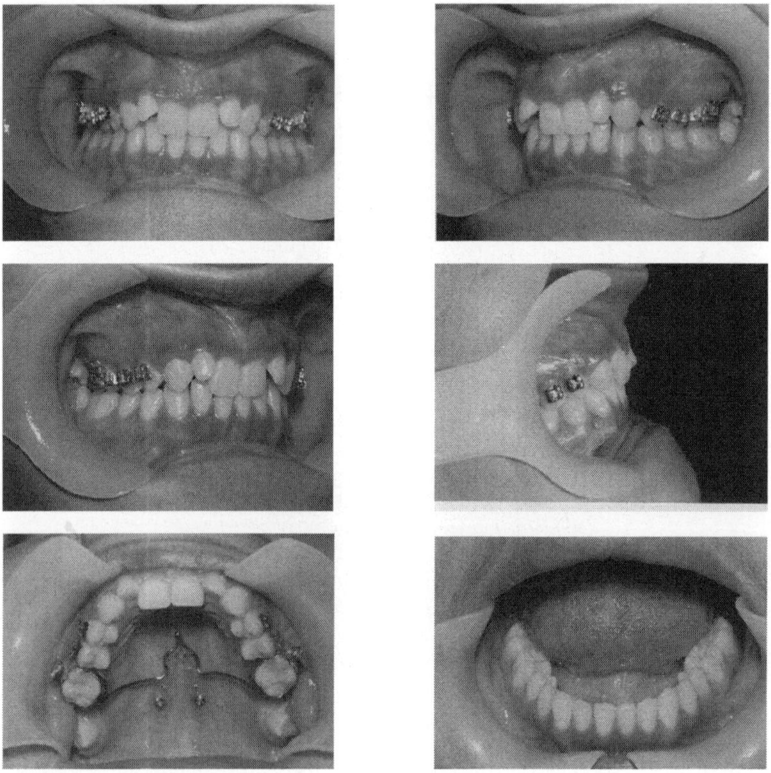

Fig. 9. Figs 9-a to 9-f, A modified version of transpalatal bar is fabricated in the maxillary arch to help distalize maxillary molars. As you see first upper molars have started to rotate.

Retraction of all posterior maxillary teeth were intended during the course of distalization, maxillary first molars started to rotate(mesial in and distal out) due to the location of mini-implants and the resultant untoward moment on them, therefore two other miniscrews were inserted in the buccal vestibule in the position of extraction of the second upper molars. The position where the miniscrews were to be inserted was critical in this case because if they were inserted too far mesially, distal root of the first molar could be cut off while they were being retracted. On the other hand, if they were inserted too far distally the third molars could not be repositioned mesially to replace the extracted second molars.

While retracting upper posterior teeth lower teeth and upper anterior teeth were not set up since it was not necessary and also the patient was sensitive on her appearance And wanted to reduce the time during which she had to bear braces in the anterior area to a minimum. Therefore, for the major part of her treatment process which included the retraction of upper posterior teeth she was free of braces in the esthetic zone. Once a class I canine and molar relationship was attained, the transpalatal bar was removed to minimize the irritation in the palatal mucosa (figures 10-a to 10-f).

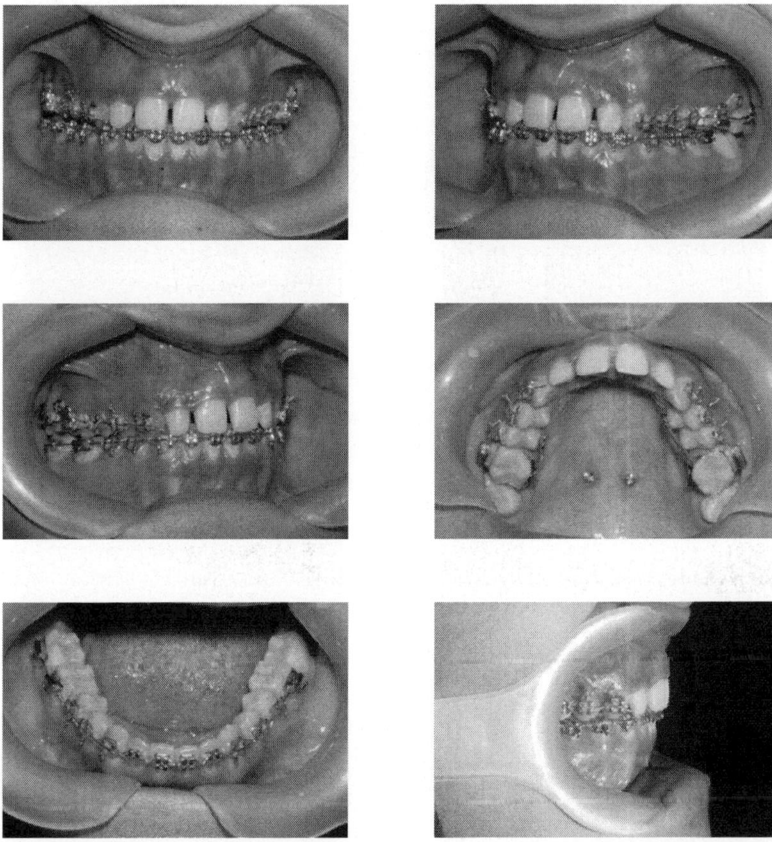

Fig. 10. Figs 10-a to 10-f, progress intraoral photographs at 6 months. A class I molar and canine relationship is maintained. Notice the miniscrews in the buccal vestibule. The transpalatal bar is removed to eliminate the irritation of soft tissue.

Upper lateral incisors were small-sized and had thus resulted in anterior Bolton discrepancy. The patient was referred for composite build up of lateral incisors to gain normal tooth size. Total treatment time was 15 months. The mini-implant and the transpalatal bar were well tolerated by the patient. The post treatment intraoral photographs show a class I canine and molar relationship. Overbite is corrected. Facial harmony is very good. The pretreatment and posttreatment superimposition of lateral cephalograms shows no backward or downward rotation of mandible. Fixed canine to canine retainers were bonded in the maxilla and mandible (figures 11-a to 11-I and figures 12-a to 12-c)

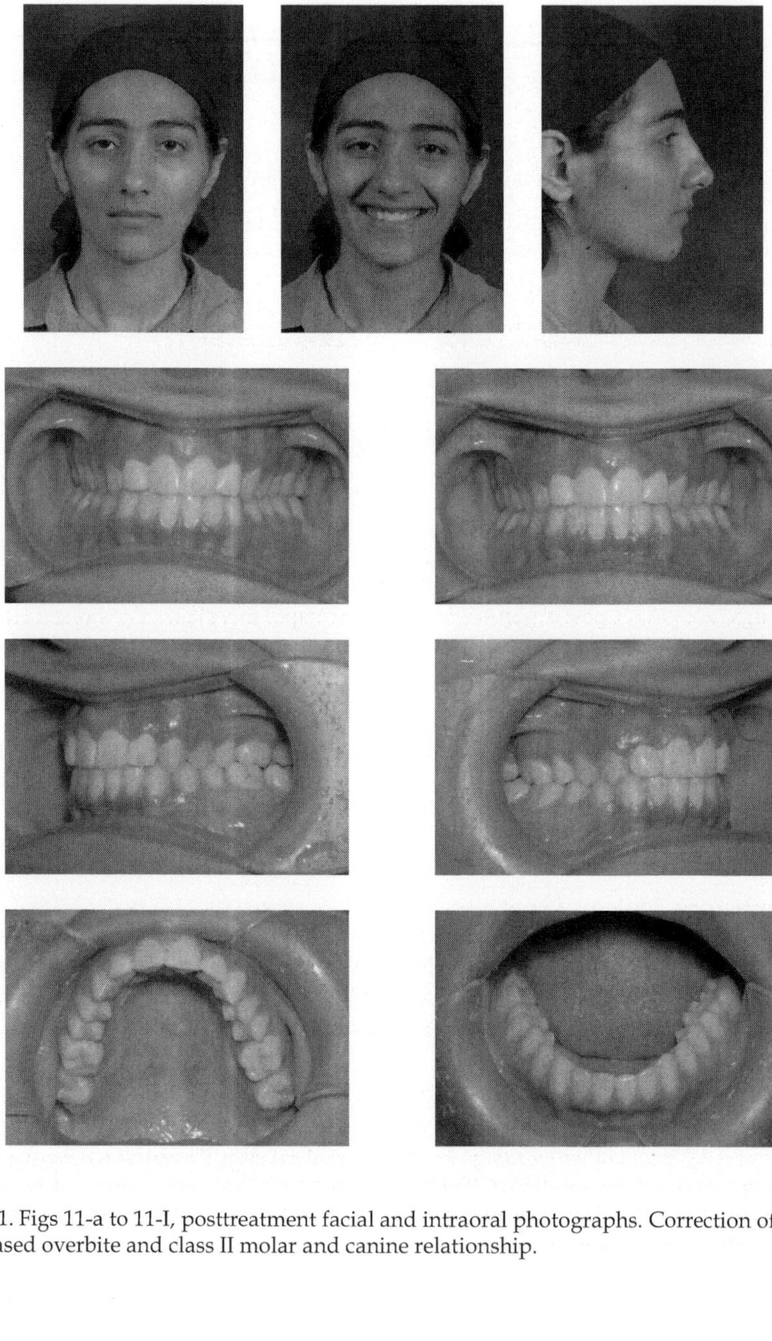

Fig. 11. Figs 11-a to 11-I, posttreatment facial and intraoral photographs. Correction of increased overbite and class II molar and canine relationship.

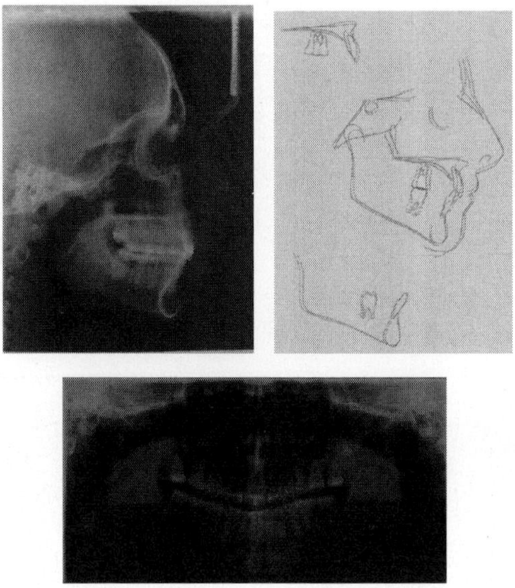

Fig. 12. figs 12-a to 12-c, post treatment cephalogram, superimposition of pretreatment (red) and post treatment (black) cephalometric tracings, and panoramic radiograph.

2.3 Case R.R.

The next patient is a 31-year-old female who was once referred to a maxillofacial surgeon with a chief complaint of gummy smile. The surgeon had performed a maxillary impaction and an advancement genioplasty on the patient without presurgical orthodontic treatment. The patient eventually was not satisfied with the results and was therefore, referred to the orthodontist. Her chief complaints were gummy smile and the present spacing.

The pretreatment facial photographs exhibit facial asymmetry along with a cant of maxillary occlusal plane. Clinical examination revealed a deviated midline (2mm). Spacing could be noticed at different areas both in maxillary and mandibular dentition. The four first premolars had already been extracted in earlier years to help alleviate crowding, but no further orthodontic treatment was carried out on the patient to consolidate the arches (figures 13-a to 13-j)

Cephalometric analysis revealed a retrusive mandible (ANB angle 7°) and an increased IMPA angle (94°). The SNA angle was within the normal limits (82°); however, SNB angle was decreased (75°). In other words, patient had a skeletal class II profile accompanied with mandibular dental compensation (figures 14-a to 14-c). The patient was not willing to undergo another orthognathic surgery to correct the existing problems and since the four first premolars had already been extracted, extracting yet another tooth was out of question.

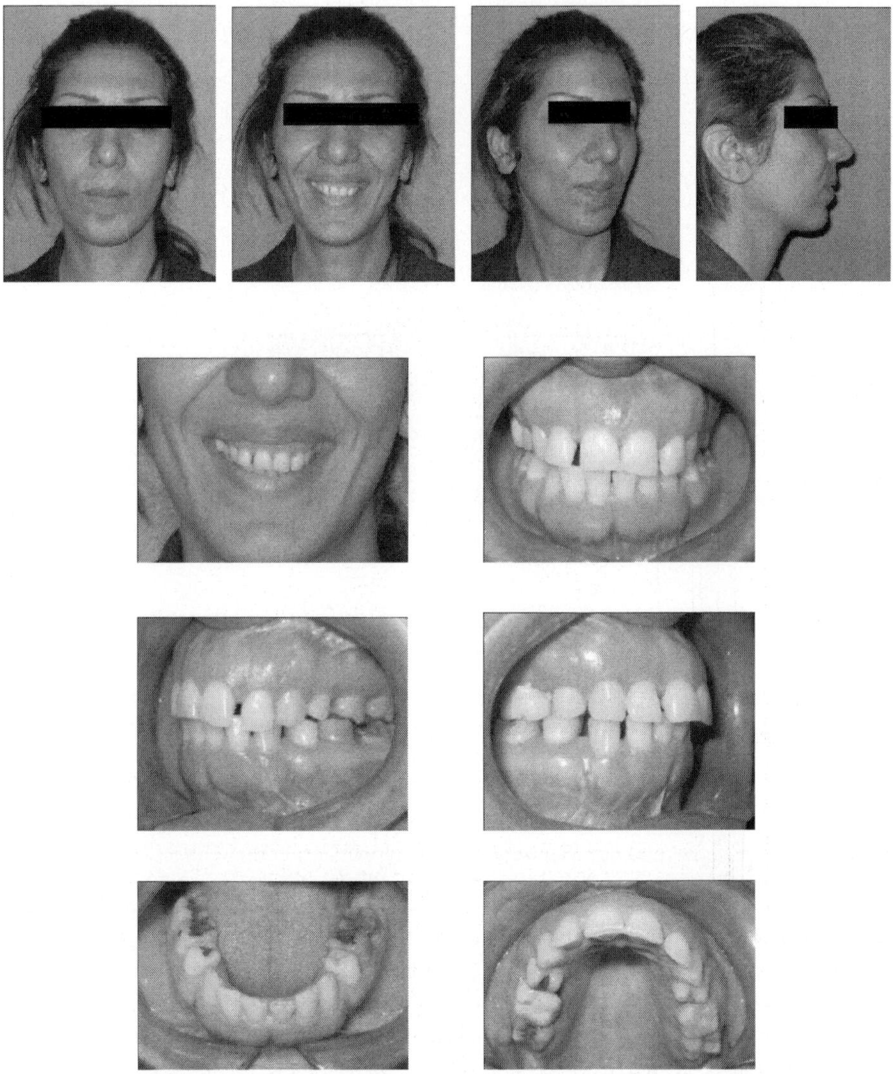

Fig. 13. Figs 13-a to 13-j pretreatment facial and intraoral photographs, the four first premolars had already been extracted; notice the canted maxillary occlusal plane and excessive gingival display.

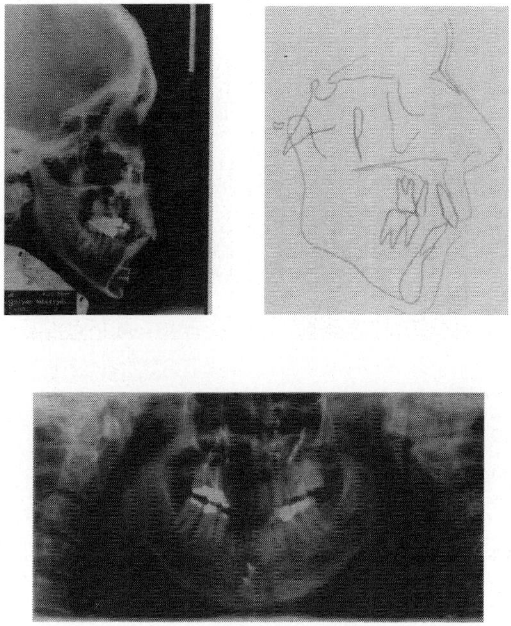

Fig. 14. figs 14-a to 14-c, pretreatment cephalogram, cephalometric tracing and panoramic radiographs.

The treatment goals were to address the patient's chief complaints, i.e correct the canted occlusal palne and close the spaces. Two mini-implants of 1.4 in diameter and 6.0 mm in length were placed between the roots of maxillary lateral incisors and canines. Initially a continuous 0.016 NiTi arch wire was placed as the initial arch wire. With the progress in the size of the arch wire, after 2 months, a 0.016×0.022-in stainless steel segmented arch wire was placed extending from left to right maxillary lateral incisors. In order to decrease the gummy smile, the patient was asked to wear $\frac{3}{16}$ - in latex elastics from the anterior segment to the mini-implants. Since, the equal use of both mini-implants would not correct the canted occlusal plane, the patient was asked to wear the latex elastic to the left mini-implant two days in a row and to the right mini-implant once every three days (figure 15-a to 15- f)

Consecutive use of latex elastics in the anterior region has the disadvantage of irritating the labial frenum, thus, decreasing the patient cooperation. After 1 month, in lieu of latex elastics, elastomeric chains were used. After intrusion of the upper anterior teeth and correction of its cant, continuous 0.016 SS arch wire was inserted in the upper and lower arches. Midline correction and space closure was carried out in both arches at this stage. Meanwhile, the upper anterior teeth were tied to the miniscrews to prevent their relapse after intrusion.

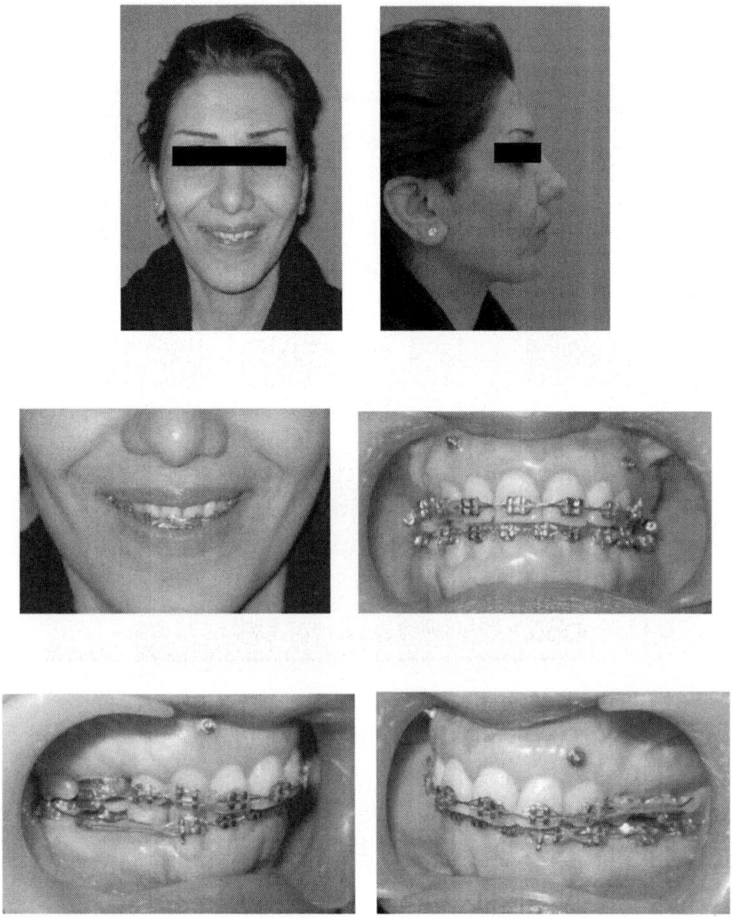

Fig. 15. Figs 15-a to 15-f, progress facial and intraoral photographs, mini-implants are placed between the roots of lateral incisor and canine to address gummy smile and canted occlusal plane.

After 13 months, the treatment was completed. The patient was very well satisfied with the changes in her appearance. The gummy smile and canted occlusal plane had resolved significantly. Fixed retainers extending from second premolar to second premolar were bonded in the maxilla and mandible (figures 16-a to 16-h). Post treatment cephalometric tracing revealed 6 mm intrusion of maxillary incisors without a significant difference in the inclination of upper incisors (upper incisors to SN angle, pretreatment : 106°, post treatment: 105°) (figures 17-a to 17-d).

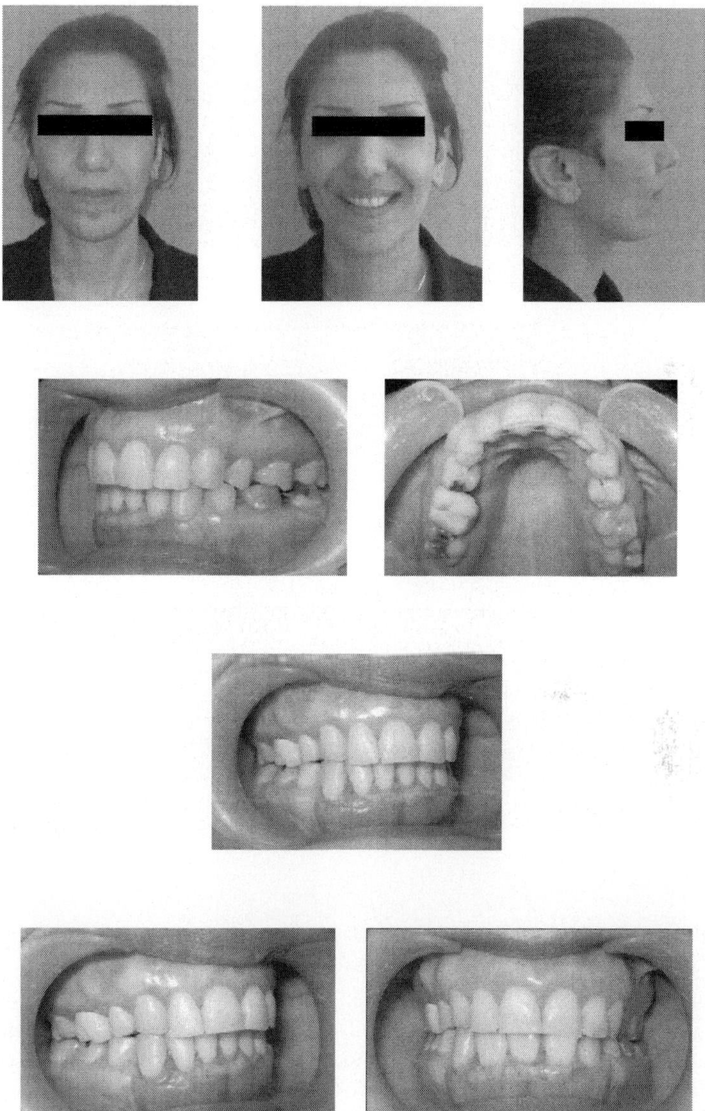

Fig. 16. Figs 16-a to 16-h, post treatment facial and intraoral photographs, notice the correction of the canted occlusal plane and gummy smile.

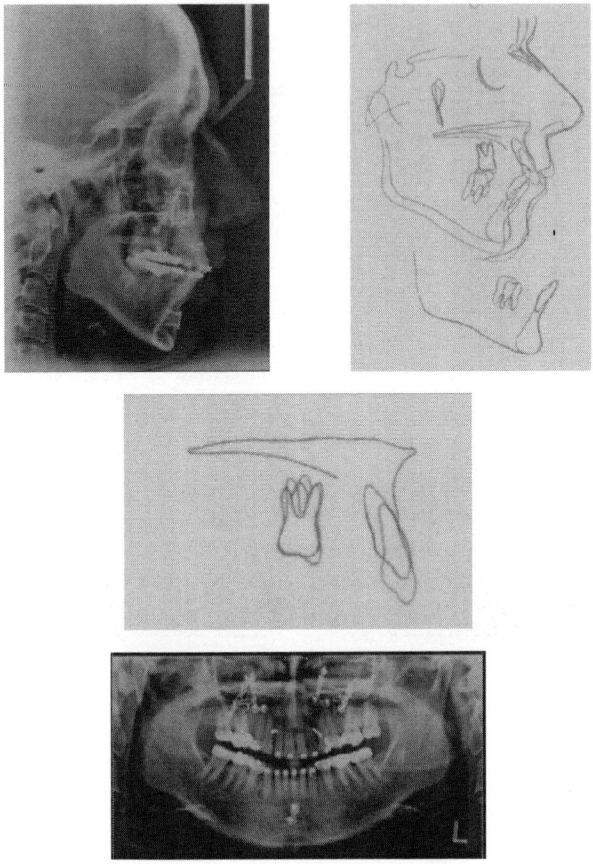

Fig. 17. Figs 17-a to 17-d. post treatment cephalogram, superimposition of pretreatment (red) and post treatment (black) cephalometric tracings and panoramic radiograph.

2.4 Case R.T.

This patient was a 31-year-old female with a class I molar and canine relationship. Her chief complaints were protrusion of her teeth and inability to bring her lips together.

Clinical examination revealed bimaxillary dentoalveolar protrusion with excessive gingival display upon rest and lip incompetence. She exhibited slight facial asymmetry with her chin deviated to the left and also a class I molar and canine relationship and spacing distal to both maxillary lateral incisors (figures 18-a to 18-h)

Cephalomettric analysis showed the A-point and B-point to be protruded (SNA angle 89° and SNB angle 85°). The upper incisor angle was increased (126°) and IMPA was also much larger than normal (105°).The interincisal angle was 97°. The ANB angle was 4°. In other words, the patient showed bimaxillary dentoalveolar protrusion (figures 19-a to 19-c).

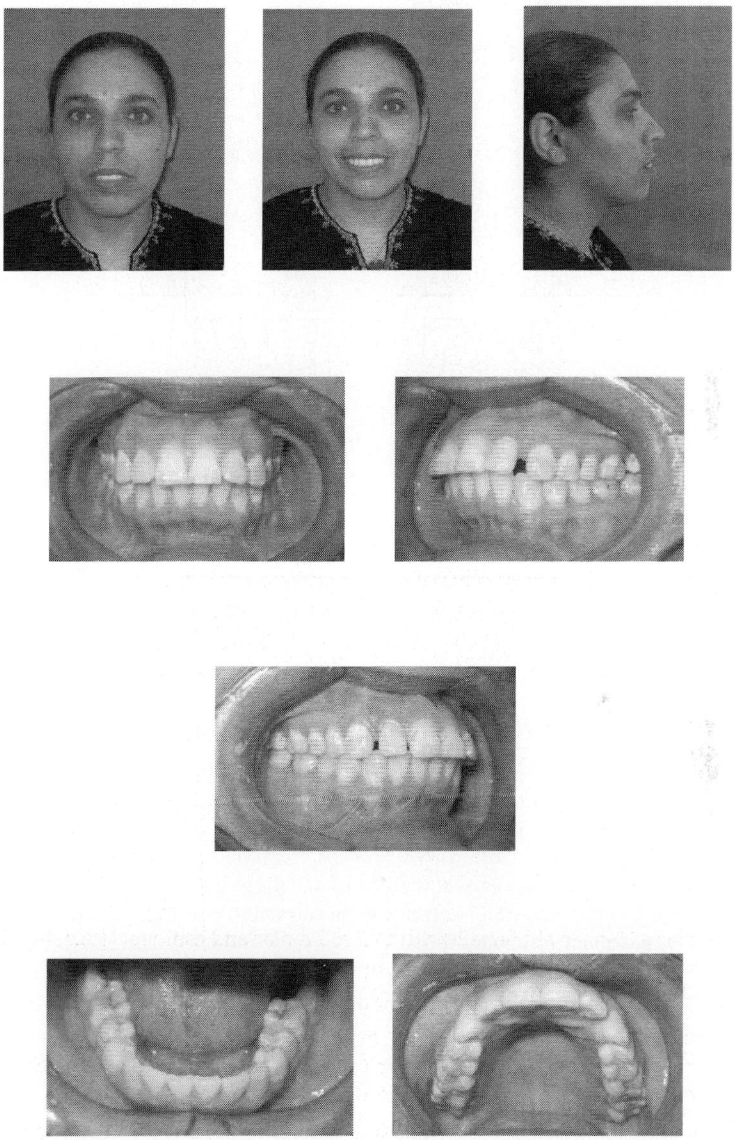

Fig. 18. Figs 18-a to 18-h, Pretreatment facial and intraoral photographs of the patient R.T.

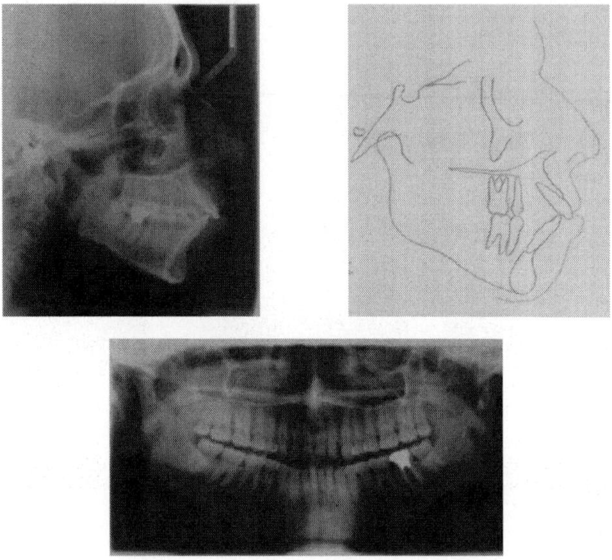

Fig. 19. Figs 19-a to 19-c, pretreatment cephalogram, cephalometric tracing and panoramic radiographic.

The best treatment approach in bimaxillary dentoalveolar protrusion is extraction of four first premolars. However, since the patient is suffering from excessive upper incisor display upon rest, extraction of premolars and retraction of anterior teeth would only exacerbate the gummy smile. In this case, the best treatment approach would probably be orthognathic surgery. The patient, however, was reluctant to undertake any type of surgery due to financial issues. The treatment alternative was to intrude the teeth and reduce the excessive gingival display with the use of mini-implants.

Two mini-implants of 1.6 in diameter and 8.0 in length were placed between the roots of maxillary lateral incisors and canines. 0.018-in slot standard edgewise brackets were bonded on the patients teeth. The four first premolars were extracted. Anchorage preparation was extremely important in this case and therefore, maxillary and mandibular second molars were added to the anchorage unit. Anterior teeth retraction was carried out in two separate stages. Initially, maxillary and mandibular canines were retracted using pull coil spring and then T-loop on 0.016×0.022-in stainless steel was used to retract the incisors during the second phase of anterior teeth retraction. Elastic chain was applied to the upper anterior teeth from miniscrews to intrude them during retraction. 0.016-in and 0.016×0.022-in stainless steel wires were inserted after space closure as ideal arch wires. Interdigitation of the teeth was achieved by a short duration of interarch elastics. [22]

After 17 months, treatment is completed. Even though the bimaxillary dentoalveolar protrusion is resolved, excessive tooth display was also corrected. Fixed retainers were bonded from the left to the right second premolars in both maxilla and mandible (figure 20-a to 20-f). cephalometric tracing revealed significant improvement in the inclination of the maxillary and mandibular incisors (upper incisors to SN angle; pretreatment: 126° and post treatment: 91°, IMPA; pretreatment: 105° and post treatment 94°, Figures 21-a to 21-e).

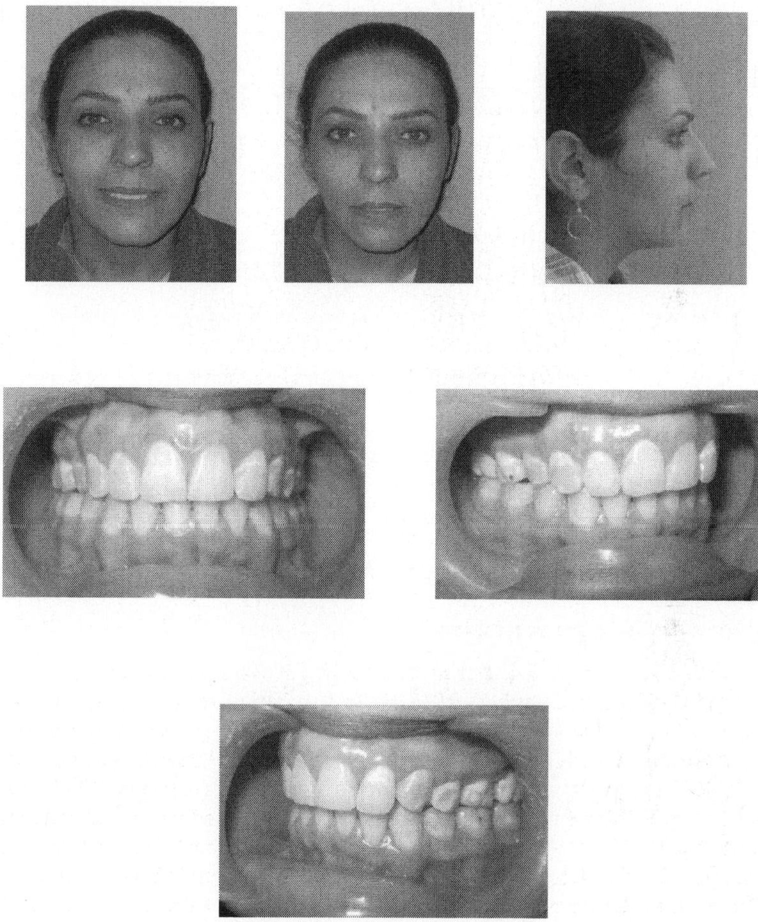

Fig. 20. Figs 20-a to 20-f, post treatment facial and intraoral photographs, notice the marked improvement in the patient's profile. Lip incompetence is resolved with no increase in upper incisor display upon rest or posed smile.

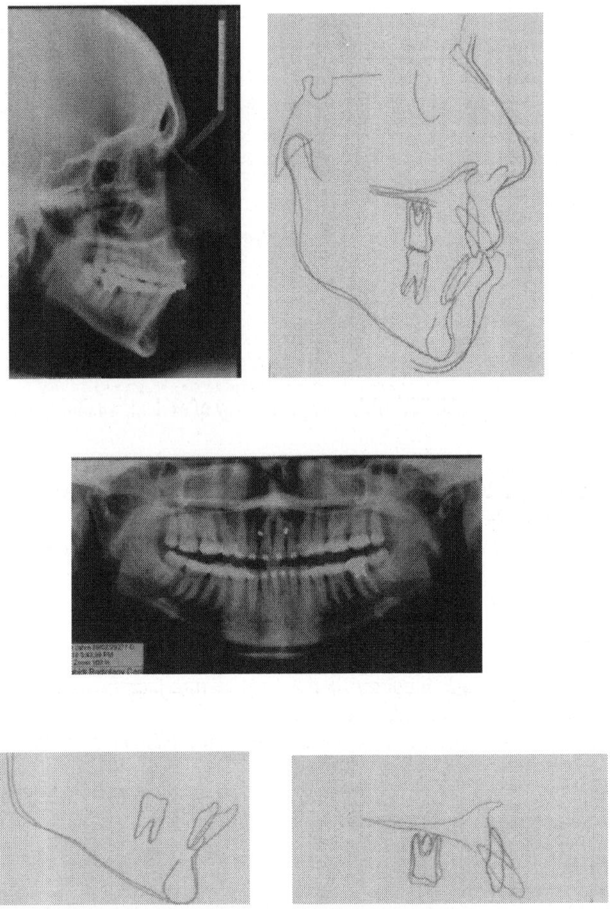

Fig. 21. Figs 21-a to 21-e, post treatment cephalogram, superimposition of pretreatment (red) and post treatment cephalometric tracings and panoramic radiograph. Notice the miniscrews in the upper arch that are not explanted yet.

3. Conclusion

The introduction of mini-implants has improved the practice of orthodontics. Treatment approaches have become available that can be an alternative to orthognathic surgery and provide acceptable results. Duration of treatment becomes shorter significantly and simpler. The envelope of tooth movement has increased to an extent that more versatile movements in three planes of space can be carried out with more success.

4. References

[1] Proffit, W.R. and J.L. Ackerman, *Orthodontic diagnosis: the developement of a problem list.* 2nd ed. Contemporary orthodontics, ed. W.R. Proffit and H.W. Fields. 1993, St Louis: Mosby.

[2] Kinzinger, G., et al., *Innovative anchorage alternatives for molar distalization- An overview.* J Orofac Orthop, 2005. 66: p. 397-413.

[3] Gedrange, T., K. Boening, and W. Harzer, *Orthodontic implants as anchorage appliances for unilateral mesialization: a case report.* Quintessence International, 2006. 37: p. 485-91.

[4] Lee, J.S., et al., *Application of orthodontic mini-implants*, ed. L.C. Bywaters. 2007, Hanover park, IL: Quintessence.

[5] Mizrahi, E. and B. Mizrahi, *Mini-screw implants (temporary anchorage devices) : orthodontic and pre-orthodontic applications.* Journal of Orthodontics, 2007. 34: p. 80-94.

[6] Linkow, L.I., *Implant orthodontics.* J Clin Orthod, 1970. 4: p. 685-690.

[7] Creekmore, T.D. and M.K. Eklund, *The possibility of skeletal anchorage.* J Clin Orthod, 1983. 17: p. 266-269.

[8] Kanomi, R., *Mini-implants for orthodontic anchorage.* J Clin Orthod, 1997. 31: p. 763-67.

[9] Gelgor, I.E., et al., *Inraosseous screw-supported upper molar distalization.* Angle Orthod, 2004. 74: p. 838-850.

[10] Nanda, R.S. and F.A. Uribe, *Temporary anchorage devices in orthodontics.* Biological response to orthodontic temporary anchorage devices, ed. J.J. DOlan. 2009, St. Louis, Missouri: Mosby.

[11] Branemark, P.I., *Osseointegration and its experimental background.* Journal of Prosthetic Dentistry, 1983. 50(3): p. 399-410.

[12] Albrektsson, T. and M. Jacobsson, *Bone-metal interface in osseointegration.* Journal of Prosthetic Dentistry, 1987. 57(5): p. 597-607.

[13] Cooper, L.F., *Biologic determinants of bone formation for osseointegration: clues for future clinical improvements.* Journal of Prosthetic Dentistry, 1998. 80(4): p. 439-49.

[14] Crismani, A.G., et al., *Miniscrews in orthodontic treatment: review and analysis of published clinical trials.* Am J Orthod Dentofacial Orthop, 2010. 137(1): p. 108-13.

[15] Chen, F., et al., *Anchorage effect of osseointegrated vs nonosseointegrated palatal implants.* Angle Orthod, 2006. 76(4): p. 660-5.

[16] Papadopoulos, M.A. and F. Tarawneh, *The use of miniscrew implants for temporary skeletal anchorage in orthodontics: a comprehensive review.* Oral Surgery, Oral Medicine, Oral Pathology, Oral Radiology and Endodontics, 2007. 103(5): p. e6-15.

[17] Nanda, R., *Correction of deep overbite in adults.* Dent Clin North Am, 1997. 41(1): p. 67-87.

[18] Burstone, C.R., *Deep overbite correction by intrusion.* Am J Orthod, 1977. 72(1): p. 1-22.

[19] Shroff, B., et al., *Simultaneous intrusion and retraction using a three-piece base arch.* Angle Orthod, 1997. 67(6): p. 455-61; discussion 462.

[20] Nanda, R., R. Marzban, and A. Kuhlberg, *The Connecticut Intrusion Arch.* J Clin Orthod, 1998. 32(12): p. 708-15.

[21] Levin, R.I., *Deep bite treatment in relation to mandibular growth rotation.* Eur J Orthod, 1991. 13(2): p. 86-94.
[22] Burstone, C.J., *The segmented arch approach to space closure.* Am J Orthod, 1982. 82(5): p. 361-78.

10

Management of Dental Impaction

Farid Bourzgui, Mourad Sebbar, Zouhair Abidine and Zakaria Bentahar
Faculty of Dentistry, University of Hassan II Ain Chok
Morocco

1. Introduction

Practitioners are frequently faced with tooth eruption anomalies during the gradual emergence of complete adult dentition, and notably disorders related to tooth impaction (Hurme et al. 1949). This process, which affects deciduous, permanent and supernumerary teeth, is thought, apart from more general causes, to stem from a breakdown in the dynamics of eruption as a result of numerous different factors (Rajic et al. 1996) among whchi we can cite the following:

- Malformation of the germ;
- Local obstacles (tumors or cysts, supernumerary teeth and odontomas);
- Inadequate available volume on the arch which can have either a primary etiology of skeletal (brachygnathism) or dental origin (macrodontia) or secondary etiology due to spontaneous mesial drift (premature loss of milk teeth due to resorption) or iatrogenic mesial drift (premature avulsions).

Agenesia of proximal teeth sometimes gives rise to tooth impaction as a result of loss of the eruption guidance function. In particular, this can affect the upper lateral incisors. And, lastly, the poorly-documented phenomenon of ankylosis occurs following the more or less total disappearance of the dental ligament associated with hypercementosis and root resorption which obstruct all physiological or provoked dental development at various stages (Chambas, 1997).

The unerupted or impacted tooth will trigger some major esthetic and/or functional disorders (Le Breton, 1997) depending on which tooth is affected; hence, the need to reposition in the arch, particularly if the impaction is located in the anterior region. With this in mind, and to achieve maximum results, treatment of tooth retention requires collaboration between surgeons and orthodontists. Consequently, the introduction of surgical-orthodontic techniques in our clinical practice has made it easier to manage dental impaction.

This chapter aims to review the current state of knowledge on management of impacted teeth in order to establish a standard protocol and thus codify the treatment of this anomaly.

2. Definition

Impacted teeth are classically defined as retained in the jaw beyond their normal date of eruption, surrounded by their coronary bag and without communication with the oral cavity (Favre, 2003).

For Izard (Izard, 1950), there is total retention tooth when the tooth is kept inside the jaw beyond the normal period of its eruption, and no tendency to make its vertical migration.

According to Lacoste (1988): a tooth that remains within bone or submucosa after the normal date of its rash is most often referred to as tooth retention.

According Bordais (1980), a tooth is said to be retained when its evolutionary potential is preserved, while a tooth is said to be included when it its evolutionary potential is lost.

Vigneul (1974) speaks of a tooth completely embedded in the bone and whose coronary bag remains unscathed. He maintains that there are two types of inclusions:

- Aphysiologicaltype, which refers to any tooth that has not erupted, and
- A pathological type, which is the topic of our study, in which the tooth can be intraosseous or submucosa.

A new classification of Dentistry Teeth (Favre, 2003) integrates data from major international reference classifications. The clinicopathological and pathophysiological classification distinguishes:

- tooth included in the way of normal eruption;
- tooth retention;
- impacted teeth, proper, or retained tooth included;
- enclosed tooth retention;
- tooth disimpaction,in its proper sense;
- tooth disimpaction at large.

3. Epidemiology

The results of different studies show variable numbers, which are not necessarily contradictory. These discrepancies come from the non-homogeneity of the samples studied. All are unanimous on the fact that the mandibular third molars are most frequently included, followed by their counterparts of maxillary and maxillary canines.

The classic distribution in order of frequency of impaction of permanent teeth can be summarized as follows : lower third molars, upper third molars, upper canines, upper and lower premolars, upper incisors, lower canines, lower incisors, upper and lower first molars and upper and lower second molars [Ericsson, 2000; Quirynen, 2000).

The position of the canines is palatal in 50% of the cases, buccal in 30%of the cases, while it occupies an intermediate position in 20% of the cases (Chambas, 1997). Its frequency is 10 times higher in Caucasians than in Chinese, while the variability in gender shows a slight prevalence in girls.

4. Etiology

Primary reasons: genetics (Vichi, 1996), endocrinologic deficiency, irradiation, palatal clefts, developmental abnormities of germs, supernumerary tooth or tooth fragments , dento-maxillary disharmony (mostly for bucal impactions), late or missing root development, growth disharmony between pre-maxilla and maxilla (concerns maxillary canines only), maxillary brachygnatia, transversal growth deficiency of the anterior maxilla (Mc Connelt, 1996).

Secondary reasons: loss of guidance of the lateral incisor (microdontia or tooth absence) (Sasakura, 1984; Ericsson, 1987; Peck, 1996), trauma, premature extraction causing space problems by mesialisation of the anterior sector (second mandibular premolar moving mesialy after extraction of the second deciduous molar), root malformation, pericoronary pathology, ectopic germ position, thick fibrous tissue (Goho, 1987), mesio-distal dimension of the nasal fossae, unerupted canine at the borderline of a palatal cleft (Benoit, 1989).

5. Diagnosis

The diagnosis of any tooth impaction should be established as early as possible in order to monitor its development and implementation of appropriate therapy in time. In the absence of a maxillary central incisor, the parents consult early for the appearance of the lateral incisor reducing the median space, thus creating an asymmetric and unsightly situation. For canines, as a rule, no functional sign would lead the patient to consult early; the discovery is almost always casual in a screening or radiological examination (presence of a late primary cuspid).

The diagnosis is based on clinical and radiographic examination. Three positions of impaction are generally possible: buccal, intermediary and palatal (in the maxilla) or lingual (in the mandible). But a very strict attitude in this subject can lead to errors in the appreciation of the precise position. Thus we know that canines whose crowns are positioned buccaly often have their root reaching out palataly behind the root-tips of the neighbouring teeth (Korbendeau, 2005).

5.1 Clinical diagnosis

5.1.1 Anamnesis

The interview will allow collecting any family predisposition to inclusions or other hereditary factors such as agenesis. The medical history should identify pathological antecedents and any counter-indications for surgical-orthodontic treatment. The patient's motivation is also an important point to consider, facing a long and difficult treatment.

5.1.2 Clinical examination

The clinical examination often allows establishing a presumption of inclusion. Two methods are used:

Inspection

- The persistence of a deciduous tooth in the arch beyond its normal replacement date;
- The absence of a permanent tooth when its normal time of eruption is exceeded;
- Reduction of the space of tooth eruption by underlying mesialization adjacent teeth;
- The malposition or malformation of the teeth adjacent to the missing tooth (versions and rotations);
- Lack of synchronization between left and right exfoliation and eruption of teeth two counterparts, are all elements for a strong presumption of inclusion or retention tooth.

Palpation

- Palpation of the buccal and lingual mucosa simultaneously using the indexes of the two hands is recommended to estimate the position of the teeth changing.
- The lack of hump canine on the arch at 10 or 11 years, coinciding with the absence of the permanent canine is also a presumption in favor of inclusion or agenesis. But only X-ray examination can establish with certainty the diagnosis of inclusion.

5.1.3 Radiological examination

In addition to clinical assessment, the protocol begins with a dental panoramic X-ray around which the complementary techniques revolve. Emphasis should be placed on simple conventional sophisticated methods and keep modern imagery to circumstances where simple tests are insufficient.

The dental panoramic X-ray or orthopantomogram (OPT)

The OPT allows practionners to:

- Give an overview of the dental arch and skeletal structures;
- Distinguish between a missing tooth in the arch, agenesis, inclusion or locoregional ectopic;
- Learn about the depth of inclusion, the general axis of the tooth, and its teeth relationship, but it cannot locate buccal or palate position.
- Identify an obstacle that blocks the development of the tooth;
- Identify possible complications;
- Discover other anomalies of the dental system.

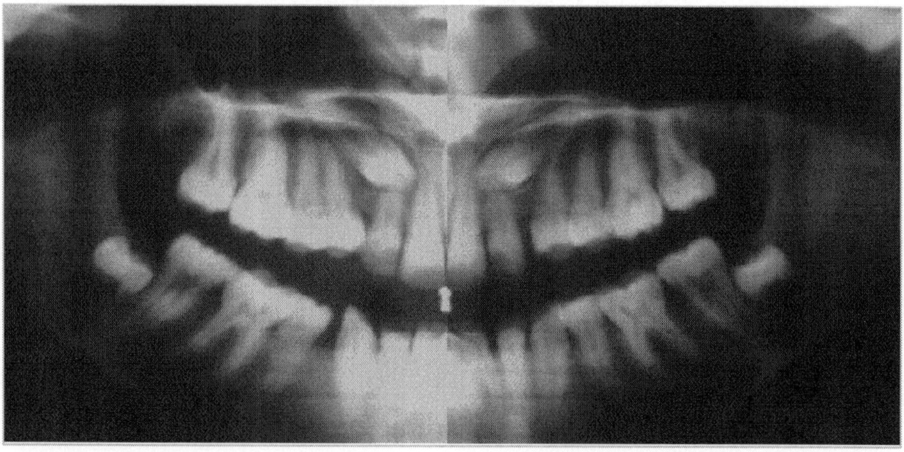

Fig. 1. The panoramic screening to determine the dental formula, which must be performed at the age of 8-9 years.

Periapical radiograph

Any x-ray is a two-dimensional representation of structures that are actually three dimensional. Therefore, it is essential to achieve at least two shots as different impacts to be able to determine the position of the canine, bothmesiodistally and vestibulo-buccally. Thus, the technique of "tubeshift" or as the "rule of Clark" is based on achieving two to three shots. The first shot is made as mesial eccentric projection, for the second shot, the central beam is positioned perpendicular to the alveolar process, the effect corresponding to the ideal axis of the canine and the third shot is made as eccentric projection distal. When the dog moves in the same direction as the source of X-rays, it is included in palatal position. It moves in the opposite direction, it is in position buccal (Crisman, 2000).

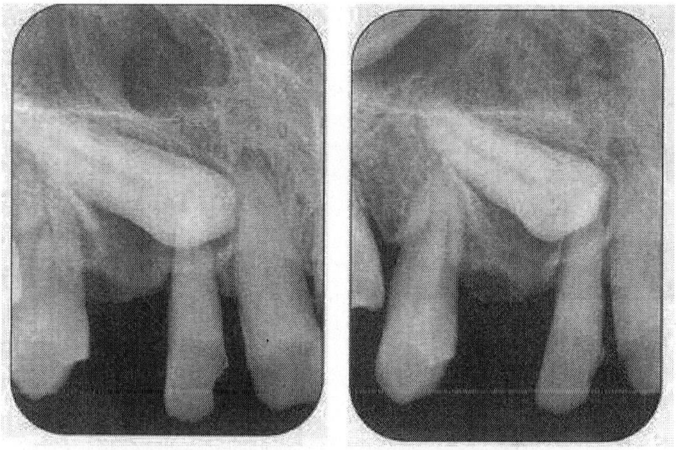

a b

Fig. 2. a) Periapical radiograph: with an orthocenter incidence. b) Periapical radiograph with a distocentric incidence. These two shots are needed to determine if the crown of the tooth is in position vestibular or buccal compared to others teeth.

Occlusal check-bit

The occlusal radiograph is very easy to use in young children because of the narrowness of the palate. Three types of effects can be used:

- The impact dysocclusale upper middle: it gives a topographic image of the hard palate and therefore precise morphology of the tooth retention,
- The impact ortho occlusion at 90 °: theory reveals the relationship of the crown of the impacted tooth with the roots of the incisors,
- The impact dysocclusale side at 60 °: this effect can view an entire canine included anteroposterior and its relationship with the incisors.

This exploration technique differentiates the position of the buccal or palatine impacted teeth by providing essential data on the transverse plane, the location of the tooth compared to the apex. It is full of orthopantomography (Korbendeau, 2005).

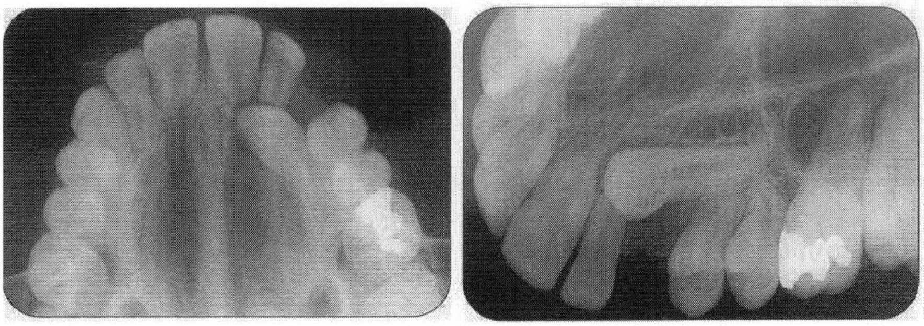

a b

Fig. 3. a) The orthoocclusal incidence reveals the palatal dystopia of 23. It allows visualizing the orientation of the impacted tooth, but it does not show the apical third of the root. The relationship with the roots of the incisors cannot be interpreted. b) The dysocclusal side to 60 ° can view the impacted tooth as a whole, and its relation with the anteroposterior incisor.

Lateral cephalometric radiographs

Orthodontic part of the record, this examination provides information in the vertical and sagittal - position - direction - height of inclusion. The superimposition of teeth from left and right arch limits the accuracy of the images (Korbendeau, 2005).

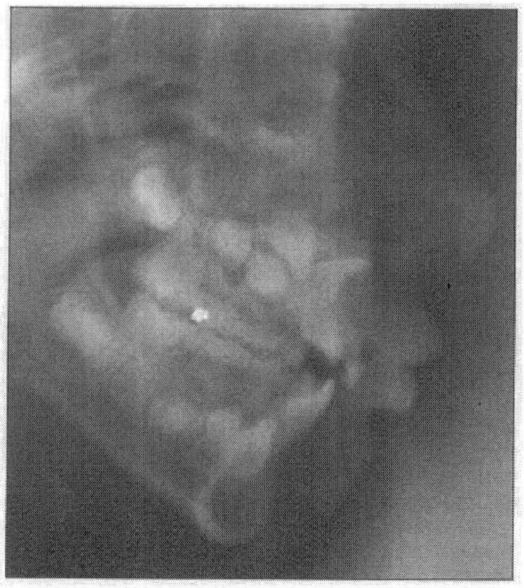

Fig. 4. the direction of the crown and the angle of the root are well highlighted in this lateral cephalometric radiograph.

CT or scanner

We realize, in the maxillary, a fine axial parallel to the palate bone; documents are provided full-scale, enabling a study and direct measurements on the photographs:

- Very precise localization of impacted teeth;
- Visualization of anatomic relationships of structures
- Neighborhood
- Location of an obstacle (odontoma, supernumerary tooth ...);
- Suspected effects on adjacent teeth (root resorption);
- Morphology of the impacted tooth (apical hooks or bends);
- Balance sheet bone abnormalities associated (cyst).

With modern software reconstruction from cuts made in all three planes of space, we will obtain three-dimensional reconstructions. These images will allow to study the position of the teeth and their relationship to adjacent anatomical structures from any angle desired and to perform distance measurements between the various structures (Nabbout, 2004; Treil, 1997).

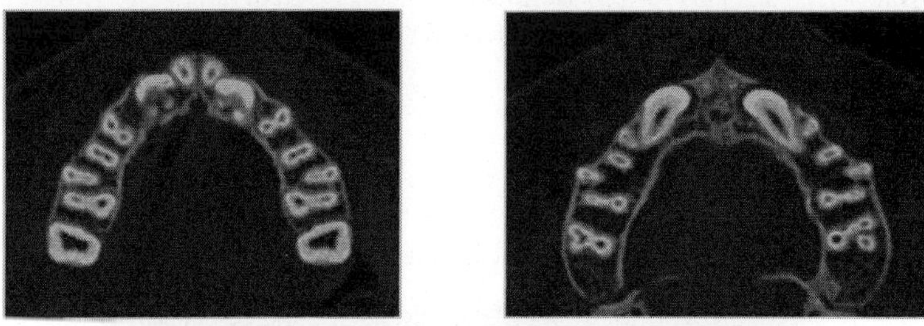

a

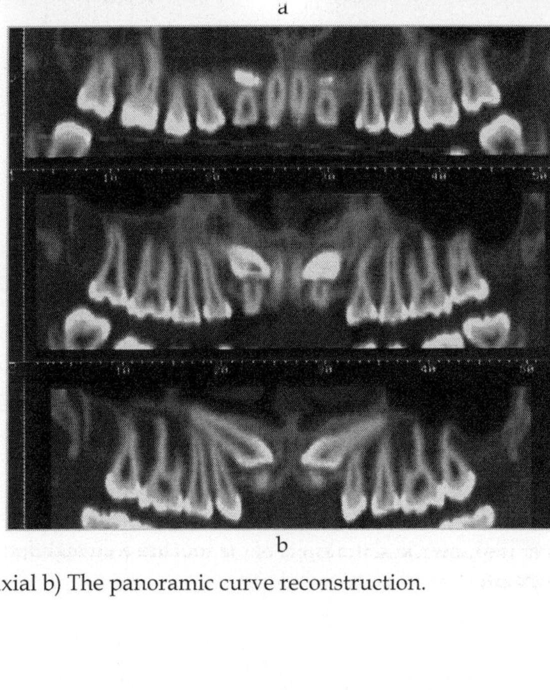

b

Fig. 5. a) Native axial b) The panoramic curve reconstruction.

CT allows a precise localization of the germ of the impacted tooth and guide the surgical approach safely. In addition, it allows the examination of the anatomical structures of neighborhood (nasal cavity, adjacent tooth), the ability to view dental resorptions, the location of a potential barrier (supernumerary teeth, follicular cyst)

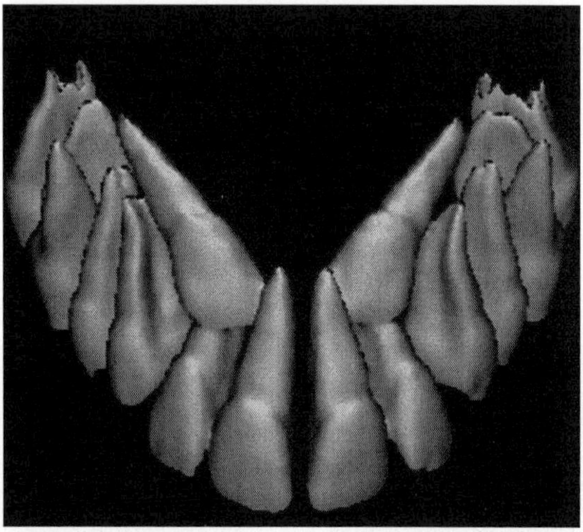

a

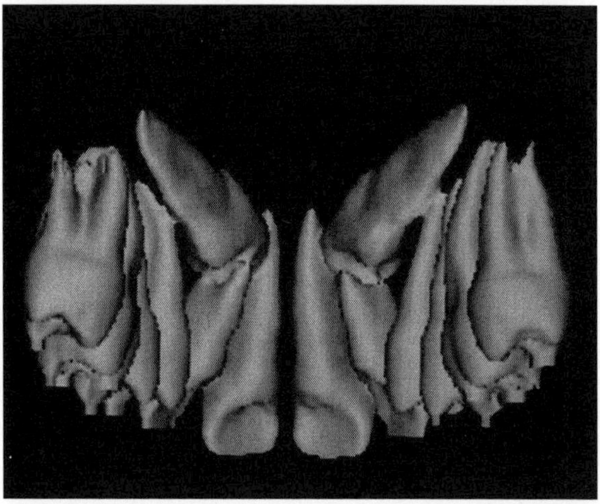

b

Fig. 6. a) b) 3D reconstruction provides a relief image of the orientation and position of teeth, and their relationship with the roots of permanent teeth. These images are very useful in the choice of operating procedures when clearing of impacted teeth deep.

6. Surgical-orthodontic management of dental impaction

After diagnosis, four types of attitudes are possible, facing impaction or missing eruption of teeth: abstention (mandibular canines close to the alveolar nerve); extraction; etiologic therapy if a deciduous tooth blocks the evolution; surgical exposure.

6.1 Abstention

The grounds for abstention may come from the patient who refuses orthodontic treatment when the impacted tooth does, by its position, represent no threat to the environment. This decision may also be related to the inability to establish the impacted tooth, because of its position or its ankylosis and the desire to avoid a too avulsion decaying in bone or adjacent teeth. In all cases, regular monitoring will be necessary to intercept any active disease of the teeth left in place.

6.2 Etiological treatment

The age of the patient is decisive when setting up preventive measures against risks of inclusion. Suspicion of impacted teeth will lead the practitioner to implement early treatment.

- Avulsion of the temporary tooth: in order to change the trajectory of eruption of the permanent tooth for a tooth-changing moves "in the path of least resistance" (Korbendeau, 2000).
- Maintenance of the space for the impacted tooth: the premature loss of deciduous tooth requires the possible establishment of a space maintainer.
- Avulsion of supernumerary teeth: the supernumerary germs and odontoma should be diagnosed early and avulsed to prevent the risk of inclusions.
- Expansion of the maxillary cross: the increase of available space by orthopedic device (palatal expander or Quad helix) (Dupont, 2001).
- Closure of a diastema therapeutic interincisal: frenotomy upper lip in front of a brake inserted deeply or avulsion of a mesiodens.

6.3 Technologies to promote spontaneous eruption of impacted teeth

6.3.1 Preventive guidance

It includes all actions necessary for the removal of barriers, but it also serves to create space for a normal development of tooth retention (Al Hussain, 1988). The goal is to awaken the potential eruption as soon as possible by lifting these barriers to have a spontaneous eruption. The avulsion of permanent or temporary teeth may be indicated to allow eruption of the impacted tooth physiological (Altounian, 1997, Langlade, 1986) but only if three conditions are met: inclusion bit old, apex not closed and canine well oriented.

6.3.2 Conductive alveolectomy

This technique, also called alveolectomy induction was established by Chatellier in 1957 (Chatellier, 1962). It creates a path of surgical eruption by releasing obstacles bone and removing the fibrous tissue periodontal (pericoronal bag). For the potential of eruption to be maximized, the conductive alveolectomy must be completed before the construction of the apical third and the apex overhangs the desired axis of extrusion (Durival, 1979). This technique has the advantage of enjoying the natural and physiological potential eruption of the tooth, however, the risk of ankylosis and / or bone resorption due to trauma of the periodontal ligament in the bone resection is not insignificant.

6.3.3 Directional osteotomy

It corrects the position of the tooth without moving its apex. It is indicated when the canine is raised, with an apex close to its normal place. A flap of the lateral incisor to first molar can expose the portal up to two thirds and a root mobilization syndesmotome is performed with a minimal apical displacement and thus a decreased risk of secondary mortification. But the risk of ankylosis still exists and the position of the canine often limits the indication of this process (Baron, 2001).

6.3.4 Autotransplantation

It is a resettlement in a newly formed alveolar at the level of the physiological eruption site of the extracted tooth. This technique is indicated when surgical-orthodontic treatment is impossible or when the impacted tooth threatens the roots of adjacent teeth. It requires sufficient space in the arch as well as mesiodistal vestibulopalatine and should be reserved for immature teeth. The major risk of this intervention is the process of ankylosis-root resorption resulting in the total resorption of the root variable within 7 to 10 years. To inhibit this process, it is necessary to follow a very strict operating procedure preserving the integrity of the periodontal ligament, and there is a differentiation of a functional periodontal ligament stable over time, putting the root transplanted immune to ankylosis phenomena (Garcia 1990).

6.4 Treatment of selected central incisors

In the absence of a maxillary central incisor, the parents consult most often after the emergence of the lateral incisor. The reduction of space further underscores the absence of the plant, because the asymmetry created is unattractive. Sometimes an early screening radiographic examination reveals the existence of inclusion.

6.4.1 Extraction of the permanent central incisor

This decision is based on therapeutic and complementary clinical examinations. The lack of a permanent central incisor is revealed after the fall of the deciduous tooth, a more or less pronounced collapse of the alveolar process in its vestibular part. Surgical-orthodontic treatment usually ensures the building of the thickness and height of the alveolar bone. Avulsion is reserved for cases of ankylosis and cases of laceration of interest to the crown or the top third root (Wong-Lee, 1985).

6.4.2 Implementation surgical-orthodontic

This is the technique of choice for positioning function of impacted teeth; it offers the best results and longevity of the tooth over time. A space to recreate the arcade is almost always necessary and this often lengthy treatment is possible at any age but requires motivation and impeccable cleanliness on the part of the patient. Several phases of treatment will succeed.

6.4.2.1 Presurgical orthodontic preparation

It aims to provide an anchor to pull the impacted tooth from its release position and to develop a surgical site on receiving the arch with an excess of up to 2 mm. This action may be obtained either by a removable appliance with resin base plate equipped with an active device (cylinder, spring ...) but it is more often preferred as a fixed multi-attachments with various accessories (coil spring, intermaxillary traction ...). This anchoring is most often offered by the entire arcade, but it can also be provided by implants or mini implants.

6.4.2.2 Surgical phase: Principle of surgical release

More than two decades ago, the surgeon used to perform a "comprehensive exhibition of the crown" of the tooth retained by making a buttonhole opening through the alveolar mucosa or attached gingiva (Archer, 1996). Other authors (Eiholtz, 1979) prepared a wider path by raising a mucoperiosteal flap to remove the bony wall, and the entire follicle to relate the crown to the anatomical neck. The mucous membrane covering the crown was then removed and the flap sutured in its original position.

Mucoperiosteal flap replaced

When the inclusion is deep, bonding intraoperatively is often difficult, so a rectangular flap provides extended release, conducive to good hemostasis. This flap is delimited by two vertical incisions, away from the impacted tooth, and a horizontal incision.

The two vertical incisions - discharge - leave the bottom of the vestibule, through the alveolar mucosa and reach the gum interdental papilla. The horizontal incision placed in the gingival sulcus, the lateral incisor, crosses the top of the edentulous ridge and follows the gingival sulcus of the contralateral central incisor to the line of the vertical incision.

This is a flap that provides a comprehensive surgery, with good visibility, and allows access to large vestibular ectopic teeth, the cystic lesions, the odontoma, ect. When the incisions are removed, hemostasis is ensured. The flap returned to its original position and ensures a rapid closure of the wound sealed. The post-operative care is reduced (Korbendeau, 1998).

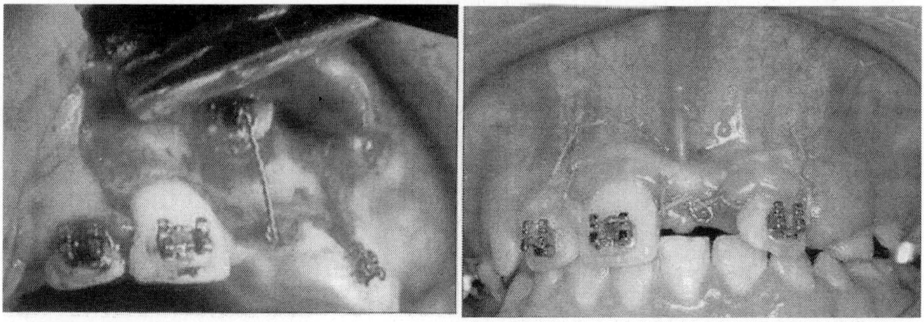

a b

Fig. 7. a) Preparation of a rectangular mucoperiosteal flap. The horizontal incision is placed at the top of the ridge, so that the pull wire reaches the axis of the arcade. b) The tissue flap is replaced in its original position. (Korbendeau, 1998).

Apically positioned flap

The apical fragment of translation is to place the gingival tissue on the labial crown of the impacted tooth to achieve a surgical emergence. The flap is delimited by two vertical incisions and a horizontal incision.

- The first vertical incision (mesial) is located along the labial frenum on the side of the tooth.
- The situation of the second vertical incision (distal) is determined so as to define an area of attached gingiva with a width at least equal to the mesiodistal crown dimension of the central incisor.
- The horizontal incision defines the height and thickness of the gum tissue to be positioned on the crown.

Apical displacement of the bottom edge of the flap provides a surgical emergence of the crown. This protocol has the advantage of seeing the crown, of picking a clip, of moving an anchor point in the weeks after surgery, and finally of leading the tooth, from the start of the pull toward eruption. Finally, the migration of the tooth, following emergent surgerical trajectory occurs spontaneously and is usually faster than if the flap is replaced (Korbendeau, 1998).

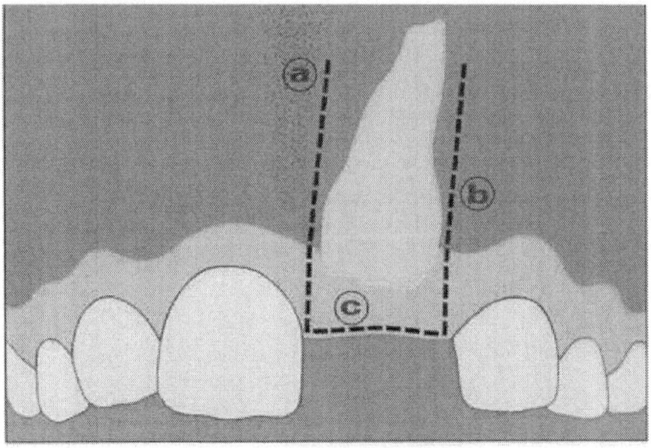

Fig. 8. The apically positioned flap is defined by three incisions: a, b and c. (Korbendeau, 1998).

6.5 Treatment of retained canines

6.5.1 Surgical techniques

Surgical exposure is undertaken only after orthodontic pre-treatment. Orthodontic preparation concerns mostly space management for the final position of the tooth. The extraction of the deciduous canine or of the premolar should only be planned after the impacted tooth has been mobilised without any sign of ankylosis (particularly in adults).

The preservation of the deciduous canine is usually not only an important question for the patients' aesthetics, but also for biomechanics and space maintenance. Nevertheless, to permit spontaneous eruption or orthodontic repositioning, disposing of sufficient keratinized tissue, extraction of the deciduous tooth may sometimes be necessary (Monnet-Corti, 2003).

Premolar extraction for space management has to be delayed until the probability of success is evaluated, and the duration of treatment and patient's motivation established (Thomine, 1995). The extraction has to be conducted to maintain the integrity of the osseous structures and particularly the bucal cortical plate, often being lost and thus reducing the buco-palatal dimension of the residual bone.

The access flaps are derived from the papers of Korbendau and Guyomard 1980 and 1998. The following techniques of surgical exposure are described: on the bucal side, gingivectomy, repositioned bucal flap, apically positioned flap and the laterally and apically repositioned flap, and the palatal side, the palatably repositioned flap in its fenestrated or not fenestrated version.

6.5.2 Gingivectomy

Gingivectomy is indicated when a big amount of keratinised tissue is found at the level of the impacted tooth. Between one third and one half of the tooth can be uncovered with a simple excision, leaving imperatively at least 3 mm of keratinised tissue on the apical side. From a periodontal point of view the application of such an excision is not indicated if only the oral mucosa is present (Archer, 1996).

6.5.3 Repositioned buccal flap

This flap is indicated when the tooth is positioned centrally to the alveolar crest or very high into the vestibulum (under the nasal spine) (Hunter, 1983; Magnusson 1990). In these very special situations apical and/or lateral translation of the keratinised tissue is impossible. It allows bone exposure and the bonding of the orthodontic device. For Boyd et al. it represents the technique of choice for any type of impaction.

6.5.4 Apically repositioned flap

This type of flap is the treatment of choice in many situations (Borghetti, 2000). It aims to create or to maintain keratinised tissue around the tooth by displacing the pre-existent keratinised tissue into the apical direction. The technique of the apically positioned flap (APF) is based on a mucosal flap (or partial thickness flap), the preservation of the existing keratinised tissue, its displacement into an apical position and its immobilisation by periostal sutures which remain in place. Access to the impacted tooth is obtained by a full thickness flap.

The dimension of the tissue to be displaced is decided according to the quality and quantity of periodontal tissue of the adjacent teeth (39). The horizontal width of the flap depends on the width of the crown of the impacted tooth (~ 7, 5-8 mm for an impacted maxillary canine) to which 1-2 mm are added if possible.

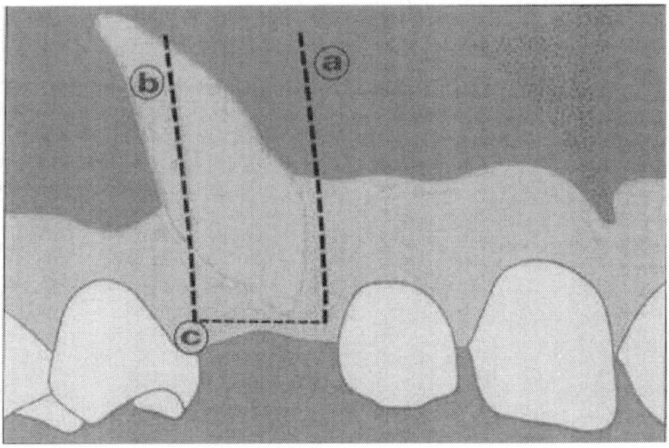

Fig. 9. The apically positioned flap is defined by three incisions a, b and c.

6.5.5 Laterally and apically positioned flap

The indications for this flap are the same as for the APF but the position of the tooth is more lateral in relation to the keratinised tissue on the crest or at the level of the adjacent teeth (Kokich, 1993).

The donor site can be the edentulous ridge (the simplest case) or the bucal tissue of the adjacent teeth. If the donor site is above a lateral or a central incisor, at least 2-3 mm of keratinised tissue have to remain over the teeth. At least 3 mm of tissue have to be displaced. Thus the donor site has to present with at least 6 mm of keratinized tissue to make sure that no dehiscence or recessions are created above the donor tooth (Kokich, 1993). The incisions permit to access the crown and to recreate a healthy periodontal environment).

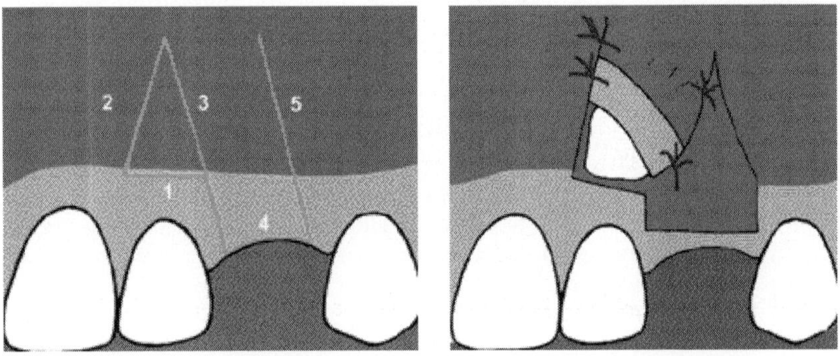

Fig. 10. Schematic drawing of laterally and apically positioned flap (from Borghetti and Monet Corti, 2000).
(a) Incision design 1: horizontal incision; 2-3: vertical incisions connecting to the first incision to remove the alveolar mucosa over the canine; 4: crestal horizontal incision and 5: vertical incision delimiting the distal part of the flap, dissected in partial thickness.
(b) Discontinuons flap sutures

6.5.6 Palatably repositioned flap

This technique is recommended for palatal inclusions. Because of the difficulties in determining the precise dimension and position of the tooth, direct access to the impacted tooth by cutting a little window into the soft tissue cannot be recommended.

Eliminating the bone, managing the bleeding and bonding the orthodontic device may present further difficulties. The intra-sulcular incisions are extending from the first premolar to the central incisor when the tooth is not deeply impacted. In cases of deep impaction near the palatal median line, the incisors can reach down to the contra-lateral premolar. No vertical incisions are made.

A full thickness flap is raised. The position of the tooth can mostly be determined by a typical convexity of the cortical bone, allowing the crown to expose. After the flap is replaced, a little window is prepared (using a new blade N° 15). The window has to be big enough to contain the rapid connective tissue proliferation, tending to close the wound (Monnet-Corti, 2003).

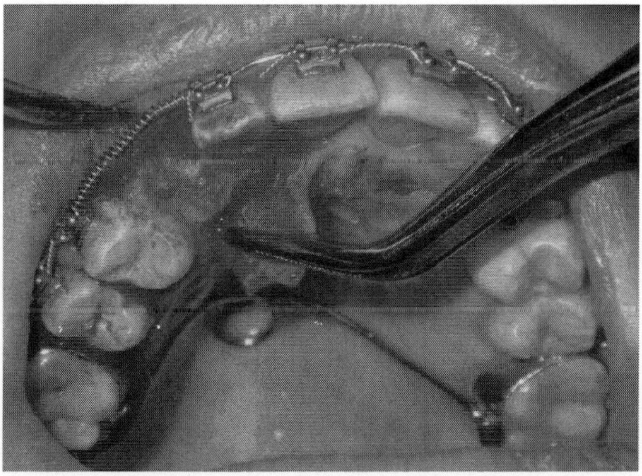

Fig. 11. Osteotomie and peri-coronary curettage disengaging the clinical crown.

7. Study conducted at the faculty of dentistry, Casablanca

The Department of Dentofacial Orthopaedics of the Faculty of Dentistry at Casablanca conducted an internal survey to review the current state of knowledge on management of impacted teeth in order to establish a standard protocol and thus codify the treatment of this anomaly (Bourzgui et al. 2009).

Our sample comprised 30 patients (24 females, 6 males) aged between 9 and 40 years. Mean age was 17 with a standard deviation of 8.141. These patients were all treated for impacted teeth by both the Surgical Dentistry Department and the Dentofacial Orthopaedics Department in Casablanca (Morocco). The clinical files included in the study comprised a clinical examination, X-rays and an iconography.

In our sample, the main reason for consultation was esthetics (54%). The discovery was made for esthetic reasons in 56.7% of the cases, for clinical examination in 16.7% of the cases, for X-ray examination and totally fortuitously in 23.3% of the cases, and delayed eruption unsuspected by the patient, but revealed by the practitioner in 3.3% of the cases.

The clinical examination was followed by X-ray examinations comprising not only a panoramic and slide-view headfilm but also a periapical radiograph and an occlusal check-bite in 36.7% of the cases, a periapical image combined xith a CT scan in 16.7% of the cases and a check-bite combined with a CT scan in 6.7% of the cases.

The number of impacted teeth varied from 1 to 6. Most often, however, only one tooth was involved (56.7%). In 66% of cases, canines were implicated, of which 9% were mandibular, 22% were incisal (all maxillary) and 12% were premolars. The impacted tooth was vestibular in 43.3% of cases, palatal in 33.3%, and in an intermediary position in 20% with 1 case with 2 impacted teeth; one vestibular, the other palatal. Level wise, distribution of dental impaction was divided into two groups: high impaction 63.3% and low impaction 36.7%.

Twenty-four patients (80%) were treated orthodontically prior to surgery. This stage aimed to prepare traction anchorage in 29.2% of cases or to open up space in 70.8%, occasionally with the assistance of extractions (41.2%). It should be noted that in 1 patient out of 30, the impacted tooth erupted spontaneously after 6 months of orthodontic preparation without course to surgery as the orthodontist had direct access to the tooth and was able to blond a bracket to it.

The surgical approach was vestibular in 17 cases, palatal in 9 cases and both vestibular and palatal in 3 cases. A replaced flap was used in 27 cases, a displaced flap in 1 case. In 1 case, a replaced flap was used on one side and a displaced flap on the other. Osteotomy was also performed to free the impacted tooth in 75.9% of cases.

An obstacle was found in 5 cases. Surgical elimination was performed in only 4 cases and the fifth case, involving a cyst, was marsupialized. Bonding was done during surgery in 27 cases and later in 2 cases. In 8 cases, a second procedure was needed following complications occurring during orthodontic traction. Treatment duration ranged from 3 to 24 months, with a mean of 11.4 months.

Twenty-one of 30 impacted teeth were correctly positioned in the arch, representing 70% success rate. Among the teeth which were not positioned, 66.6% were upper canines, 22.2% were upper central incisors and 11.1 were upper first premolars.

8. Discussion

The diagnosis of tooth impaction is made at different stages in the clinical examination and is then confirmed by radiological documents. In the course of our study, we looked most specifically into the reason for consulting which, in some cases, can lead the orthodontist to suspect the presence of an impacted tooth.

Dental impaction can be associated with various accidents, whether infectious, mechanical, or other, or with clinical silence. In the latter case, the practitioner should look carefully for revelatory clinical signs such as diastemas, swelling, teeth loss, etc. which can confirm any suspicion the patient may have had during the pretreatment history-taking (Roberts-Harry et al. 2004). Apart from the fairly uncommon cases of impaction which are easily detected from symptoms, the orthodontist should also use X-ray in order to localize unerupted teeth. According to the British body which deals with the use of radiographic imagery for orthodontic diagnosis, any tooth which has not yet erupted and which has not been felt on palpation should necessarily be X-rayed (Isaacson and Thom 2001)

A number of potential complications can occur and disrupt treatment leading inevitably to failure. Some of these complications may require a second surgical procedure. This is the case, for instance, when soft tissue covers the site which is deliberately left open and thus prevents clinical access to the impacted tooth (Burden et al. 1999) or when the orthodontic attachment detaches during traction mechanics (Pearson et al.1997).

Other complications can occur in which no second procedure can be of assistance, notably resorption (Blair et al. 1998), necrosis and ankylosis (Roberts-Harry et al. 2004). This last instance presents the worst scenario. Encountered in one of our patients, it was treated by extraction.

Enhanced management of impacted teeth can be achieved in daily practice by implementing the dental impaction charter which we submit in conclusion to our study. The charter comprises three items:

- Prevention: by means of awareness campaigns, early screening and interceptive treatment (extraction of the temporary tooth at the site of impaction);
- A scale of difficulty: this would allow practitioner to take the appropriate treatment decision according to the level of difficulty presented by each clinical situation as determined by a number of factors;
- A global treatment protocol: information is gathered during the initial history-taking and the clinical examination and complemented by radiological examinations including a panoramic, an occlusal check-bite, and even a CT-scan, depending on the case.

If surgical-orthodontic treatment is scheduled, it is essential to coordinate the appointments with both the orthodontist and the surgeon. The following considerations should be taken into account:

- space opening if space is inadequate;
- preferably a closed eruption technique with the least aggressive osteotomy possible;
- orthodontic traction with alignment of the tooth in the arch;
- gingivoplasty if the periodontal tissue is of unsatisfactory quality.

Furthermore, the practitioner should consider the benefit/risk ratio as well. In some instances, it is advisable to refrain from treatment.

9. Clinical cases

Clinical case 1

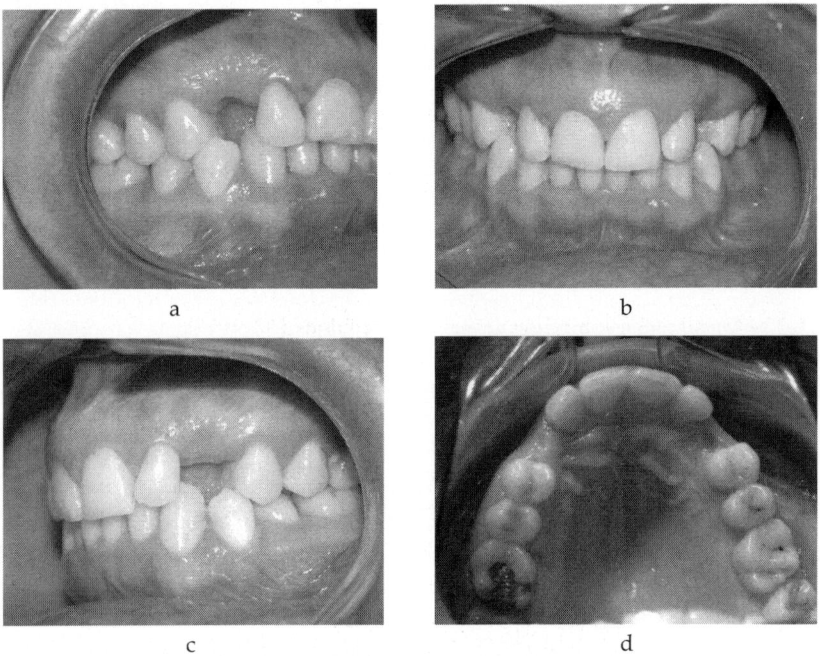

Fig. 12. a, b, c, d: Views buccal, right, front and left at the start of treatment. We note the absence of 13 and 23 with persistence of their spaces on the arcade. On palpation, we note the presence of palatal voussoirs.

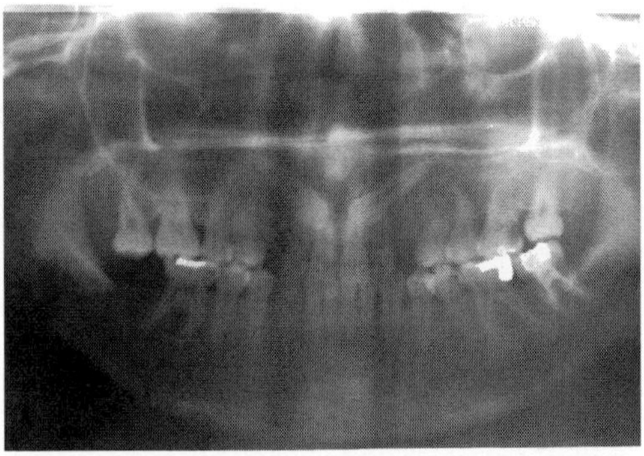

Fig. 13. The panoramic photograph shows the presence of 13 and 23 which have an inclination mesially and whose images are superimposed with those of the roots of the maxillary incisors.

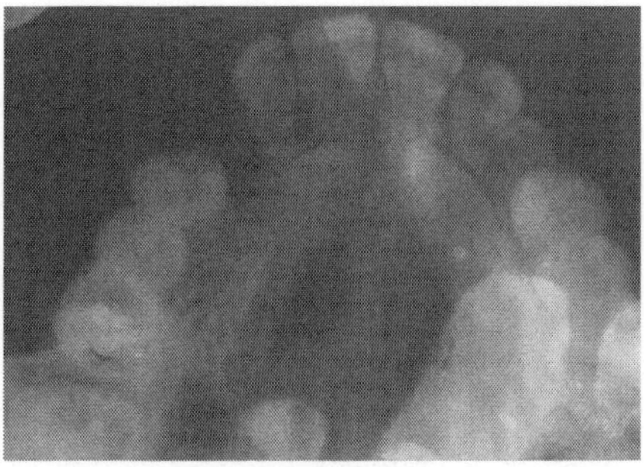

Fig. 14. The Occlusal check-bit shows the palatal position of 13 and 23.

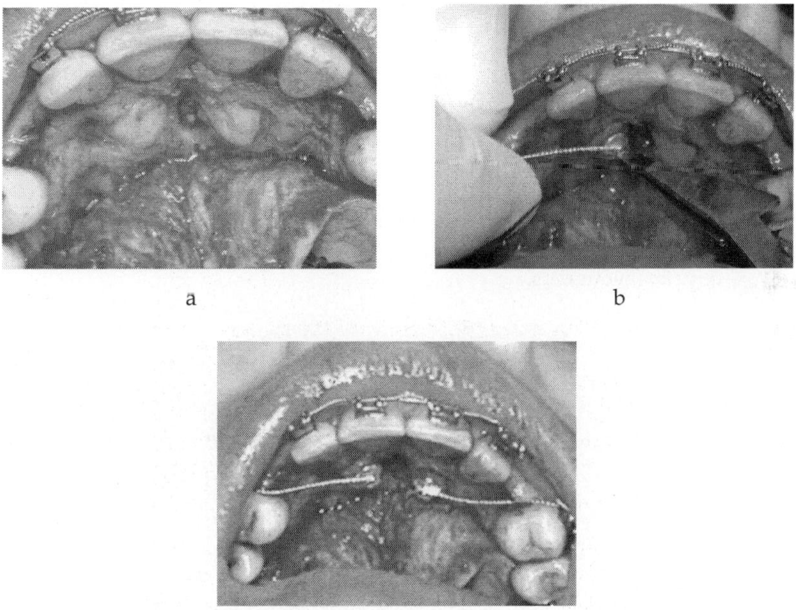

a b

c

Fig. 15. a, b, c: a palatal flap ranging from 14 to 24 is off. After the release bone, the palatal surfaces of 13 and 23 are exposed. The clip provided with a tie wire is attached during surgery.

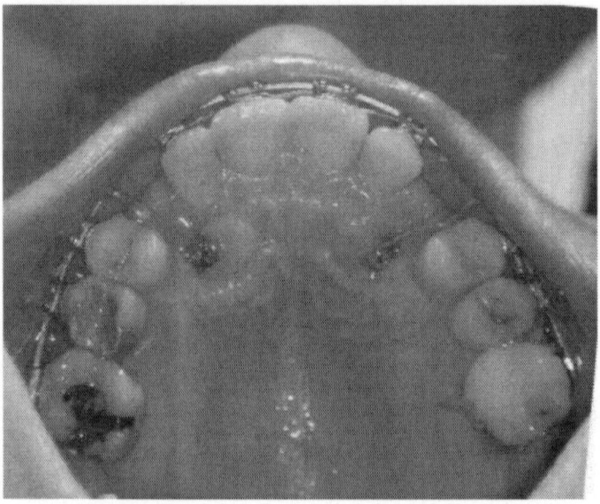

Fig. 16. The traction of 13 and 23 is made using elastic. A window gum can be achieved to facilitate the orthodontic traction.

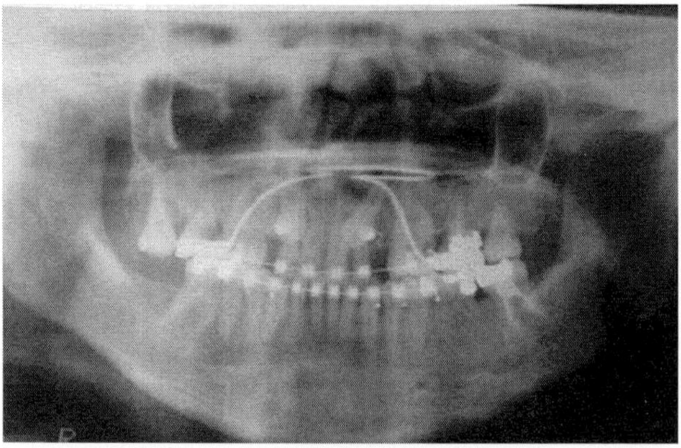

Fig. 17. The panoramic photograph shows the favorable axis of 13 and 23.

Clinical case 2

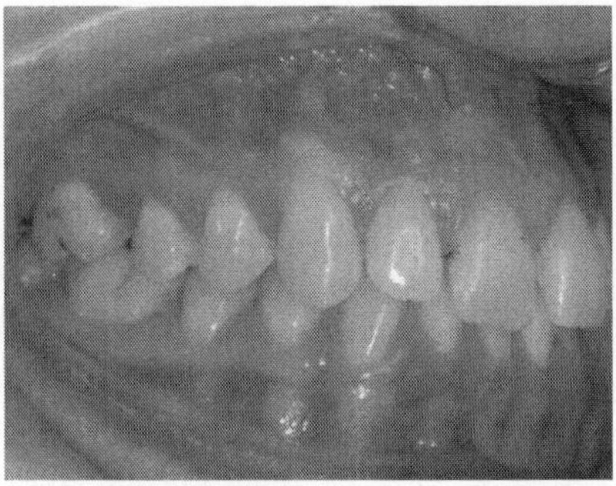

a

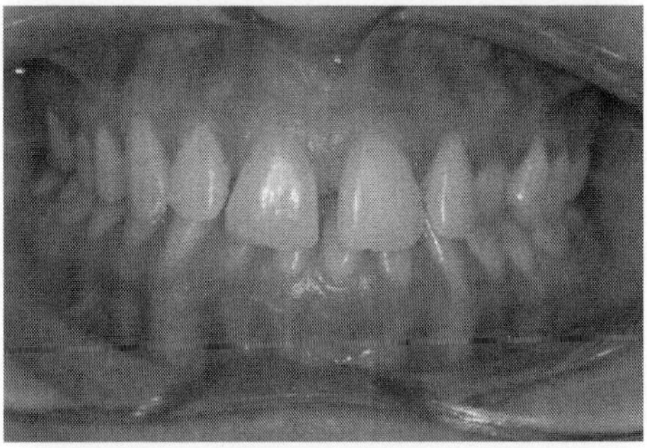

b

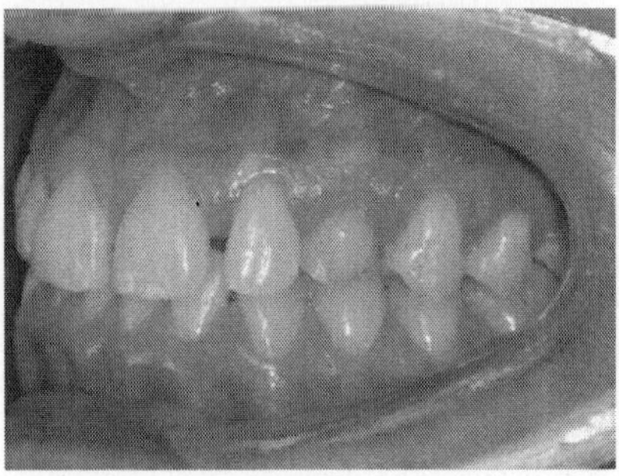

c

Fig. 18. a; b ;c : Views of buccal, right, front and left at the start of treatment. We note the absence of the 23 with persistence of 63 on the arcade.

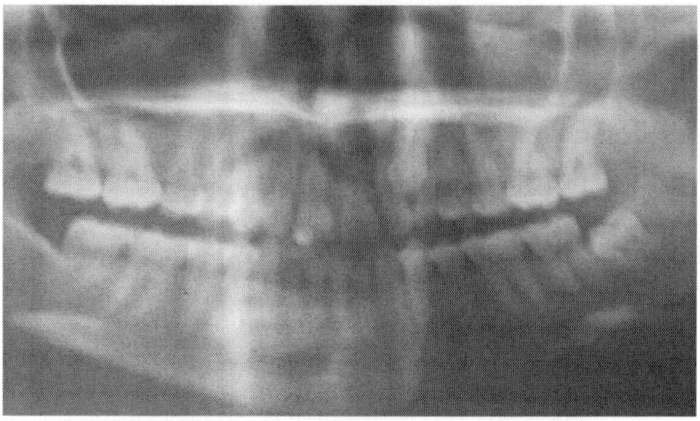

Fig. 19. The panoramic photograph shows the presence of 23 which is inclined mesially and whose axis is favorable for an attempt to orthodontic traction.

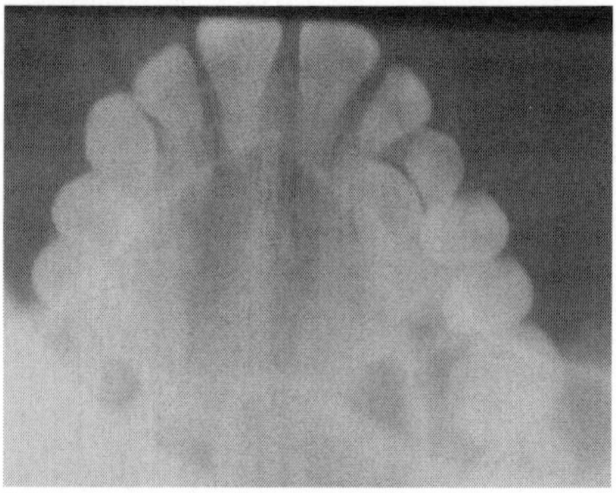

Fig. 20. The Occlusal check-bit shows an intermediate position of 23, the crown appears in buccal position and the root in palatal position.

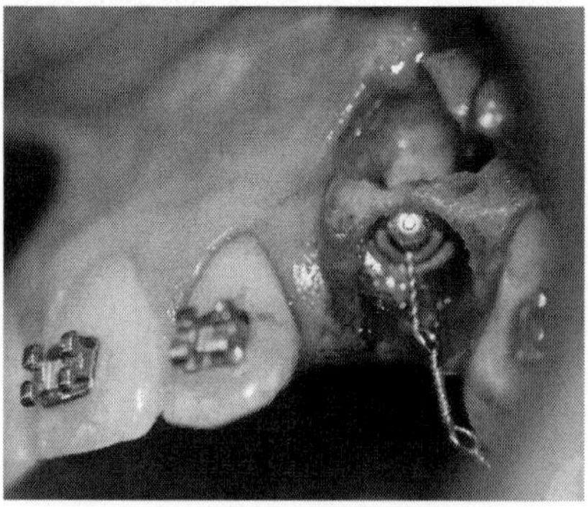

Fig. 21. Apically positioned flap was performed. The clip was bonded to the buccal surface of 23.

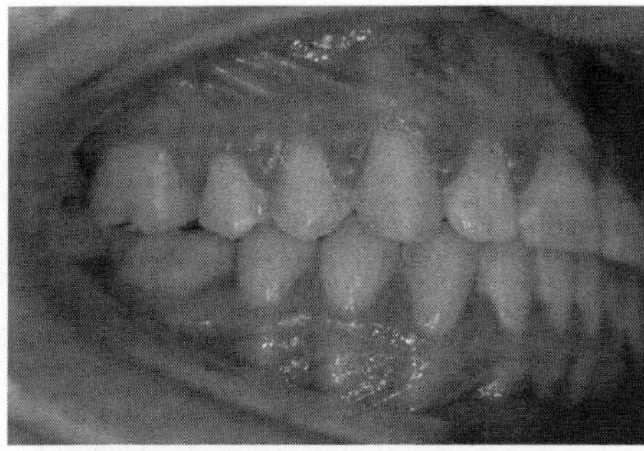

a

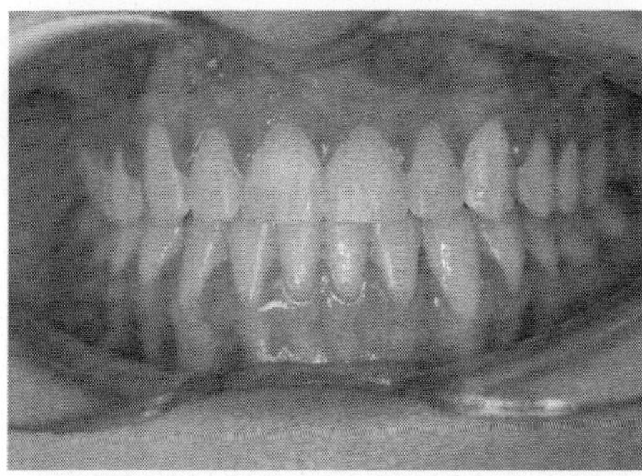

b

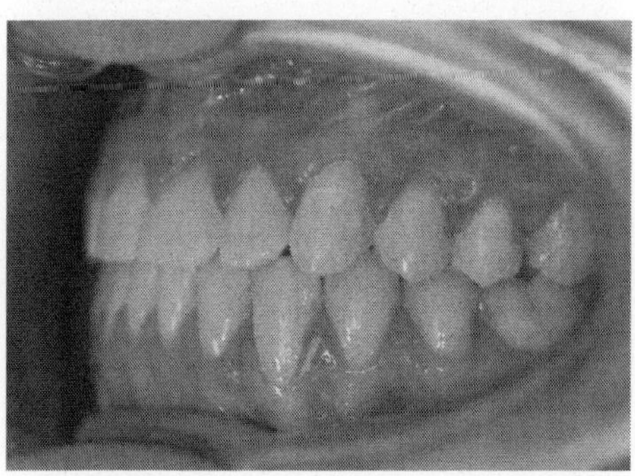

c

Fig. 22. a; b ;c : Views of buccal, right front and left at the end of treatment. We note the establishment of 23 that seems built on both the aesthetic and functional.

Clinical case 3

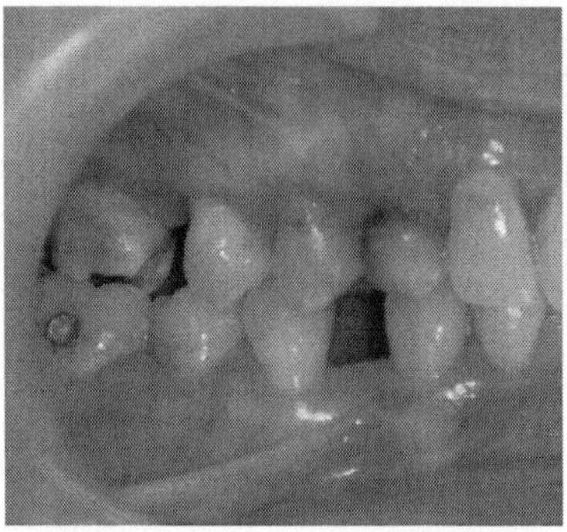

Fig. 23. Intraoral labial view of right at the start of treatment. We note the absence of the 13 with persistence of 53 on the arcade.

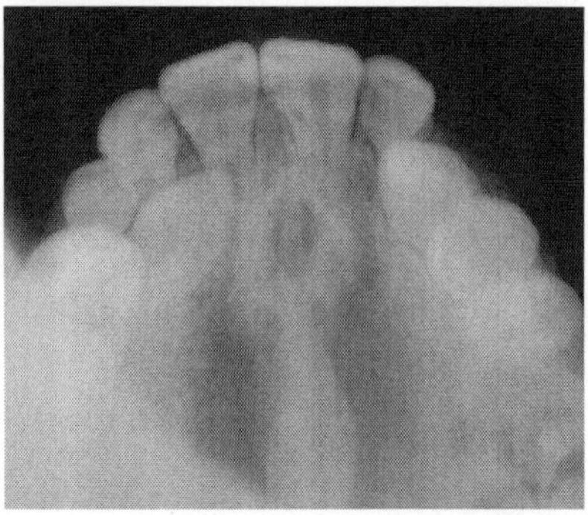

Fig. 24. The Occlusal check-bit shows palatal position of the 13.

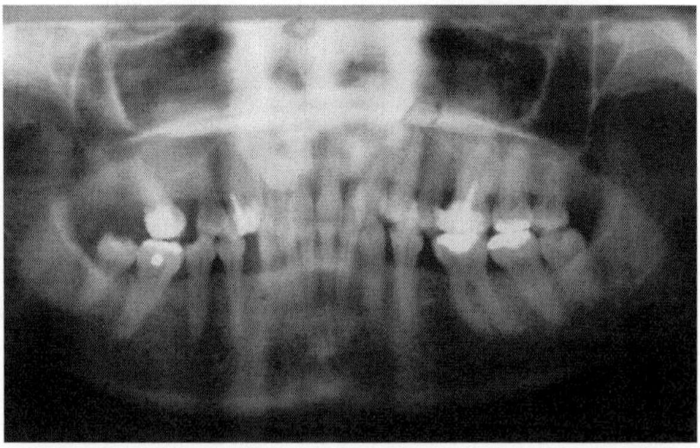

Fig. 25. The panoramic photograph shows the presence of 23 which is inclined mesially and whose axis is favorable for an attempt to orthodontic traction.

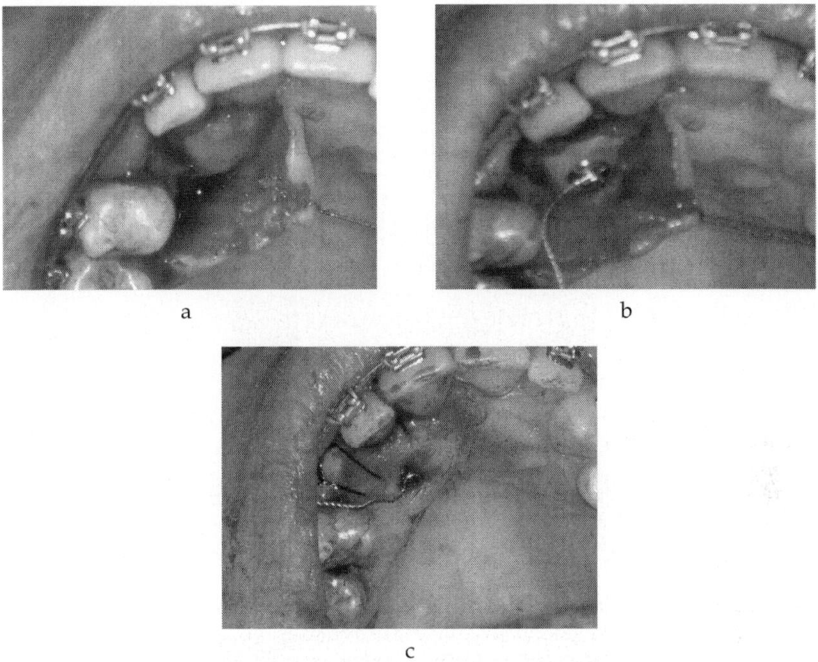

Fig. 26. a, b, c: a palatal flap is lifted off. The palatal surface of 13 is exposed. The clip provided with a tie wire is attached during surgery.

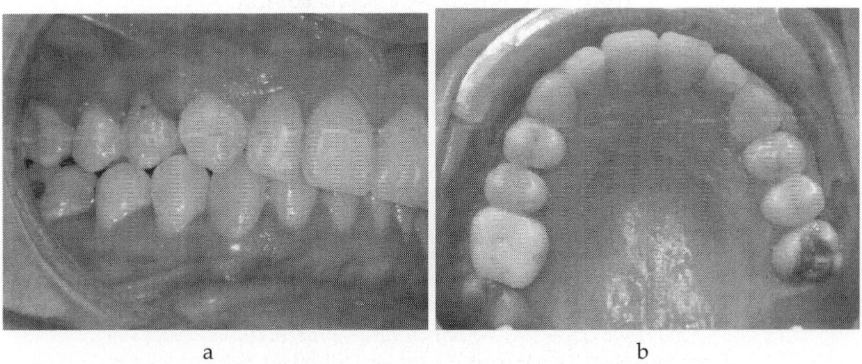

Fig. 27. a; b: View vestibular intraoral right, and view of occlusal jaw at the end of treatment. We note the establishment of 13.

10. Conclusion

Dental impaction confronts the practitioner with a serious challenge. Failure of the various approaches can be highly frustrating.

Treatment for dental impaction is a complex procedure on account of the wide range of cases encountered and the difficulty involved in making a precise and, most importantly, an early diagnosis and adequate treatment plan. Nevertheless, the treatment of choice for the placement of the unerupted tooth in the arch will involve close collaboration between orthodontists and surgeons.

The 70% success rate achieved on the 30 cases treated in our study is the result of a close partnership between the two specialties. Nevertheless, this figure can be improved still further by following the threefold strategy described above for the management of impacted teeth.

11. Acknowledgment

I would like to express my gratitude to my colleague Pr. Samir Diouny for his big help with the translations.

12. References

Al Hussain I. Contribution à l'étude de la canine maxillaire incluse. [these 3e cycle], Strasbourg, 1988. 128p.

Altounian G. Mise en place de la canine maxillaire en ectopie palatine. Orthod Fr 1997; Vol 68:291-6.

Archer WH. Oral surgery. 4th ed. Philadelphia: WB Saunders Co, 1996.

Baron P. Désinclusion orthodontico-magnétique des canines. J Edge 2001; Vol 43:59-71.

Benoit R., Leduc J.P., Genon P. Considérations orthodontiques et parodontales pour la mise en place des canines en bordure des fentes labio-alvéolaires. J Parodont 1989; Vol 8:139-154.

Blair GS, Hobson RS, Leggat TG. Posttreatment assessment of surgically exposed and orthodontically aligned impacted maxillary canines. Am J Orthod Dentofacial Orthop. 1998; Vol 113:329-32.

Bordais P. ET AL. Les dents incluses. Encycl. Med. Chir. Paris, Odontologie ; 22032 G10, 10-1980.

Borghetti A., Monnet-Corti V. Chirurgie Plastique Parodontale. Ed: CdP Paris, 2000.

Bourzgui F, Belhaj S, Tazi H, Hamza M, Khazana MM. Int Orthod. 2009 Sep;7(3):257-67

Burden DJ, Mullally BH, Robinson SN. Palatally ectopic canines: closed eruption versus open eruption. Am J Orthod Dentofacial Orthop. 1999;Vol 115:640-4.

Chambas C. Désinclusion et mise en place des dents retenues. Encycl Méd Chir (Elsevier SAS, Paris), Odontologie, 23-492-A-10,1997.

Chatellier J, Chateau M, Kolf J, Landart L. Notes sur le traitement chirurgico-orthodontique des dents retenues et incluses. Actual Odontostomatol (Paris) 1962; Vol 59:293-318.

Crismani AG, Freudenthaler JW, Weber, Bantleon RH. Canines supérieures incluses – méthodes conventionnelles de diagnostic radiologique et de traitement. Rev Mens Suisse Odontostomatol 2000,Vol 110:1264-1268.

Dupont S, Durand B.Approche préventive et orthopédique des canines maxillaires incluses dans les cas de brachygraphie maxillaire. J Edge 2001;Vol 43:85-99.

Durivaux S, Viennet D, Demetz P. Alvéolectomie conductrice de la canine supérieure permanente. Rev Odontostomatol (Paris) 1979; Vol 8:91-3.

Eiholtz B, Salaun R, Brethaux J, Allain P, Huard JL. Conduite à tenir devant la rétention de l'incisive centrale supérieure. Actual Odonto Stomatol 1979;Vol 128:751-65.

Ericson S, Kurolj. Radiographic examination of ectopically erupting maxillary canines. Am J Orthod Dentofac Orthop 1987, Vol 91:483-492.

Ericsson S, Kurol J. Resorption of incisors after ectopic eruption of maxillary canines: a CT study. Angle Orthod 2000; Vol 70:415-23.

Favre de Thierrens C, Cantaloube D, Delestan C, Goudot P, Predine- Hug F, Torres JH. Nouvelle classification médicochirurgicale odontostomatologique des dents incluses. Encycl Méd Chir (Elsevier SAS,Paris), Odontologie, 23-400-A-19, 2003.

Favre de Thierrens C, Moulis C, Bigorre M et De la Chaise S. Inclusion dentaire (I). Aspects biologiques, odontogéniques, physiologiques et pathologiques. Encycl Méd Chir (Elsevier SAS), Stomatologie, 22-032-A-15, Odontologie, 23-400-A-16, 2003.

Garcia R. Canine quand tu nous tiens! Rev Orthop Dentofac 1990; Vol 24: 359-66.

Goho C. Delayed eruption due to overlying fibrous connective tissue: case reports. J Dent Child 1987; Vol 54:359-360.

Hunter S. Treatment of the unerupted maxillary canine. Brit dent J 1983; Vol 154:294-296.

Hurme VO. Ranges of normalcy in the eruption of permanent teeth. J Dent Child. 1949; Vol 16:11-5.

Isaacson K G, Thom A R. Guidelines for the use of radiographs in clinical orthodontics. British Orthodontic Society, London 2001.

Izard G. Orthodontie Masson et Cie .;édit. ;Paris,1950

Korbendau JM, Guyomard F. Apport de la chirurgie parodontale à la mise en place des canines en dystopie vestibulaire. Rev Ortho Dent Fac 1980; Vol 14:459-477.

Korbendau JM, Guyomard F. Chirurgie parodontale orthodontique. Editions CdP 1998.

Korbendau JM, Pajoni D. Canines maxillaires, inclusions profondes, diagnostic : choix du protocole opératoire. J Parodontol Implantol Orale 2000; Vol 19:279-89.

Korbendeau JM., Patti A. Le traitement orthodontique et chirurgical des dents incluses Quintessence Internationale, Paris, 2005.

Lacoste J.L. Désinclusion et mise en place des dents retenues. Encycl. Med .Chir. , Paris, odontologie 23492 A10, 1-1988,9.

Langlade M. Thérapeutique orthodontique. Paris: Maloine; 1986 (863p).

Le Breton G. Traité de sémiologie et clinique odonto-stomatologique. Paris CdP 1997:100-109.

Magnusson H. Saving impacted teeth. J Clin Ortho 1990;24:246-249.

Mc Connelt. L., Hoffman D.L., Forbes D.P., Janzen E.K., Weintraub N.H. Maxillary canine impaction in patients with transverse maxillary deficiency. J dent Child 1996;63:190-195.

Monnet-Corti V, Borghetti A. Canines incluses et chirurgie plastique parodontale. Rev Odont Stomat 2003;32:259-277.

Nabbout F, Faure J, Baron P, Braga J, Treil J. L'ancrage dentaire en orthodontie : les données du scanner. Int Orthod 2004; Vol 2:241-56.

Pearson MH, Robinson SN, Reed R, Birnie DJ, Zaki GA. Management of palatally impacted canines: the findings of a collaborative study. Eur J Orthod. 1997; Vol 19, N°5:511-5.

Peck S., Peck L., Katajam. Site specificity to tooth agenesis in subjects with maxillary canine malpositions. Angle Orthodontist 1996; Vol 66:473-476.

Quirynen M, Opheij DG, Andriasens A, Opdebeek HM, Van Steenberghe D. Periodontal health of orthodontically extruded impacted teeth. Asplit mouth, long-term clinical evaluation. J Periodontol 2000; Vol 71:1708-14.

Rajic S, Muretic Z, Percac S. Impacted canine in a prehistoric skull. Angle Orthod. 1996;66:477 -80.

Roberts-Harry D, Sandy J. Orthodontics. Part 10: Impacted teeth. Br Dent J. 2004; Vol 196:319-27; quiz 362.

Sasakura H., Xoshida T., Murxama S., Hamadak., Makajima T. Root resorption of upper permanent incisor caused by impacted canine. An analysis of 23 cases. Int J Oral Surg 1984; Vol 13:299-306.

Thomine F., Korbendau J.M., Martineau C. - Mise en place chirurgico-orthodontique des dents retenues. Réalités Clin 1995;6:351-369.

Treil J, Casteigt J, Madrid C, Borianne P. Une nouvelle construction céphalométrique tridimensionnelle. Un nouveau paramétrage d'analyse tridimensionnelle : les axes d'inertie. Un nouveau concept de l'équilibre maxillo-facial. Orthod Fr 1997; Vol 68:171-81.

Vichi M., Franchi L. Eruption anomalies of the maxillary permanent cuspids in children with cleft lip and or palate. J Clin Pedia Dent 1996; Vol 20:149-53.

Vigneul J.C. Extraction chirurgicale des canines incluses Act. Odonto-Stomatol. 1974; Vol 105 :53-78

Wong-Lee TK, Wong FC. Maintaining an ideal tooth-gingiva relationship when exposing and aligning an impacted tooth. Br J Orthod. 1985; Vol 12:189-92.

11

Uprighting of the Impacted Second Mandibular Molar with Skeletal Anchorage

Stefano Sivolella, Michela Roberto, Paolo Bressan, Eriberto Bressan, Serena Cernuschi, Francesca Miotti and Mario Berengo
University of Padua, Departments of Oral Surgery and Orthodontics
Italy

1. Introduction

Eruption disorder of the mandibular second permanent molars is quite rare, but it does need to be treated early.

There are many functional, periodontal, hygienic and prosthetic reasons which justify retrieving a second molar with eruption problems.

In terms of occlusion, the patient is assured of the proper arch length, with obvious functional and masticatory advantages, and any extrusion of the antagonist is avoided, especially when the eruption of third molars is unpredictable. (McAboy et al., 2003)

Oral hygiene at home becomes more straightforward and effective, thanks to the elimination of the pseudo-pocket. The incidence of caries is much higher in impacted teeth, and there is often radiographic evidence of severe damage to the crown or root of the first permanent molar. (Shellhert & Oesterle, 1999)

Adult and elderly patients often present with molars which are over-erupted and mesially inclined. Tipping of the first molar may initiate a vicious cycle of traumatic occlusion and periodontal problems mesial to the tipped tooth

1.1 Epidemiology and causes

The permanent teeth most often affected by eruption problems are the mandibular and maxillary third molars, maxillary canines, central incisors and, more rarely, second mandibular premolars. (Aitasalo et al., 1972)

The incidence of eruption disorder involving the second molars is quite rare, ranging in the literature between 0.03-0.04% of all impacted teeth. (Mead, 1930), (Grover & Norton, 1985). The problem is encountered more frequently in the mandible, often only on one side, and with a predilection for the female gender. (Frank, 2000)

Because second-molar impaction is a relatively rare clinical problem, there is only a limited amount of literature regarding case management.

The main cause of second molar eruption anomalies is shortage of space. (Mead, 1930) The space required for the second molar to erupt in the mandible derives from resorption-apposition processes typical of normal growth, which lead to remodeling of the anterior border of the mandibular ramus. During the normal growth and development of the lower jaw, the molar tooth buds distal to the first permanent mandibular molar have a mesial inclination, which is usually self-correcting as the anterior border of the mandibular ramus resorbs. In addition to this, the mesial drift of the first permanent molar creates approximately 2.7 mm of space per side for angular adjustment. (Majourau & Norton, 1995)

Functional impairment of this natural process leads to molar eruption problems, due to inadequate arch length. A further increase in the available space stems from the mesial migration of the first mandibular molar into the leeway space. (Majourau & Norton, 1995) Orthodontic treatment designed to prevent such migration, e.g., using the lingual arch or lip bumper, may increase the risk of eruption anomalies. (Kokich & Mathews, 1993)

Other important iatrogenic factors include an incorrectly fitted band cemented on the first mandibular molar, or of the first maxillary molar previous orthodontic sagittal expansion. (Eckhart, 1998)

Another reason for impaction is sometimes an excessive amount of space, because the eruption of the second molar needs to be guided by the roots of the first molar. (Shapira et al., 1998) This may give rise to eruption problems even though there is too much space between the two teeth, g.e. when orthodontic expansion of the maxillary arch occurs. The molar may also sometimes undergo spontaneous eruption anomalies, due to excessive mesioversion of the tooth germ or the presence of the third molar. Other problems may be due to premature extraction of the first permanent molar, molar ankylosis, odontogenic cysts, or odontomas. (Frank, 2000)

1.2 Surgical options

Extraction of an impacted mandibular second molar which appears to have no chance of uprighting itself may allow the third molar to erupt into the second molar position. This requires precise manipulation by the oral surgeon, who must carefully consider the unpredictability of these eruption patterns. (Tinerfe & Blakey, 2000)

Surgical methods vary from simply uncovering the tooth to third molar extraction and surgical second molar repositioning, with or without bone grafts in the medullar space. Surgical uprighting and repositioning of the mandibular second molar, with or without extraction of the third molar, is a possible option.

When a molar tooth is severely impacted, surgical uprighting may provide a quick and easy solution, particularly when orthodontic treatment is contraindicated. (Johnson & Quirk, 1987)

Typical orthodontic treatment for these molars may not be an option if patient commitment is minimal, or if the position of the tooth does not provide the proper environment for bonding a bracket.

When the decision has been made to perform surgical uprighting and repositioning second molars, Tinerfe and Blakey (Tinerfe & Blakey, 2000) recommend that certain criteria be considered.

These include ascertainment of root length/form, available space within the dental arch, arc of rotation, occlusion, periodontal status and jaw development. The optimal root length should be one-third to half of the eventual length of the fully formed root, to enhance revascularization after tipping and bodily movement. As adequate space must be available in the arch, third molars may need to be prophylactically removed.

Ideally, the tooth to be uprighted should not be buccally or lingually inclined, since the buccal and lingual cortical plates are needed for primary stabilization once the second molar is surgically uprighted.

The angle of rotation for uprighting the second molar should not exceed 90° because, as Pogrel suggested (1995), uprighting teeth by more than 90° causes them to behave like transplants, thus diminishing the chance of future vitality.

Once the molar has been uprighted, any occlusion should be carefully checked for interferences which may lead to occlusal trauma. The uprighted tooth also should be positioned in a manner which allows healthy soft tissue attachment and ease of access for appropriate hygiene. Careful handling and positioning of the keratinized gingiva during the procedure are critical for the long-term periodontal health of uprighted molars.

It is also important that vertical jaw growth should be nearly complete, to achieve ideal occlusion and prevent tooth submersion during growth. If these criteria are met, surgical second molar uprighting has been shown to be a predictable procedure and a viable option when other types of treatment are not possible. (McAboy et al., 2003)

1.3 Orthodontic treatment

The best timing for treating impacted second molars is between 11 and 14 years of age, when the root is still not fully developed. The type of treatment depends on the slant of the tooth and the amount of orthodontic movement required.

Minor malpositioning can be corrected by placing an elastic separator between the two teeth. (Moro et al., 2002)

More severe malpositioning demands the use of surgical methods or orthodontically assisted eruptions, with or without surgical disinclusion of the tooth.

Mesially inclined molars should be differentiated not only by degree of impaction, but also by the types of tooth movement required for correction in all three spatial planes. For any particular tooth movement, it is very difficult to plan a correct force system with respect to the center of resistance. In the sagittal plane, the appropriate combination of vertical movement and uprighting must be determined. (Melsen et al., 1996)

A good treatment option is orthodontically assisted eruption, with or without surgical uncovering. The general approach is an attachment bonded to the surgically uncovered buccal or distobuccal surface of the second mandibular molar, followed by application of an uprighting force delivered by tip-back cantilever (Melsen et al., 1996), (Sawicka et al., 2007), NiTi-coil spring (Aksoy & Aras 1998), super-elastic NiTi wire (Going & Reyes-Lois, 1999), a variety of uprighting springs (Shapira & Borell 1998), (Park, 1999), (Majourau & Norton 1995), a fixed appliance (Carano et al. 1996), (Miao & Zhong, 2006) or a sectional arch wire (Alessandri Bonetti et al., 1999), (Kogod M & Kogod HS.,1991).

Molar uprighting may be secured by pure rotation obtained by applying a couple force system with a high moment-to-force ratio (so that the center of rotation is very close to the center of resistance). A long cantilever gives a high moment-to-force ratio, which results in a clinical effect very close to that of pure rotation. The magnitude of the moment required to rotate a molar has been suggested to be 800–1500 g/mm. (Romeo & Burstone, 1977)

The cantilever produces effects on the tooth in three planes, mainly in the mesiodistal (distal crown tipping) and vertical directions (molar extrusion). Determining the forces on teeth also requires defining the forces delivered to the cantilever inserted in the molar tube. The activation force is directed to the occlusal plane and is opposed by the apically directed force which the molar tube exerts on the wire. Mesial and distal aspects of the molar tube also exert forces on the wire which oppose the counterclockwise rotation resulting from activation forces. The forces acting on the teeth are of the same magnitude as, but of opposite direction to, those acting on the wire. Thus, the intrusive force is on the anterior segment and the extrusive force on the molar, and the couple distally rotates. (Sawicka et al., 2007)

In traditional orthodontic biomechanics, when the molar is to be extruded, uprighting is often performed with simple tipback mechanics. If significant extrusion is needed, the force delivered to the bracket should be relatively large compared with the moment. If little or no extrusion is desired, the moment should be larger and the cantilever as long as possible. (Melsen et al., 1996)

Melsen et al. believe that, when molar intrusion is required, the biomechanics become more complex. The law of equilibrium states that the moment added to the molar must be smaller than the moment added to the anterior unit. This force system corresponds to what Burstone and Koenig defined as a geometry V, and can be obtained by proper activation of a root spring, as described by Roberts and colleagues. (Roberts et al., 1982)

It is also important to consider the force system generated in the horizontal plane. Although both the root spring and the V bend act parallel to the dental arch, in close proximity to the center of resistance, the cantilevers may have their point of force application on either side of the center of resistance, and thus generate tipping in either the buccal or the lingual direction. (Melsen et al., 1996)

The difficulty of managing these complex biomechanics has led many authors to seek easier alternative solutions, such as appliance design specifications.

The distal jet appliance, modified for use in the lower arch (uprighter-jet), is an example of a fixed appliance associated with an open-coil spring for proper lower molar uprighting. (Carano et al., 1996) The appliance design involves soldering an 0.036" tube to the premolar band, parallel to the occlusal plane but below the level of the edentulous ridge, so as not to interfere with the occlusion. The tube is oriented so that a wire with a bayonet bend can be slid into the tube from the distal end. A loop is bent into the distal end of this wire and attached to the molar band with a screw. Thus, wire and molar band are held together but are free to rotate around a common axis.

An adjustable screw-clamp and a 150g nickel titanium open-coil spring is placed over the tube. The two premolars are connected with a soldered lingual wire to form the anchorage unit. As the clamp is moved distally, the coil spring is compressed and a distalizing force is applied. Because the connection of the molar band to the wire is not rigid, the line of action of this force is at the molar crown and the point of force application is at the screw. The molar crown will therefore be tipped distally.

Often, however, these stages of treatment are impossible, due to the severe mesio-inclination angle and the gingival position of the element which does not permit proper bonding. Many techniques have therefore been proposed involving, for example, segmented TMA (Majourau & Norton 1995) to avoid the problem or for pre-positioning the element.

Miao et al. (Miao & Zhong, 2006) proposed using a fixed appliance composed of a mini-hook and a push-spring (arrow) to move the crown of an impacted molar distally.

The mini-hook is made of 0.014" stainless steel wire and is conventionally bonded to the distal surface of a horizontally impacted molar or the occlusal surface of a mesially impacted molar, so that the hook opens mesially. Surgical exposure is needed only if horizontal impaction is so severe that the molar has not erupted at all. In such a case, the distal surface of the impacted tooth should be exposed just enough to bond the mini-hook.

A stainless steel wire, about 60 mm long, is soldered to the middle of the lingual surface of the mesially adjacent molar band. The wire is bent at the distolingual corner of the band, extended 2-3 mm buccally, and then turned distally, making a double- or triple-bend push-spring. The band with the push-spring is cemented to the mesially adjacent molar. The spring is stretched 4-5 mm distally and attached to the open mesial end of the mini-hook. The push-spring will then exert a distalizing and uprighting force. It should be reactivated monthly until the impacted molar is upright.

All these techniques present complex biomechanics which require careful evaluation to avoid side-effects such as extrusion or loss of anchorage.

Placing placing titanium miniscrews in the retromolar area for molar uprighting has been recommended as the most predictable and easiest method to manage. (Park et al., 2002), (Giancotti et al, 2003, 2004), (Nęcka et al., 2010)

2. Skeletal anchorage

The most common problem of classical distalization techniques is the frequent loss of anchorage and adverse effect on adjacent teeth.

Anchorage is a direct consequence of Newton's Third Law, i.e., "For every action there is an equal and opposite reaction", and is defined as the resistance to unwanted tooth movement. (Daskalogiannakis, 2000)

Orthodontic anchorage can also be defined as the "amount of movement allowed to the reactive unit", where the latter is composed of tooth/teeth acting as anchorage units during movement of the active unit, and the active unit is composed of tooth/teeth undergoing movement. (Cope, 2007)

Orthodontists often have inadequate mechanical systems to control anchorage, which leads to loss of anchorage in the reactive unit and thus incomplete correction of malocclusion. To avoid this kind of side-effect, clinicians often associate acrylic or extraoral appliances which, when combined with the ever-challenging problem of uncooperative patients, are often futile attempts at best. As even a small reactive force can cause undesirable movements, it is important to ensure that anchorages are solidly based. (Pilon et al., 1996)

Absolute or infinite anchorage is defined as no movement of the anchorage unit (zero anchorage loss) as a consequence to the reaction forces applied to move teeth. (Daskalogiannakis, 2000)

This kind of anchorage can only be obtained with ankylosed teeth or dental implants as anchors, both of which rely on bone to inhibit undesired movement.

The need to check anchorage during orthodontic treatment has led clinicians to develop many types of Temporary Anchorage Devices (TAD). These may be defined as devices which are temporarily fixed to bone for the purpose of enhancing orthodontic anchorage by supporting the teeth of the reactive unit (indirect anchorage) or by obviating the need for the reactive unit altogether (direct anchorage) and are subsequently removed after use. (Cope, 2007).

The idea of using screws fixed to bone to obtain absolute anchorage goes back to 1945, when Gainsforth and Higley (Gainsforth & Higley, 1945) placed Vitallium screws in the ascending ramus of six dogs to retract their canines. The first clinical use reported in the literature came in 1983, when Creekmore and Eklund (Creekmore & Eklund,1983) used a Vitallium bone screw inserted in the anterior nasal spine to treat a patient with a deep overbite. However, miniscrew implants for orthodontic anchorage were not immediately popular. Thereafter, a number of papers focused on other means of obtaining skeletal anchorage for orthodontic tooth movement, such as dental implants, onplants and palatal implants. (Papadopulos et al., 2009)

In 1997, Kanomi (1997) described a mini-implant specifically made for orthodontic use and, in 1998, Costa et al. (1998) presented a screw with a bracket-like head requiring a simplified procedure: only local anesthesia, placement of a drill-free screw, and immediate loading.

Labanauskaite et al. (2005) suggested the following classification of implants for orthodontic anchorage:

1. according to shape and size:
   - conical (cylindrical)
   - miniscrew implants
   - palatal implants
   - prosthodontic implants
   - mini-plate implants
   - disc implants (onplants);
2. according to implant bone contact
   - bone-integrated
   - not bone-integrated;
3. according to application
   - used only for orthodontic purposes (orthodontic implants)
   - used for prosthodontic and orthodontic purposes (prosthodontic implants).

With the exception of the Orthodontic Mini-Implant, which is made of stainless steel, all other above-mentioned systems are made of medical type IV or type V titanium alloy.

Miniscrew implants can be used as anchorages for tooth movements which could not otherwise be achieved, as in patients with insufficient teeth for conventional anchorages to be applied, when the forces on the reactive unit would generate adverse side-effects, in patients requiring asymmetrical tooth movements in all spatial planes and, in some cases, as an alternative to orthognathic surgical procedures. (Melsen B. 2005)

Using the retromolar area to position orthodontic implants was proposed by Roberts et al. in 1990. The authors used an experimental titanium bone-integrated implant to obtain absolute anchorage for second and third molar protraction after a first extracted molar replacement.

The retromolar area is particularly suitable for screw insertion, due to the presence of compact cortical bone tissue which immediately provides excellent primary stability (Figures 1 and 2).

The side-effects of positioning screws in this area are the risk of inflammation and hypertrophy of the movable mucosa, which may coverthe screw entirely, resulting in difficult case management and the need for additional gingivectomy. Care must be taken in evaluating the position of the mandibular canal, in order to avoid neurological complications (e.g., damage to the inferior alveolar nerve).

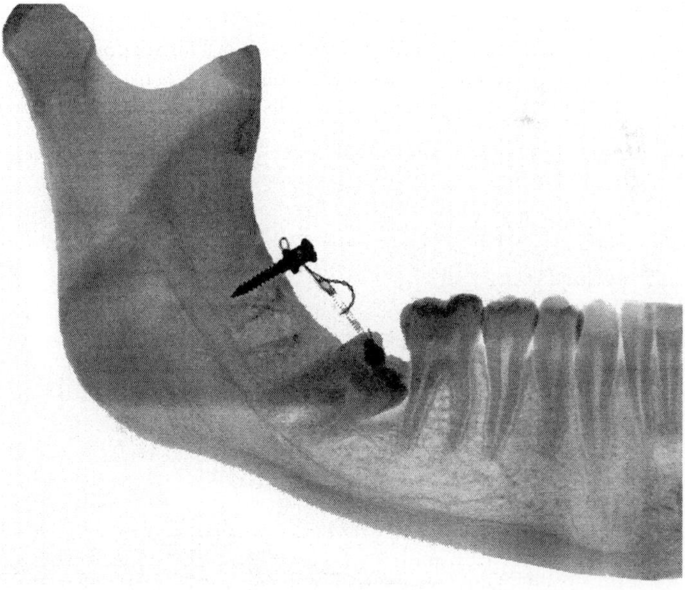

Fig. 1. Example of screw positioning in retromolar area. Lateral view.

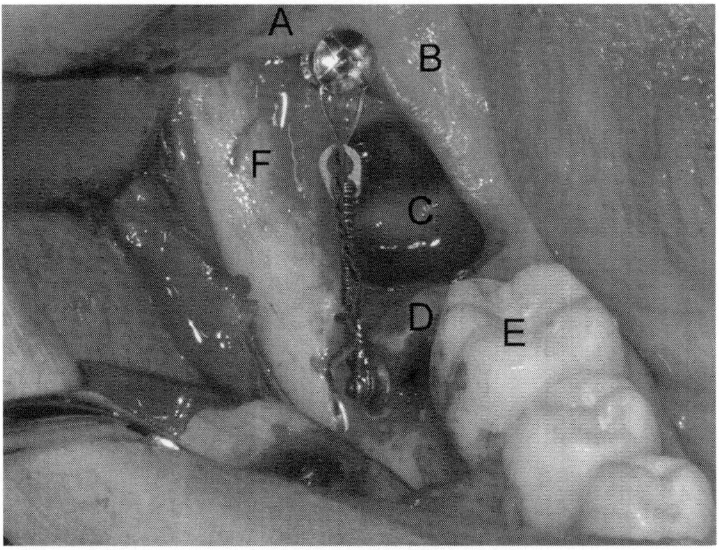

Fig. 2. Example of screw positioning in retromolar area. (A) Retromolar area. (B) Screw and device in place. (C) Third molar extraction socket. (D). Impacted second molar. (E) First molar. (F) Oblique external line.

Using implants as a method of skeletal anchorage for second lower molar uprighting was first proposed by Shellhart et al. These Authors placed a bone-integrated implant in an edentulous site, from which the first molar had previously been extracted. (Shellhart et al., 1996)

Park, first proposed the use of orthodontics implants for uprighting of the second molar by placing miniscrews in retromolar area. (Park H.S., 2002) The distalizing force is exerted through the use of elastomeric threads using perhaps rather low forces, about 50-80g. Other authors (Giancotti, 2003, 2004), (Nęcka et al., 2010) propose a very similar method, involving elastomeric chains, with monthly reactivations, or 50g-force closed Ni-Ti coil springs. The average treatment time in all these case reports was 7-9 months.

In an adolescent patient with a developing third molar, however, it is difficult to insert a miniscrew in the retromolar area unless the third molar is extracted. Thick overlying soft tissue and poor accessibility of the insertion site can also hinder miniscrew insertion. In such cases, the miniscrew can be inserted into the buccal alveolar bone on the mesial side to generate a "pushing" force. Lee et al. proposed to position the microscrew in interradicular area between second premolar and first molar and the use of a 0.016" or 0.016"x0.022" stainless steel wire with welded hook and open-coil spring for force delivery. (Lee et al., 2007)

Other Authors (Sohn et al., 2007) proposed a mesial positioning, using the screw as an anchor for the indirect stabilization of the first molar and second premolar. A 0.016"x0.022" stainless steel wire directly bonded with composite on teeth surface was used to connect dental elements and microscrews.

3. Combined surgical and orthodontic treatment using a distal screw as skeletal anchorage

This chapter describes a multidisciplinary surgical and orthodontic procedure for the treatment of second lower molar impaction.

3.1 Materials and methods

A brief and schematic description of the materials and methods is given in this section.

1. Orthodontic evaluation of the patient and diagnosis of second molar inclusion. If the patient is still not in orthodontic treatment, before surgical disinclusion, a bracket is placed on the buccal surface of the lower first molar ipsilateral to facilitate the stabilization of the metal ligature wire and to improve patient comfort; (Figure 3-6)
2. Surgical workup to define the procedure;
3. Surgical procedure. A full-thickness flap is performed with distal extension, the third molar ipsilateral to the impacted tooth is extracted and, at the same time, in the site distal to the extracted tooth, a surgical steel screw for orthodontic traction with a head complete with a slot and holes is inserted. During the same session, the crown of the impacted second molar is surgically exposed and one or more orthodontic bracket are placed in position; the second molar is connected to the screw by means of two metal ligatures with eyelets for attaching the intermediate traction module or an NiTi closed coil-spring. The flap is repositioned and sutured; (Figure 7-15)
4. Sutures are removed and an early orthodontic traction element emplaced;
5. Follow-up is carried out every 3 weeks, according to patient requirements (including any intermediate gingivectomies, and adjusting the position of the bracket on the tooth as necessary) until the tooth has been uprighted; (Figure 16-19).
6. A further orthodontic step may be necessary to complete the process and finalize occlusion.

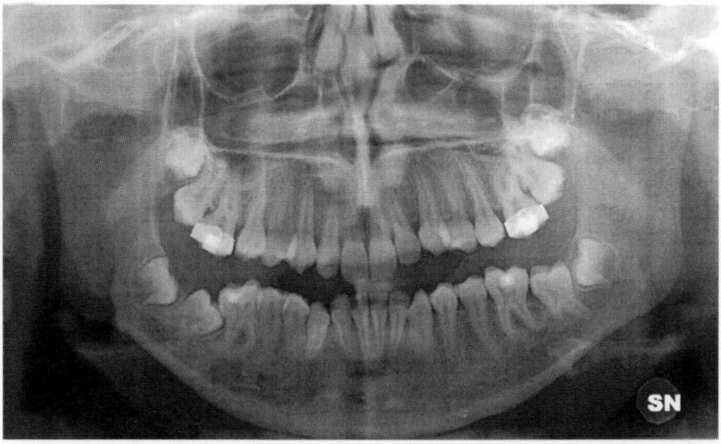

Fig. 3. Patient MF, aged 14 at the beginning of the therapy, had the following Orthodontic characteristics: I skeletal class with a normal vertical dimension, mild II molar and canine class, increased overjet, moderate anterior-inferior and anterior-superior crowding, cross bite 1.6-4.6, 2.6-3.6, eruption disorder of the right second lower molar with complete gingival inclusion.

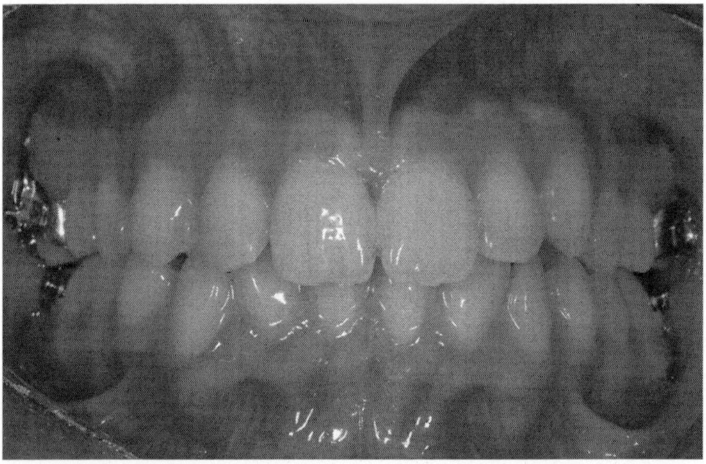

Fig. 4. Intraoral frontal view before treatment. The patient was treated by the use of criss-cross elastic for the correction of XB and EOT for the correction of molar Class II.

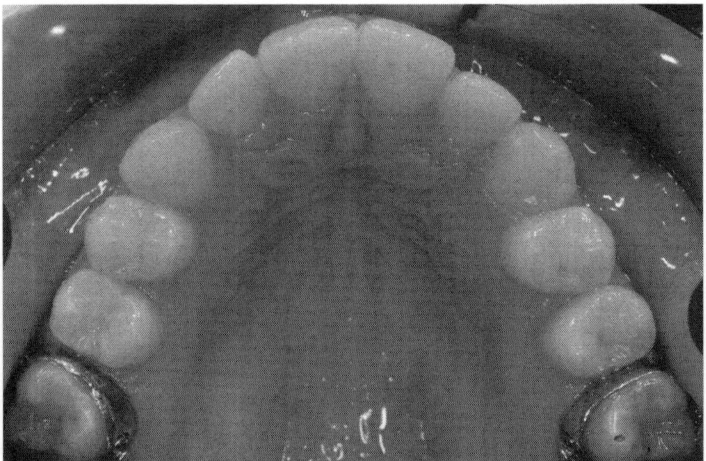

Fig. 5. Upper dental arch after distalization.

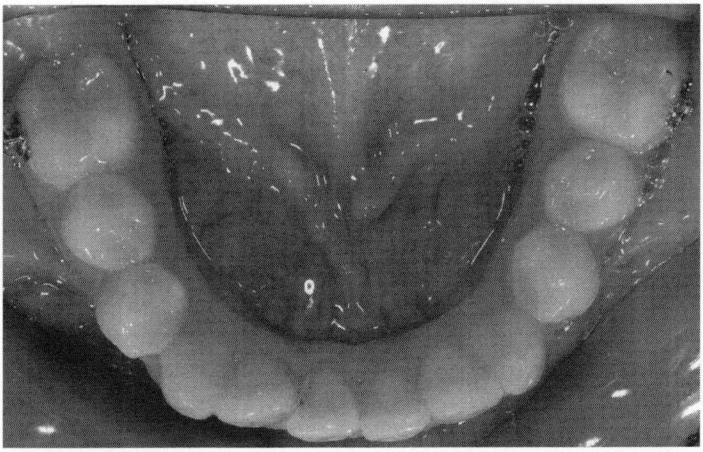

Fig. 6. Lower dental arch before surgical-orthodontic treatment. Patient simultaneously underwent the procedure for the surgical-orthodontic disinclusion of the element 47, during the last phase of interceptive treatment.

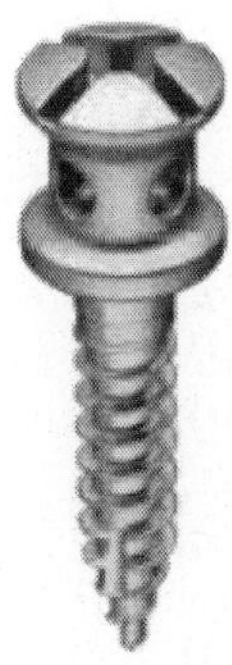

Fig. 7. The screw used in the proposed case has the following features: 2.0mm screws, 8-12mm thread lengths, made of 316L extra-hard stainless steel for maximum strength; self-drilling, self-tapping for one-step insertion; groove under screw-head secures wires or elastics; cruciform head design; two cross-holes with align cruciform head slots; a 4-mm capstan-style head to hold the wire away from the mucosa (Synthes, West Chester, Pennsylvania).

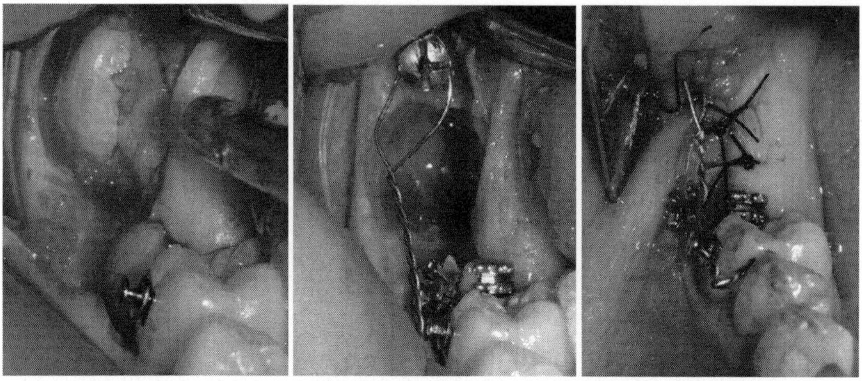

Fig. 8, 9 and 10. Surgical phases. The left mandibular third molar was extracted (germectomy), and a skeletal anchorage (2.0mm diameter/12mm length screw, Synthes, West Chester, Pennsylvania) was immediately applied. Two brackets, Roth Prescription slots 0.22, were positioned on the second molar (vestibular and occlusal) to optimize traction direction. Second molar was immediately connected to the screw by means of two metal ligatures with eyelets to attach intermediate traction elastic module. Eyelet to anchor the screw was modeled with 0.010" metallic ligature wire.

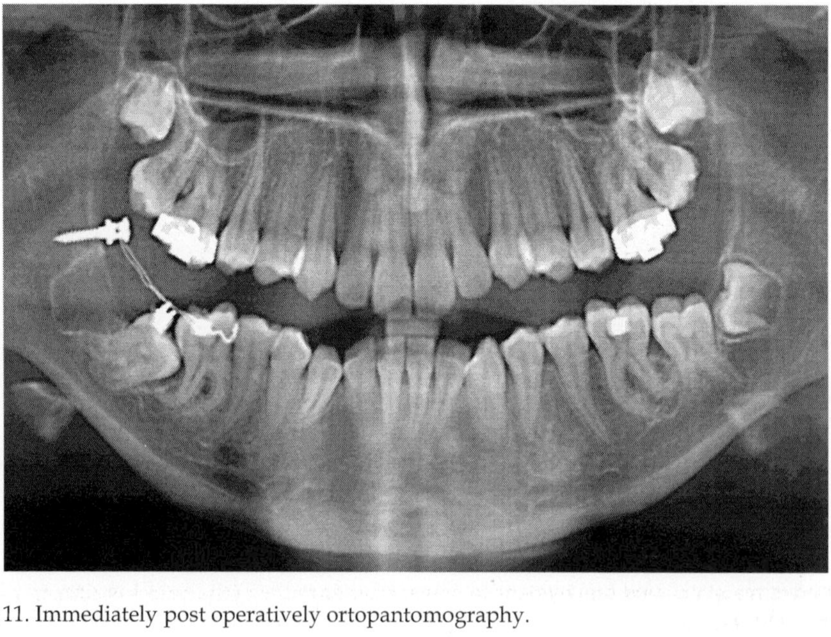

Fig 11. Immediately post operatively ortopantomography.

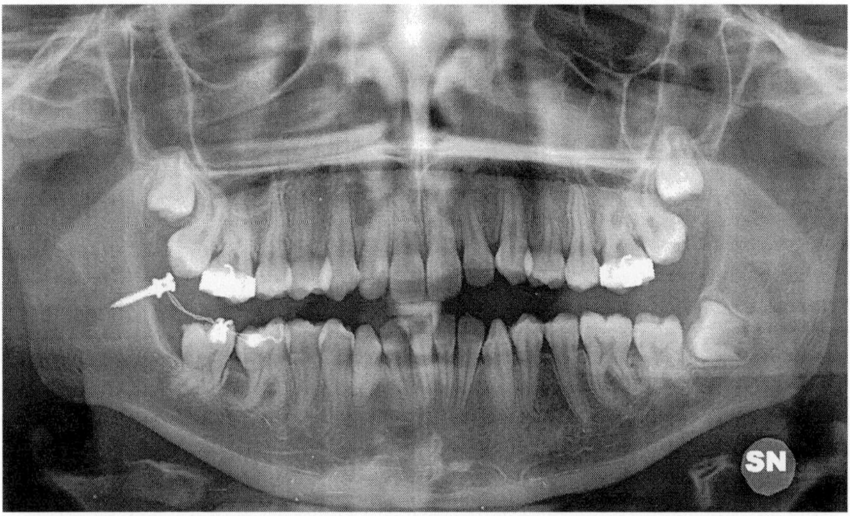

Fig. 12. Radiological check taken approximately 11 months later. The second left mandibular molar is in the correct position, the screw is still in place with no signs of bone inflammation. The time of treatment to achieve uprighting: about 9 months.

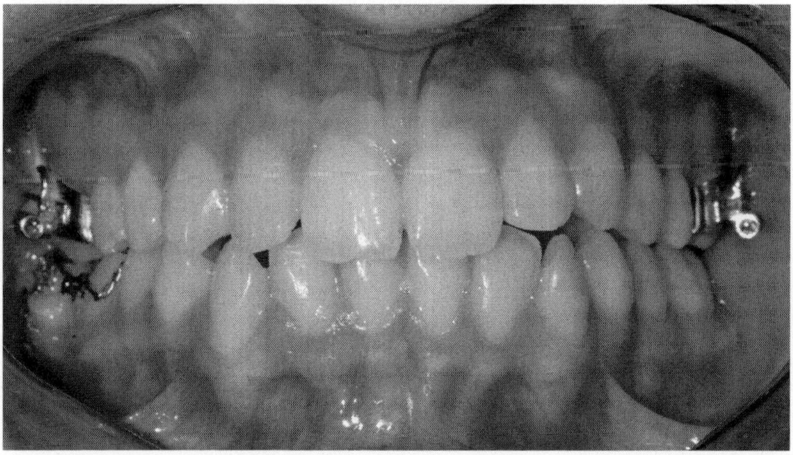

Fig. 13. Intraoral frontal view after treatment. The periodic checks to reactive the elastic traction, performed monthly at patient's request, rather than twice a week, caused a lengthening of time required to achieve the therapeutic effects. The patient was often advised to maintain good oral hygiene to prevent hypertrophy of the mucosa in the area of screw insertion.

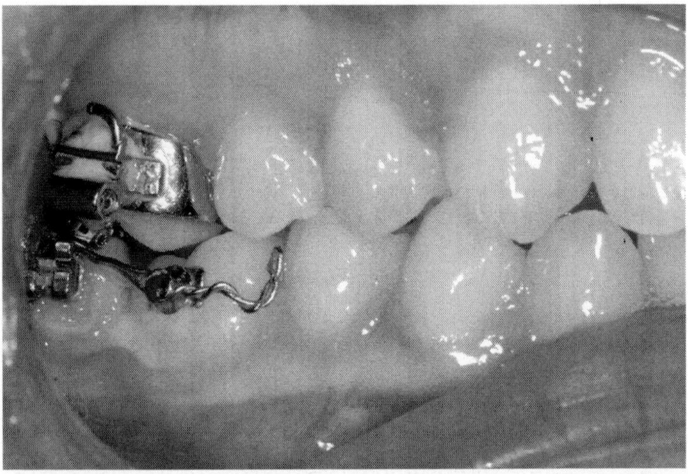

Fig. 14. Intraoral right lateral view after treatment. Passive ligature metallic wire still anchored on element 46. Only one gingivectomy was necessary during treatment, to set bracket in better position.

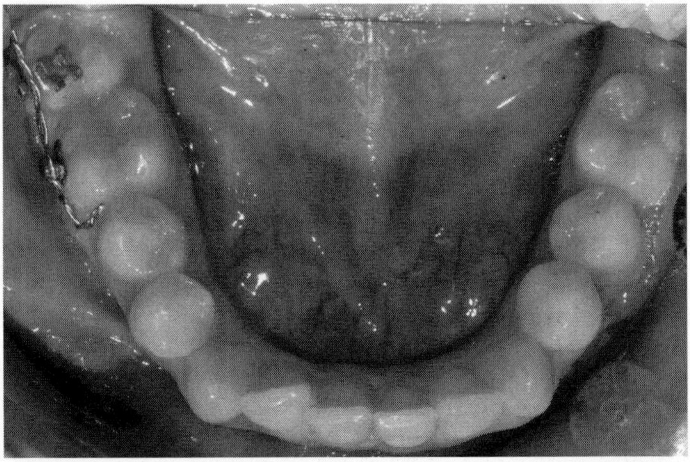

Fig. 15. Lower dental arch after treatment. Case will conclude with fixed orthodontic treatment to correct and finalize the occlusion.

4. Cases presentation

Until now, the Authors successfully treated five cases of eruptive disorder of the second lower molar with the described technique (table 1).

Patients' mean age was 15.8 years; only one was female. When present, the third molar was always extracted. No damage to the inferior alveolar nerve or other major complications were encountered. Patients' compliance was crucial: oral hygiene at home and relatively frequent clinical checks (about every 3 weeks) were important to prevent inflammation, hypertrophy of soft tissues and pain. When present, these minor complications did not affect the outcome of the procedure. The average duration of treatment for uprighting was 10.4 months. Results remained stable over 5 year follow-up.

Patient number	1	2	3	4	5
Age at start of treatment	14	16	15	18	16
Gender	F	M	M	M	M
Tooth	4.8	4.8	3.8	4.8	3.8
Type of inclusion	Mucosa inclusion	Bone inclusion	Mucosa inclusion	Partial bone inclusion	Mucosa inclusion
Presecne of third molar	Yes	No	Yes	Yes	Yes
Duration of therapy	9 months	14 months	10 months	11 months	10 months
Undesired effects	Low compliance	None	Low hygiene	Mucosa hypertrophy	None

Table 1. Patients treated with Combined Surgical and Orthodontic treatment using a distal screw as skeletal anchorage.

5. Discussion and conclusions

This chapter discusses the application of a skeletal anchorage device to achieve a very complex orthodontic movement such as second lower molar uprighting, an issue relatively little discussed in the literature due to the low prevalence of this kind of malocclusion.

The method described is minimally invasive, as the surgery needed to expose the impacted tooth and emplace the screw is quite simple and can be completed in a single session, together with extraction of the third molar, which is necessary in most cases. It also seems that the creation of a cortico-medullar void distal to the second molar, after third molar extraction or appositely surgically performed (Finotti et al, 2009), is important in shortening treatment time.

The dimensions of the device are minimal. It only requires one miniscrew and a single bracket or button attachment, and is more comfortable for the patient than complex segmental biomechanics.

Miniscrew insertion, preparation of the appliance and delivery can all be done during a single appointment, unlike conventional treatment which requires impressions and laboratory work. The simple design reduces chair time compared with more complex indirect anchorages. This system guarantees the utmost respect of periodontal tissues, soft tissues and bone. The method allows absolute control of the anchorage and no unwanted movement of adjacent teeth. (Park et al., 2002), (Giancotti et al, 2003, 2004), (Nęcka et al., 2010)

The direct application of force to the target tooth eliminates any unwanted movement of the anchorage unit, which may occur even with indirect miniscrew anchorage as a result of technical errors in passive bracket placement or weak attachment between miniscrew and anchor tooth.

Removing the anchoring screw is straightforward, with negligible risks and consequences for the patient. The use of miniscrews and their success rate are predictable. (Degichi et al., 2003), (Motoyoshy et al., 2007), (Yanosky & Holmes, 2008), (Moon et al., 2008), (Manni et al., 2010).

Temporary skeletal anchorage devices enable orthodontic movements that were previously considered difficult, if not impossible, without consequences for the other teeth (e.g., anchorage loss, unwanted extrusion). Treatment involving skeletal anchorage requires interdisciplinary collaboration and planning with regular interaction, ongoing education, improvement of materials and continual reviews of the latest literature.

6. References

Aitasalo K., Lehtinen R., Oksala E. (1972). An orthopantomographic study of prevalence of impacted teeth. *International Journal of Oral Surgery*, Vol 1, No. 3, (1972), pp.117–120.

Aksoy A., Aras S. (1998). Use of nickel titanium coil spring for partially impacted second molars. *Journal of Clinical Orthododontics*. Vol. 32, (1998), pp. 479– 482.

Alessandri Bonetti G., Pelliccioni G.A., Checchi. L. (1999). Management of bilaterally impacted mandibular second and third molars. *Journal of the American Dental Association*. Vol. 130, No. 8, (August 1999), pp. 1190-1194.

Carano A., Testa M., Siciliani G. (1996). The Distal Jet for Uprighting Lower Molars. *Journal of Clinical Orthodontics*, Vol. 30, No. 12, (1996), pp. 707-710

Cope, J. (2007). *ORTHOTADs. The clinical Guide and Atlas,* Under Dog Media, ISBN 978-0-9776301-0-3, Dallas, Texas

Costa A., Raffaini M., Melsen B. (1998). Miniscrews as orthodontic anchorage: a preliminary report. *International Journal Adult Orthodontics & Orthognathic Surgery,* Vol. 13, (1998), pp. 201-209.

Creekmore TD, Eklund MK. The possibility of skeletal anchorage. J Clin Orthod 1983;17:266-9.

Daskalogiannakis J. *Glossary of orthodontic terms*. (2000). Leipzig: Quintessence Publishing Co.

Deguchi T., Takano-Yamamoto T., Kanomi R., Hartsfield J.K., Roberts W.E., Garetto L.P. (2003). The use of small titanium screws for orthodontic anchorage. *Journal of Dental Research*, Vol. 82, (2003), pp. 377-381.

Eckhart J.E. (1998). Orthodontic uprighting of horizontally impacted mandibular second molars. *Journal of Clinical Orthodontics*. Vol. 32, (1998), pp. 621– 624.

Finotti M., Del Torre M., Roberto M., Miotti F.A. Could the distalization of the mandibular molars be facilitated? A new therapeutic method. *Orthodontie Francaise*. Vol. 80, No. 4, (December 2009), pp. 371-378.

Frank C. (2000). Treatment options for impacted teeth. *Journal of the American Dental Association*, Vol. 131, (2000), pp. 623-32.

Gainsforth BL, Higley LB. A study of orthodontic anchorage possibilities in basal bone. Am J Orthod Oral Surg 1945;31:406-17.

Giancotti A., Muzzi F., Santini F., Arcuri C. (2003). Miniscrew treatment of ectopic mandibular molar. *Journal of Clinical Orthodontics*. Vol. 37, (2003), pp. 380–383.

Giancotti A., Arcuri C., Barlattani A., (2004). Treatment of ectopic mandibular second molar with titanium miniscrews. *American Journal of Orthodontics and Dentofacial Orthopedics*, Vol. 126, No. 1 (July 2004), pp. 113-117

Going R.E., Reyes-Lois D.B. (1999). Surgical exposure and bracketing technique for uprighting impacted mandibular second molars. *Journal of Oral Maxillofacial Surgery*. Vol. 57, (1999), pp. 209–212.

Grover P.S., Norton L. (1985). The incidence of unerupted permanent teeth and related clinical cases. *Oral Surgery, Oral Medicine, Oral Pathology, Oral Radiology and Endodontology*, Vol. 59, (1985), pp. 420–425.

Johnson J.V., Quirk G.D. (1987). Surgical repositioning of impacted second molar teeth. *American Journal of Orthodontics and Dentofacial Orthopedics*. Vol. 91, (1987), pp. 242–251

Kanomi R. (1997). Mini-implant for orthodontic anchorage. *Journal of Clinical Orthodontics*; Vol. 31, (1997), pp. 763-767.

Kogod M., Kogod H.S. (1991). Molar uprighting with the piggyback buccal sectional arch wire technique. *American Journal of Orthodontics and Dento-facial Orthopedics*. Vol. 99, (1991), pp. 276–280.

Kokich V.G., Mathews D.P. (1993). Surgical and orthodontic management of impacted teeth. *Dental Clinics of North America*. Vol. 37, (1993), pp.198-201

Labanauskaite B., Jankauskas G., Vasiliauskas A., Haffar N. (2005). Implants for orthodontic anchorage. Meta-analysis. *Stomatologija*, Vol. 7 (200), pp. 128-32.

Lee KJ, Park Y.C., Hwang W.S., Seong E.H. (2007). Uprighting mandibular second molars with direct miniscrew anchorage. *Journal of Clinical Orthodontics*, Vol. 41, No. 10 (October 2007) Oct, pp. 627-35.

Majourau A., Norton L.A. (1995). Uprighting impacted second molars with segmented springs. *American Journal of Orthodontics and Dentofacial Orthopedics*, Vol. 107, (1995), pp. 235–238.

Manni A., Cozzani M., Tamborrino F., De Rinaldis S., Menini A. (2011). Factors influencing the stability of miniscrews. A retrospective study on 300 miniscrews. *European Journal of Orthodontics*. Vol. 33, No. 4, (August 2011), pp. 388-395.

McAboy C.P., Grumet J.T., Siegel E.B., Iacopino A.M. (2003). Surgical uprighting and repositioning of severely impacted mandibular second molars. *Journal of American Dental Association*. Vol. 134, (2003), pp. 1459- 1462.

Mead S. (1930). Incidence of impacted teeth. *International J Orthodontics*, Vol. 16, (1930), pp. 885–890.

Melsen B., Fiorelli G., Bergamini A. (1996). Uprighting of lower molars. *Journal of Clinical Orthodontics*. Vol. 30, No. 11, (November 1996), pp. 640-645.

Melsen B. (2005). Mini-implants: where are we? *Journal of Clinical Orthodontics, Vol. 39,* (2005), pp. 539-47.

Miao Y.Q., Zhong H. (2006). An uprighting appliance for impacted mandibular second and third molars. *Journal of Clinical Orthodontics*, Vol. 40, No.2 (February 2006), pp. 110-116.

Moon C.H., Lee D.G., Lee H.S., Im J.S., Baek S.H. (2008). Factors associated with the success rate of orthodontic miniscrews placed in the upper and lower posterior buccal region. *Angle Orthodontics*. Vol. 78, No. 1 (January 2008), pp. 101-106.

Moro N., Murakami T., Tanaka T., Ohto C. (2002). Uprighting of im-pacted third molars using brass ligature wire. *Australian Orthodontic Journal,* Vol. 18, (2002), pp. 35–38

Motoyoshy M., Yoshiba T., Ono A., Shimizu N. (2007). Effect of cortical bone thickness and implant placement torque on stability of orthodontic mini-implants. *International Journal of Oral & Maxillofacial Implants,* Vol. 22, No. 5, (September-October 2007) pp. 779-84

Nęcka A., Skrzypczyński J., Antoszewska J. (2010). Miniscrew-Anchorage in Treatment of Impacted Second Molar in Mandible - Case Report. *Dental and Medical Problems,* Vol. 47, No. 3, (2010) 379–383

Papadopoulos M.A., Papageorgiou S.N., Zogakis I.P. (2009). Clinical effectiveness of orthodontic miniscrew implants: a meta-analysis. *Journal of Dental Research,* Vol. 90, No. 8, (Aug 2011), pp. 969-76.

Park D.K. (1999). Australian uprighting spring for partially impacted second molars. *Journal of Clinical Orthodontics,* Vol. 33, (1999), pp. 404–405.

Park H.S., Kyung H.M., Sung J.H. (2002). A simple method of molar uprighting with micro-implant anchorage. *Journal of Clinical Orthodontics,* Vol. 36, (2002) pp. 592-6

Pilon J.J., Kuijpers-Jagtman A.M., Maltha J.C. (1996). Magnitude of orthodontic forces and rate of bodily tooth movement. An experimental study. *American Journal of Orthodontics and Dentofacial Orthopedics,* Vol. 110, No.16, (1996), pp. 16-23.

Pogrel A. (1995). The surgical uprighting of mandibular second molars. *Amercian Journal of Orthodontics and Dento- facial Orthopedics,* Vol. 108, (1995), pp. 180-183.

Roberts W.E., Marshall K.J., Mozsary P.G. (1990). Rigid endosseous implant utilized as anchorage to protract molars and close an atrophic extraction site. *Angle Orthod*ontics. Vol. 60, No. 2, (Summer 1990), pp. 135-152.

Roberts W.W., Chacker F.M., Burstone C.J. (1982). A segmental appproach to mandibular molar uprighting. *American Journal of Orthodontics.* Vol. 81, (1982), pp. 177–184.

Romeo D.A., Burstone C.J. (1977). Tip-back mechanics. Am J Orthod. 1977; 72:414–421.

Sawicka M., Racka-Pilszak B., Rosnowska-Mazurkiewicz A. (2007). Uprighting partially impacted permanent second molars. *Angle Orthodontics.* Vol. 77, No. 1, (January 2007), pp. 148-154.

Shapira Y., Borell G., Nahlieli O., Kuftinec M.M. (1998). Uprighting mesially impacted mandibular permanent second molars. *Angle Orthodontics.*;No. 68, (1998), pp. 173–178.

Shellhart W.C., Moawad M., Lake P. (1996). Case report: implants as anchorage for molar uprighting and intrusion. *Angle Orthodontics,* Vol. 66, No. 3, (1996), pp. 169-72

Shellhert W.C., Oesterle L.J. (1999). Uprighting molars without extrusion. *Journal of American Dental Association. Vol.* 130, (1999), pp. 381–385.

Sohn B.W., Choi J.H., Jung S.N., Lim K.S. (2007). Uprighting mesially impacted second molars with miniscrew anchorage. *Journal of Clinical Orthodontics.* Vol. 41, No. 2, (February 2007), pp. 94-97

Tinerfe T.J., Blakey G.H. (2000). *Oral and maxillofacial surgery.* (2000) Saunders, Philadelphia

Yanosky M.R., Holmes J.D. (2008). Mini-implant temporary anchorage devices: orthodontic applications. *Compendium of Continuing Education in Dentistry* (January-February 2008), Vol. 29, No. 1, pp. 12-21

12

Guidelines for "Surgery First" Orthodontic Treatment

Jeong Hwan Kim[1], Niloufar Nouri Mahdavie[2] and Carla A. Evans[2]
[1]*Private Practice, Seoul*
[2]*University of Illinois at Chicago, Chicago*
[1]*Korea*
[2]*USA*

1. Introduction

Pre-surgical orthodontic preparation was uncommon for patients requiring orthognathic surgery until the 1960's. However, as surgical techniques advanced and the number of patients choosing an orthognathic approach increased, the patients' and clinicians' desire for optimal esthetic and occlusal results led to the most common current treatment approach. This approach involves pre-surgical orthodontic decompensation of the occlusal relationships and attainment of normal dental alignment. As most orthognathic treatment is planned now, there are two phases of orthodontic tooth movement, namely before and after orthognathic surgery. The disadvantages of having orthodontic interventions both before and after orthognathic surgery include a long treatment time and temporary worsening of facial appearance. Many patients become discouraged.

In recent years, a trend toward implementing treatment plans that achieve immediate facial change has arisen. In "Surgery First" treatment plans, the presurgical orthodontic treatment phase is eliminated or greatly reduced, the jaws are surgically repositioned into the desired locations, and orthodontic tooth movement follows. Patients appreciate the immediate improvement in facial appearance while the orthodontist can utilize the increased bone turnover to achieve accelerated tooth movement.

Caution is important when embarking on a "Surgery First" course of treatment. Even for the highly experienced orthodontist and surgeon, it is difficult to identify the occlusal relationship that will accompany an ideal facial and functional result. The planning process is time-consuming and requires choosing the desired appearance and skeletal relationships, mounting the casts in the position determined by the skeletal change, and then planning the post-operative orthodontic tooth movements. The surgical movement must be sufficient to allow dental decompensation after the surgical procedure. Surgical splints are fabricated on the articulated study models. Generally, the teeth are bonded/banded and a passive archwire is placed pre-surgically. Active orthodontic tooth movement begins within a relatively short period of time after the jaw(s) are repositioned to capitalize on the potential for accelerated tooth movement.

This chapter illustrates step-by-step concepts for "Surgery First" treatment with case records of increasing complexity. Surgical fixation and skeletal anchorage are discussed as well.

1.1 Background

Ever since the first orthognathic surgery procedure was performed by Hullihen in 1848, many new techniques and methods have been introduced. The introduction of orthognathic surgery widened the possibilities for treatment of severe malocclusions which could not be treated by orthodontics alone. As shown by Kondo and her colleagues (2000, 2005), the limits of orthodontic treatment alone for severe malocclusions are broadening, but the underlying skeletal imbalances remain. Until the 1960's, orthognathic surgeries were usually performed without any pre-surgical orthodontic treatment. In fact, when Hullihen performed the first mandibular sub-apical osteotomy on a burn victim, he was able to correct the prognathism but created an edge-to-edge occlusion anteriorly (Aziz, 2004).

The three stage philosophy of orthognathic surgery was later adapted and is still valid today in the majority of cases. These stages involve pre-orthognathic orthodontic treatment to relieve the dental compensations followed by the orthognathic surgical procedure and finally post-surgical orthodontics to finish the case and settle the occlusion.

1.2 Challenges associated with conventional orthognathic surgery cases

The pre-surgical orthodontic treatment of patients requiring orthognathic surgery has been criticized to be the most time consuming stage of treatment (O'Brien et al., 2009). The mean length of this stage has been reported anywhere between 7 to 47 months (Luther et al., 2003). The longer pre-operative treatment phase can potentially aggravate the dental caries and periodontal problems and negatively influence patient compliance.

The worsening of facial profile prior to surgery which results from dentoalveolar decompensation is also a great disadvantage. This is even more so noticeable in Class III patients. The removal of natural dental compensation in these patients often results in advancement of the lower lip as well as retrusion of the upper lip which together accentuate the soft tissue disharmony. Considering the fact that patients who desire to undergo orthognathic surgery are often very concerned about facial esthetics, the long pre-surgical orthodontic preparation delays addressing the patient's chief complaint.

1.3 "Surgery First" orthognathics

The challenges involved with the conventional three stage model of orthognathic surgery have given rise to new concepts such as what is known as "Surgery First" orthognathics. In 1991 Brachvogel proposed this approach with the goal of reducing some of the disadvantages and inconveniences of pre-surgical orthodontics (Brachvogel et al., 1991). In that article the advantages of post-surgical orthodontics are outlined as follows: 1) Orthodontic movement does not interfere with compensatory biological responses, 2) Dental movements can be based on an already corrected skeletal pattern, and 3) Some surgical relapse can be managed during treatment. Informative case reports have been published by Tsuruda et al. (2003) and Sugawara et al. (2008).

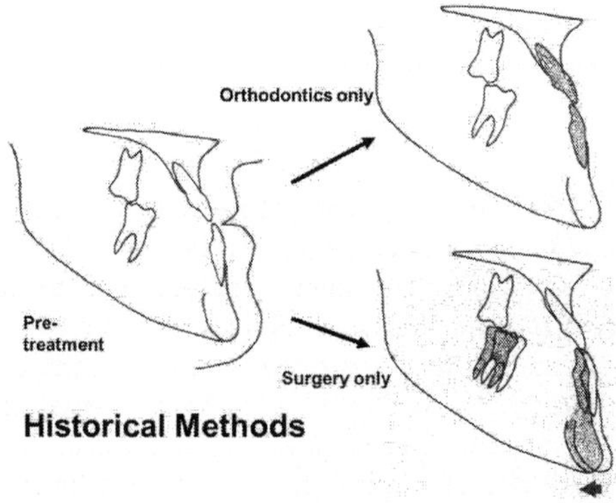

A.

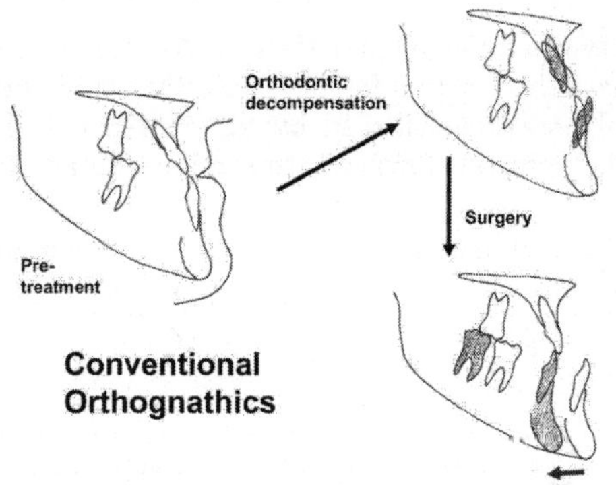

B.

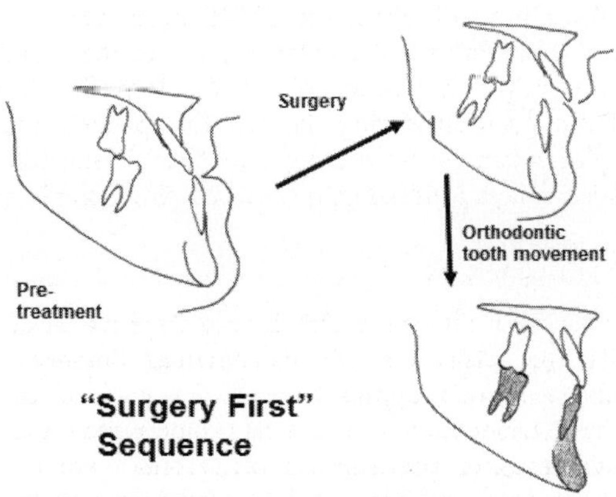

C.

Fig. 1. Various approaches to the treatment of severe skeletal disharmonies. A. Historical methods. B. Conventional orthognathics. C. "Surgery First" sequence.

A major driving motive for performing surgery first orthognathics has been the reduced treatment time reported in the literature (Yu et al., 2010; Villegas et al., 2010; Liou et al., 2011a, 2011b). Traditionally, a number of studies have focused on accelerated orthodontics as a result of corticotomy procedures with or without bone augmentation. It has been shown that orthodontic treatment time decreases by using alveolar osteotomy procedures (Wilcko et al., 2001; Wilcko et al., 2009). The proposed mechanism for this decrease in treatment time is the increase in cortical bone porosity which translates to decreased resistance to tooth movement (Wilcko et al., 2009). The same concept can be applied to performing orthognathic surgery before orthodontic treatment begins, but actual supporting data are sparse.

It has been shown that during the healing process after orthognathic surgery, there is an increase in blood flow above the pre-surgical levels (Justus et al., 2001). The increase in blood flow facilitates the healing process and stimulates bone turnover which can potentially speed up orthodontic tooth movement. Despite the postulated hypothesis, there is very limited information about the molecular basis for accelerated tooth movement. Moreover, the decrease in treatment time has only been documented as case reports. As knowledge becomes available about the reasons for increased bone turnover after osteotomies of the jaws (Iliopoulos et al., 2010), new surgical techniques will improve treatment options for the patients.

In recent years, more attention has been given to the subject and more and more cases are being treated with the "Surgery First" approach. The basic concept that underlies surgery first orthognathics is the elimination of the pre-surgical orthodontic phase and elimination of soft tissue imbalance accompanying the dentofacial deformity. The most important consideration in using this technique is the fact that it is a complicated approach that requires close cooperation of a highly experienced orthodontist and the orthognathic surgeon. Prediction of the desired final occlusion is a very difficult task. Also, the surgeon must be able to arrange the skeletal components to match the predicted skeletal positions and occlusion precisely. More importantly, the advent of rigid fixation was the key which allowed the surgery first approach to be implemented. With the conventional wire fixation, the mobility of the bony segments would not allow for a stable position of bone post surgically. Hence, any attempted movement could potentially result in movement of the skeletal components. Skeletal relapse caused by occlusal instability can be partially overcome with rigid fixation (Liao et al., 2010). In a series of case studies, it seems that the postoperative skeletal changes are similar between surgery first and conventional treatment of Class III malocclusions (Baek et al, 2011; Liao et al, 2010). Postoperatively in both types of treatment there was some forward superior movement of the mandible, but overall the needed posterior movement of the mandible was achieved and preserved.

The following segmental osteotomy case demonstrates the concepts of surgery first technique before getting into conventional one or two-jaw orthognathic surgery cases. Figure 2 shows the initial presentation of a patient with a chief complaint of unattractive smile and broken front teeth. On examination it was revealed that the bimaxillary protrusion could be resolved by extraction of upper and lower first premolars and segmental osteotomy procedures to retract the maxillary and mandibular dentoalveolar segments. After model surgery was performed (Figure 3), it was decided to remove the teeth at the time of surgery and utilize the surgery first approach. Maxillary and mandibular first premolars were extracted at the time of surgery and the anterior dentoalveolar segments were set back before any orthodontic treatment was initiated. An advancement genioplasty was done simultaneously; bony continuity between the right and left sides of the mandible could be maintained because the vertical dimension of the mandibular symphysis was large.

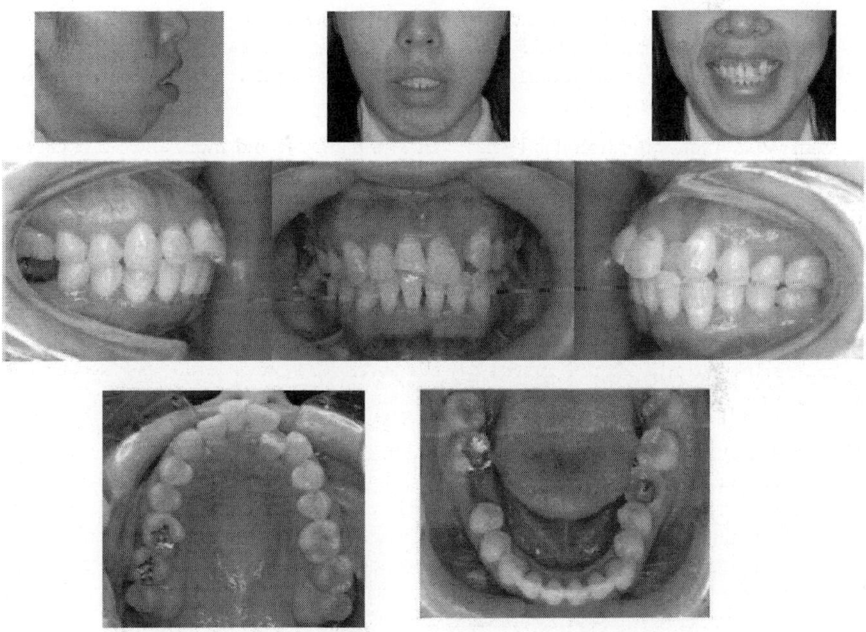

Fig. 2. Initial Presentation.

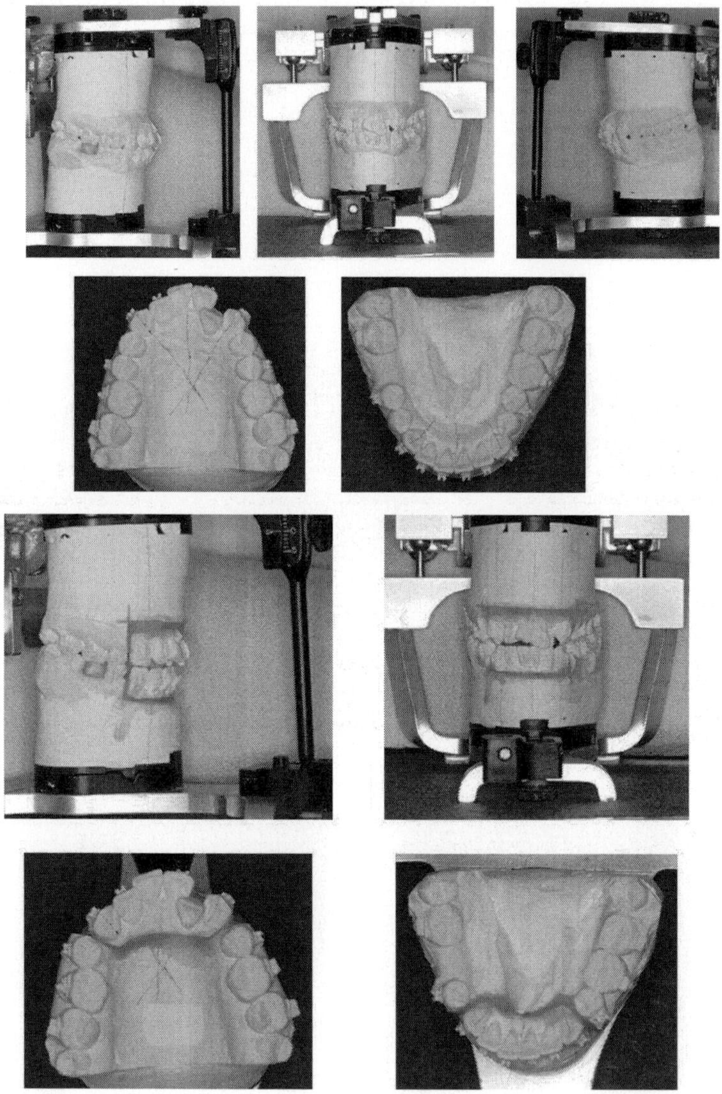

Fig. 3. A) Initial Models B) Model Set-up.

Figure 4 shows the patient immediately following the procedure. The occlusion immediately following surgery shows the same occlusion as was predicted in the model surgery. Orthodontic treatment was initiated 3 weeks after surgery and case was finished in 15 months. The treatment time in this case was longer than typical anterior segmental osteotomy cases due to the need for Class II correction. Subsequently the maxillary anterior teeth were restored for better esthetics. The final intra-oral and extra-oral pictures are shown in Figure 5.

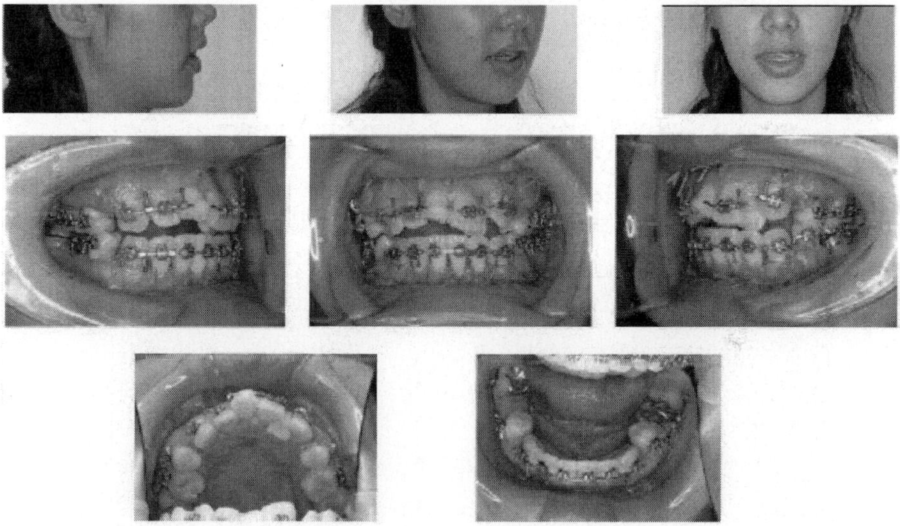

Fig. 4. Records immediately after surgery.

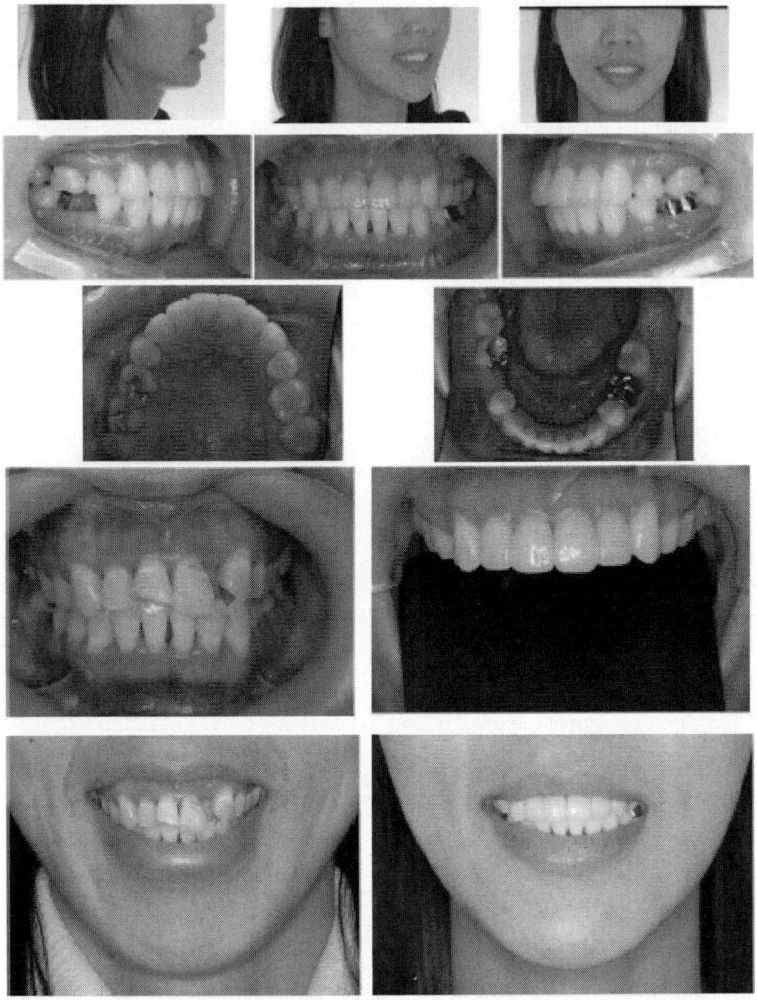

Fig. 5. Final Presentation.

By performing surgery first, patient was very satisfied with the reduction in protrusion as soon as the surgery was performed. The reduced treatment time also was an advantage.

2. Surgery first orthognathics indications

The surgery first approach can be used to treat a variety of cases depending on the specific characteristics of the malocclusion and the dentofacial deformity. Nonetheless, there are certain criteria which can make a case the ideal surgery first case.

In the ideal situation, the malocclusion accompanying the skeletal deformity represents mild to moderate crowding, normal to mild proclination and retroclination of upper and lower incisors, and minimal transverse discrepancies (Liou et al., 2011a, 2011b).

Even though the surgery first technique can be applied to Class II as well as Class III malocclusions, the majority of cases treated using this approach have been cases with Class III malocclusion meeting the above criteria. A possible explanation is that a Class III skeletal relationship results in a more pronounced soft tissue imbalance. Often, Class II skeletal deformities can be masked as the patient shifts the mandible forward, but the equivalent backward shift of the mandible to mask Class III deformities is physically impossible. In the traditional approach, decompensation of the arches results in an even more disfiguring profile for Class III patients. Hence, these patients seem to see the benefit of the surgery first approach to a greater extent than Class II cases and possibly seek this new approach more. It is also likely that for Class II patients, advancing a retrognathic mandible into the correct position will create an anterior crossbite temporarily worsening the patient's appearance until orthodontic treatment can upright and retract the lower incisors; this occurrence doesn't fit with surgery first concepts.

Figure 6 illustrates an ideal case which was treated using the surgery first approach. Patient presented at the age of 22. After the case was treatment planned and the model surgery was performed, the surgery first approach was indicated. Teeth were bonded and passive stainless steel arch wires were placed a few days prior to surgery. A two-jaw orthognathic surgery was performed and the patient returned five weeks after surgery for the initiation of orthodontic treatment. As it will be discussed later in this chapter, immediately after surgery there was a lateral open bite as can be seen in Figure 7. This transitional malocclusion was predicted during the model surgery procedure. Since the skeletal discrepancy was no longer present, the case could subsequently be treated as a Class I skeletal case. Figure 7 shows the occlusion at the start of orthodontic treatment followed by settling of the bite and improvement of overbite and overjet after eight months of orthodontic movement. The case was finished after a total treatment time of 20 months (19 months of orthodontic treatment) with lateral incisor restorations and satisfactory results in terms of facial aesthetics and occlusion as evident in the final records (Figure 8).

3. Advantages of surgery first orthognathics

In most cases, patients who receive orthognathic surgery in order to correct a dento-skeletal deformity present to the orthodontist's office with a chief complaint that includes dissatisfaction with their facial appearance. Hence, the main concern of the patient must be addressed during the course of treatment. The conventional three-stage approach in orthognathic surgery requires decompensation of the teeth which often results in worsening of the facial profile especially in patients with Class III malocclusion. The improvement in facial aesthetics in these patients does not occur until months later when the actual surgery is performed. Having surgery first eliminates the unsightly pre-surgical profile and allows the chief complaint of the patient to be addressed at the beginning of treatment. With the conventional approach, it is very difficult for the patient and the orthodontist to predict the exact time of surgery. Since the surgical procedure precedes orthodontic treatment, the patient has the opportunity to choose the timing of surgery to allow for the postoperative healing period.

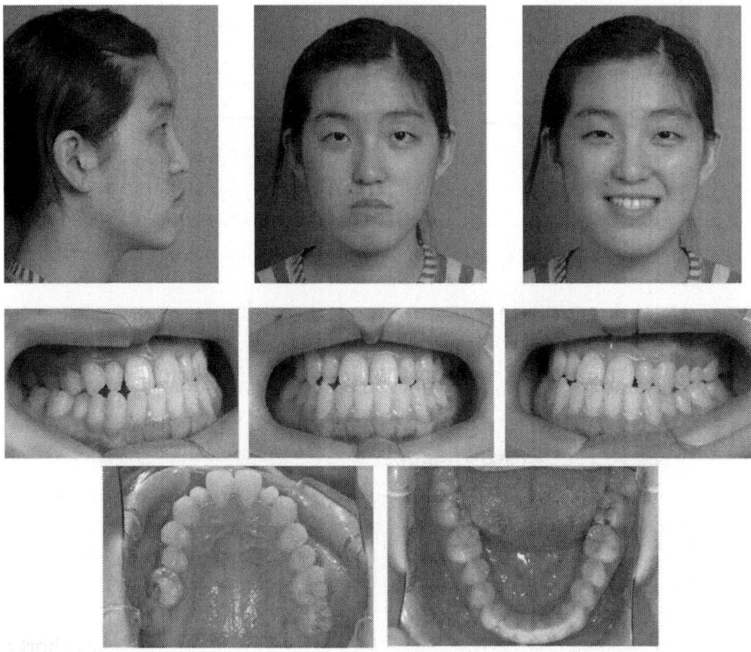

Fig. 6. Initial Presentation.

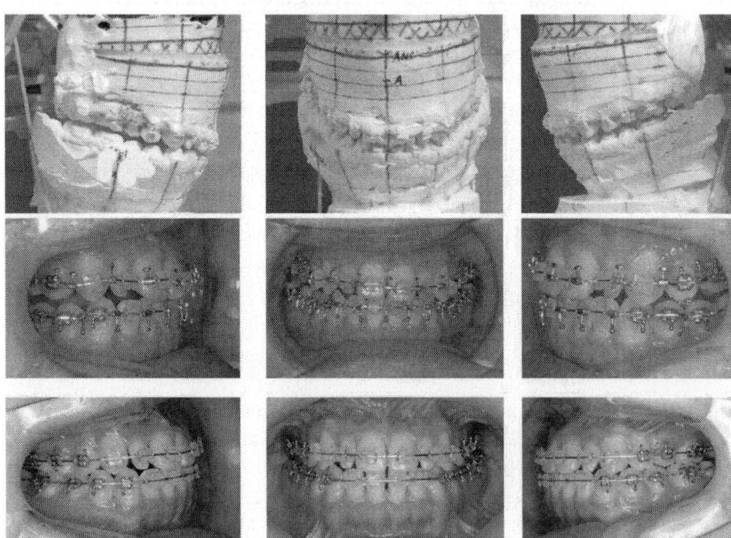

Fig. 7. A) Model Surgery B) Progress records at the start of orthodontic treatment and C) Progress records 8 months into orthodontic treatment.

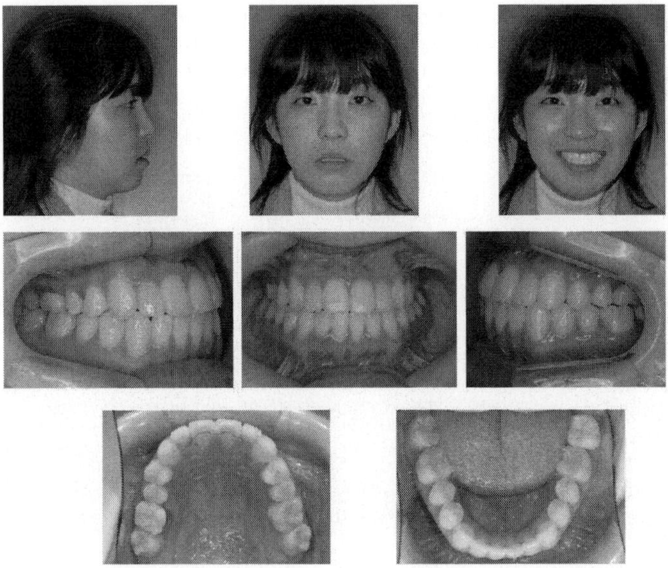

Fig. 8. Final Presentation.

The total treatment time in surgery first cases is reduced. Treatment times as short as seven months have been reported in the literature (Villegas et al., 1997). The pre-surgical orthodontic phase in conventional three-step orthognathic surgery cases is the most time consuming step. Bypassing this step results in an overall shortened treatment time to 1 to 1.5 years or less (Liou et al., 2011a, 2011b). The treatment time varies depending on the treating orthodontist's experience and the orthodontist's standard for finishing.

Immediate resolution of the soft tissue and skeletal imbalance is an added advantage in surgery first approach (Baek et al, 2010; Nagasaka et al, 2009). Dentoalveolar decompensation which is performed in conventional pre-surgical orthodontics works against the physiological compensatory dentoalveolar processes. In other words, the orthodontist tries to achieve a pre-operative occlusion which is against what the soft tissue and skeletal components dictate. This has been thought of as one of the challenges in decompensating the arches prior to surgery. When surgery is completed first, the skeletal and soft tissue discrepancy is relieved and the teeth can be aligned without the need to fight with the physiological limitations.

3.1 Reduced treatment time in surgery first orthodontics

The reduced treatment time in surgery first approach can be attributed to two main factors: 1) the resolution of skeletal and soft tissue imbalance prior to initiation of tooth movement and 2) the regional acceleratory phenomenon.

As mentioned previously, the resolution of skeletal and soft tissue imbalance through surgery allows the orthodontist to move the teeth in a normal skeletal and soft tissue envelope which facilitates the orthodontic movement. For example, in a Class III skeletal pattern, the relationship between the upper and lower jaw is not ideal. The imbalance between the two jaws results in dentoalveolar compensation which throughout an individual's lifetime, attempts to minimize and mask the skeletal deformity by maintaining contact between the teeth. This often results in proclination of upper incisors and retroclination of lower incisors in an attempt to minimize the negative overjet.

Figure 9 illustrates the initial presentation of a male patient. The skeletal Class III relationship in this patient was camouflaged by proclined upper incisors as well as slightly

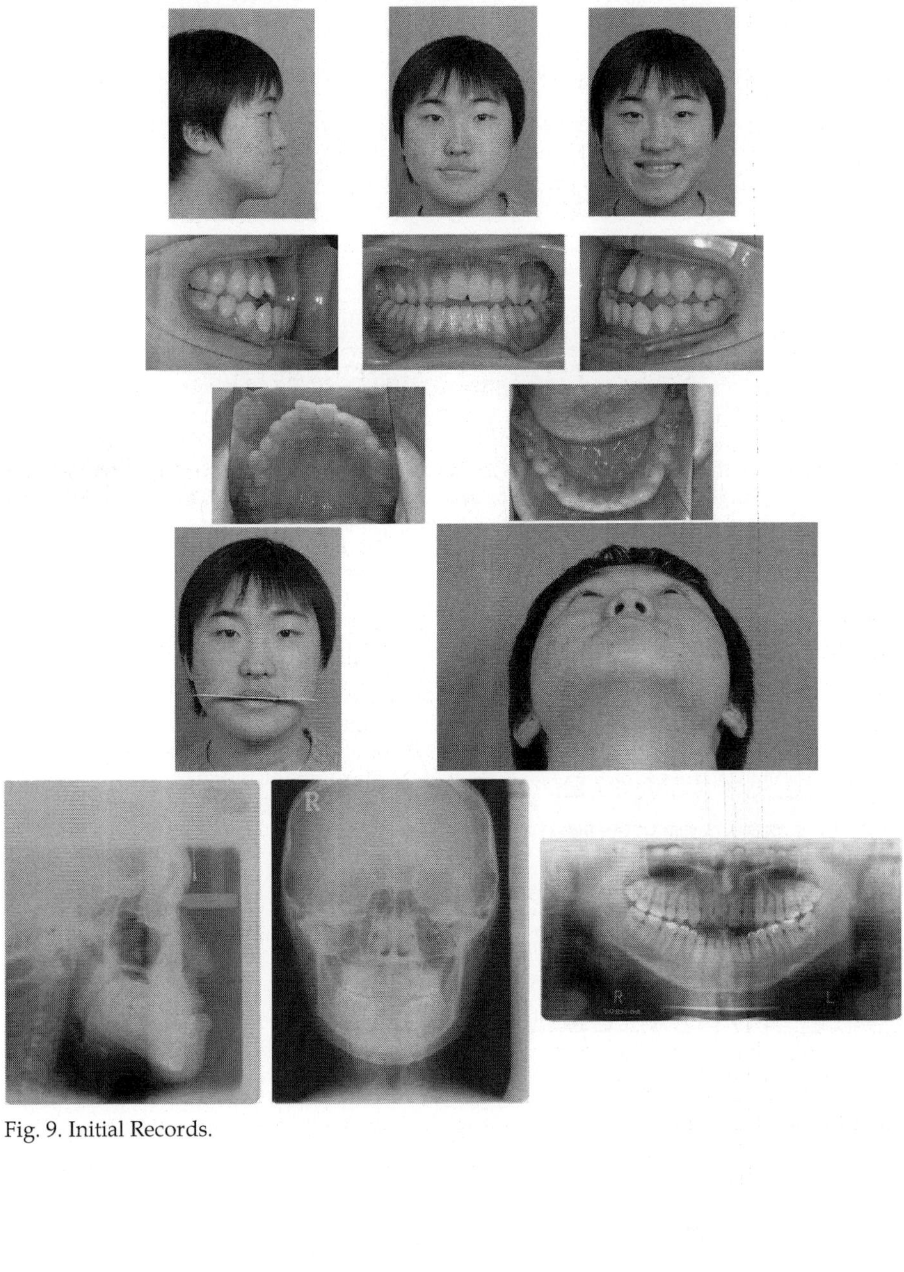

Fig. 9. Initial Records.

retroclined lower incisors. Anterior open bite was present and the chin was deviated to the right side. Such compensation had given him the best possible soft tissue profile and occlusion biologically possible with such skeletal disharmony. If this case was to be treated with the conventional protocol for orthognathic surgery, the upper incisors would need to be retroclined and the lower incisors would need to be proclined in order to de-compensate the upper and lower arches, achieve sufficient negative overjet, and finally perform the orthognathic surgical procedure. This decompensation would place the teeth in a position which is not "natural" for the current skeletal relationship and is against the compensatory mechanisms which have been at work for many years. The price would have been paid by a relatively long pre-surgical treatment time.

Figure 10 shows the model surgery and fabrication of the intermediate splint to position the maxilla which is then followed by prediction of the final occlusion and preparation of the final splint. The final occlusion is predicted on the models.

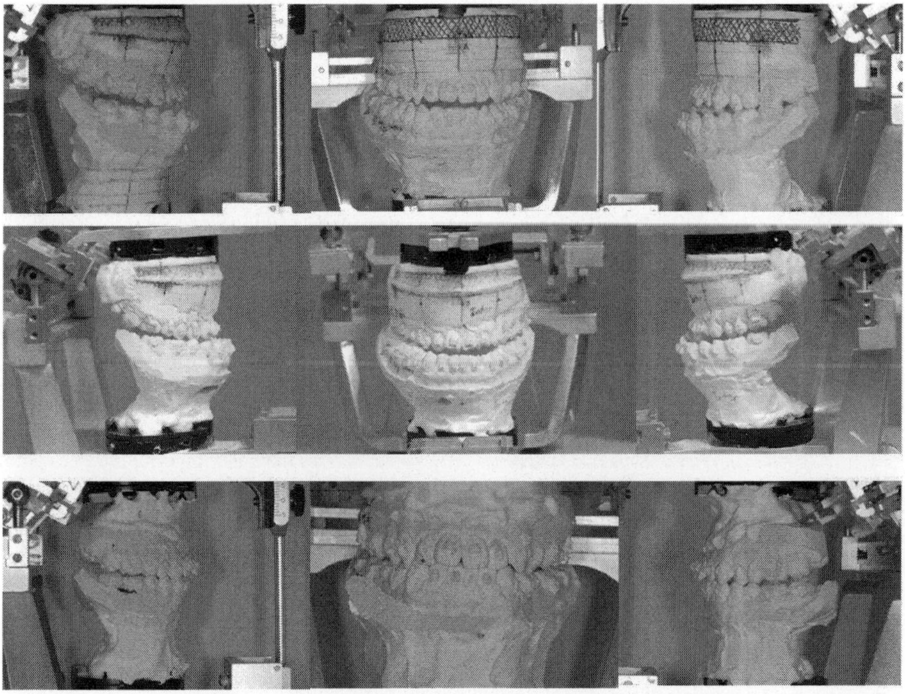

Fig. 10. Progress Records.

The surgery first approach was instead utilized in treating this patient. Brackets were bonded three days prior to surgery and passive arch wires were placed. A two-jaw surgical procedure was performed and orthodontic treatment was started in six weeks. Figure 11 shows the bonding of brackets before surgery followed by progress records of the patient. The bite settled as the teeth were aligned and decompensated. Patient was debonded after finishing and detailing. The total treatment time was eighteen months. Figure 12 shows the final records of the patient at the time the appliances were removed.

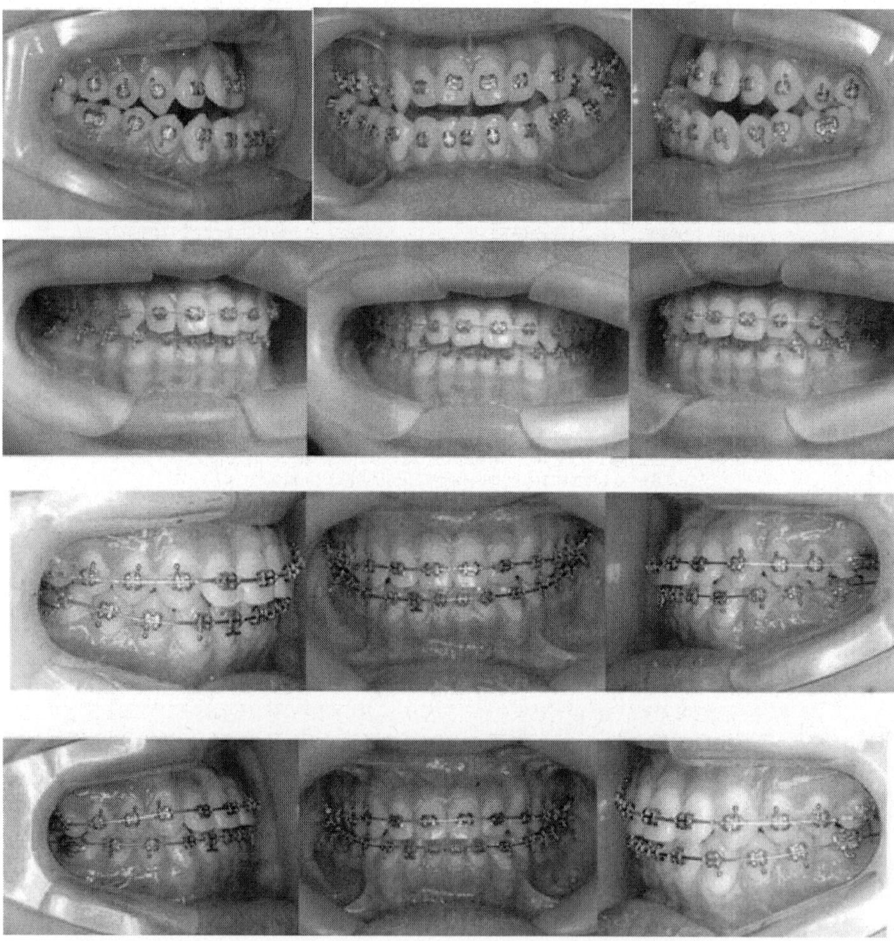

Fig. 11. Progress Records A) Bracket position before placement of passive arch wires, B) 4 months after surgery, C) 9 months after surgery, D) 11 months after surgery.

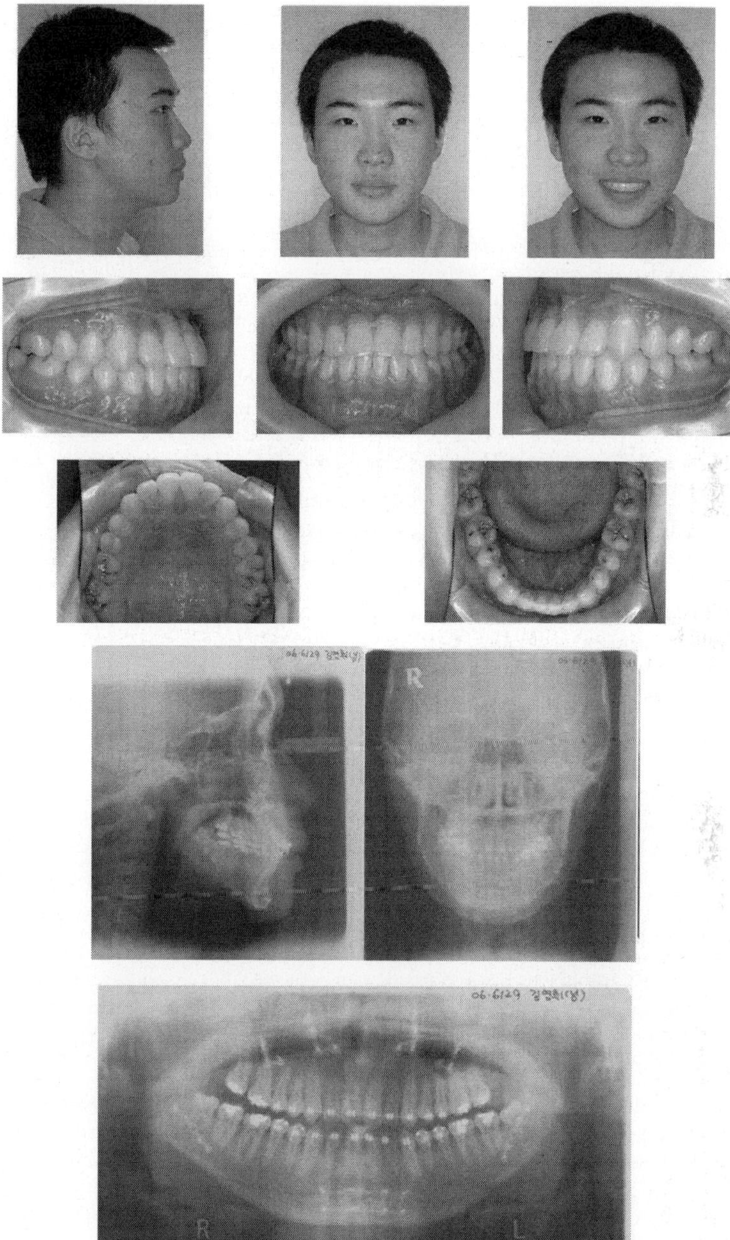

Fig. 12. Final Records

3.2 Regional Acceleratory Phenomenon (RAP)

The regional acceleratory phenomenon (RAP) was well described by Frost in 1993. After an osteotomy, bone remodeling around the healing tissue facilitates the healing process. This regional acceleratory phenomenon can be utilized by the orthodontist following orthognathic surgery to accelerate tooth movement. By performing surgery first, this period of rapid metabolic activity within the tissues can be harvested for efficient orthodontic treatment.

The extent and duration of this window of opportunity becomes an important issue in these cases. In order to answer this question, the by-products of bone metabolism have been measured in patients' blood samples following orthognathic surgery. Alkaline phosphatase and C-terminal telopeptide of type I collagen are two bone markers which have been studied. The former is associated with osteoblastic activity while the latter is a by-product of osteoclastic breakdown of bone. The results of one such study show that orthognathic surgery triggers three to four months of higher osteoclastic activities and metabolic changes in the dentoalveolus (Liou et al., 2011a, 2011b). This short period of regional acceleratory phenomenon is a possible explanation for shortened treatment time in surgery first orthodontics.

The regional acceleratory phenomenon is not exclusive to surgery first approach. In the conventional approach, this phenomenon is seen after decompensation has been accomplished and patient has had the surgical procedure completed. The surgery first approach however, utilizes this golden opportunity to speed up the decompensation process which occurs after the surgery unlike the traditional approach. Since the decompensation of the arches is the most time consuming step of the way, the regional acceleratory phenomenon is used when it is needed the most.

Despite the findings demonstrated as case reports on shortened treatment time, the actual duration of the window of time during which the regional acceleratory phenomenon can be utilized for orthodontic tooth movement is still unknown. Various studies have shown different lengths of accelerated tooth movement. Hence, more studies are required at the time being to give sufficient evidence on the actual molecular basis for the accelerated tooth movement as well as the duration of this phenomenon after surgical procedures.

4. Treatment planning considerations

Careful planning is the key to the success of any orthognathic surgery case especially when the surgical procedure is to be performed prior to orthodontic treatment. As with any orthodontic treatment, obtaining high quality records including intraoral and extra-oral pictures, models, and radiographs is the first step.

Multiple treatment planning considerations must be taken into account when orthognathic surgery is being performed without prior orthodontic treatment. The orthodontist plans the surgery on the pre-operative models in such a way that a relatively stable occlusion can be achieved during surgery. The teeth will be decompensated to normal positions and angulations following surgery; therefore, the transitional occlusion must allow for post surgical movement of teeth. Since the incisors cannot be used as a guide to predict the final occlusion in surgery first cases, the molar relationship can be utilized as a starting point to come up with a temporary occlusion.

The inclination of upper incisors is important in determining the need for possible extractions. If the upper incisor is excessively proclined, extractions may be considered to allow retraction of upper incisors post-operatively. As a rule of thumb, if the upper incisor to occlusal plane angulation is less than 53 to 55 degrees (Liao et al., 2010), extraction must be considered. Another possibility involves changing the position of the whole maxilla so that the occlusal plane is steeper and producing more upright maxillary incisors. Also, one might distalize the maxillary posterior segments using zygomatic plates as shown by Nagasaka et al. (2009) and Villegas et al. (2010) thus opening space to retrocline the maxillary incisors.

When placing upper and lower models into occlusion, the transverse dimension of the arches in many cases does not allow perfect interdigitation. Hence, the transverse dimension often poses a special challenge when performing model surgery in surgery first cases. The midlines must be coincident or close to it after surgery and proper buccal overjet must be established bilaterally. Depending on the degree of discrepancy between the two arches, the orthodontist can resolve this issue by planning for segmental osteotomies in more severe cases or possibly plan on resolving the issue post-surgically by arch coordination and elastics.

The most challenging and time consuming step in preparing for surgery first orthodontics is the prediction of the final occlusion based on the current position of teeth. The experience of the orthodontist plays a very important role in the process. The term intended transitional malocclusion (ITM) is used to describe the occlusion which will be used to fabricate the surgical splint and is the surgeon's guide during surgery (Park et al., 2011). The ITM must be stable enough to allow predictable splint fabrication and skeletal movement. Therefore, at least a three-point contact must be established between the upper and lower models when deciding on the ITM. In cases where such temporary occlusion cannot be established, it is advisable to initiate some orthodontic movement in order to relieve some of the interferences and allow for a more stable transitional malocclusion to be established. In a Class III skeletal malocclusion after surgery, a Class I or II malocclusion with the characteristic dental compensations of a Class III malocclusion is established. The decompensation of the teeth is performed following surgery. The following cases demonstrate the importance of meticulous treatment planning in surgery first orthodontics.

Figure 13 demonstrates the initial records of a 24 year old female patient who presented with chief complaints of a long face, strong chin, and difficulty in pronunciation (lisping sound).

Upon initial examination, the patient had a Class III malocclusion with anterior open bite. The upper second premolars were displaced palatally and the upper right first premolar was restored with an ill-fitting full coverage crown due to lack of sufficient space which compromised the tooth esthetically and periodontally. It was determined that extractions in the maxillary arch will be needed to allow for decompensation of teeth after surgery. Model surgery was performed allowing upper second premolar extraction during surgery. The concept behind extraction of upper second premolars can be explained in terms of conventional decompensation procedure as well. If the case was being treated with orthodontic decompensation of teeth prior to surgery, one way to achieve sufficient negative overjet would have been to extract the upper premolars to allow retraction and retroclination of upper incisors. In surgery first approach, extracting the premolars during surgery provides for the space needed to decrease the overjet and retract the incisors after surgery. Careful planning and precise surgical delivery is of utmost importance in such cases due to the added complexity of simultaneous extractions. Figure 14 shows the model surgery and set-up of the case during surgical planning.

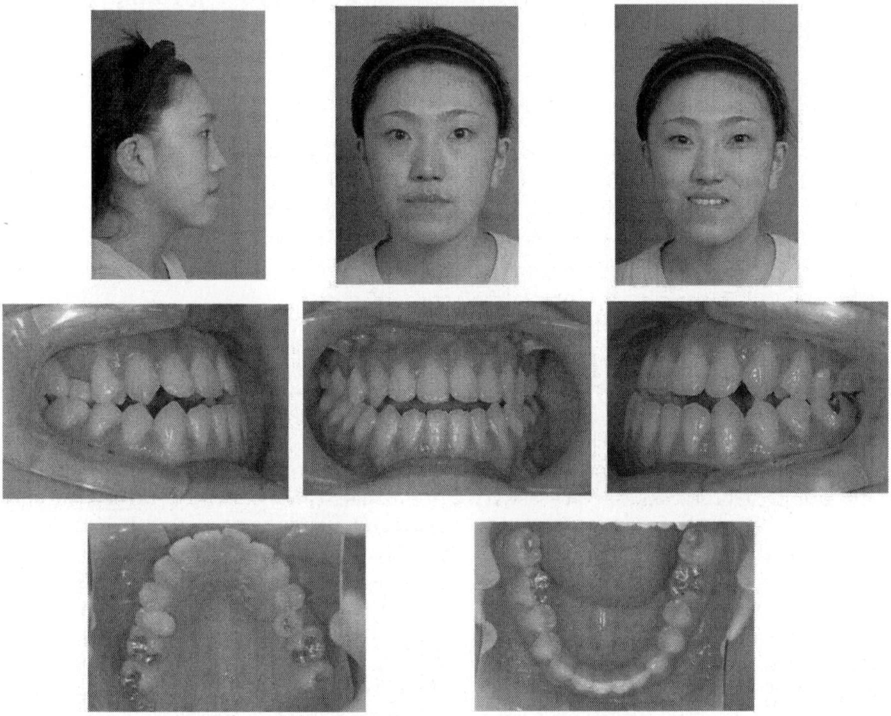

Fig. 13. Initial Records.

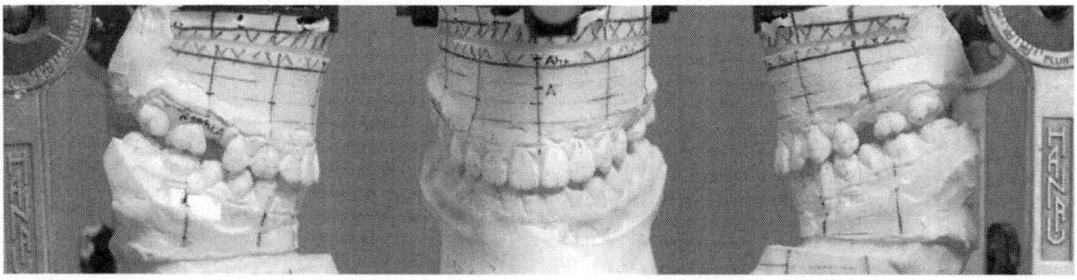

Fig. 14. Model Surgery.

The indirect bonding technique was used in this case which allowed the bending of stainless steel passive arch-wires on the models. The bonding of brackets, placement of the wire, and splint try-in were done at the same visit a few days prior to surgery. Orthodontic movement was initiated 7 weeks after the surgical procedure was completed (Figure 15).

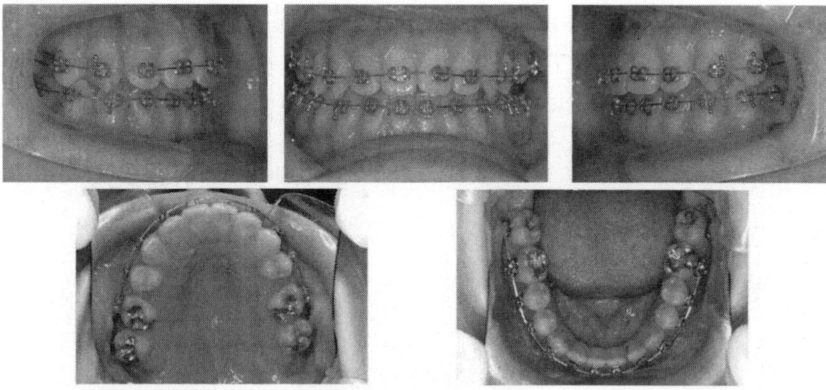

Fig. 15. Initiation of orthodontic movement.

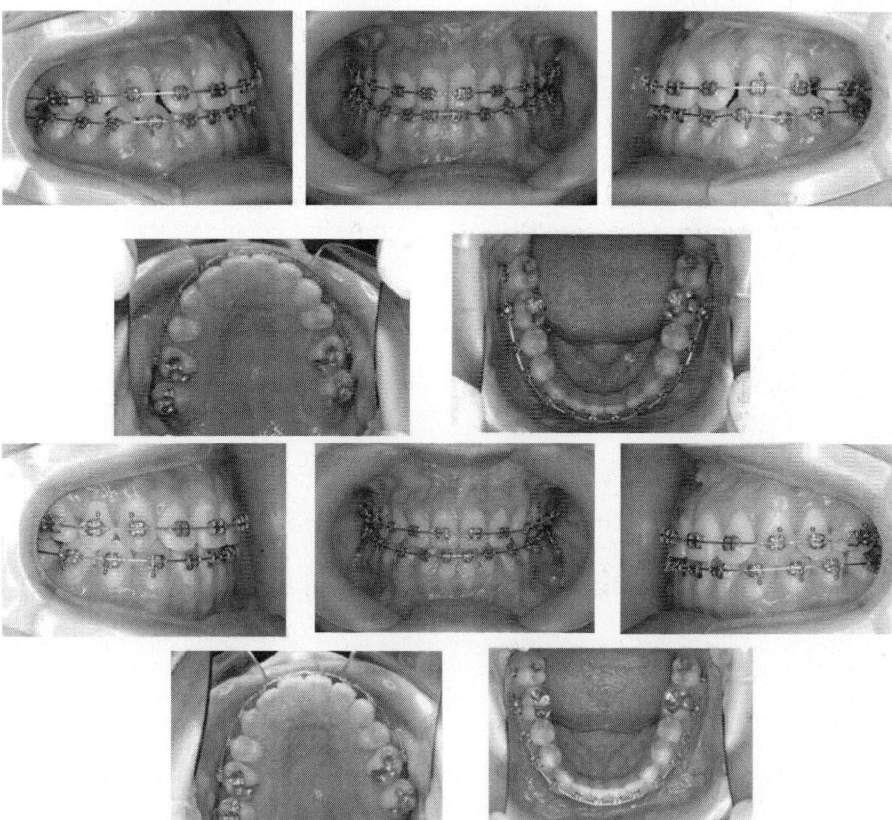

Fig. 16. Orthodontic Treatment in Progress A) 5 months B) 13 months into treatment.

Case was debonded after 16 months of active orthodontics. Figure 17 shows the final records with good occlusion and esthetics.

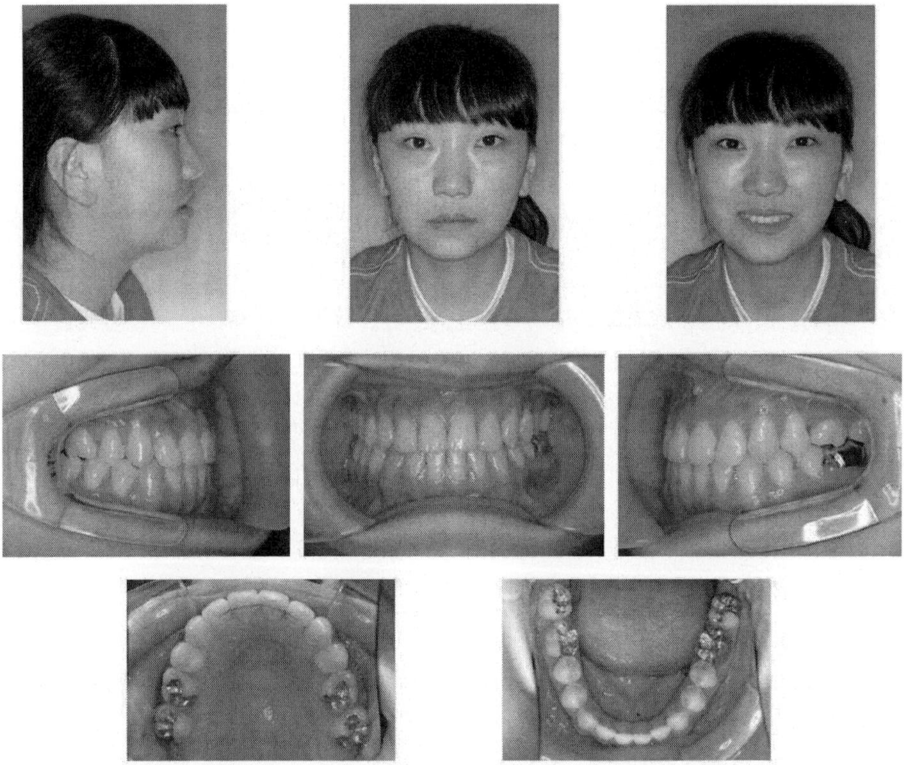

Fig. 17. Final Records.

The results of this particular case were stable over a two year retention period. Figure 18 shows the intraoral images at two years after removal of the orthodontic appliances.

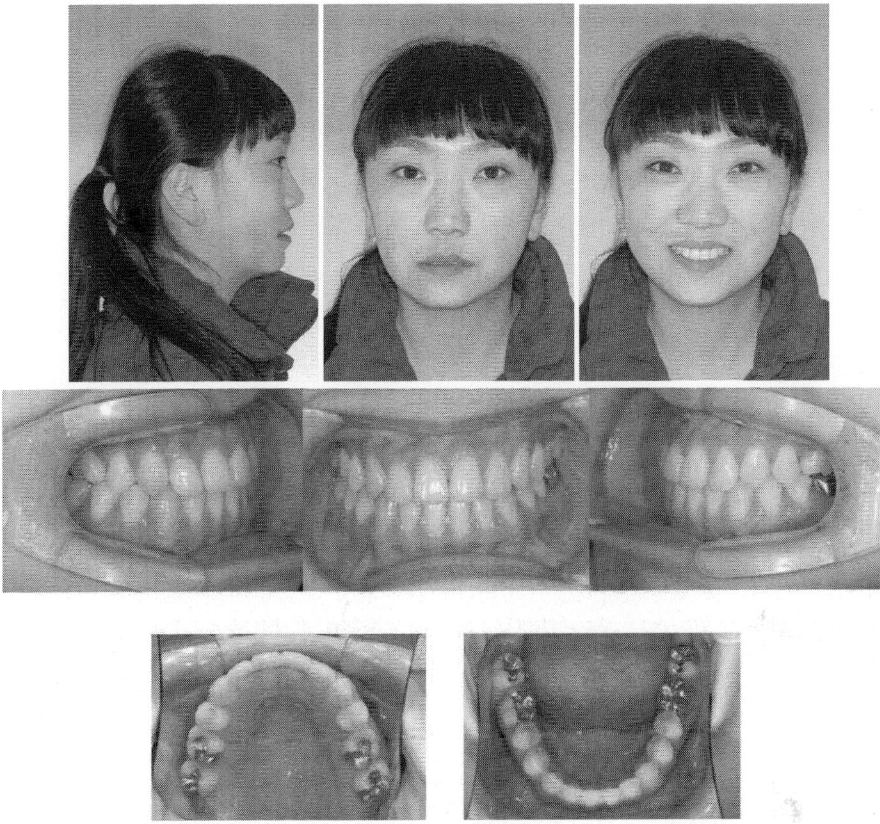

Fig. 18. Retention after two years.

4.1 Protocol variations

While the sequence of treatment is similar, different protocols are being used to prepare the patient for surgery, perform the surgical procedure, and initiate orthodontic treatment. Orthodontists often have their own customized preferences which have developed in their years of practice.

In most cases, the brackets and the wires are placed right before surgery. While some clinicians prefer to bond the wire directly to the surface of teeth, others choose to utilize the conventional orthodontic attachments. Although bonding the wire directly to the teeth is very fast, it makes post-surgical orthodontics a problem since teeth need to be bonded at that point. Given the healing period after surgery, it is very difficult to place brackets on teeth while minimizing patient discomfort.

Different types of wires are being used by orthodontists across the globe prior to surgery. Contrary to conventional orthognathic surgery cases, in surgery first treatments leveling and aligning have not yet been performed which makes it very difficult to place the wire.

Some orthodontists prefer to place a passive stainless steel wire which has been bent and adapted to each tooth to prevent any tooth movement. The first author's preference is to use 0.022 slot brackets as well as passive stainless steel wires of 0.017 inch x 0.025 inch dimensions. Other orthodontists who use the surgery first approach have opted to use nickel-titanium wires at time of surgery. Finally, a few orthodontists prefer not to place any wires at the time of surgery.

The use of nickel-titanium wires translates into immediate tooth movement after surgery which can be an advantage. However, in doing so, the orthodontist loses the opportunity to observe the stability of the surgical correction prior to starting the tooth movement. The rapid acceleratory phenomenon not only affects the tooth movement but also can affect the alveolar bone. Hence, it is the first author's preference not to use these wires or elastics immediately after surgery to prevent unwanted movement of the alveolar process and rather wait for about 4 to 6 weeks after surgery.

The use of surgical splint during and after surgery also varies between different orthodontists. While some advocate the use of the splint only during surgery, other groups have advocated its use anywhere between one to four weeks after surgery. Nagasaka et al. have used removable Gelb-type splints post operatively (Nagasaka et al., 2009). The first author's preference is to leave the splint in for about 4 to 6 weeks after surgery and if an open bite is observed, to use elastic between the splint and the mini-screws or to leave the splint for a longer period of time. The use of mini-screws will further be discussed in the following section. Also, during the post-surgical period, the first author tries to avoid vertical elastics and allows the bite to settle as the dental compensations resolve. Table 1 summarizes the first author's protocol in comparison to other existing protocols.

First Author's Protocol	Other Protocol Variations
.022 bracket slots	0.018 brackets No brackets (wires bonded directly to teeth)
0.017 x 0.025 stainless steel passive wires prior to surgery	Nickel titanium wires No wires
Heavy intermaxillary elastics full time for 2-3 weeks, then check if teeth go into splint smoothly without elastics Release splint from maxilla but patient continues to use splint and simple elastics	No use of splints after surgery (splints only used during surgery) Use of splint 4 weeks after surgery
If mandible is stable, at 5-7 weeks start moving teeth with NiTi or copper NiTi	Start moving teeth soon after surgery (less than 1 month)

Table 1. Comparison of first author's protocol with other protocol variations.

4.2 Use of skeletal anchorage in conjunction with surgery first approach

In recent years, temporary anchorage devices have become very popular in orthodontics. The use of skeletal anchorage has provided for more predictable orthodontic movements while minimizing the undesirable side effects. Some authors have placed great emphasis on the use of mini plates and mini screws to control the inclination of the upper incisors and to prevent the relapse of an anterior crossbite in Class III cases (Liao et al., 2010).

The surgery first approach requires meticulous treatment planning and collaboration between the orthodontist and the orthognathic surgeon. The model surgery is based on the orthodontist's vision on what is achievable post orthodontically based on previous experience. Hence, many uncertainties remain at the time the patient is sent to surgery. By utilizing the temporary anchorage devices, many orthodontists try to have a "back-up" system which can be used to help in post-surgical orthodontic phase. These devices are anywhere from single mini-implants to titanium plates which can be placed at the time of surgery.

Nagasaka et al. have advocated the use of zygomatic plates as temporary anchorage devices to aid in post-operative orthodontic movement (Nagasaka et al., 2009). In one case report, a Class III surgery first case was corrected surgically to a Class I skeletal relationship with a Class II dental tendency. Since the teeth were not decompensated prior to surgery, after the surgery the occlusion was expected to exhibit excessive overjet. During orthognathic surgery zygomatic plates were placed. The plates were then used to distalize the upper arch post-operatively to achieve Class I canines and ideal overjet (Nagasaka et al., 2009).

Figure 19 shows the initial presentation of a female patient. The skeletal Class III pattern was accompanied by open bite and mild crowding in both arches. the upper incisors had previously been restored with full coverage crowns.

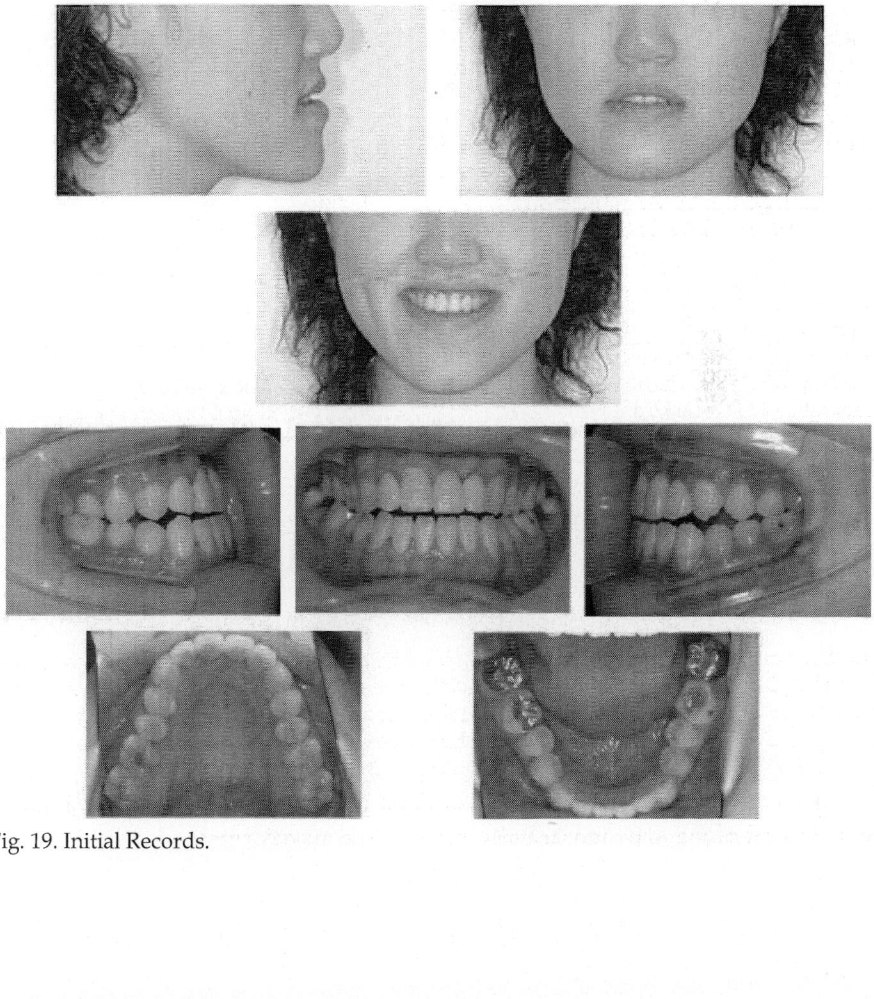

Fig. 19. Initial Records.

After careful treatment planning, model surgery was performed to predict the final position of teeth and fabricate the splint. Prior to surgery, teeth were bonded and stainless steel arch wires were passively engaged (Figure 20). Patient underwent a two-jaw surgical procedure and at the time of surgery four mini-implants were placed mesial to upper and lower canines. The mini-implants were used after surgery to settle the bite with elastics. Figure 21 shows the progress of the case and the use of temporary anchorage devices in settling the bite.

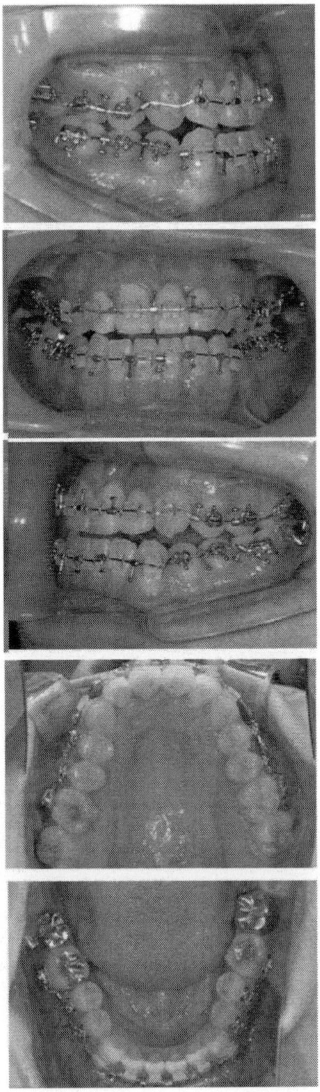

Fig. 20. Placement of passive stainless steel wires prior to surgery.

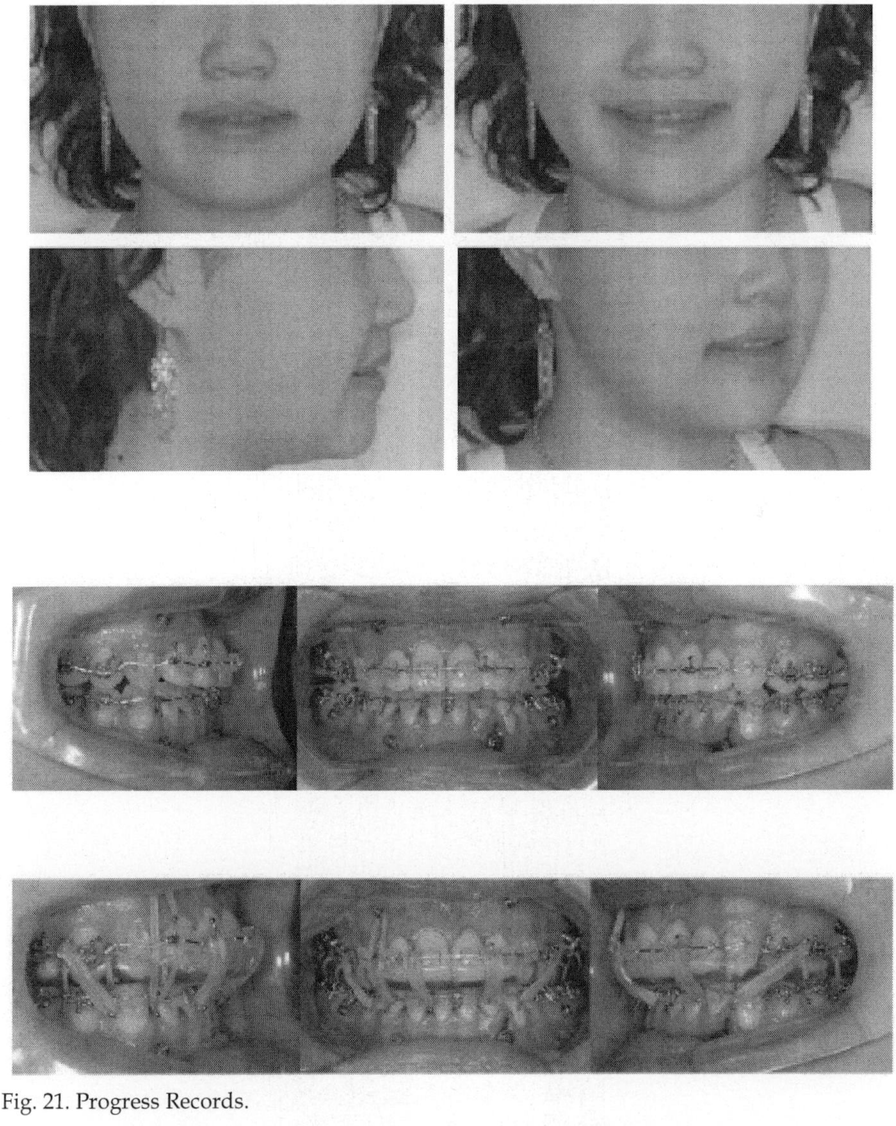

Fig. 21. Progress Records.

Case was finished in nineteen months with acceptable occlusion and facial aesthetics achieved. Figure 22 shows the final records.

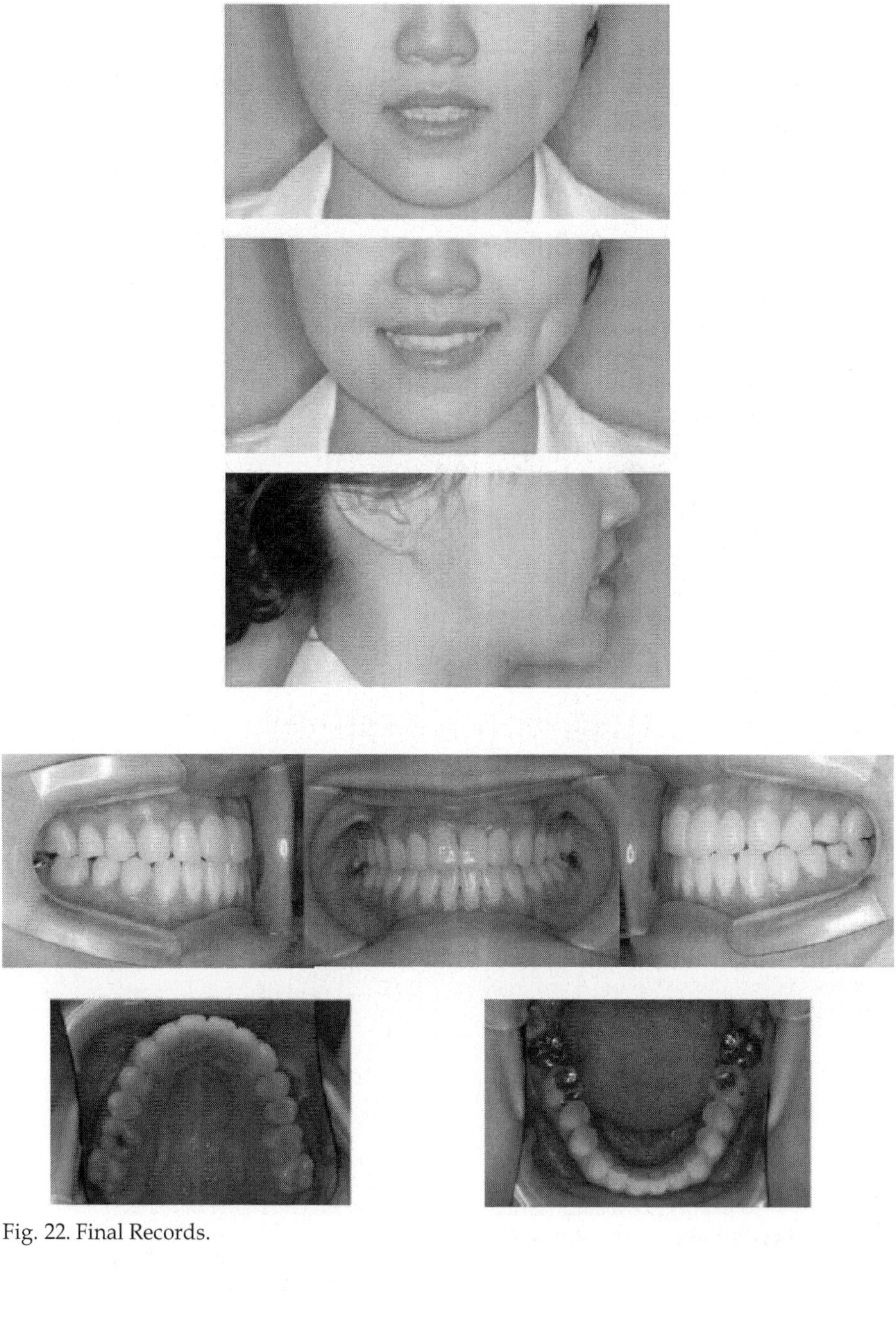

Fig. 22. Final Records.

The use of temporary anchorage devices becomes more crucial in more complicated cases that are attempted with the surgery first approach. When extractions or segmented osteotomies are planned, prediction of the final occlusion is far more challenging and placement of mini-implants during the surgery allows for efficient mechanics post- surgically. Figure 23 shows the initial presentation of a female patient who was treatment planned for three-piece maxillary osteotomy and mandibular set-back procedures due to a severe transverse discrepancy between the upper and lower jaws and excessive proclination of upper incisors.

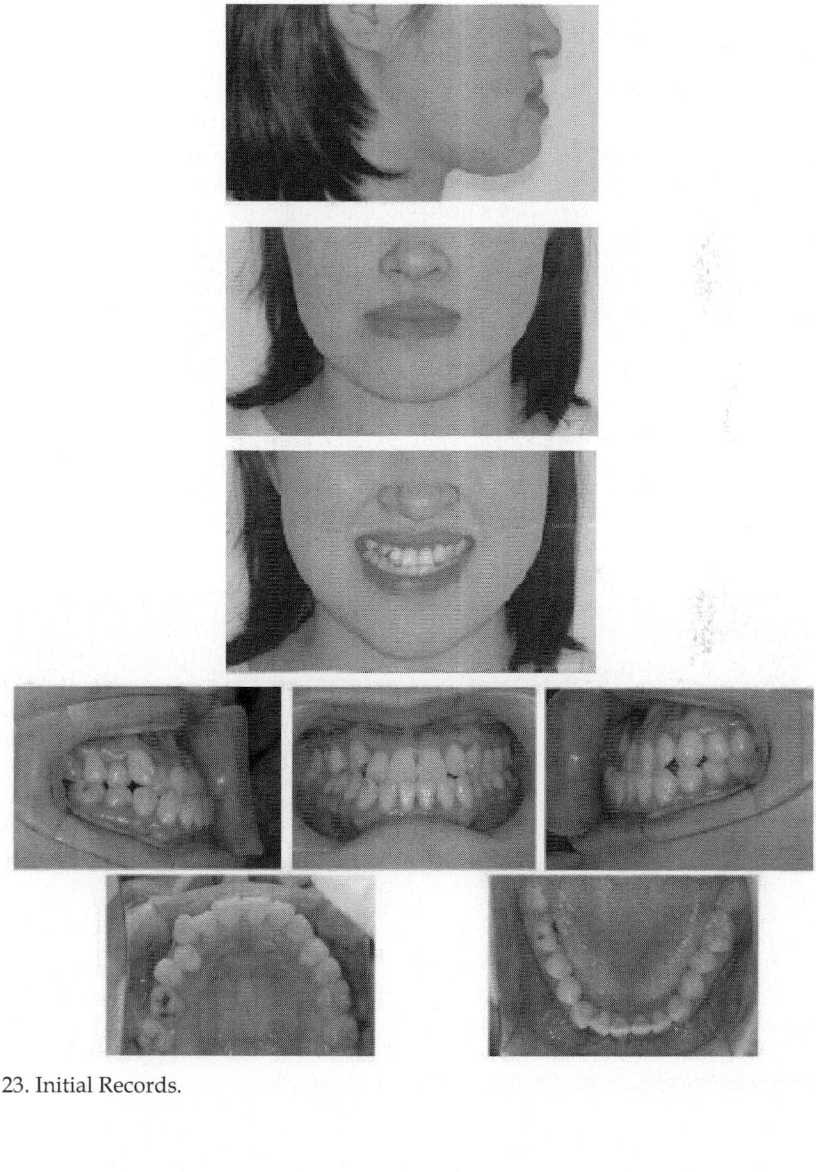

Fig. 23. Initial Records.

Upper first premolars were extracted during the surgical procedure and at the same time eight mini-implants were placed. Figure 24 shows the progress of the case immediately after surgery and in weeks that followed.

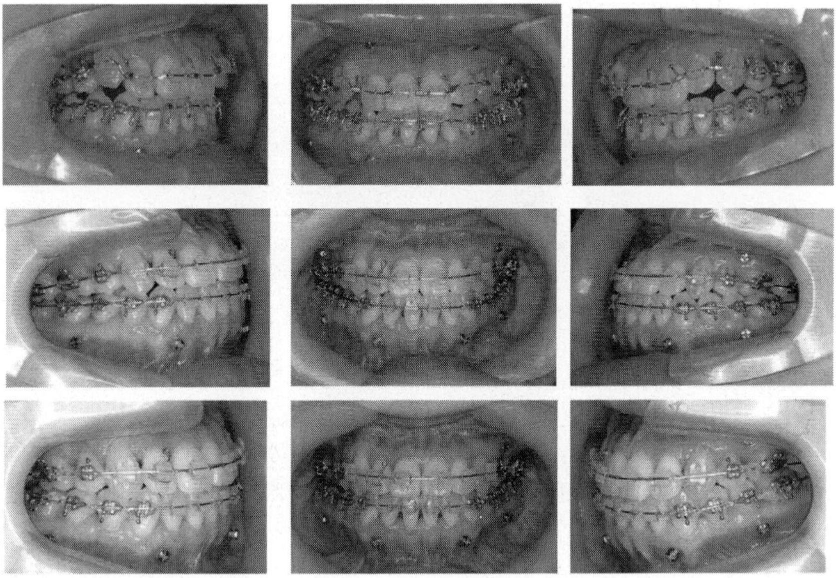

Fig. 24. Progress Records.

The case was finished in nineteen months and the patient was very pleased with the results. Figure 25 illustrates the final records of the patient at the time of appliance removal. Considering the complexity of the case, the treatment time was significantly reduced. However, the upper left canine showed discoloration as treatment continued possibly indicating necrosis as a result of the segmental osteotomy procedure.

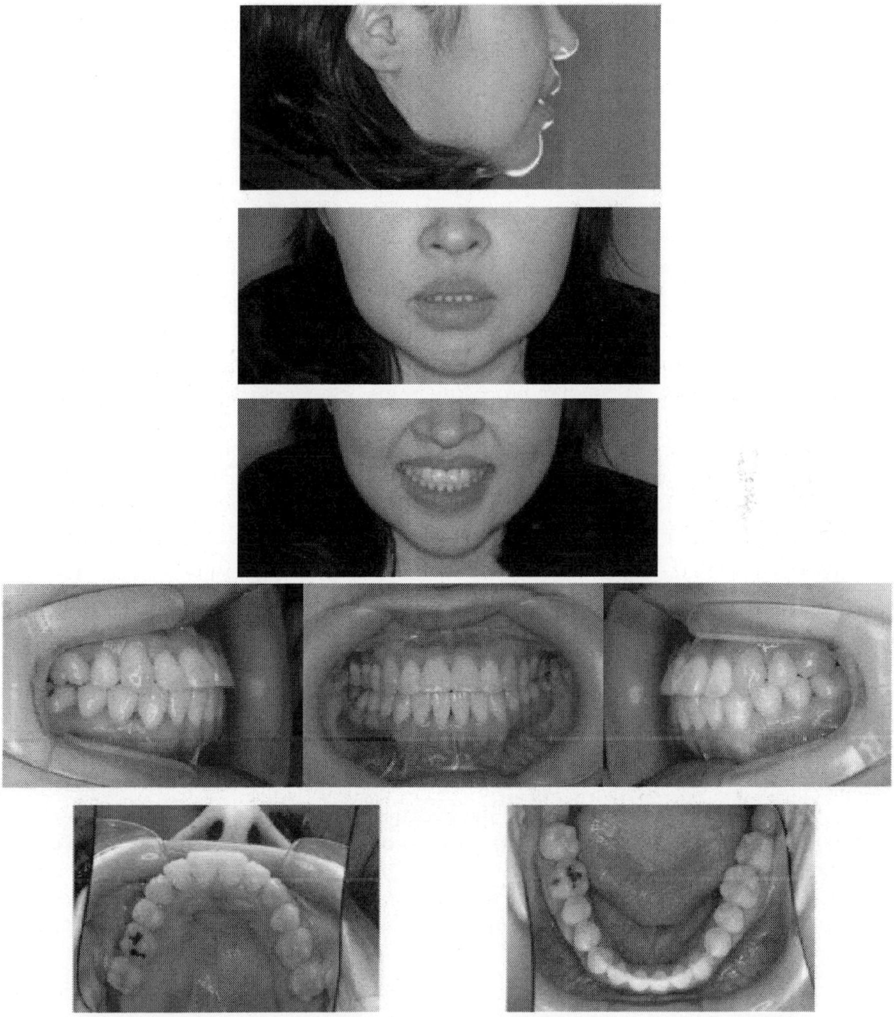

Fig. 25. Final Records.

5. Disadvantages and potential problems

Performing the surgical procedure prior to orthodontic treatment has multiple advantages, particularly the shortened treatment time. However, there are many drawbacks to this approach which should be taken into consideration.

Predicting the final occlusion is the hardest challenge with surgery first approach. In many cases, the upper and lower models cannot be placed in an ideal occlusion due to multiple dental interferences. If the predicted final occlusion is not achievable or is not planned accurately, the result will be far from ideal. Cases requiring extractions are especially very difficult to plan when performing surgery first. Thus, case selection is of utmost importance.

Even when the final occlusion has been determined carefully by the orthodontist, the surgical procedure must be performed meticulously since any minor surgical error can compromise the result. Hence, the treating orthodontist and orthognathic surgeon must be experienced enough to be able to know the limitations and possibilities.

The planning process is very time consuming in contrast to the total treatment time which is usually shortened. This becomes a financial issue for the treating orthodontist in many cases. Increasing the treatment fee is one solution but it should be reasonable to the patient.

When passive stainless steel wires are placed prior to surgery each wire must be bent to rest passively on the surface of each tooth. This is also another challenging and time consuming procedure for the orthodontist especially when teeth are severely rotated and misaligned. To simplify the pre-surgical bonding procedure, some orthodontists bond the wires directly to the surface of teeth without using any brackets. Even though this can simplify the pre-surgical appointment, the authors note that there is a higher failure rate during surgery and the need for another bonding appointment at the initiation of orthodontic treatment. Indirect bonding technique can be utilized to allow for accurate bracket positioning as well as bending the passive arch wires beforehand.

To utilize the maximum potential of the regional acceleratory phenomenon, two jaw surgeries are preferred. Also, severe transverse discrepancies sometimes lead to two-piece or three-piece Le Fort I osteotomies. The increase in the number and complexity of osteotomy procedures poses a greater risk to the patient.

6. A look into the future of "Surgery First" approach

Despite the many challenges associated with performing the orthognathic surgery prior to decompensation of the arches, the basics of this approach can be incorporated into treatment planning other surgical cases to reduce the pre-surgical treatment time. Careful treatment planning and prioritizing the steps that are absolutely necessary prior to the surgical procedure while leaving other steps until the surgery is performed can speed up the process. In doing so, the patient will be able to have the surgery sooner than the traditional approach and the orthodontist will be able to use the rapid acceleratory phenomenon when it is needed the most.

Figure 26 shows the initial presentation of a patient who presented with severe skeletal Class III malocclusion and anterior open bite. The upper incisors were proclined and the lower incisors were severely retroclined. The lower right lateral incisor was lingually blocked out and the lower arch was constricted with lingually tipped teeth.

The complexity of the case called for starting the orthodontic treatment before performing surgery. However, during the treatment planning process the emphasis was placed on doing minimal orthodontic preparation for surgery to reduce the time spent in pre-surgical orthodontics. The decompensation process in this case would have otherwise taken a very long time if the conventional approach was utilized.

One month after placement of brackets on the upper arch, a lower Schwartz expansion appliance was used to expand the lower arch and upright the lower posterior segments. The expansion screw was activated two times per week. Figure 27 shows the progress of the case at 1 month, 2 months, and 6 months after the initiation of orthodontic treatment.

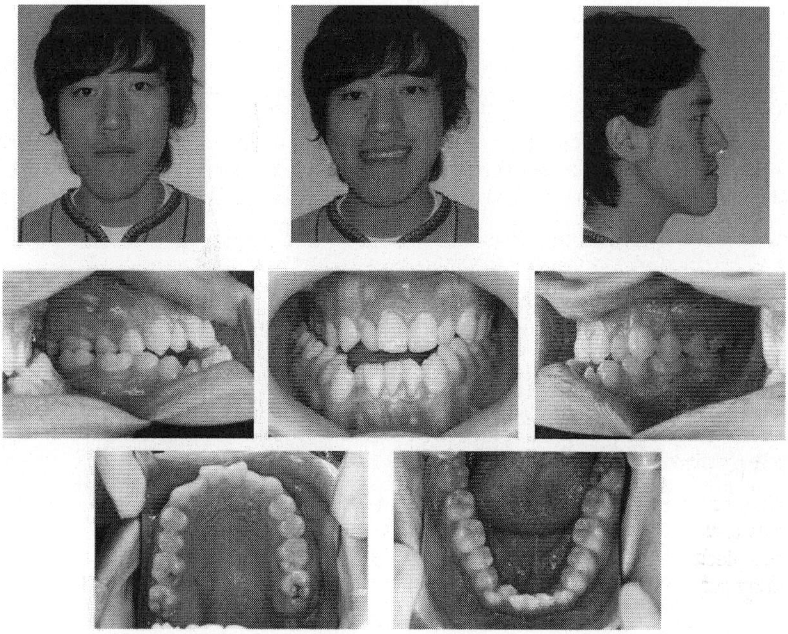

Fig. 26. Initial Records.

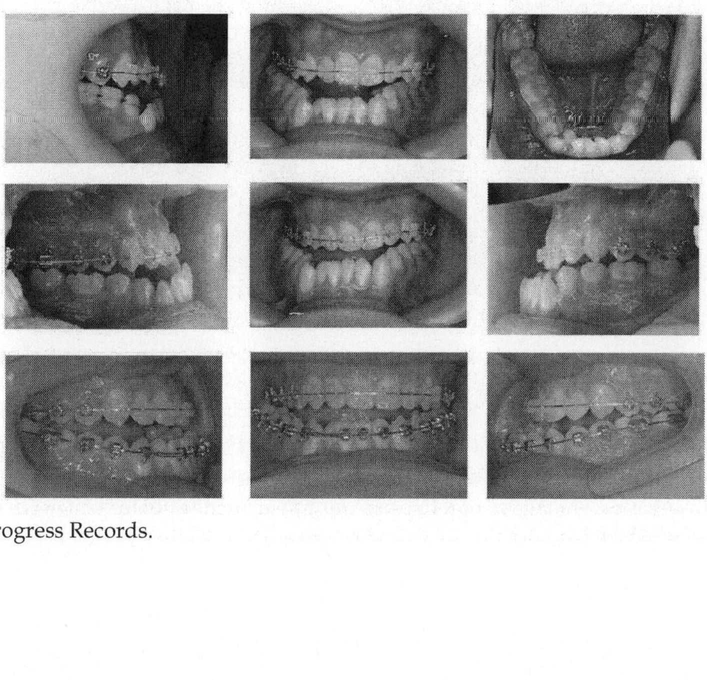

Fig. 27. Progress Records.

The upper right second molar required a significant amount of buccal root torque in preparation of surgery. A temporary anchorage device was placed palatally between the upper right first and second molars and a power chain was used from the screw to achieve ideal torque. After eight months of orthodontic preparation, the case was ready for orthognathic surgery. Note that the alignment of the arches was not complete but the model surgery performed at this point indicated that the surgical procedure could be performed and the remainder of orthodontic tooth movements could be finished after surgery utilizing the regional acceleratory phenomenon. Figure 28 shows the model surgery and the intraoral pictures at the time of placement of passive archwires for surgery.

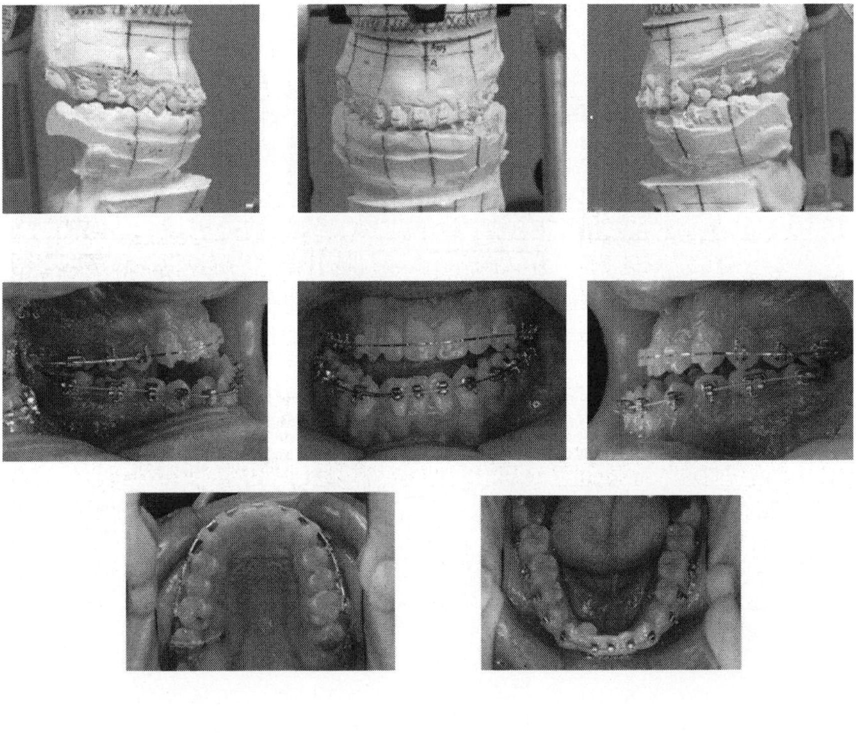

Fig. 28. Model surgery and records right before surgery.

After the operation was performed, the leveling, alignment, and the decompensation were completed in one year. Figure 29 shows the progress of the case immediately after, one month, four months, and twelve months after surgery. Note the use of temporary anchorage devices post-surgically.

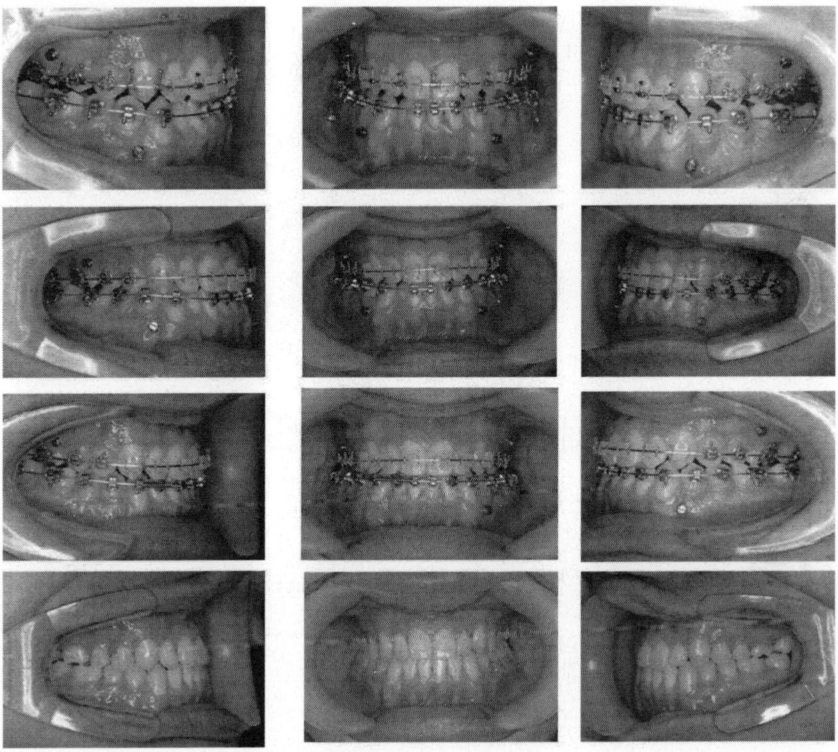

Fig. 29. Progress records A) immediately after, B) one month C) four months D) twelve months after surgery.

The case was debonded after a total treatment time of 22 months which included 8 months of presurgical orthodontics. Figure 30 shows the final records of the patient at the time of appliance removal.

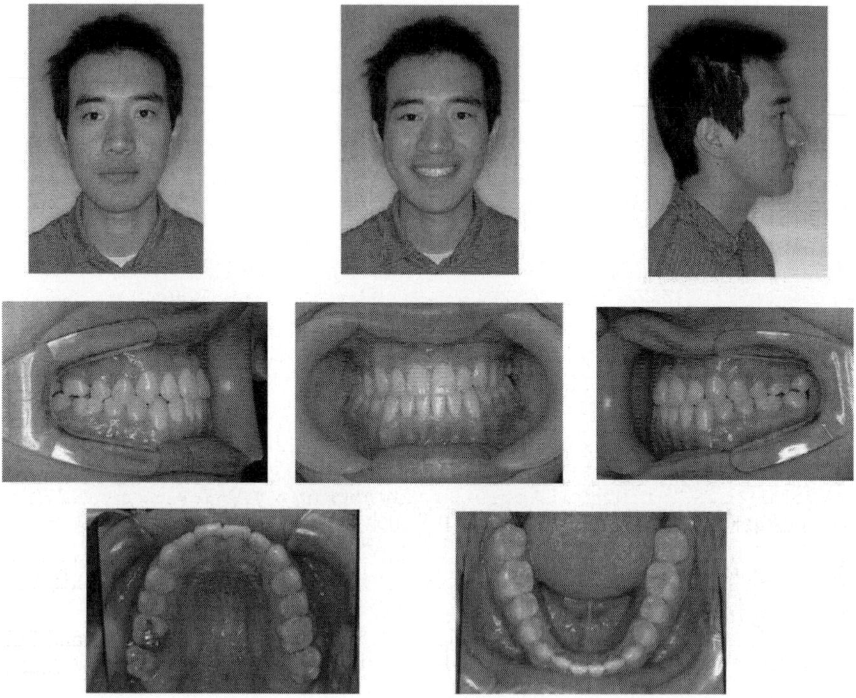

Fig. 30. Final Records.

This case illustrates that the surgery first approach concepts can be modified to fit the specific needs of the patient. The main principle to keep in mind is not to spend countless months to achieve the absolute ideal presurgical decompensation and leveling. The surgical procedure should be performed as soon as the occlusion allows for a stable post-surgical transitional occlusion. Once again, the experience of the orthodontist and the surgeon are extremely important in treating these cases.

7. Conclusion

Performing orthognathic surgery before orthodontic treatment has multiple advantages including but not limited to shortened treatment time, increased patient acceptance, and the utilization of the regional acceleratory phenomenon. If the cases are selected carefully, the orthodontist and the surgeon are experienced enough to predict the final occlusion beforehand, and the level of cooperation between the clinicians is high, the results are very promising. However, even the slightest error during the treatment planning, surgical, and post-surgical orthodontic steps can be very difficult to correct. By utilizing the principles of surgery first technique, the pre-surgical orthodontics period can be shortened even if it is not eliminated. As with any other surgical procedure, the patient's well-being and chief complaint should always be the first priority. The future of orthognathic surgery is geared toward minimizing the overall treatment time without compromising the final results.

8. Acknowledgments

Jeong Kim thanks Dr. Sang H. Park for his collaboration and Dr. Barry Grayson for guidance.

9. References

Aziz, S.R. (2004). Simon P. Hullihen and the Origin of Orthognathic Surgery. *Journal of Oral and Maxillofacial Surgery*, Vol.62, No.10, (October, 2004), pp. 1303-1307, ISSN 0278-2391

Baek, S.H.; Ahn, H.W.; Kwon, Y.H. & Choi, J.Y. (2010). Surgery First Approach in Skeletal Class III Malocclusion Treated with 2-Jaw Surgery: Evaluation of Surgical Movement and Postoperative Orthodontic Treatment. *Journal of Craniofacial Surgery*, Vol.21, No.3, (March, 2010), pp. 332-338, ISSN 1049-2275

Brachvogel, P.; Berten, J.L. & Hausamen, J.E. (1991). Surgery before orthodontic treatment: a concept for timing the combined therapy of skeletal dysgnathias. *Deutsche Zahn-, Mund-, und Kieferheilkunde mit Zentralblatt*, Vol.79, No.7, (July, 1991), pp. 557-563, ISSN 0940-855X

Frost, H.M. (1983). The Regional Acceleratory Phenomenon: a Review. *Henry Ford Hospital Medical Journal*, Vol.31, No.1, (January, 1983), pp. 3-9, ISSN 0018-0416

Iliopoulos, C.; Zouloumis, L. & Lazaridou, M. (2010). Physiology of Bone Turnover and Its Application in Contemporary Maxillofacial Surgery. A review, *Hippokratia*, Vol.14, No.4, (October-December, 2010), pp. 244–248, ISSN 1108-4189

Justus, T.; Chang, B.I.; Bloomquist, D. & Ramsay D.S. (2001). Human Gingival and Pulpal Blood Flow During Healing After Le Fort I Osteotomy. *Journal of Oral and Maxillofacial Surgery* Vol. 59, No.1, (January, 2001), pp. 2-7, ISSN 0278-2391

Ko, E.W.; Hsu, S.S.; Hsieh, H.Y.; Wang, Y.C.; Huang, C.S. & Chen YR. (2011). Comparison of Progressive Cephalometric Changes and Postsurgical Stability of Skeletal Class III Correction With and Without Presurgical Orthodontic Treatment, *Journal of Oral and Maxillofacial Surgery*, Vol.69, No.5, (May, 2011), pp. 1469-1477, ISSN 0278-2391

Kondo E. & Aoba, T.J. (2000). Nonsurgical and Nonextraction Treatment of Skeletal Class III Open Bite: Its Long-Term Stability. *American Journal of Orthodontics and Dentofacial Orthopedics*, Vol.117, No.3, (March, 2000), pp. 267-287, ISSN 0889-5406

Kondo E. & Arai, S. (2005). Nonsurgical and Nonextraction Treatment of a Skeletal Class III Adult Patient with Severe Prognathic Mandible. *World Journal of Orthodontics*, Vol.6, No.3, (Fall, 2005), pp. 233-247, ISSN 2160-2999

Lee, R.T. (1994). The Benefits of Post-Surgical Orthodontic Treatment. *British Journal of Orthodontics*, Vol.21, No.3, (August, 1994), pp. 265-274, ISSN 0301-228X

Liao, Y.F.; Chiu, Y.T.; Huang, C.S.; Ko, E.W. & Chen, Y.R. (2010). Presurgical Orthodontics Versus No Presurgical Orthodontics: Treatment Outcome of Surgical Orthodontic Correction For Skeletal Class III Open Bite, *Plastic and Reconstructive Surgery*, Vol.126, No.6, (December 2010), pp. 2074-2083, ISSN 0032-1052

Liou, E.J.; Chen, P.H.; Wang, Y.C.; Yu, C.C.; Huang, C.S. & Chen, Y.R. (2011). Surgery-First Accelerated Orthognathic Surgery: Orthodontic Guidelines and Setup For Model Surgery, *Journal of Oral and Maxillofacial Surgery*, Vol.69, No.3, (March, 2011), pp. 771-780, ISSN 0278-2391

Liou, E.J.; Chen, P.H.; Wang, Y.C.; Yu, C.C.; Huang, C.S. & Chen, Y.R. (2011). Surgery-First Accelerated Orthognathic Surgery: Postoperative Rapid Orthodontic Tooth Movement, *Journal of Oral and Maxillofacial Surgery*, Vol.69, No.3, (March, 2011), pp. 781-785, ISSN 0278-2391

Luther, F.; Morris, D.O. & Hart, C. (2003). Orthodontic Preparation for Orthognathic Surgery: How Long Does It Take and Why? A Retrospective Study. *British Journal of Oral and Maxillofacial Surgery*, Vol.41, No.6, (December, 2003), pp. 401-406, ISSN 0266-4356

Nagasaka, H.; Sugawara, J.; Kawamura, H. & Nanda, R. (2009). "Surgery First" Skeletal Class III Correction Using the Skeletal Anchorage System. *Journal of Clinical Orthodontics*, Vol.43, No.2, (February, 2009), pp. 97-105, ISSN 0022-3875

O'Brien, K.; Wright, J.; Conboy, F.; Appelbe, P.; Bearn, D.; Caldwell, S.; Harrison, J.; Hussain, J.; Lewis, D.; Littlewood, S.; Mandall, N.; Morris, T.; Murray, A.; Oskouei, M.; Rudge, S.; Sandler, J.; Thiruvenkatachari, B.; Walsh, T. & Turbill, E. (2009). Prospective, Multi-Center Study of the Effectiveness of Orthodontic/Orthognathic Surgery Care in the United Kingdom, *American Journal of Orthodontics and Dentofacial Orthopedics*, Vol.135, No.6, (June, 2009), pp. 709-714, ISSN 0889-5406

Park, S.; Hyon, W.L.; Lee, J.G.; Lee, S.; Lee, Y. & Shin, S. (2011). Increasing Efficiency and Improving Patient Compliance/Affordability/Orthognathic Surgery With Surgery First Orthognathic Approach (SFOA) . Abstract from *Proceedings of the 3rd William H. Bell Lectureship Symposium*, "Accelerated Orthognathic Surgery and Increased Orthodontic Efficiency," March 18-20, 2011, Houston, Texas

Sugawara, J.; Aymach, Z.; Nagasaka, D.H.; Kawamura, H. & Nanda, R. (2010). "Surgery First" Orthognathics to Correct a Skeletal Class II Malocclusion with an Impinging Bite. *Journal of Clinical Orthodontics*, Vol.44, No.7, (July, 2010), pp. 429-438, ISSN 0022-3875

Tsuroda, H. & Miyamoto, Y. (2003). None or Minimum Pre-operative Orthodontic Treatment for Orthognathic Surgery in Answer to Patient's Request of Immediate Facial Aspect Change. *Journal of Japan Society of Aesthetic Plastic Surgery*, Vol.25, No.2, (February, 2003), pp. 79-86, ISSN 0288-2027

Villegas, C.; Uribe, F.; Sugawara, J. & Nanda, R. (2010). Expedited Correction of Significant Dentofacial Asymmetry Using a "Surgery First" Approach. *Journal of Clinical Orthodontics*, Vol.44, No.2, (February, 2010), pp. 97-103, ISSN 0022-3875

Wilcko, W.M.; Wilcko, T.; Bouquot, J.E. & Ferguson, D.J. (2001) Rapid Orthodontics With Alveolar Reshaping: Two Case Reports of Decrowding. *International Journal of Periodontics & Restorative Dentistry*, Vol.21, No.1, (February, 2001), pp. 9-19, ISSN 0198-7569

Wilcko, M.T.; Wilcko, W.M.; Pulver, J.J.; Bissada, N.F. & Bouquot, J.E. (2009) Accelerated Osteogenic Orthodontics Technique: a 1-Stage Surgically Facilitated Rapid Orthodontic Technique With Alveolar Augmentation. *Journal of Oral Maxillofacial Surgery*, Vol.67, No.10, (October, 2009), pp.2149-2159, ISSN 0278-2391

Yu, C.C.; Chen, P.H.; Liou, E.J.; Huang, C.S. & Chen, Y.R. (2010). A Surgery-First Approach in Surgical-Orthodontic Treatment of Mandibular Prognathism – A Case Report, *Chang Gung Medical Journal*, Vol.33, No.6, (November-December, 2010), pp. 699-705, ISSN 2072-0939

13

Spectrum of Factors Affecting Dental Arch Relationships in Japanese Unilateral Cleft Lip and Palate Patients

Mohammad Khursheed Alam[1,*], Takashi S. Kajii[2] and Junichiro Iida[2]
[1]*Orthodontic Unit, School of Dental Sciences, Health Campus, Universiti Sains Malaysia, Kelantan,*
[2]*Department of Oral Functional Science, Section of Orthodontics, Hokkaido University, Graduate School of Dental Medicine,*
[1]*Malaysia*
[2]*Japan*

1. Introduction

Cleft lip and palate care involves multidisciplinary management of affected anatomical structures and functions. These include speech, hearing, and social integration. Maxillary growth retardation and high incidence of Class III malocclusion are the major problems in patients with cleft lip and palate (Ross and Johnston, 1972; Ross, 1987c; Mars and Houston, 1990; Mars et al., 1992; Ishikawa et al., 2002). Orthodontic anomalies such as crowding, rotation and malposition of the teeth are also common in cleft lip and palate patients. In children with cleft lip and palate, abnormalities in number, size, shape and timing of tooth formation are more frequent than in the general population (Ranta R, 1986). The development of methods to detect levels of treatment outcomes is necessary if surgeons are to have a sound basis on which they can justify modifications of their timing or techniques (Atack et al., 1997) Dental arch relationships are important parameters for facial growth and are thus an important indicator for the quality of cleft treatment outcome (Hathorn et al., 1996). This Cleft lip and palate is a congenital anomaly. The etiology has been thought to be multifactorial in nature with genetic and environmental factors contributing to its presence (Berkowitz, 2006). This congenital anomaly affects approximately 1.41 per 1000 live births in Japanese (nonsyndromic clefts) and 1.25 in the other Asian populations (Cooper et al., 2006).

Several methods have been proposed to evaluate dental arch relationships in patients with cleft lip and palate. To evaluate the occlusion in patients with cleft lip and palate, measurement of dental arch length and width (Keller et al., 1988) and examination on the prevalence of crossbite (Pruzansky and Aduss, 1967; Bergland and Sidhu, 1974; Dahl et al., 1981) have been used in many previous studies. Although these methods are useful to

*Corresponding Author

evaluate individual parameters, an overall estimate of the dental arch relationship is not obtained. To address this problem, Huddart and Bodenham (1972) developed a numerical scoring system of the crossbite in deciduous dentition and estimated the overall degree of the malocclusion. The degrees of crossbite for individual teeth were calculated to give a total score. Recently, Mossey et al. (2003) proposed a modified method to apply to the mixed dentition. However, these methods take time to rate individual models.

The dental arch relationship in patients with unilateral cleft lip and palate (UCLP) can be assessed using the Goslon Yardstick (Mars et al., 1987), the 5-Year-old index (Atack et al., 1997a, b) and the GOAL Yardstick (Friede et al., 1991). The Goslon Yardstick was developed for late mixed or early permanent dentition, and the 5-Year-old index was developed for the deciduous dentition to allow early assessment of the primary surgery. The GOAL Yardstick defined the condition of crossbite more strictly and has been used for mixed dentition. The Goslon (Great Ormond Street, London and Oslo) Yardstick was first described by Mars et al. (1987). This Yardstick rates the dental arch relationships in the late mixed and early permanent dentition of patients with unilateral cleft lip and palate (UCLP) into five categories: excellent, good, fair, poor, and very poor. The Goslon Yardstick proved to be capable of discerning dental arch relationships and inference of facial morphology outcomes between different centers (Mars et al., 1992; Hathorn et al., 1996; Morris et al., 2000; Williams et al., 2001). The Yardstick has been verified as an easy and practical evaluation to discriminate between the qualities of dental arch relationships during all stages of dental development (Noverraz et al., 1993). Moreover, the Goslon Yardstick can be used to predict surgical outcome as early as 5 years of age (Atack et al., 1997). 5-Year-Old Index was developed for the deciduous dentition to allow earlier assessment of the primary surgery. However, the Eurocleft study (Mars et al., 1992; Shaw et al., 1992a, 1992b) documented that it is possible to detect differences in outcome as early as 10 years of age by assessing the dental arch relationships with the Goslon yardstick. We used the Goslon Yardstick, the 5-Year-Old Index because these are robust, (Mars et al., 1987) reproducible (Mars et al., 1987, Atack et al., 1997b), and reliable (Atack et al., 1997b).

The effect of factors such as using a presurgical orthopedic plate or not (Hotz and Gnoinski, 1976, 1979; Mishima et al., 1996; Prahl et al., 2001, 2006; Bongarts et al., 2006), type of cheiloplasty (Dahl et al., 1981; Ross, 1987a; Mars et al., 1992; Molsted et al., 1992; Kuijpers-Jagtman and Long, 2000), and type of palatoplasty (Dahl et al., 1981; Ross, 1987b; Mars et al., 1992; Molsted et al., 1992; Noverraz et al., 1993; Leenstra et al., 1995; LaRossa, 2000; Kuijpers-Jagtman and Long, 2000) on occlusion, are controversial. However, there are no clinical studies with large number of sample size using all these factors.

The contemporary use of preoperative orthopedics in the habilitation of children born with UCLP has been a controversial issue since it was first introduced by McNeil (1956). Preoperative orthopedics was introduced as a treatment to improve maxillary arch form and the position of alar base to prevent crossbites and to facilitate surgery (McNeil. 1956). Many specialists believe that orthopedic manipulation of the maxillary segments facilitates closure of the cleft lip and palate and improve the esthetic outcome of primary nasolabial repair (LaRossa, 2000). The efficacy of the Hotz plate plate in the improvement of feeding, growth and configuration of the maxillary segments, has been previously described (Huddart, 1979; Mishima et al., 1996). Other advantages reported in the literature are straightening of the nasal septum, normalization of the deglutition process, prevention of twisting and positioning of the tongue in the cleft and better speech development (Hotz and Gnoinski, 1976, 1979; Huddart, 1987; Gnoinski, 1990; Kramer et al., 1994; Mishima et al., 1996a). Ishii et al., (2000) reported UCLP subjects with two-stage palatoplasty combined with Hotz plate was better than that in UCLP subjects with one-stage palatoplasty, and relatively similar to that of subjects with normal occlusion.

Although disadvantages mentioned in literature include maxillary growth restriction, negative influences on speech because of delayed palate closure, the costs of the treatment, and its complexity (Pruzansky and Aduss, 1964; Huddart and Bodenham, 1972; Ross, 1987; Kramer et al., 1992; Prahl et al., 2001). But preoperative orthopedics has been criticized as being unnecessary and in some cases viewed as positively harmful, as it can restrict maxillary growth (Ross, 1987). Furthermore, it is difficult to come any firm conclusions, when so many variables affect the subsequent growth pattern. Many different appliances, both active and passive, have been described (Berkowitz, 2006). The so-called Zurich approach, using a passive plate of soft and hard acrylic, has had a major influence on treatment by the European cleft teams (Gnoinski, 1990).

For several decades, an abundance of research on cleft lip and palate has been published from a variety of specialties. Clearly, the malformation due to cleft lip and palate presents tremendous challenges for the patients, their families, and health care teams who provide treatment. The team approach for the management of cleft lip and palate patients involves the service of specialists like the plastic surgeon, oral and maxillofacial surgeon, pediatrician, otolaryngologist, pedodontist, orthodontist, speech therapist and prosthodontist. Generally, the orthodontist examines cleft lip and palate patients at 5 or 6 years of age for starting orthodontic treatment. Cleft lip and palate patients often show underdevelopment of the maxilla in the sagittal, vertical, and transverse dimensions following surgical repair of the cleft (Tindlund et al., 1993). Numerous investigations and discussions on the influence of primary surgery have been reported (Ross and Johnston, 1972; Kuijpers-Jagtman and Long, 2000; Berkowitz, 2006), but the cause of retrusion is still controversial. Many of the orthodontic problems of cleft lip and palate children in the late and early mixed dentition result not from the cleft itself, but from the effects of surgical repair. Closure of the cleft lip inevitably creates some constriction across the anterior part of the maxillary arch, and closure of the cleft palate causes at least some degree of lateral constriction, though the techniques for repair of cleft lip and palate have improved tremendously in recent years. As a result, surgically treated cleft lip and palate patients have a tendency toward both anterior and lateral crossbite, which is not seen in patient with untreated clefts (Ross and Johnston, 1972). The aims of this study were to determine the treatment outcome based on the dental arch relationship of Japanese patients with nonsyndromic unilateral cleft lip and palate (UCLP) and to assess the various congenital and environmental factors that affect dental arch relationship in UCLP patients using multivariate statistical analyses.

2. Materials and methods

2.1 Subjects

Among the 450 Japanese cleft lip and palate patients who visited the orthodontic clinic at Hokkaido University Hospital from 1996 to 2005 (10 years), 164 nonsyndromic UCLP subjects were finally included in this study.

The inclusion criteria were;

1. Non syndromic UCLP,
2. Lip surgery and palatoplasty had been performed at Hokkaido University Hospital
3. No previous orthodontic treatment.
4. No alveolar bone graft.

The Exclusion criteria were;

1. Syndromic UCLP
2. Lip surgery and palatoplasty had not been performed at Hokkaido University Hospital
3. Previous orthodontic treatment
4. Insufficient clinical records

The average gestation period and weight at birth of these subjects were 276 days and 3020 grams, respectively. Among these, 31 subjects had a family history of skeletal Class III (maxillary growth retardation and/or excessive mandibular growth). There were 93 males and 71 females. Fourty seven patients had right-sided UCLP. Eighty nine subjects had not received any presurgical orthopedic treatment (Psot) while 41 subjects had received Hotz plate (Figure 1) and 34 subjects had received an active plate (Figure 2). Though there were subjects who had received a Hotz plate and subjects who had received an active plate, we compared the subjects who had received Psot (Hotz plate and active plate) with those who had not received any treatment in this study. Treatment with Hotz plate according to a modified Zurich approach was usually initiated within 24 to 48 hours after birth (Hotz and Gnoinski, 1976, 1979). The active plate was an active, pin-retained device that moved the maxillary alveolar segments by screw activation (Latham, 1980).

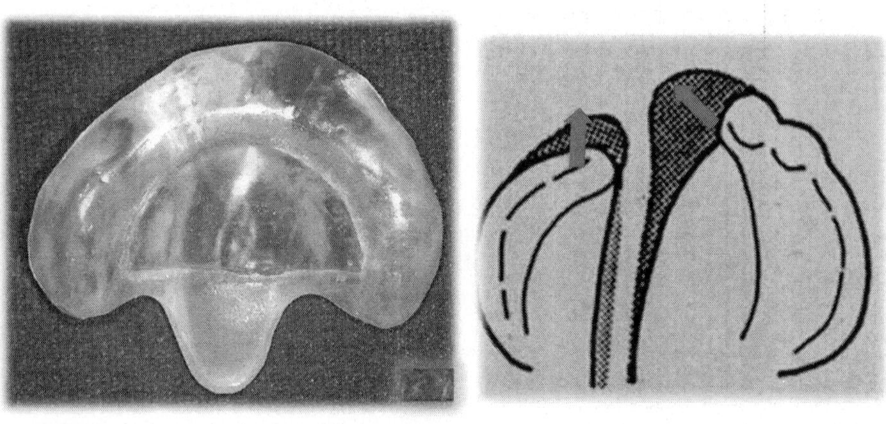

Fig. 1. Hotz plate.

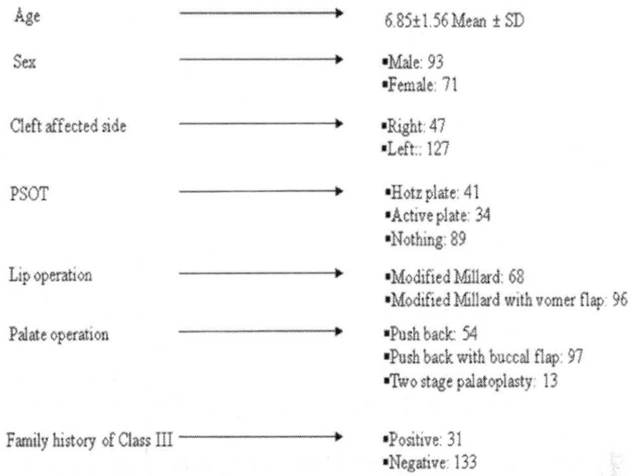

Psot: presurgical orthopedic treatment.

Fig. 2. Distribution of subjects with variable factors.

All subjects had undergone cheiloplasty at the Department of Plastic Surgery, Hokkaido University Hospital. In 68 subjects, modified Millard technique for lip closure (Figure 3) had been performed and in 96 subjects, modified Millard technique with anterior palate closure by vomer flap had been performed.

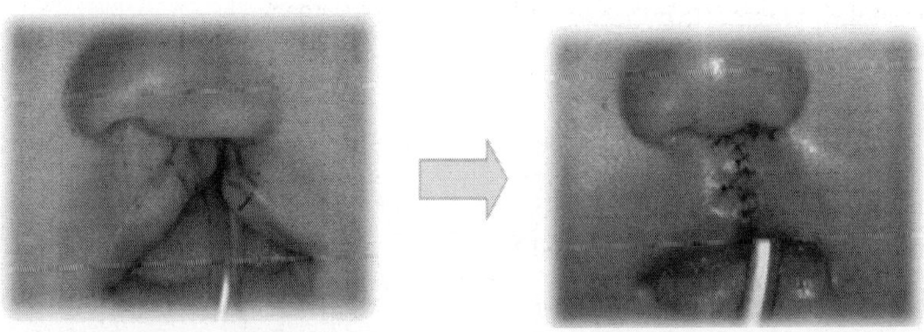

Fig. 3. Modified Millard technique for lip closure.

Subjects had undergone cheiloplasty at the average age of 5 months. All subjects underwent palatoplasty at the 1st or 2nd Departments of Oral and Maxillofacial Surgery or the Department of Plastic Surgery of Hokkaido University Hospital. Regarding palatoplasty, 54 subjects underwent pushback method (Figure 4a) at the average age of 20 months, 97 subjects underwent palatoplasty using pushback with buccal flap at the average age of 18 months. Pushback with buccal flap and two-stage palatoplasty (Figure 4b and 4c) were carried out to decrease the raw surface. The remaining 13 subjects underwent two-stage palatoplasty (using Furlow or Perko technique for closing the soft palate and then closing hard palate) at the average age of 20 months and 56 months. In this study, we compared subjects who received pushback only (palatoplasty with exposed raw surface) with subjects who received pushback with buccal flap or two-stage palatoplasty (palatoplasty with decreased raw surface).

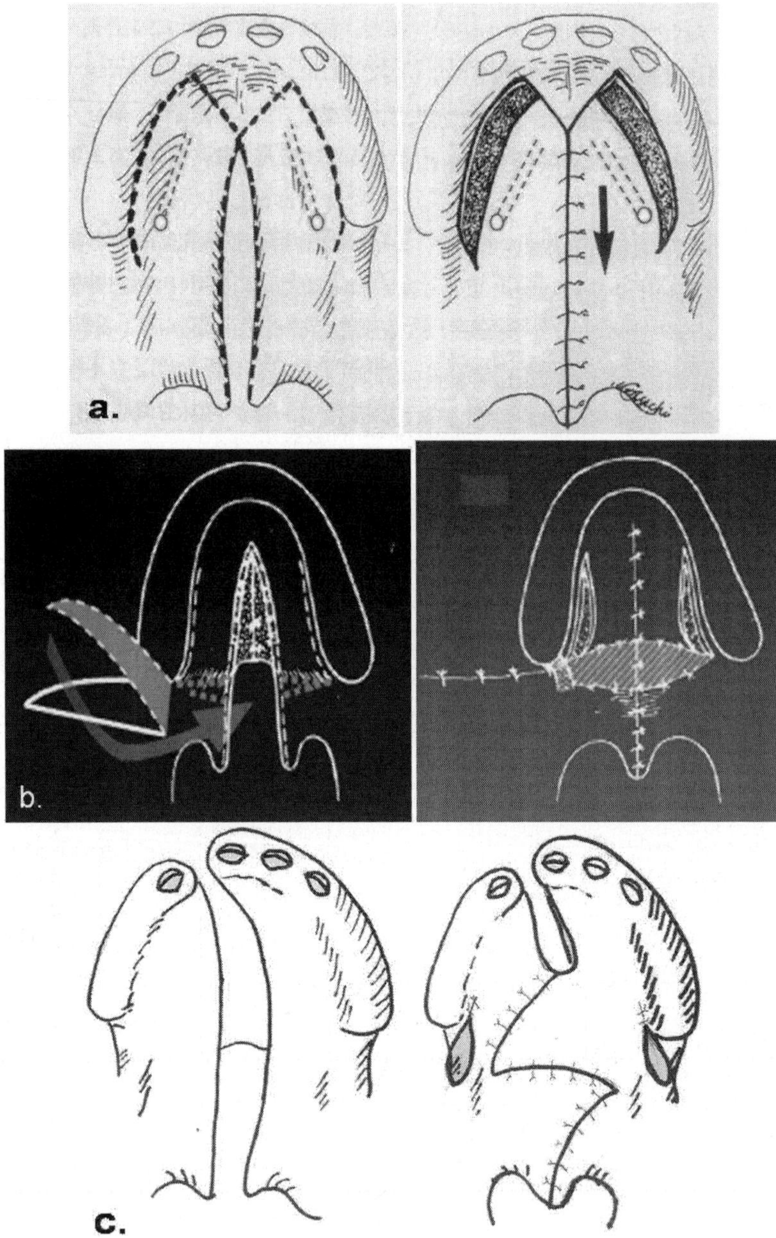

Fig. 4. a,b and c: a. Palatoplasty using pushback method, b. pushback with buccal flap and c. two-stage palatoplasty.

2.2 Assessment

Dental models taken at the initial examination (Mean age 6.85 ± 1.56 years) at the orthodontic clinic of Hokkaido University Hospital, were used for evaluating dental arch relationships. Dental arch relationships of these patients were assessed using the 5-year-old index (Atack et al., 1997a, b; Bongaarts et al., 2004) or the Goslon Yardstick (Mars et al., 1987, 2006; Morris et al., 2000; Chan et al., 2003) which have five-category ratings namely, 1: excellent, 2: good, 3: fair, 4: poor, and 5: very poor. The 5 year-old-index and the Goslon Yardstick are presented in tables in a simplified manner for assessment (Table 1 and 2).

The 5-year-old Index	Anterior OverJet (OJ)	Unilateral Cross Bite (CB) (Minor segment)	Unilateral Cross Bite (Major segment)	Open Bite (Around Cleft side)	Upper Incisor Procli-nation	Special feature
1 (Excellent)	+	- ~ ± (1 or 2 teeth)	-	-	- ~ ±	Good maxillary shape and palatal vault
2 (Good)	+	± ~ +	-	+	± ~ +	Edge to edge bite in the front plus no unilateral CB
3 (Fair)	± or – (with retrocline d upper central incisor)	+	-	±	± ~ +	Edge to edge bite with average inclined or proclined incisors.
4 (Poor)	-	+	±	±	± ~ +	
5 (Very poor)	-	+	+		+	Poor maxillary shape and palatal vault

Table 1. General features of the models in the 5-year-old Index (+: positive, –: negative, ±: tendency, and ~: to) Alam et al., 2008.

1 (Excellent)	Favorable Advantageous skeletal form Positive overjet and overbite Exhibit Angle Class II division 1	Straightforward Ortho Tx or none at all
2 (Good)	Favorable relationship Class I dental relationship	Straightforward Ortho Tx or none at all
3 (Fair)	Edge to edge dental relationship (Class III malocclusion) In case of borderline case between 3 and 4: Deep overbite - group 3	Complex Orthodontic Tx
4 (Poor)	Unfavorable facial growth Reverse overjet of 3 to 5 mm case belong to group 4 In case of borderline case between 3 and 4: anterior openbite – group 4	Borderline Tx
5 (Very poor)	Significant Class III Reverse overjet of 3 to 5 mm but marked proclination of upper incisors and retroclination of lower incisor	Surgical Tx

Table 2. General features of the models in the Goslon yardstick (Tx: treatment) Alam et al., 2008.

Three examiners rated the 164 models of subjects four times, twice for the 5 year-old-index and for the Goslon Yardstick on different days. Taking together the data in each model, we generated a mean score (Mars et al., 1992). Based on the 5-year-old index and the Goslon Yardstick, the subjects were divided into two groups, favorable (category ratings 1-3) and unfavorable (category ratings 4 and 5) groups. This grouping was carried out because the patients in the favorable groups could be treated with conventional orthodontics, whereas patients in the unfavorable groups sometimes required surgical correction (Chan et al., 2003).

2.3 Statistical analysis

The kappa statistics has been used previously to determine inter-examiner agreement of the 5-year-old index or the Goslon Yardstick scores (Mars et al., 1992; Noverraz et al., 1993; Atack et al., 1997a; Morris et al., 2000; Chan et al., 2003; Bongaarts et al., 2004). The intra- and interexaminer agreements of the 5-year-old index and the Goslon Yardstick scores were carried out with the weighted kappa statistic. According to Altman (1991), the kappa values of the intra- and interexaminer agreements were interpreted (Table 3).

Logistic regression analysis was performed using the dichotomous dependent variable, favorable and unfavorable groups (Hosmer, 1989). Both crude and backward stepwise logistic regression analyses were done to determine which factors affect the dental arch relationship in UCLP patients (Kleinbaum, 1994). These analyses were carried out using the statistical package SPSS Ver. 8.0 (SPSS Inc, Chicago, I11), with a probability level of 0.05 considered statistically significant. Hosmer-Lemeshow tests were used for assessment of goodness-of-fit of the overall model.

Kappa Value	Strength of Agreement
<0.20	Poor
0.21–0.40	Fair
0.41–0.60	Moderate
0.61–0.80	Good
0.81–1.00	Very good

Table 3. Interpretation of Kappa Values (Altman, 1991).

3. Results

The dental arch relationships (degree of malocclusion) of 164 Japanese patients with UCLP were evaluated at Hokkaido University Hospital and to assess the factors that affect the dental arch relationship using multivariate statistical analyses.

Intra- and Interexaminer Agreement for the 5 Year-Old-Index and the Goslon Yardstick: Intraexaminer agreements for examiners A, B, and C were 0.778, 0.744, and 0.762, respectively. The kappa scores ranged from 0.679 to 0.871 for the interexaminer agreement among all examiners. A kappa value >0.6 indicates good agreement and >0.8 represents very good agreement (Table 3, Altman, 1991). The kappa scores for the 5-year-old index thus indicated sufficient intra- and interexaminer agreement.

Intraexaminer agreements for examiners A, B, and C were 0.798, 0.674, and 0.879. The kappa scores ranged from 0.718 to 0.876 for the interexaminer agreement among all examiners. The kappa scores for the Goslon Yardstick thus indicated sufficient intra- and interexaminer agreement.

3.1 Score distributions

The distribution of subjects based on the five-category ratings of the 5-year-old index and the Goslon Yardstick were showed in Figure 5. Mean scores of the 5-year-old index and the Goslon Yardstick were 3.16 and 3.12, respectively.

The mean scores of the 5-year-old index of different countries, and the present study studies were showed in figure 6 (Atack et al., 1997a, b, Boongarts et al., 2004, 2006, William et al., 2001, William et al., 2001). The mean scores of the Goslon Yardstick of different countries, Eurocleft center and different Japanese studies were showed in figure 7 (Mars et al., 1987, 1990, 1992, 2006, Morris et al., 2000, Molsted et al., 1992, Nollet et al., 2005, Okazaki et al., 2002, Susami et al., 2006).

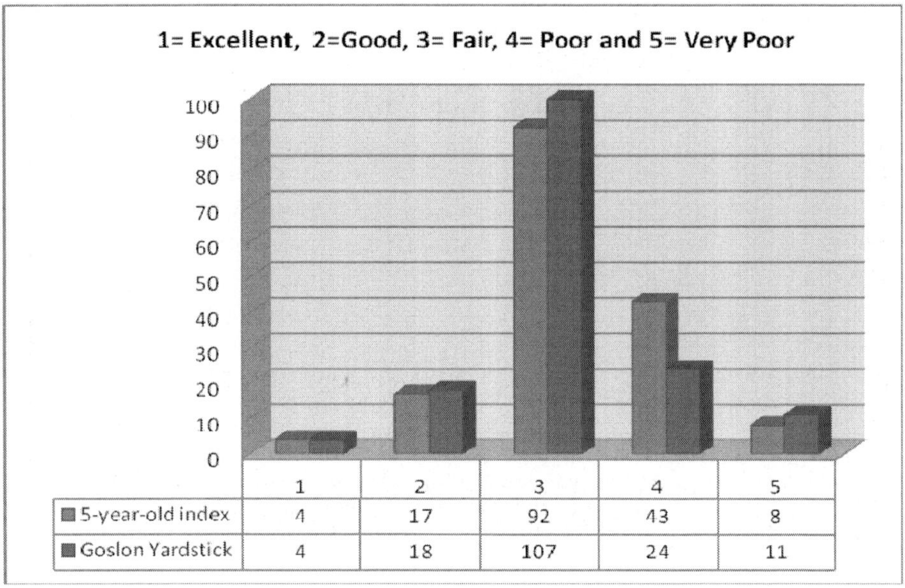

Fig. 5. Score distribution (percentages) for 164 UCLP subjects at Hokkaido University Hospital: The 5-year-old index and the Goslon yardstick.

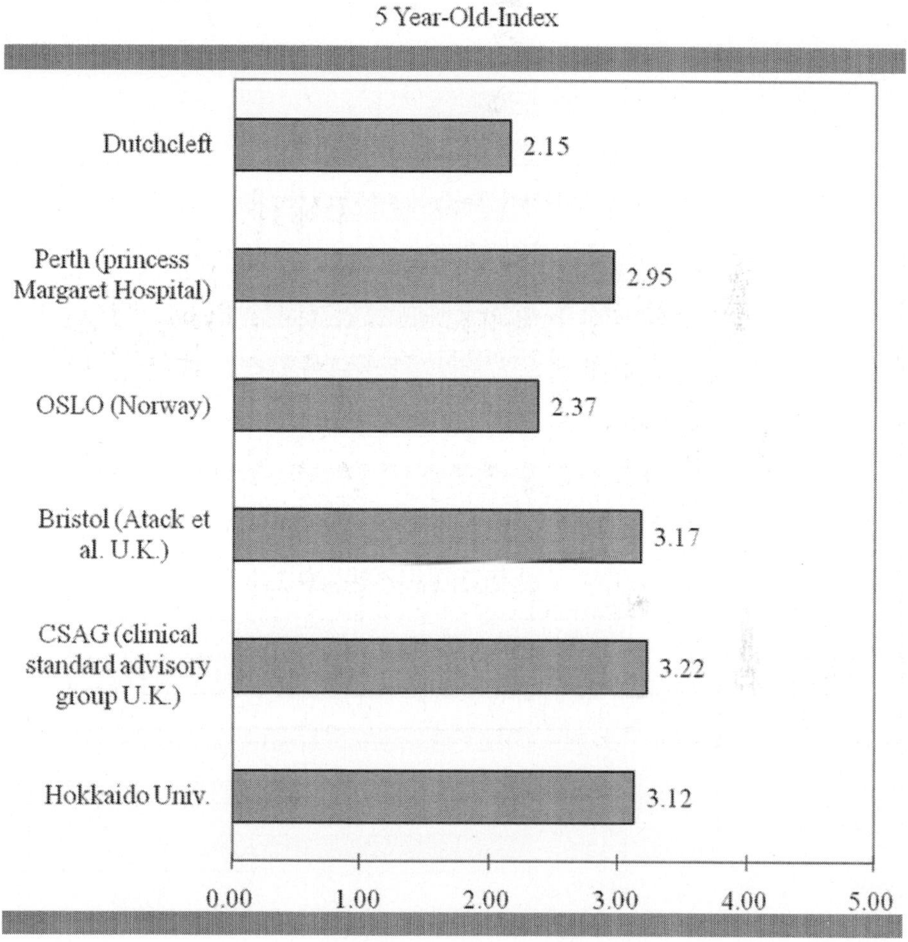

Fig. 6. Mean 5 Year-Old-Index score of other countries and present study.

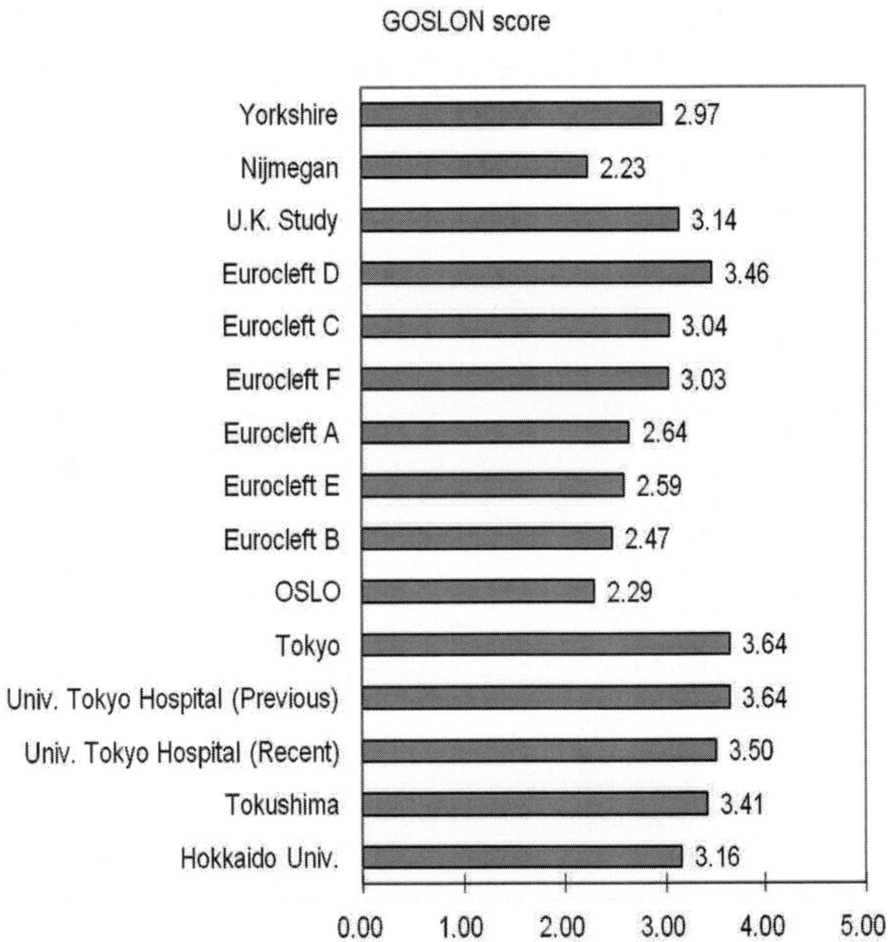

Fig. 7. Mean Goslon Yardstick score of other countries, Eurocleft centers. different Japanese studies and present study.

3.2 Comparisons of factors between favorable and unfavorable groups

Using the 5-year-old index and the Goslon yardstick presented in Table 4.

Variables		The 5-year-old index Favorable %	The 5-year-old index Unfavorable %	The Goslon Yardstick Favorable %	The Goslon Yardstick Unfavorable %
Family history of skeletal Class III	Positive	16	20	15	27
	Negative	84	80	85	73
Gender	Male	55	52	55	50
	Female	45	48	45	50
UCLP affected side	Right	30	20	29	20
	Left	70	80	71	80
Psot	Nothing	51	53	51	54
	Wearing Psot	49	47	49	46
Cheiloplasty	Modified Millard with vomer flap	53	66	54	70
	Modified Millard	47	34	46	30
Palatoplasty	Pushback with exposed raw surface	27	41	27	47
	Pushback with decreased raw surface	73	59	73	53

Table 4. Distribution of subjects with variable factors in favorable and unfavorable groups using the 5-year-old index (the number of subjects in favorable and unfavorable groups was 113 and 51, respectively) and the Goslon Yardstick (the number of subjects in favorable and unfavorable groups was 129 and 35, respectively).

3.3 Crude logistic regression analysis using the 5-year-old index scores

Table 5 shows the results of the crude logistic regression analysis that estimated the associations between various factors (independent variable) and dental arch relationships (dependent variable). Odds ratio, 95% confidence interval, and p value for the various factors are presented. Although no significant associations were found among various factors, the methods of cheiloplasty (odds ratio of modified Millard with vomer flap for anterior hard palate closure = 1.716) and palatoplasty with exposed raw surface (odd ratio of pushback only = 1.874) were slightly correlated with the dental arch relationship.

Variables	Odds Ratio	95% Confidence Interval	*P* Value
Family history of skeletal Class III	1.269	0.567-3.462	0.463
UCLP affected side (right)	0.591	0.244-1.346	0.221
Psot	0.897	0.456-1.844	0.862
Cheiloplasty (modified Millard with vomer flap)	1.716	0.812-3.569	0.148
Palatoplasty with exposed raw surface	1.874	0.876-3.938	0.101

Psot: presurgical orthopedic treatment.

Table 5. Crude odds ratios: Favorable vs unfavorable group using the 5-year-old index.

Note: An odds ratio greater than 1 indicates that the respective independent factor associates with unfavorable dental arch relationship and less than 1 indicates that the respective independent factor associates with favorable dental arch relationship.

3.4 Stepwise logistic regression analysis using the 5-year-old index scores

Table 6 shows the results of the stepwise logistic regression analysis that estimated the associations between various factors and dental arch relationships. Although no significant associations were found among various factors, the method of palatoplasty with exposed raw surface (odd ratio of pushback only = 1.987) was slightly correlated with dental arch relationship.

Hosmer-Lemeshow tests were used for assessment of goodness-of-fit of the overall model. The probability value was 0.725 (by the 5-year-old index). Thus, these models fitted well.

Variables	Odds Ratio	95% Confidence Interval	*P* Value
Family history of skeletal Class III	1.659	0.588-4.057	0.364
UCLP affected side (right)	0.513	0.204-1.263	0.139
Palatoplasty with exposed raw surface	1.987	0.919-4.154	0.071

Table 6. Adjusted odds ratios (Stepwise regression analysis: backward method): Favorable vs unfavorable group using the 5-year-old index.

3.5 Crude logistic regression analysis using the Goslon Yardstick scores

Table 7 shows the results of the crude logistic regression analysis that estimated the associations between various factors and dental arch relationships. Significant associations were found between palatoplasty with exposed raw surface (odd ratio of pushback only = 2.328) and dental arch relationship. Family history of skeletal Class III (odds ratio = 2.146) and method of cheiloplasty (odds ratio of modified Millard with vomer flap for anterior hard palate closure = 2.014) also seemed to be correlated with dental arch relationship.

Variables	Odds Ratio	95% Confidence Interval	*P* Value
Family history of skeletal Class III	2.146	0.811-5.520	0.114
UCLP affected side (right)	0.610	0.225-1.622	0.319
Psot	0.807	0.396-2.033	0.714
Cheiloplasty (modified Millard with vomer flap)	2.014	0.848-4.794	0.109
Palatoplasty with exposed raw surface	2.328	1.014-5.355	0.047 *

* $P < 0.05$

Psot: presurgical orthopedic treatment.

Table 7. Crude odds ratios: Favorable vs unfavorable group using the Goslon Yardstick.

Note: An odds ratio greater than 1 indicates that the respective independent factor associates with unfavorable dental arch relationship, and less than 1 indicates that the respective independent factor associates with favorable dental arch relationship.

3.6 Stepwise logistic regression analysis using the Goslon Yardstick scores

Table 8 shows the results of the stepwise logistic regression analysis that estimated the associations between various factors and dental arch relationships. Significant associations were found between palatoplasty with exposed raw surface (odd ratio of pushback only = 2.465) and dental arch relationship. Family history of skeletal Class III (odds ratio = 2.491) was also correlated with dental arch relationship.

Hosmer-Lemeshow tests were used for assessment of goodness-of-fit of the overall model. The probability value was 0.322 (by the Goslon Yardstick). Thus, these models fitted well.

Variables	Odds Ratio	95% Confidence Interval	*P* Value
Family history of skeletal Class III	2.491	0.867-6.943	0.081
UCLP affected side (right)	0.465	0.144-1.277	0.134
Palatoplasty with exposed raw surface	2.465	1.056-5.849	0.039 *

* $P < 0.05$

Table 8. Adjusted odds ratios (Stepwise regression analysis: backward method): Favorable vs unfavorable group using the Goslon yardstick.

4. Discussion

In this field no large-scale Japanese intercenter comparisons or randomized control trials have been performed. However, it is highly desirable that the standards of Japanese cleft surgery be evaluated in a global context. A six-center comparative study of the treatment outcome in Japan (Japancleft) was recently proposed (Asahito et al., 2003), and continuing research along these lines should reveal the general standard of cleft care in Japan.

In this study, we analyzed 164 non-syndromic UCLP subjects. The sample size was comparatively much higher than the number of subjects in the previous studies (Mars et al., 1992; Mishima et al., 1996; Atack et al., 1997a, b; Morris et al., 2000; Prahl et al., 2001; Chan et al., 2003; Bongaarts et al., 2004; Susami et al., 2006).

We used the 5-year-old index and the Goslon Yardstick for evaluation of dental arch relationship (degree of malocclusion) because these were reproducible (Mars et al., 1987, 1992; Atack et al., 1997a, b), and reliable methods (Mars et al., 1992; Atack et al., 1997a, b). Our subjects had a mean age of 6.85 ± 1.56 (Mean ± SD) years. The 5-year-old index was used to evaluate the primary dentition (Atack et al., 1997a, b). Initially, the Goslon Yardstick was used in the late mixed and early permanent dentition (Mars et al., 1987), but the Goslon Yardstick can be used to predict the surgical outcome as early as 5 years of age (Atack et al., 1997a, b). The Goslon Yardstick can also be used for all stages of dental development (Noverraz et al., 1993). Consequently, we used the Goslon Yardstick for primary and early mixed dentition in this study. The 5-year-old index and the Goslon Yardstick are thought to be the best-known clinical tools available to qualitatively assess dental arch relationships in UCLP patients. The future treatment plan can also be predicted using these indexes. In addition, these indexes are also closely related with cephalometric analysis (Morris et al., 2000).

In this study, intra- and interexaminer agreements were evaluated using the weighted kappa statistics and determine the repeatability and reproducibility of the of the five category ratings. The kappa scores for the 5 Year-Old-Index and the Goslon Yardstick were good to very good for both in the present study. The intraexaminer agreement for the

Goslon Yardstick was similar to that of the study reported by Susami T et al., (2006). Stepwise logistic regression analysis was used to explore the associations between precise factors (among various factors) and dental arch relationships. Crude logistic regression analysis was used to estimate associations between each congenital and environmental factor and dental arch relationships. Stepwise logistic regression analysis is used in the exploratory phase of research (Kleinbaum, 1994). Backward stepwise regression appears to be the preferred method of exploratory analyses, in which the analysis begins with a full model and variables are eliminated one by one using the largest p value (Kleinbaum, 1994). The final model is the last step model, in which eliminating another variable would not improve the model significantly (Kleinbaum, 1994).

Since it was first introduced by McNeil (1956), the contemporary use of preoperative orthopedics for treatment of children born with UCLP has been a controversial issue. Many different appliances, both active and passive, have been described (Berkowitz, 2006). The effect of infant orthopedics (IO) on maxillary arch dimensions in unilateral cleft lip and palate (UCLP) has been studied for decades, but controversy regarding the effect of IO on the maxillary arch still exists. Advocates of IO claim that the presurgical orthopedic plate molds the alveolar segments into a better arch form and prevents the tongue from positioning in the cleft. In this way, the dentomaxillary development would improve (McNeil, 1956; Hotz and Gnoinski, 1976, 1979; Gnoinski, 1990; Kramer et al., 1994; Berkowitz, 1996). Opponents of this therapy claim that lip surgery alone has the same effect and that the presurgical orthopedic plate is only an expensive appliance used to comfort the parents by starting treatment at the earliest moment possible (Pruzansky and Aduss, 1967; Ross, 1987; Kramer et al., 1992; Mars et al., 1992; Shaw et al., 1992a, 1992b; Prahl et al., 2001).

The results of the present study suggest that Psot does not so much correlate with the dental arch relationship. Use of the Hotz' plate during the first 18 months improves anterolateral growth of the tip of the alveolus on the cleft sides, shaping the alveolar arch towards ideal morphology (Ono et al., 1995) thus, facilitating the lip closure. Furthermore, by continuing use of the plate after lip closure, it increasingly reduces the pressure exerted by this newly surgically closed lip on the alveolar bone of the premaxilla. Then, by also closing the soft palate, the anterior hard palate cleft width is reduced by 55% and the posterior part by 50% of that at the time of velar closure (Ono et al., 1996). This facilitates hard palate closure. From this time onwards, the patient must continue to wear the plate, until closure of the hard palate at 6 years. In our hospital, this is done mainly by vomer flaps, also using artificial dermis made of atelocollagen to cover the raw surface and reduce surgical damage and produce fewer postoperative fistulae and less scar tissue (Iida et al., 1998). The scarring is believed to retard maxillary growth (Blocksma et al., 1975). By postponing closure of the hard palate to a later age, less growth is affected and better final growth of the maxilla will result (Friede and Enemark, 2001). However, it is possible that Psot correlates with other phenomena such as recovery of maxillary alveolar width/length and ease for palatoplasty (Mishima et al., 1996).

In the present study, it was speculated that cheiloplasty with vomer flap resulted in unfavorable dental arch relationship than cheiloplasty alone using crude logistic regression analysis, although this variable did not remain as a precise factor in the stepwise regression analysis using the 5-year-old index and the Goslon. Bardach and Kelly (1988) reported that closure of the lip defect with anterior palate resulted in more significant growth aberration than lip repair alone in a study using beagles. Anterior palate closure with vomer flap was carried out due to the ease of the palatoplasty procedure. Modified Millard cheiloplasty with anterior hard palate closure showed unfavorable maxillary protrusion, unfavorable midface (facial vertical proportion), and small total maxillary area (horizontal and vertical development of anterior nasal spine) (Ross, 1987a).

In an intercenter study by Ross (1987a, 1987b, 1987c), 1600 cephalometric radiographs from males with complete UCLP were examined to discern the effects of surgical and orthopedic treatment on facial growth. Among other things, Ross concluded that simple treatment protocols produced the most favorable results, and similar to the suggestion made by Dahl et al., that surgical expertise was found to be a major determinant of overall success. Presurgical orthopedics was found to provide no long-term benefits. Despite the obvious significance of this large study, the fact that its design was limited to cephalometric analysis made the analysis of many occlusal relationships impossible. These dental and arch-form factors often play an important role in treatment considerations. In contrast, Mars et al. (1987) used dental casts and a new form of arch relation analysis called the Goslon Yardstick to compare outcomes between various clinics. The rating process is based on the Goslon reference models, which are divided into five groups. Depending on the amount of maxillary protrusion present, and to a lesser extent on transverse and vertical variables, the groups are ordered from the best arch relationships to the worst. "Ones" are considered the best, and conversely, "fours" and "fives" are considered severe enough to likely require surgical maxillary advancement during end-stage treatment. The dental casts to be studied are compared with these reference groups and are assigned a score. Simpler means of arch assessment have been suggested, such as crossbite evaluation (Huddart and Bodenham, 1972) and incisal overjet measurement (Morris et al.,); these techniques, however, are not as sensitive and do not predict facial morphology outcomes as accurately as the Goslon Yardstick. The Yardstick is a practical means of evaluating malocclusion severity and associated treatment difficulty, and was used in the Mars et al. (1987) study to compare outcomes between a sample from Oslo and two samples from Greater Ormond Street (only one of which received presurgical orthopedics). Although the Oslo ratings were superior to those of Greater Ormond Street, no significant difference was found between the two subgroups of the latter. Presurgical orthopedics was therefore reported as having no major effect in this study. The Eurocleft study, published in 1992 as a series of five papers (Shaw et al., 1992a, 1992b; Mølsted et al., 1992; Mars et al., 1992; Asher-McDade et al., 1992) expanded the scope of intercenter research by comparing treatment outcomes of 8- to 10-year-olds with UCLP from six European cleft centers using cephalometric radiographs, dental casts evaluated with the Goslon Yarsdstick, and nasolabial photographs to evaluate craniofacial form, arch relationships, and nasolabial appearance.

Our study suggests that palatoplasty with exposed raw surface caused significantly unfavorable dental arch relationship than the palatoplasty with decreased raw surface (using the Goslon Yardstick). Pushback palatoplasty is generally thought to have more advantage in improving speech than the two-stage palatoplasty.

When we evaluated the dental arch relationship using the 5-year-old index, odds ratio of the palatoplasty with exposed raw surface failed to reach a significant level, but was still quite higher than that of the other factors. Over recent years, much attention has been given to the adverse effects of surgery in infants with cleft palate, with a number of reports indicating that the growth and development of the maxillary arch may be inhibited as a result of the nature of the primary repair (Ross, 1987c; Mars and Houston, 1990; Mars et al., 1992). Pushback palatoplasty showed a higher degree of maxillary and dentoalveolar deformity (Ross, 1972), although it is generally thought to have more advantage in improving speech than the two-stage palatoplasty. In an animal study, it was reported that the type of surgical repair may have an influence on the lateral constriction of the upper arch, particularly the use of surgical flaps in which palatal bone is denuded of mucoperiosteum (Leenstra et al., 1995; Kim et al., 2002). These reports coincide with our results.

The degree of constriction of the maxillary arch in patients with repaired UCLP is an important factor when considering the merits of different surgical techniques (Joos, 1995; Kramer et al., 1996). The information available from many of these studies has been in the mixed and permanent dentitions with less information available about the primary dentition.

In untreated adult UCLP arches,there is certainly some narrowing of the maxillary arch (da Filho Silva et al., 1992). However, there is some evidence that the type of surgical repair may have an influence on the lateral constriction of the upper arch, particularly the use of surgical flaps in which palatal bone is denuded of mucoperiosteum (Leenstra et al., 1995). This is an area that requires further investigation.

Follow-up investigation of the push-back palatoplasty has shown deleterious effects on transverse maxillary arch growth (Ross, 1970). However, institution of alternative surgical regimes does not necessarily minimize adverse effects on maxillary growth (Friede et al., 2000).

In the present study, subjects who had a family history of skeletal Class III (maxillary growth retardation and/or mandibular excessive growth) were more likely to fall into an unfavorable dental arch relationship, especially using the Goslon Yardstick. The results suggest that cleft patients tend to develop Class III malocclusion not only as an effect of primary surgery but also due to the genetic influence of family history. Our results also revealed that patients who have right-sided UCLP were slightly correlated with favorable dental arch relationship using stepwise logistic regression analysis, although the correlation was not significant. It is interesting to note that patients who have a right-sided UCLP had favorable dental arch relationship. Future studies are needed to determine the cause.

5. Conclusion

Treatment outcome based on dental arch relationships among Japanese children born with nonsyndromic complete UCLP seems to be intermediate (the mean scores of the 5-year-old index and the Goslon Yardstick were 3.16 and 3.12, respectively). This study provided evidence that there was a significant association between palatoplasty with exposed raw surface and dental arch relationship using crude and stepwise logistic regression analysis (judged by the Goslon Yardstick). Early palatal closure may negatively affect the outcome, but a factor of craniofacial differences between ethnic groups should be taken into consideration. The results suggest that cleft patients tend to develop Class III malocclusion not only as an effect of primary surgery but also due to the genetic influence of family history.

6. Acknowledgement

The authors would like to express gratitude to Mino Koshikawa-Matsuno (Instructor), Yuki Sugawara-Kato (Assistant Professor), Yoshiaki Sato (Associate Professor), of the Department of Oral Functional Science, Section of Orthodontics, Dr. Satoru Sasaki (Associate Professor, Plastic Surgery, Hokkaido University Hospital), Dr. Motonori Kudou, Dr. Tadashi Mikoya (Associate Professors, Oral and Maxillofacial Surgery, Hokkaido University Hospital) and Professor Manabu Morita (Preventive dentistry, Hokkaido University Hospital) for their valuable contributions to this study.

7. References

Alam MK, Kajii TS, Koshikawa-Matsuno M, Sugawara-Kato Y, Sato Y, Iida J. Multivariate analysis of factors affecting dental arch relationships in Japanese unilateral cleft lip and palate patients at Hokkaido University Hospital. *Orthodontic Waves.* 2008;67:45-53.

Altman DG. Practical statistics for medical research. London: Chapman and Hall; 1991:325-364, 404–408.

Asahito T, Hanada K, Ono K, Morita S, Mohri T, Takagi R, Terao E, Ishii K, Kouchi S, Ohtsuka S, Susami T, Negoro T, Kitai N, Tachimura T. Intercenter comparison studies for patients with cleft lip and palate in Japan. In: *Program and Abstracts. The 62nd Annual Meeting of the Japanese Orthodontic Society.* Tokyo: The Japanese Orthodontic Society; 2003:268.

Asher-McDade C, Brattstrom V, Dahl E, Mars M, McWilliam J, Mølsted K, Plint DA, Prahl-Andersen B, Semb G, Shaw WC, The RPS. A six-center international study of treatment outcome in patients with clefts of the lip and palate: part 4. Assessment of nasolabial appearance. *Cleft Palate Craniofac J.* 1992;29:409–412.

Atack N, Hathorn I, Mars M, Sandy J. Study models of 5 year old children as predictors of surgical outcome in unilateral cleft lip and palate. *Eur J Orthod.* 1997a;19:165–170.

Atack NE, Hathorn IS, Semb G, Dowell T, Sandy JR. A new index for assessing surgical outcome in unilateral cleft lip and palate subjects aged five: reproducibility and validity. *Cleft Palate Craniofac J.* 1997b;34:242–246.

Bardach J and Kelly KM. The influence of lip repair with and without soft-tissue undermining on facial growth in beagles. *Plast Reconstr Surg.* 1988;82:747-755.

Bergland O, Sidhu SS. Occlusal changes from the deciduous to the early mixed dentition in unilateral complete clefts. *Cleft Palate J.* 1974;11:317–326.

Berkowitz S. Cleft lip and palate. 2nd ed. Springer-Verlag Berlin Heidelberg; 2006:285-299, 395-404.

Blocksma R, Leuz CA, Mellerstig KE: A conservative program for managing cleft palates without the use of mucoperiosteal flaps. Plast Reconstr Surg 55: 160–169, 1975

Bongaarts CAM, Kuijpers-Jagtman AM, Vanthof MA, Prahl-Andersen B. The Effect of Infant Orthopedics on the Occlusion of the Deciduous Dentition in Children With Complete Unilateral Cleft Lip and Palate (Dutchcleft). *Cleft Palate Craniofac J.* 2004; 41:633-641.

Bongaarts CAM, van 't Hof MA, Prahl-Andersen B, Dirks IV, Kuijpers-Jagtman AM. Infant Orthopedics Has No Effect on Maxillary Arch Dimensions in the Deciduous

Dentition of Children With Complete Unilateral Cleft Lip and Palate (Dutchcleft). *Cleft Palate Craniofac J.* 2006;43:665–672.

Chan K T, Hayes C, Shusterman S, Mulliken J B, Will L A. The effects of active infant orthopedics on occlusal relationships in unilateral complete cleft Lip and palate. *Cleft Palate Craniofac J.* 2003;40:511–517.

Cooper ME., Ratay JS., Marazita ML. Asian Oral-Facial Cleft Birth Prevalence. *Cleft Palate Craniofac J.* 2006; 43:580-589.

da Silva Filho OG, Ramos AL, Abdo RCC. The influence of unilateral cleft lip and palate on maxillary dental arch morphology. *Angle Orthod.* 1992;62:283–290.

Dahl E, Hanusardo´ttir B, Bergland O. A comparison of occlusions in two groups of children whose clefts were repaired by three different surgical procedures. *Cleft Palate J.* 1981;17:122–127.

Friede H, Enemark H, Semb G, Paulin G, Abyholm F, Bolund S, Lilja J, Ostrup L. Craniofacial and occlusal characteristics in unilateral cleft lip and palate patients from four Scandinavian centres. *Scand J Plast Reconstr Surg Hand Surg.* 1991;25:269–276.

Gnoinski WM. Infant orthopedics and later orthodontic monitoring for unilateral cleft lip and palate patients in Zu¨rich. In: Bardach J, Morris HL, eds. *Multidisciplinary Management of Cleft Lip and Palate.* Philadelphia: WB Saunders; 1990:578–585.

Hathorn I, Roberts-Harry D, Mars M. The Goslon yardstick applied to a consecutive series of patients with unilateral clefts of the lip and palate. *Cleft Palate Craniofac J.* 1996;33:494–496.

Hosmer DW and Lemeshow S. Applied logistic regression. Wiley series in probability and mathematical statistics;1989.

Hotz MM and Gnoinski WM. Comprehensive care of cleft lip and palate children at Zurich University: a preliminary report. *Am J Orthod.* 1976;70: 481–504.

Hotz MM, Gnoinski WM. Effects of early maxillary orthopaedics in coordination with delayed surgery for cleft lip and palate. *J Maxillofac Surg.* 1979;7:201–210.

Huddart AG, Bodenham RS. The evaluation of arch form and occlusion in unilateral cleft palate subjects. *Cleft Palate J.* 1972;9:194–209.

Iida A, Ohashi Y, Takagi R, Ono K, Imai N, Kannari Y, Hayatsu M: Hard palate closure in two-stage palatoplasty. J Jpn Cleft Palate Assoc 23: 68–74, 1998

Ishii N, Deguchi T, Hunt NP. Craniofacial differences between Japanese and British Caucasian females with a skeletal class III malocclusion. *Eur J Orthod.* 2002;24:493–499.

Ishikawa H, Kitazawa S, Iwasaki H, Nakamura S. Effects of Maxillary Protraction Combined with Chin-Cap Therapy in Unilateral Cleft Lip and Palate Patients. *Cleft Palate Craniofac J.* 2000;37:92-97.

Joos U. Skeletal growth after muscular reconstruction for cleft lip, alveolus and palate *Br J Oral Maxillofac Surg.* 1995;33:139–144.

Keller BG, Long RE, Gold ED, Roth MD. Maxillary dental arch dimensions following pharyngeal-flap surgery. *Cleft Palate J.* 1988;25:248–257.

Kim T, Ishikawa H, Chu S, Handa A, Iida J, Yoshida S. Constriction of the maxillary dental arch by mucoperiosteal denudation of the palate. *Cleft Palate Craniofac J.* 2002;39:425-31.

Kleinbaum DG. Logistic regression. Springer;1994.

Kramer GJC, Hokesma JB, Prahl-Anderson B. Early palatal changes after initial palatal surgery in children with cleft lip and palate. *Cleft Palate Craniofac J*. 1996;33:104–111.

Kuijpers-Jagtman AM, Long RE. The influence of surgery and orthodontic treatment on maxillofacial growth and maxillary arch development in patients treated for orofacial cleft. *Cleft Palate Craniofac J*. 2000;37:527.

LaRossa D. The state of the art in cleft palate surgery. *Craniofac J*. 2000;37:225–228.

Latham RA. Orthopedic advancement of the cleft maxillary segment: a preliminary report. *Cleft Palate J*. 1980;17:227-233–322.

Leenstra TS, Kuijpers AM, Maltha JC, Freihofer HPM. Palatal surgery without denudation of bone favours dentoalveolar development in dogs. *Int J Oral Maxillofac Surg*. 1995;24:440–444.

Mars M, Plint DA, Houston WJ, Bergland O, Semb G. The Goslon Yardstick: a new system of assessing dental arch relationships in children with unilateral clefts of the lip and palate. *Cleft Palate J*. 1987;24:314–322.

Mars M. and Houston WJ. A preliminary study of facial growth and morphology in unoperated male unilateral cleft lip and palate subjects over 13 years of age. *Cleft Palate Craniofac J*. 1990;27:7–10.

Mars M, Asher-McDade C, Brattstrom V, Dahl E, McWilliam J, Molsted K, Plint DA, Prahl-Andersen B, Semb G, Shaw WC, The RPS. A six-center international study of treatment outcome in patients with clefts of the lip and palate. Part 3. Dental arch relationships. *Cleft Palate Craniofac J*. 1992;29:405–408.

Mars M, Batra P. Complete Unilateral Cleft Lip and Palate: Validity of the Five-Year Index and the Goslon Yardstick in Predicting Long-Term Dental Arch Relationships. *Cleft Palate Craniofac J*. 2006;43:557–562.

McNeil CK. Congenital oral deformities. *Br Dent J*. 1956;18:191–198.

Mishima K, Sugahara T, Mori Y, Sakuda M. Three-dimensional comparison between the palatal forms in complete unilateral cleft lip and palate with and without Hotz plate from cheiloplasty to palatoplasty. *Cleft Palate Craniofac J*. 1996;33:312–317.

Morris DO, Roberts-Harry D, Mars M. Dental arch relationships in Yorkshire children with unilateral cleft lip and palate. *Cleft Palate Craniofac J*. 2000;37:453–462.

Mossey PA, Clark JD, Gray D. Preliminary investigation of a modified Huddart/ Bodenham scoring system for assessment of maxillary arch constriction in unilateral cleft lip and palate subjects. *Eur J Orthod*. 2003;25:251–257.

Molsted K, Asher-McDade C, Brattstrom V, Dahl E, Mars M, McWilliam J, Plint DA, Noverraz AE, Kuijpers-Jagtman AM, Mars M, van't Hof MA. Timing of hard palate closure and dental arch relationships in unilateral cleft lip and palate patients: a mixed-longitudinal study. *Cleft Palate Craniofac J*. 1993;30:391–396.

Okazaki M, Yokozeki M, Miki Y, Horiguchi S, Inokuma K, Yuasa K, Liu J, Kawakami S, Hirose K, Hiura K, Moriyama K. Evaluation for malocclusion of 37 Japanese patients with unilateral cleft lip and palate by Goslon Yardstick. *J Jpn Cleft Palate Assoc*. 2002;27:47–57.

Ono K, Ohashi Y, Takagi R, Nagata M, Iida A, Imai N, Kannari Y, Hayatsu M: Spontaneous narrowing of residual hard palate cleft after velar closure in two-stage palatoplasty. J Jpn Cleft Palate Assoc 21: 126–141, 1996

Nollet PJPM, Katsaros C, Hof MAV, Kujpers-Jagtman. Treatment outome in unilateral cleft lip and palate evaluated with the GOSLON Yardstick: A meta-analysis of 1236 patients. Plast Reconstr Surg. 2005;116:1255-1262.

Prahl-Andersen B, Semb G, Shaw WC, The RPS. A six-center international study of treatment outcome in patients with clefts of the lip and palate: part 2. Craniofacial form and soft tissue profile. *Cleft Palate Craniofac J.* 1992;29:398–404.

Prahl C, Kuijpers-Jagtman AM, van 't Hof MA, Prahl-Andersen B. A randomized prospective clinical trial into the effect of infant orthopaedics on maxillary arch dimensions in unilateral cleft lip and palate (Dutchcleft). *Eur J Oral Sci.* 2001;109:297–305.

Prahl C, Prahl-Andersen B, van 't Hof MA, Kuijpers-Jagtman AM. Infant orthopedics and facial appearance: A randomized clinical trial (Dutchcleft). *Cleft Palate Craniofac J.* 2006;43:659-664.

Pruzansky S, Aduss H. Arch form and the deciduous occlusion in complete unilateral clefts. *Cleft Plate J.* 1964;1:411–418.

Ranta R. A review of tooth formation in children with cleft lip/palate. *Am J Orthod Dentofacial Orthop.* 1986;90:11-18.

Ross RB, Johnston MC. *Cleft Lip and Palate.* Baltimore: Williams & Wilkins; 1972:121-205, 227–288.

Ross RB. Treatment variables affecting facial growth in complete unilateral cleft lip and palate. Part 4: repair of the cleft lip. *Cleft Palate J.* 1987a;24:45–53.

Ross RB. Treatment variables affecting facial growth in complete unilateral cleft lip and palate. Part 6: techniques of palate repair. *Cleft Palate J.* 1987b;24:64–70.

Ross RB. Treatment variables affecting facial growth in complete unilateral cleft lip and palate. Part 7: an overview of treatment and facial growth. *Cleft Palate J.* 1987c;24:71–77.

Shaw WC, Asher-McDade C, Brattstrom V, Dahl E, McWilliam J, Mølsted K, Plint DA, Prahl-Andersen B, Semb G, The RP. A six-center international study of treatment outcome in patients with clefts of the lip and palate: part 1. Principles and study design. *Cleft Palate Craniofac J.* 1992a;29:393–397.

Shaw WC, Dahl E, Asher-McDade C, Brattstrom V, Mars M, McWilliam J, Mølsted K, Plint DA, Prahl-Andersen B, Roberts C, The RP. A six-center international study of treatment outcome in patients with clefts of the lip and palate: part 5. General discussion and conclusions. *Cleft Palate Craniofac J.* 1992b;29:413–418.

Susami T, Ogihara Y, Matsuzaki M, Sakiyama M, Takato T, Shaw WC, Semb G. Assessment of Dental Arch Relationships in Japanese Patients With Unilateral Cleft Lip and Palate. *Cleft Palate Craniofac J.* 2006;43:96–102.

Tindlund RS, Rygh P, Boe OE. Intercanine widening and sagittal effect of maxillary transverse expansion in patients with cleft lip and palate during the deciduous and mixed dentitions. *Cleft Palate Craniofac J.* 1993;30:195–207.

Williams AC, Bearn D, Mildinhall S, Murphy T, Sell D, Shaw WC, Murray JJ, Sandy JR. Cleft lip and palate care in the United Kingdom—the Clinical Standards Advisory Group (CSAG) study. Part 2: dentofacial outcomes and patient satisfaction. *Cleft Palate Craniofac J.* 2001;38:24–29.

William Ac, Jhonson NC, Singer S, Southall P, Mildinhall S, Semb G, Sell D, Thomas S, Sendy JR. Outcome of cleft care in western Australia: A pilot study. Aust Dent Jour. 2001;46:32-36.

Part 4

Temporomandibular Disorder and Orthodontic

14

Occlusion, Orthodontic Treatment and Temporomandibular Disorders: Myths and Scientific Evidences

Ephraim Winocur and Alona Emodi-Perlman
Department of Oral Rehabilitation, the Maurice and Gabriela Goldschleger School of Dental Medicine, Tel Aviv University, Tel Aviv, Israel

1. Introduction

Temporomandibular joint (TMJ) disorders and related masticatory muscle pain represent the most common chronic orofacial pain condition, and are the main cause of pain of non dental origin in the oro-facial region including head ,neck and face (de Leeuw 2008). The etiology of temporomandibular disorders (TMD) is multifactorial. One of historical proposed factors was improper occlusion (Egermark-Eriksson et al 1990, Kirverskari et al 1992, Pullinger 1993).

In the late 1980s the attention of the orthodontic community regarding TMD was awakened following litigation involving orthodontic treatment as the cause of TMD in an orthodontic patient in the US court. The orthodontist at cause lost the case only because at that time there was a lack in evidence based medicine literature (Pollack 1988).

In 1987 the Board of Trustees of the American Association of Orthodontists (AAO) passed a motion "that the AAO immediately initiate a program to conduct documented studies for the purpose of determining the relationship, or lack thereof, between orthodontic treatment and temporomandibular joint disorders." They also moved to form a new task-oriented committee, the Scientific Studies Committee, to conduct the program. Early in 1988, the committee was formed, consisting of persons with recognized knowledge in this area but with differing backgrounds: a prosthodontist, an oral pathologist, a general practitioner, and two orthodontists. Their conclusion was that orthodontic treatment generally is not a primary factor in TMD (Behrents and White 1992).

Since then many important investigations have been conducted, but still the possible association between orthodontic therapy and TMD signs and symptoms is a matter of debate among orthodontists, orthognatic surgeons, dentists and dental patients.

With the development of new aesthetic orthodontic techniques (lingual orthodontics, invisaline etc.) more adults seek orthodontic treatments, and therefore there appears to be an increased likelihood of orthodontic patients having TMD. Orthodontist should be capable to recognize the signs and symptoms of TMD already during the anamnestic appointment, to inform the patient of the finding, to point it out in the patient file, and if necessary to refer the patient to an Orofacial/TMD specialist.

The objective of this chapter is to discuss the effectiveness of orthodontic intervention in reducing symptoms in people with temporomandibular disorders and to establish if there is any evidence based data that proves that active orthodontic intervention leads to TMD.

In order to fulfill these objectives the following questions should be asked:

1. Does occlusal interferences cause TMD?
2. Does malocclusion cause TMD?
3. Does orthodontic treatment cause TMD?
4. Does orthodontic treatment cure or prevent TMD?

2. Temporomandibular disorders

Temporomandibular disorder (TMD) is a collective term that embraces a number of clinical problems that involve the masticatory muscles, the TMJs and its associated structures, or both. TMD is considered a musculo-skeletal disorder. It is the most prevalent clinical entity affecting the masticatory apparatus, and is the main cause of pain of non dental origin in the oro-facial region (de Leeuw 2008). The main TMD symptom is pain in the masticatory muscles, preauricular area and/or TMJ. As usual in all the musculo-skeletal disorders, pain increases during masticatory function. Other common signs or symptoms are limited or altered jaw movements, joint noises (eg. clicks, crepitus, etc), earache, headache, non specific dental tooth pain etc (Carlsson and de Boever 1994; Dworkin and LeResche 1992). For details regarding the guidelines for classification, assessment and management of TMD please refer to de Leeuw 2008.

The prevalence of TMD signs (e.g. abnormal jaw movements, joint noises, and tenderness on palpation) in the general population, as demonstrated by epidemiologic studies ranges up to 75% of the population. Approximately 33% of the population has at least one symptom (e.g. facial pain, joint pain) (Rugh 1985;Schiffman 1988; Friction and Schiffman 1995).

It is important to state that symptoms and signs are not real muscular or articular compound temporomandibular disorders. A single symptom or sign from the masticatory system is not synonymous with TMD, or automatically leads to a TMD diagnosis. In order to diagnose TMD formal diagnostic criteria should be fulfilled. For more details regarding the diagnosis of TMD, please refer to the AAOP guidelines (de Leeuw 2008), or to the Research Diagnostic Criteria for TMD (Dworkin and Le Resche 1992).

The aetiology and the pathophysiology of TMD are poorly understood. It is generally accepted that it is a multifactorial phenomenon. Contributing factors (central, peripheral, behavioral psychological, physical, etc) may predispose, initiate, or perpetuate temporomandibular disorders. Normally great physiologic and external forces are absorbed in the masticatory system with no consequence. But, if the forces exceed the individual genetic- physiologic tolerance the system may undergo detrimental changes. When the structural tolerance is exceeded breakdown will occur in the weakest structure of the system (teeth, muscles or joints) (Okeson, 2003). In the past occlusion was considered to be the most important contributing factor in TMD, but more recent studies concluded that occlusal factors play no role in the developing of TMD (see below) .

3. Occlusion and occlusal adjustment

Occlusion is defined as "the static relationship between the incising or occlusal surfaces of the maxillary or mandibular teeth or tooth analogues. The occlusion should be balanced and as stress free as possible" (The glossary of prosthodontics terms, 2005)

When occlusion was recognized as the main etiologic factors of bruxism and TMD, one of the main therapies used was occlusal adjustment that tried to eliminate all "tooth contacts that inhibit the remaining occluding surfaces from achieving stable and harmonious contacts (occlusal interferences) and may produce pathologic changes in the stomatognathic system (Bakke et al 1992). With time more and more evidenced based data accumulated against this invasive, irreversible technique. We should keep in mind that the prevalence of malocclusion is high: 42 % of the population exhibit Angle class 1, 23 % is class 2 malocclusion and 4% have class 3 malocclusion (Gremillion 1995). In other words, only 31% of the population has a normo-occlusion ("ideal occlusion") according to Angle's classification. Does 69% of the population suffer from TMD, and need to be treated? The answer is definitively NO!

4. Temporomandibular disorders & occlusion

The possible relationship between malocclusion and TMD was first reported in1934 by the otorhinolaryngologist Costen (Costen 1934). After analyzing 11 patients Costen hypothesized that dental changes (e.g. loss of vertical dimension and deep bite) led to anatomical changes in the temporomandibular joints, creating a syndrome composed of impaired hearing, tinnitus, dizziness, burning sensation in the throat and pain of unknown origin on side of face. The treatment proposed by Costen was "correction of the overbite, renewal of molar support to take pressure off the condyle....". The Costen's syndrome converted the temporomandibular disorders into another dental discipline. Dentists started treating patients suffering from "Costen syndrome" with bite raising appliances that augmented the vertical occlusal dimension of the face.

Old myths regarding the relationship between orthodontics treatment and TMD were twofold: In one hand, the myths that orthodontic treatment when done according to specific functional occlusion guidelines (gnathologic principles) reduces the likelihood of subsequently developing temporomandibular disorders, was rebutted. On the other hand the fact that the use of certain traditional orthodontic procedures and/or appliances may increase the likelihood of subsequently developing temporomandibular disorders could not be evidence proved (Rinchuse and Kandasamy , 2009). Many common myths among orthodontists were discussed and declined (Rinchuse and Kandasamy, 2009).The myths were that people with certain types of untreated malocclusion (eg. class II Division 2, deep overbite, and crossbite), excessive incisal guidance or people with gross maxilla - mandibular disharmonies are more likely to develop TMD. Other myths discussed were that pre-treatment radiographs of both TMJs should be taken before starting orthodontic treatment since the position of each condyle in its fossa should be assessed and corrected. They myth rebutted was that adult patients who have some type of occlusal disharmony along with the presence of temporomandibular disorder symptoms will probably require some form of occlusal correction. Finally, they could not found any evidence that retrusion of the mandible (because of natural causes or after treatment procedures) may cause the articular disc to slip off the front of the condyle and become a major factor in the aetiology of temporomandibular disorders. The assumption that premolar extractions in the upper arch can cause a posterior displacement of the condyle which in turn could be associated with increased risk of joint dysfunction was also refuted (Bonilla et al 1999; Keshvad and Winstanley 2001; Gallo et al 2005). It can be concluded that since none of the above was ever proven, and accordingly cannot stand as evidence based medicine, clinicians should refrain from adopting therapeutic procedures based on it.

Micheloti et al (2005) investigated the effect of an acute occlusal interference on habitual muscle activity. Each individual was monitored for 6 weeks in 4 different conditions: 1.interference free at the beginning, 2.active interference, 3.dummy interference, 4. interference free at the end .The activity of the masseter muscle ipsilateral to the interference side was recorded by a portable EMG recorder. The response of the masticatory system to active occlusal interferences was a reduction in daytime habitual activity of the masseter muscle. None of the subjects reported signs and/or symptoms of TMD. It should be kept in mind that this study was performed on healthy subjects (without present or passed history of TMD). It may be possible that patients suffering already from TMD react differently to an experimentally introduced occlusal interference due to a deficiency in their adaptation capacity (Le Bell et al 2002). This hypothesis is also based in the observation that TMD patients do keep their teeth in contact more often during daytime (Chen, 2005) and therefore are more likely to feel the interference as a disturbing factor (Le Bell et al, 2006; Cao et al 2009). To test this assumption Le Bell et al (2002) performed a randomized double-blind clinical set-up that included healthy women without TMD as well as women with an earlier TMD history. Both groups were randomly divided into true and placebo interference groups. The subjects without a TMD history showed fairly good adaptation to the interferences, but the subjects with a TMD history and true interferences showed a significant increase in clinical signs compared to the other groups. The authors suggest that the etiological role of occlusal interferences in TMD may not have been correctly addressed in previous studies with artificial interferences and allow no conclusions as regards TMD etiology. Bell's group further analyzed the subjective reactions of these individuals. They found that the most prominent symptoms were occlusal discomfort and chewing difficulties. The group reached the conclusion that difference in outcome between the groups with and without a TMD history suggests that there are individual differences in vulnerability to occlusal interferences (LeBell 2006). In a third study (Niemi et al, 2006) the group tested the psychological factors and responses to artificial interferences in subjects with and without a history of TMD. They concluded that psychological factors appear significant for the symptom responses to artificial interferences, and they seem to play a different role in responses in subjects with an earlier TMD history compared to those without.

An occlusal interference animal model was conducted on rats (Cao 2009) by directly bonding crowns of different heights on their molars. The rats showed bilateral mechanical hyperalgesia in the masticatory muscles. The induced hyperalgesia remained 6 days after removal of the crowns and was reduced by injecting N-meyhyl-D-aspartate antagonist, suggesting a central sensitization mechanism. The animal model described mimics clinical masticatory muscle pain and provided a method to further investigate mechanisms of occlusion - related muscle hyperalgesia, and to explore possible pain management strategies.

Christensen and Rassouli (1995) placed a rigid unilateral intercuspal interference in 12 subjects, and obtained bipolar surface electromyograms from the right and left masseter muscles during brisk and forceful clenching on the interference. On the side opposite the interference, myoelectric clenching activity was significantly reduced. Correlation analyses showed that the interference elicited a non-linear (complex) co-ordination of the amplitude, but not the duration, of bilateral masseteric clenching activity, i.e. frequently there was significant motor facilitation on the side of the interference, and significant motor inhibition on the side opposite the interference. The author further performed theoretical considerations that predicted that the observed contraction patterns would easily lead to frontal plane rotations of the mandible.

This was further supported by Clark et al (1999). The conclusion of their literature review was that experimental occlusal interferences may induce transient local tooth pain, loosening of the tooth, a slight change in postural muscle tension levels, chewing stroke patterns, and sometimes a clicking joint. They were of the opinion that since such findings are present in relatively asymptomatic patients, these data do not prove that occlusal interferences are causally related to a chronic jaw muscle pain or TMD.

Finally it could be hypothesized that subjects who are occlusally hypervigilant and or predisposed to suffer from TMD may be disturbed by occlusal interferences and increase the activity of the masticatory muscles which leads to pain and dysfunction as demonstrated by McDermid et al (1996); Raphael et al (2000);Hollins et al (2009).In some cases a very serious intractable disorder may be induced by occlusal changes. This disorder was term by Clark (2003) occlusal dysesthesia and is defined as "a persistent uncomfortable sense of maximum intercuspation after all pulpal, periodontal, muscle and TMJ pathologies have been ruled out and a physically obvious bite discrepancy cannot be observed". This serious disorder is was previously termed by Marbach et al (1983) "phantom bite syndrome".

5. Temporomandibular disorders & orthodontics

An article by McNamara et al (1995) represents the evolution of a solicited manuscript first presented at the International Workshop on the TMDs and Related Pain Conditions, sponsored by the National Institute of Health (Hunt Valley, Md., April 17 to 20, 1994).

Its conclusions were:"(1) signs and symptoms of TMD may occur in healthy persons; (2) signs and symptoms of TMD increase with age, particularly during adolescence, until menopause, and therefore TMDs that originate during orthodontic treatment may not be related to the treatment; (3) in general, orthodontic treatment performed during adolescence does not increase or decrease the chances of development of TMD later in life; (4) the extraction of teeth as part of an orthodontic treatment plan does not increase the risk of TMD; (5) there is no increased risk of TMD associated with any particular type of orthodontic mechanics; (6) although a stable occlusion is a reasonable orthodontic treatment goal, not achieving a specific gnathologic ideal occlusion does not result in signs and symptoms of TMD; and (7) there is little evidence that orthodontic treatment prevents TMD, although the role of unilateral posterior crossbite correction in children may warrant further investigation." (McNamara et al,1995;McNamara and Turp 1997).

Pullinger et al (1993) used a multiple logistic regression analysis to compute the odds ratios for 11 common occlusal features for asymptomatic controls vs. five temporomandibular disorder groups. They found that the following features did not increase the odds to develop TMD: retruded contact position (RCP) to intercuspal position (ICP) occlusal slides < 2 mm, slide asymmetry, unilateral RCP contacts, deep overbite, minimal overjet, dental midline discrepancies, < 4 missing teeth, and maxillo-mandibular first molar relationship or cross-arch asymmetry. They found that groupings of a minimum of two to at most five occlusal variables contributed to the TMD patient groups. On the other hand, significant increases in risk occurred selectively with anterior open bite, unilateral maxillary lingual crossbite overjets> 6-7 mm > 5-6 missing posterior, and RCP-ICP slides > 2 mm. The authors were of the opinion that certain features such as anterior open bite in osteoarthrosis patients were considered to be a consequence of rather than etiological factors for the disorder. They concluded "that occlusion cannot be considered the unique or dominant factor in defining TMD populations".

The hypothesis that different orthodontic techniques such as functional appliances class I/II elastics , chin-cup , headgear , fixed or removable appliances as aetiological factors for TMD has been tested in many studies. Dibbets and Van der Weele (1992) compared children treated with different procedures. Patients were monitored for a 20 year period after the start of orthodontic treatment. Although signs and symptoms of TMD increased with age, after 20 years neither orthodontic treatment showed a causal relationship with signs and symptoms of TMD. Henrikson and Nilner (2000) compared class II division 1 treated and untreated females with normal occlusion (11-15 years old) monitored for 2 years. They reported individual fluctuations of TMD symptoms in all 3 groups. Orthodontic treatment did not increase the risk for aggravating pre-treatment signs of TMD. On the contrary subjects with class II and TMD of muscular origin seemed to improve. Rey et al (2008) compared a sample of class III patients treated with mandibular cervical headgear and class I patients treated orthodonticaly and no treated subjects. No difference in TMD prevalence was found between the 3 groups after 2-3 years. Regarding orthognatic surgery, Farella et al (2007), reported that bi-maxillary osteotomy did not initiate or aggravate signs and symptoms of TMD. A 20 year cohort longitudinal study by MacFariane et al (2009) investigated the relationship between orthodontic treatment and TMD concluded that orthodontic treatment neither causes nor prevents TMD and that participants with a history of orthodontic treatment did not have higher risk of new or persistent TMD .

Henrikson and Nilnerl (2000), prospectively and longitudinally studied signs of TMD and occlusal changes in girls with Class II malocclusion receiving treatment, compared to subjects with untreated Class II malocclusion and with normal occlusion subjects. They concluded that orthodontic treatment does not increase the risk for TMD or for worsen pre-treatment signs. On the contrary, they found that subjects with Class II malocclusion and signs of muscular TMD seem to benefit from the orthodontics treatment.

6. Conclusions & clinical aspects

A recent Cochrane systematic review was published (Luther et al 2010). Its objective was to establish the effectiveness of orthodontic intervention in reducing symptoms in patients with TMD (compared with any control group receiving no treatment, placebo treatment or reassurance) and to establish if active orthodontic intervention leads to TMD. The authors identified 284 records from all databases, but only four demonstrated any data that might be of value with respect to TMD and orthodontics. After further analysis of the full texts of the four studies identified, none of the retrieved studies met the inclusion criteria and all were excluded from this review. The authors' conclusions were: "1.There is insufficient research data on which to base our clinical practice on the relationship of active orthodontic intervention and TMD; 2. There is an urgent need for high quality randomized controlled trials in this area of orthodontic practice; 3. When considering consent for patients it is essential to reflect the seemingly random development/alleviation of TMD signs and symptoms.

7. Summary and conclusions

The main articles reviewed in this chapter are summarized in table 1.

Study Reference*	Study design	Conclusions & Comments
Al-Riyami et al (part 2) 2009	Systematic Review	Although orthognatic surgery should not be advocated solely for treating TMD, patients having orthognatic treatment for correction of their dento-facial deformities and who are also suffering from TMD appear more likely to see improvement in their signs and symptoms than deterioration
Behrents & White 1992	Viewpoint intended to recount a research program initiated by the American Association of Orthodontists	(1) Consistently significant associations between structure (dental and osseous) and TMD have not been demonstrated. (2) The development of TMD cannot be predicted. (3) No method of TMD prevention has been demonstrated. (4) The prevalence of TMD symptoms increases with age; thus TMD may originate during orthodontic treatment, but not be related to the treatment. (5) Orthodontic treatments per se do not initiate TMD. (6) Evidence favors the beneficial nature of orthodontic treatment; orthodontics, as a part of the regimen of care, may assist in the lessening of symptoms. (7) Once TMD is present, TMD cures cannot be assumed or assured.
Dibbets &Van der Weele 1992	Prospective-longitudinal	Based upon the finding of similar prevalences after 20 years of observation, it appears that neither orthodontic treatment nor extraction has a causal relationship with the signs and symptoms of TMD

Study Reference*	Study design	Conclusions & Comments
Egermark-Eriksson et al 1990	Longitudinal	No differences in prevalences of occlusal interferences, or in signs or symptoms of TMD were found between subjects that had corrective orthodontic treatment and those without such treatment. The associations between TMD and different morphological malocclusions were low. Nevertheless, in a long-term perspective cross-bite, both uni- and bilateral, anterior open bite, post-, and prenormal occlusion had some association with the development of CMD.
Farella et al 2007	Longitudinal	Pressure pain thresholds of the masseter and temporalis muscles did not change significantly from baseline values throughout the whole study period. The occurrence of signs and symptoms of TMD fluctuates with an unpredictable pattern after orthognathic surgery for class III malocclusions.
Gremillion 2006	Review article	Scientific literature has not convincingly demonstrated a definitive relationship between static occlusal factors and TMD.
Henrikson et al 2000	Prospective-longitudinal	Orthodontic treatment do not increase the risk for TMD or for worsen pre-treatment signs. On the contrary, they found that subjects with Class II malocclusion and signs of muscular TMD seem to benefit from the orthodontics treatment.
Le Bell et al 2002	Randomized double-blind clinical set-up	Since subjects with a TMD history and true interferences showed a significant increase in clinical signs compared to the other groups. The authors suggest that the etiological role of occlusal interferences in TMD may not have been correctly addressed in previous studies with artificial interferences and allow no conclusions as regards TMD etiology
Le Bell et al 2006	Randomized double-blind clinical set-up	The most prominent symptoms following the introduction of artificial occlusal interferences were occlusal discomfort and chewing difficulties. The difference in outcome between the groups with and without a TMD history suggests that there are individual differences in vulnerability to occlusal interferences.

Study Reference*	Study design	Conclusions & Comments
Luther et al 2010	Systematic Review (COCHRANE)	(1) There are insufficient research data on which to base the clinical practice on the relationship of active orthodontic intervention and TMD. (2) There is an urgent need for high quality randomized controlled trials in this area of orthodontic practice. (3) When considering consent for patients it is essential to reflect the seemingly random development/alleviation of TMD signs and symptoms.
Macfariane et al 2009	Prospective	Orthodontic treatment neither causes nor prevents TMD. Female sex and TMD in adolescence were the only predictors of TMD in young adulthood.
McNamara, Jr 1997	Review Article	(1) signs and symptoms of TMD may occur in healthy persons; (2) signs and symptoms of TMD increase with age, particularly during adolescence, until menopause, and therefore TMDs that originate during orthodontic treatment may not be related to the treatment; (3) orthodontic treatment performed during adolescence does not increase or decrease the chances of development of TMD later in life; (4) the extraction of teeth as part of an orthodontic treatment plan does not increase the risk of TMD; (5) there is no increased risk of TMD associated with any particular type of orthodontic mechanics; (6) although a stable occlusion is a reasonable orthodontic treatment goal, not achieving a specific gnathologic ideal occlusion does not result in signs and symptoms of TMD; and (7) thus far, there is little evidence that orthodontic treatment prevents TMD, although the role of unilateral posterior crossbite correction in children may warrant further investigation
Michelotti & Iodice. 2010	Review Article	(1) TMD is a multifactorial pathology, and it is difficult to demonstrate a direct correlation between one of the causes, such as occlusion, and TMD. (2) Dysfunctional patients have a lower adaptive capability to occlusal changes because they seem to be more vigilant on their occlusion and are easily disturbed by occlusal instability. (3) When severe pain is present, occlusal treatments (such as orthodontics and prosthodontics) have to be postponed until symptoms are improved.

Study Reference*	Study design	Conclusions & Comments
Niemi et al 2006	Randomized double-blind clinical set-up	Psychological factors appeared significant for the symptom responses to artificial interferences, and they seem to play a different role in responses in subjects with an earlier TMD history compared to those without.
Pullinger et al 1993	A multiple logistic regression analysis to compute the odds ratios for 11 common occlusal features for asymptomatic controls (n = 147) vs. five temporomandibular disorder groups (n=413).	Occlusion cannot be considered the unique or dominant factor in defining TMD populations.
Rey et al 2008	Retrospective Comparative	Subjects with Class III malocclusions treated with mandibular cervical headgear and fixed appliances do not have greater prevalence of TMD symptoms than do Class I subjects treated with fixed appliances or untreated subjects.
Rinchuse & Kandasamy 2009	Special Review Article	(1) Orthodontic gnathologists have proved no health benefit to justify the many perfunctory exercises of the philosophy. (2) The view that occlusion and condyle position are the primary causes of TMD, and that diagnoses and treatments should be based on these notions, has been discredited. (3) There is little to no evidence that treating subjects with TMJ ID will prevent or mitigate future TMD.

* References has been arranged alphabetically according to the first author

Table 1. Summary of main articles reviewed.

The main conclusions are the following:

1. TMD is a collective term embracing a number of clinical problems that involve the masticatory muscles and the TMJs.
2. The pathogenesis of TMD is not dental - related but rather is a part of a wider family of orofacial pain disorders which account for the need to consider neurologic, endocrine and psychosocial factors during the diagnostic process. Occlusion, condyle position, and lack of canine guidance are not the primary causes of TMD (Manfrendini and Nardini 2010).
3. TMD treatments are no longer dental, but are based on biopsychosocial approach (Rinchuse and Kandasamy 2009). Treatment options are: patient education , cognitive behavior therapy (CBT) (Turk et al 1996; Turk 1997), bio feedback, physiotherapy(Stholer 1999) , acupuncture(List et al 1993), transcutaneous nerve stimulation (TENS), low intensity laser , splint therapy (Greco et al 1997; List and Axelsson 2010), drug therapy, surgical intervention (Al-Riyami et al 2009), but not occlusal definitive;

4. TMD signs and symptoms are often resolved by conservative and reversible therapies.
5. No scientific evidence exists that orthodontic treatment will prevent or mitigate the development of future TMD, or cure an existing disorder.
6. Orthodontic treatment performed during adolescence does not increase or decrease the risk of developing TMD in later life.

The authors' clinical recommendations are the following:

1. An attentive orthodontist should always identify and document findings of the TMJ and related structures. TMD signs and symptoms may occur before, during and after orthodontic treatment even though these findings may not necessarily lead to treatment.
2. Inform the patient of his/her temporomandibular situation and discuss the prognosis. Ask a signed informed consent.
3. Inform the patient that his/her occlusion will undergo changes and that it is essential to avoid parafunctional, constant auto-checking of the bite in order to prevent the possible development of occlusal dysesthesia.
4. If the patient presents TMD symptoms BEFORE treatment:
   a. Insignificant symptoms such as painless clicking or movement limitation due to prolonged periods of gum chewing or deviations in opening closing pattern should not delay the beginning of orthodontic treatment.
   b. If pain and severe dysfunction are present the patient should be referred to a TMD specialist before orthodontic therapy is initiated .
5. If the patient develops symptoms DURING treatment :
   a. Temporarily stop active orthodontics treatment.
   b. Perform basic pain management and supportive therapy in order to reduce the symptoms, after which orthodontic treatment may continue.
   c. If the symptoms persist, the treatment plan should be reconsidered because the patient might become hypervigilant and of poor adaptation capability. An alternative treatment plan should be considered.
6. If the patient develops symptoms AFTER treatment :
   a. If the patient was informed before treatment about a possible development of TMD, there should not be a problem explaining that TMD was probably not a result of the orthodontics.
   b. As TMD sign and symptoms tend to be observed between 20 to 30 years old (De Kanter et al 1993;Mohlin et al 2004) there is a possibility of an orthodontic patient developing symptoms after treatment based only on his/her age.

8. References

Al-Riyami S, Cunningham SJ, Moles DR. A systematic review of TMD and orthognatic treatment. Part 2. Signs and symptoms and meta-analyses. Am J Orthod Dentofacial Orthop 2009;136:626.e1-626.e16

Al-Riyami S, Moles DR, Cunningham SJ. A systematic review of TMD and orthognatic treatment. Part 1. A new quality-assessment technique and analysis of study characteristics and classifications. Am J Orthod Dentofacial Orthop 2009;136:624.e1-624.e15

Bakke M, Michler L, Moller E. Occlusal control of mandibular elevator muscles. Scand J Dent Res 1992;100:284-91.

Behrents R.G. , White RA . Am J Ortho & Dentofac Orthop , Vol 101 ; no 1 Jan 1992 .

Bonilla-Aragon H, Talents RH, Katzberg RW, Kirkanides S, Moss ME. Condyle position as a predictor temporomandibular joint internal derangement. J Prosthet Dent. 1999;82:205-208.

Cao Y , Xie QF, Li K, Light AR , Fu KY. Experimental occlusal interferences induce long-term masticatory muscle hyperalgesia in rats. Pain. 2009;144:287-293.

Carlsson GE , DeBoever JA. Epidemiology. In : Zarb GA ,Carlsson GE ,Sesle BJ , Mohl ND (eds.) Temporomandibular joint and Masticatory Muscle Disorders , ed 2 . Copenhagen : Munnksgaard , 1994 : 171-187.

Chen YJ, Gallo LM, Meler D, Palla S. Individualized oblique-axial magnetic resonance imaging for improved visualization of mediolateral TMJ disc displacement. J Orofac Pain. 2000;14:128-139.

Chen YJ. Frequency of non-functional tooth contacts in normal subjects and patients with a myoarthropathy of the masticatory system. Thesis . University of Zurich . Zurich: Medical faculty ,2005.

Christensen LV , Rassouli NM . Experimental occlusal interferences . Part II . Masseteric EMG responses to an intercuspal interference. J Oral Rehabil . 1995;22:521-531.

Christensen LV, Rassouli NM. Experimental occlusal interferences. Part I. A review. J Oral Rehab . 1995; 22 :515-520.

Clark G, Simmons M. Occlusal Dysesthesia and temporomandibular disorders. Is there a link? Alpha Omegan,3003, Vol 96(2), 33-39

Clark G, Tsukiyama Y, Baba K, Watanabe T. Sixty-eight years of experimental occlusal interference studies . What have we learned? J Prosthet Dent . 1999;82:704-713.

Costen JB. A syndrome of ear and sinus symptoms dependent upon disturbed function of the temporomandibular joint. Ann Ortol Rhinol Laryngol. 1934;43:1-15.

De Kanter RJ, Truin GJ, Burgersdijk RC, Van't Hop MA,Battistuzzi PG, Kalsbeek H et al. Prevalence in the Dutch adult population and a meta-analysis of signs and symptoms of temporomandibular disorder. J Dent Res 1993;72:1509-1518.

De Leeuw R (ed) Orofacial pain; guidelines for assessment, diagnosis, and management. 4th ed. Chicago: Quintessence pub. Co; 2008, 129-204.

Dibbets JM, Van der Weele LT. Long- term effects of orthodontic treatment, including extraction, on signs and symptoms attributed to CMD. Eur J Orthod.1992;14:16-20.

Dworkin S , LeResche L. Research diagnostic criteria for temporomandibular disorders: review, criteria, examinations and specifications, critique. J Craniomandib Disord Fac Oral Pain 1992; 6: 301-355.

Egermark-Eriksson I ,Carlsson GE ,Magnusson T , Thillander B. A longitudinal study on malocclusion in relation to signs and symptoms of cranio-mandibular disorders in children and adolescents. Eur J Orthod 1990; 12: 399-407.

Farella M, Michelotti A, Bocchino T, Cimino R, Laino A, Steenks MH. Effects of orthognatic surgery for class III malocclusion on signs and symptoms of temporomandibular disorders and on pressure pain thresholds of the jaw muscles. Int J Oral Maxillofac Surg.2007;36:583-587.

Friction JR , Schiffman EL. Epidemiology of temporomandibular disorders . in : Fricton JR , Dubner R (eds). Orofacial Pain and Temporomandibular Disorders. New York : Raven Press, 1995 ; 1-14.

Gallo LM, Gossi DB, Colombo V, Palla S. Relationship between kinematic center and TMJ anatomy and function. J Dent Res. 2008;87:726-730.

Greco CM, Rudy TE, Turk DC, Andrew H, Zaki HS. Traumatic onset of temporomandibular disorders. Positive effects of a standardized conservative treatment program. Clin J Pain 1997;13:337-347.

Greene CS. Laskin DM. Long-term status of TM clicking in patients with myofacial pain and dysfunction. J Am Dent Assoc. 1988;117:461-465.

Greene CS. Orthodontists and TMD. Orthodontic Products 2007;14:12.

Gremillion HA. The relationship between occlusion and TMD: an evidence based discussion. J.Evid Based Dent Pract 2006;6:43-47.

Gremillion HA. TMD and maladaptive occlusion : does a link exist ? J Craniomandib Pract 1995; 13(4): 205-6.

Henrikson T, Nilner M. Temporomandibular disorders and the need for stomatognathic treatment in orthodontically treated and untreated girls. Eur J Orthod. 2000;22:283-292.

Hollins M, Harper D, Gallagher S, Owings EW, Lim PF, Miller V et al. Perceived intensity and unpleasantness of cutaneous and auditory stimuli: an evaluation of the generalized hypervigilance hypothesis. Pain. 2009;141:215-221.

Keshvad A, Winstanley RB. An appraisal of the literature on centric relation. Part III. J Oral Rehab. 2001;28:55-63.

Kirveskari P , Alanen P , Jamsa T . Association between craniomandibular disorders and occlusal interferences in children. JProsthet Dent 1992 ; 67 : 692-6.

Le Bell Y , Niemi PM , Jamsa T, Kylmala M, Alanen P. Subjective reactions to intervention with artificial interferences in subjects with and without a history of temporomandibular disorders. Acta Odontol Scand. 2006;64:59-63.

Le Bell Y, Jamsa T, Korri S , Niemi PM , Alanen P . Effect of artificial occlusal interferences depends on previous experience of temporomandibular disorders. Acta Odontol Scand 2002; 60:219-222.

List T, Axelsson S. Management Of TMD : evidence from systemic reviews and meta-analyses. J Oral Rehabil. 2010:37:430-451.

List T, Helkimo M, Karlsson R: Pressure pain thresholds in patients with craniomandibular disorders before and after treatment with acupuncture and occlusal splint therapy: a controlled clinical study.Journal Of Orofacial Pain [J Orofac Pain] 1993 Summer; Vol. (3), 7: 275-282.

Luther F, Layton S, McDonald F. Orthodontics for treating temporomandibular joint (TMJ) disorders (review). Cochrane review;Cochrane library 2010, Issue 7.

Macfariane T, Kenealy P, Kingdon A, Mohlin B, Pilley R, Richmond S et al. Twenty-year cohort study of health gain from orthodontic treatment: temporomandibular disorders. AmJ Orthod Dentofacial Orthop. 2009;135:692.e1-692.e8.

Manfrendini D, Nardini LG. Daniele Manfrendini, TMD Classification and epidemiology.Current concepts on Temporomandibular Disorders.2010 Quintessence Publishing ;Chap 2:25-39.

Marbach JJ, Varoscak JR, Blank TR, Lund P. "Phantom bite": Classification and treatment. J. Prosthetic Dentistry. 1983 Vol. 49 (4), 556-559

McDermid AJ, Rollman GB, McCain GA. Generalized hypervigilance in fibromyalgia: evidence of perceptual amplification. Pain 1996;66:133-144.

McNamara JA Jr, Seligman DA, Okeson JP. Occlusion, orthodontic treatment, and temporomandibular disorders : a review . J Orofac Pain. 1995;9:73-90.

McNamara JA Jr, Turp JC. Orthodontic treatment and temporomandibular disorders:is there a relationship? Part 1: Clinical studies. J Orofac Orthop. 1997;58:74-89.

McNamara JA Jr. Orthodontic treatment and temporomandibular disorders. Oral Surg Oral Med Oral pathol Oral Radiol Endod. 1997;83:107-117.

Michelotti A, Farella M, Gallo LM , Veltri A , Palla S, Martina R . Effect of occlusal interferences on habitual activity of human masseter. J Dent Res. 2005;84:644-648.

Michelotti A, Iodice G . The role of orthodontics in temporomandibular disorders: J Oral Rehabilitation;vol 37:411-429 june 2010.

Mohlin BO, Derweduwen K, Pilley R, Kingdon A, Shaw WC, Kenealy P. Malocclusion and temporomandibular disorder a comparison of adolescents with moderate to severe dysfunction with those without signs and symptoms of temporomandibular disorders and their further development to 30 years of age. Angle Orthod 2004;74:319-327.

Niemi PM, Le Bell Y, Kylmälä M, Jämsa T, Alanen P: Psychological factors and responses to artificial interferences in subjects with and without a history of temporomandibular disorders. Acta Odontologica Scandinavica, 2006; 64: 300-305.

Okeson JP (editor): Management of Temporomandibular Disorders and Occlusion .5th edition, 2003, Mosby, St Louis, Missouri, page 159.

Pollack B . Cases of note. Michigan jury awards $ 850,000 on ortho case : a tempest in a teapot . Am J Orthod Dentofacial Orthop . 1988 ; 94:358-360.

Pullinger AG, Seligman DA, Gornbien JA. A multiple logistic regression analysis of the risk and relative odds of temporomandibular disorders as a function of common occlusal features. J Dent Res. 1993;72:968-979.

Raphael KG, Marbach JJ, Gallagher RM. Somatosensory Amplification and Affective Inhibition are elevated in Myofascial face Pain. Pain Med.2000;1:247-253.

Rey D, Oberti G, Bacceti T. Evaluation of temporomandibular disorders in class III patients treated with mandibular cervical headgear and fixed appliances. Am J Orthod Dentofacial Orthop.2008;133:379-381.

Richuse DJ, Kandasamy S. Myths of orthodontic gnathology. Am J Orthod Dentofacial Orthop. 2009;136:322-330.

Rudy TE, Turk DC, Kubinski JA, Zaki HS. Differential treatment response of TMD patients as a function of psychological characteristics. Pain 1995;61:103-112.

Rugh JD, Solberg WK. Oral health status in the United States. Temporomandibular disorders. Journal of Dental Education 1985;49:398-404.

Schiffman E, Fricton J, Haley D, Tylka D, A pressure algometer for myofascial pain syndrome; reliability and validity testing. In: Dubner, Gebhart CF, Bond MR (eds.). Proceedings of Vth World Congress on Pain. New York Elsevier Science, 1988:407-413.

Sphai TJ, Witzig JW. The clinical management of basic maxillofacial orthopedic appliances I. mechanics, lIttleton (MA): PSG publishing 1987.

Stholer CS, Zarb GA. On the management of temporomandibular disorders : a plea for a low-tech , high-prudence therapeutic approach. J Orofac Pain 1999;13:255-61.

The glossary of prosthodontic terms . J Prosthet Dent 2005 ;94:10-92.

Turk DC, Rudy TE, Kubinski JA, Zaki HS, Greco CM. Dysfunctional patients with temporomandibular disorders: evaluating the efficacy of a tailored treatment protocol. J Consult Clin Psychol 1996;64:139-146.

Turk DC, Zaki H, Rudy T. Effects of intraoral appliance and biofeedback/stress management alone and in combination in treating pain and depression in TMD patients. J Prosthet Dent 1993;70:158-164.

Turk DC. Psychosocial and behavioral assessment of patients with temporomandibular disorders: diagnostic and treatment implication. Oral Surg Oral Med Oral Pathol Oral Radiol Endod 1997;83:65-71.

15

Orthodontic Treatment and Temporomandibular Disorders

Ticiana Sidorenko de Oliveira Capote, Silvana Regina Perez Orrico, Juliana Álvares Duarte Bonini Campos, Fernanda Oliveira Bello Correa and Carolina Letícia Zilli Vieira
Araraquara School of Dentistry,
São Paulo State University, UNESP
Brazil

1. Introduction

Temporomandibular disorders (TMD) are characterized by dysfunctions involving the muscles related to chewing, the temporomandibular joint (TMJ) and associated structures.

The most frequent symptom is pain, generally located in the chewing muscles, preauricular area and/or TMJ. In addition to pain, patients often experience limited or asymmetric mandibular movements and TMJ sounds most frequently described as snapping, cracking, gnashing or crepitating and headaches may also occur (Okeson, 1998).

Some studies have demonstrated that morphological malocclusions and occlusal interferences alone may not be considered as etiological factors for the development of TMJ dysfunctions (Vanderas, 1993; Perry, 1995). They may be considered as predisposing factors of TMD because currently psychological aspects are more associated with the appearance of the dysfunction.

However according to Mongini (1977), the occurrence of dysfunctional problems of the stomatognathic system may be related to the termination of orthodontic treatment. Other authors have demonstrated the need for occlusal therapy after termination of orthodontic treatment in order to eliminate the risk of bone reabsorption, muscular pain and TMJ disorders resulting from occlusal trauma (Salzman, 1974; Runge et al., 1989; Gianelly, 1989, Kundinger et al., 1991).

Abd Al-Hadi (1993) showed a high dependence between the frequency of TMD and malocclusion class II division I of Angle, function in group, high values of horizontal overlap and a larger number of contacts on the balancing-side. However Kahn et al. (1999), studying the relationship between occlusion and TMD, suggested the lack of any specific difference in the type of occlusal contacts that distinguish symptomatic from asymptomatic patients.

Winocur et al. (2001), assessing the contribution of some parafunctional activities in the appearance of TMD symptoms, concluded that jaw play was the characteristic most associated to deleterious habits and that the chronic use of chewing gum was an important contributor to noises and pain in the joints.

Considering the multifactorial etiology of TMD, its understanding, treatment and possible prevention becomes one of the greatest challenges for practitioners and their patients. So in view of the need for more studies that correlate TMD and predisposing factors, the objective of this study was to analyze the interaction among TMD, orthodontic treatment and some occlusal characteristics.

2. Materials and methods

The study was submitted and approved by the Human Research Ethics Committee of the Araraquara School of Dentistry, UNESP (no. 112/2000) and all patients signed an informed consent for participating in the study.

Seventy three patients were selected, 40 women and 33 men, ranging from 15 to 25 years of age and with no race distinction. Thirty six individuals had been submitted to orthodontic treatment with a fixed apparatus during periods ending from 6 months to 2 years prior to the study (experimental group). Thirty seven patients who never received orthodontic treatment had normal occlusion (control group). The selected patients had 24 to 32 completely erupted teeth with few dental restorations, no prostheses, no occlusal adjustments and no TMD treatment was conducted prior to the study.

The presence of signs and symptoms of TMD was evaluated by means of a questionnaire providing an anamnestic index (Fonseca, 1994), with a variation ranging from the absence of TMD (0 to 19), to mild TMD (20 to 44), moderate TMD (45 to 69), and severe TMD (70 to 100).

For occlusal evaluation, contacts were analyzed in maximum habitual intercuspal position, with the odontological chair positioned at 180° (lying down position) and at 90° (sitting position). The contacts were marked with the aid of a film for occlusal recording.

The mandible was guided to perform lateral movements to the right and left, mapping contacts and interferences on the balancing and working-sides. The lateral disocclusion was classified as canine guidance (contact between canines on the working side, disoccluding the teeth on the balancing side), partial (contact between canines and premolars on the working side, disoccluding the teeth on the balancing side), in group (contact between canines, premolars and molars on the working side, disoccluding the teeth on the balancing side), or atypical (lateral guidance differing from those mentioned above, such as eccentric movement with disocclusion caused by the incisors and the presence of contacts on the balancing side).

All data were collected by a single previously trained and calibrated examiner and noted on an odontogram designed for this study.

2.1 Statistical analysis

The interaction among the variables temporomandibular disorder (TMD) (absent, present) and orthodontic treatment (Yes, No) with the variables right lateral type of disocclusion, left lateral type of disocclusion and gender (male, female), being assessed separately, was estimated with a log-linear analysis with a Poisson probability model.

In order to compare the average of occlusal contacts and the number of interferences, according to the absence or presence of TMD and orthodontic treatment, the two-factor Analysis of Variance was applied. The hypothesis of normality and homoscedasticity of the dependent variables were assessed by using Shapiro-Wilk's and Levene's test, respectively.

3. Results

Seventy-three individuals participated, from whom 54.8% were female, 50.7% had not been submitted to orthodontic treatment, and 89% presented some degree of temporomandibular disorder. The average age was 20.03±3.38 years old.

The distribution of the participants according to gender, temporomandibular disorder and orthodontic treatment can be found in Table 1.

Variable	**Orthodontic Treatment**	
Temporomandibular Disorder (TMD)	Without	With
Absent	18 (48.6)	22 (61.1)
Mild	14 (37.8)	11 (30.6)
Moderate	5 (13.5)	3 (8.3)
Gender		
Male	16 (43.2)	17 (47.2)
Female	21 (56.8)	19 (52.8)

Table 1. Distribution of individuals according to gender, temporomandibular disorder and orthodontic treatment.

The interaction among the variables temporomandibular disorder (TMD) (absent TMD=0, present TMD=1) and orthodontic treatment (Yes, No) with the variable right lateral type of disocclusion is shown in Table 2.

	No orthodontic treatment		**Orthodontic treatment**		
Right lateral disocclusion	**TMD=0**	**TMD=1**	**TMD=0**	**TMD=1**	**Total**
Canine	10	6	17	6	39
Partial	2	4	3	1	10
In group	1	4	-	3	8
Atypical	5	5	2	4	16
Total	18	19	22	14	73

Table 2. Distribution of individuals according to orthodontic treatment, presence (TMD=1) or absence (TMD=0) of temporomandibular disorder and right lateral disocclusion.

The pattern of total independence between the variables reproduces, appropriately, the scores observed (G^2=18.153; p=0.078). There is evidence that the variables are independent (χ^2=16.852; p=0.112).

The interaction among the variables temporomandibular disorder (TMD) (absent TMD=0, present TMD=1) and orthodontic treatment (Yes, No) with the variable left lateral type of disocclusion is shown in Table 3.

	No orthodontic treatment		Orthodontic Treatment		
Left lateral disocclusion	**TMD=0**	**TMD=1**	**TMD=0**	**TMD=1**	**Total**
Canine	8	9	12	9	38
Partial	3	2	5	1	11
In group	2	5	2	1	10
Atypical	5	3	3	3	14
Total	18	19	22	14	73

Table 3. Distribution of individuals according to orthodontic treatment, presence (TMD=1) or absence (TMD=0) of temporomandibular disorder and left lateral disocclusion.

In the same way as previously, the variables left lateral type of disocclusion, orthodontic treatment and temporomandibular disorder reproduce, appropriately, the scores observed (G^2=7.534; p=0.674). There is evidence that the variables are independent (χ^2=8.083; p=0.621).

The interaction among the variables temporomandibular disorder (TMD) (absent TMD=0, present TMD=1) and orthodontic treatment (Yes, No) with the variable gender is shown in Table 4.

	No orthodontic treatment		Orthodontic treatment		
Gender	**TMD=0**	**TMD=1**	**TMD=0**	**TMD=1**	**Total**
Male	9	7	9	8	33
Female	9	12	13	6	40
Total	18	19	22	14	73

Table 4. Distribution of individuals according to orthodontic treatment, presence (TMD=1) or absence (TMD=0) of temporomandibular disorder and gender.

The variables gender, orthodontic treatment and temporomandibular disorder reproduce appropriately, either, the scores observed (G^2=2.825; p=0.588). There is evidence that the variables are independent (χ^2=2.778; p=0.596).

The interaction among the variables temporomandibular disorder (TMD) (absent TMD=0, present TMD=1), orthodontic treatment (Yes, No) with the variables number of contacts in sitting position, number of contacts in lying down position, age, number of occlusal interferences on the right side, number of occlusal interferences on the left side is shown in Table 5.

The individuals who were not submitted to orthodontic treatment were significantly older and showed a higher number of sitting contacts and a higher number of left lateral interferences. The individuals without TMD showed a number of sitting and lying down contacts, significantly higher than those individuals with TMD.

	No orthodontic treatment		Orthodontic treatment		ANOVA (p)		
Variable	TMD=0	TMD=1	TMD=0	TMD=1	ortho	TMD	interaction
Sitting P.	30.33±7.68	21.37±6.17	26.27±9.05	18.29±3.43	0.040	<0.001	0.775
Lying P.	28.06±10.29	18.16±8.87	29.86±10.99	24.64±7.50	0.076	0.002	0.313
Age	21.28±2.14	22.16±1.46	17.64±3.66	19.29±3.71	<0.001	0.069	0.577
R Inter.	0.28±0.46	0.47±0.70	0.18±0.39	0.14±0.36	0.077	0.511	0.327
L Inter.	0.44±0.62	0.42±0.77	0.14±0.35	0.07±0.27	0.013	0.734	0.873

Table 5. Distribution of individuals according to orthodontic treatment, presence (TMD=1) or absence (TMD=0) of temporomandibular disorder, number of contacts in sitting position, number of contacts in lying down position, age, number of occlusal interferences on the right side and number of occlusal interferences on the left side.

4. Discussion

Many etiological factors had been related to TMD among which may be cited arthritis, tumors, congenital malformation, traumatic injuries, degenerative and neurological alterations, muscular diseases, cerebrovascular diseases, occlusal interferences and psychological aspects. According to Okeson (1998) a specific and unique etiologic factor has not been detected.

Over the years, much was discussed about the role of occlusal factors in the etiology of TMD.

Although Schwartz & Chayes (1968) believe that dental occlusion is a secondary factor in the development of TMD, other studies (Stuart, 1964; Guichet & Niles, 1970) have indicated occlusal interference as the primary etiological factor.

On the other hand, Mohlin & Kopp (1978) and Seligman et al. (1988), evaluating patients regarding the presence of dysfunction and pain in the masticatory muscles, concluded that there was no significant correlation between occlusal interferences and these alterations.

To evaluate the distribution of occlusal contacts in individuals with TMD, Ciancaglini et al. (2002) developed a study with 25 students, of both genders aged 19 to 30, that presented signs and symptoms of TMD and 25 subjects in the control group. No difference was found regarding the total number, distribution and intensity of the contacts between the groups. However, intraindividual analysis demonstrated that there was a significant bilateral asymmetry in the number of contacts in both groups. Ciancaglini et al. (2003) verified the existence of a weak correlation between unilateral TMD and the number of occlusal contacts.

According to our results, the individuals without TMD showed a number of sitting and lying down contacts significantly higher than those individuals with TMD.

The importance of occlusal factors in the complex and controversial concept of TMD etiology cannot be totally neglected. Weak, but still significant associations were found between long-term development of TMD, and some malocclusions like a lateral forced bite between retruded contact position and intercuspal position, as well as unilateral crossbite, may be a potential risk factor in this respect (Egermark et al., 2003).

The possible relationship of orthodontic treatment with signs and symptoms of TMD has also been studied lately.

He et al. (2010) verified centric relation-maximum intercuspation discrepancy in 107 pre-treated orthodontic patients with signs and symptoms of TMD and concluded that this discrepancy may be a contributory factor to the development of TMD in these patients.

Karjalainen et al. (1997) evaluated 123 healthy adolescents who had undergone orthodontic treatment regarding the presence of TMD signs and symptoms. The experimental group (patients that presented signs and symptoms of TMD) received occlusal adjustment at base line and repeated every 6 months thereafter, as needed. After 3 years, 96% of the patients returned for revaluation and the number of individuals with muscular pain and signs of TMD diminished significantly in the experimental group but not in the control group. The authors concluded that a therapy of occlusal adjustment may prevent the occurrence of signs of TMD in healthy adolescents that have had orthodontic treatment.

Conti et al. (2003) evaluated the prevalence of temporomandibular disorders in 200 individuals with 9 to 20 years of age, before and after orthodontic treatment. When the TMD anamnestic index for the whole sample was considered, 34% of the subjects had mild TMD, 3.5% had moderate TMD, and 62.5% were considered TMD free. The presence and severity of TMD have not shown any relationship with type of orthodontic mechanics, so the authors concluded that orthodontic treatment was not associated with presence of signs and symptoms of TMD.

In our study, it was found 61.1% of the orthodontic treated individuals had TMD free, 30.6% had mild TMD and 8.3% had moderate TMD. As well as in the study of Conti et al. (2003), no subjects presented severe TMD. Comparing the orthodontically treated and not treated groups according to the presence of TMD, it was observed that in both groups a higher percentage of the sample was associated with absence of TMD and with mild TMD, and no significant interaction between TMD and orthodontic treatment was verified in the different scores.

As such, recommendations concerning the need for occlusal adjustments after orthodontic therapy as a measure to prevent the appearance or aggravation of signs and symptoms of TMD are not conclusive.

In agreement with other studies (Sadowsky & Begole, 1980; Rendell et al., 1992) no significant correlation between TMD and orthodontic treatment was verified in the different scores.

Sadowsky & Polson (1984) reported that orthodontic treatment performed during adolescence does not generally increase or decrease the risk of developing TMD in later life. Similar results were found by Egermark et al. (2003). After a 20-year follow up of the influence of orthodontic treatment on signs and symptoms of TMDs, the authors verified that subjects who have received orthodontic treatment do not run a higher risk of developing signs and symptoms of TMD later in life.

Thus, the present study showed no difference between the orthodontically treated and nontreated groups in terms of the different TMD scores, although the treated group had not been evaluated regarding the presence or absence of TMD before orthodontic therapy.

Other authors (Ricketts, 1966; Roth, 1973) disagree and have demonstrated that orthodontic treatment is a possible cause of TMD. Roth analyzed patients of both genders submitted to orthodontic treatment and others not submitted, regarding signs and symptoms of TMD and concluded that in the female patients who had orthodontic treatment presented a significant correlation with facial symptoms of dysfunction.

In this study, it was observed no significant interaction between gender and presence or signs and symtoms of TMD. Some authors agree (Wigdorowicz-Makowerowa et al., 1979; Ludeen et al., 1986; Abd Al-Hadi, 1993) while others (Seligman et al., 1988; Mello & Araújo, 1997; Teixeira et al., 1999; Conti et al., 2003) demonstrate a predominance of the female over the male gender in young patients.

Abd Al-Hadi evaluated 600 asymptomatic students, of both genders ranging from 22 to 28 years of age. The authors verified a significant correlation between TMD and chewing side preference. In addition, as the number of contacts on the non-working side increased, the association with TMD also increased. Nevertheless, no association with gender was observed.

According to the results of this study, no significant interactions were found among occlusal characteristics (type of disocclusion and occlusal interferences) and TMD.

Kahn et al. evaluated the association between molar relationship, lateral movement, and nonworking side contacts with intraarticular TMD. The results demonstrated that symptomatic patients presented a higher prevalence of class II, division 1 related to the left side when compared to the control group. There was a higher prevalence of canine guidance on the right side of symptomatic patients with disk displacement. Asymptomatic patients had a higher prevalence of one or more non-working side contacts compared with symptomatic patients with normal joints and symptomatics with disc displacement. As such the authors were unable to demonstrate a relation between the characteristics studied and intraarticular TMD.

Henrikson & Nilner (2003) observed that orthodontic treatment either with or without extractions did not increase the prevalence or worsen pre-treatment symptoms and signs of TMD, however, the authors verified that type of occlusion may play a role as a contributing factor for the development of TMD. Valle-Corotti et al. (2007) also found that some occlusal characteristics (non-working side contacts) can be factors of risk of TMD, and verified that Class III orthodontic treatment was not associated with the presence of TMD signs and symptoms.

No relationship was found between orthodontic treatment and TMD, but a positive association between TMD and parafunctional habits and reported emotional tension was verified in the study of Conti et al., 2003. According to the authors, the emotional tension is a very frequent complaint in our days, can affect general health and can predispose and cause muscle contractions and parafunctional habits, increasing the risk of initiating TMD symptoms.

It was verified no relationship between TMD and orthodontic treatment in the most of cases, but discussions are still relevant. Although the parafunctional habits and emotional factors are closely related to the etiology of TMD, occlusal characteristics can't be neglected since some studies still find occlusal risk factors for TMDs.

5. Conclusion

According to the results of our study, it was observed no relationship between TMD and orthodontic treatment, and there was no interaction among TMD and characteristics such as gender, lateral type of disocclusion and number of occlusal interferences.

6. References

Abd Al-Hadi, L. (1993). Prevalence of temporomandibular disorders in relation to some occlusal parameters. *The Journal of Prosthetic Dentistry*, Vol. 70, pp.(345-350), ISSN 0022-3913

Ciancaglini, R; Gherlone, EF; Redaelli, S; Radaelli, G. (2002). The distribution of occlusal contacts in the intercuspal position and temporomandibular disorder. *Journal of Oral Rehabilitation*, Vol. 29, pp.(1082-1090), ISSN 0305-182X

Ciancaglini, R; Gherlone, EF; Redaelli, G. (2003). Unilateral temporomandibular disorder and asymmetry of occlusion contacts. *Journal of Oral Rehabilitation*, Vol. 89,pp. (180-185), ISSN 0305-182X

Conti, A; Freita, M; Conti, P; Henriques, J; Janson, G. (2003). Relationship between signs and symptoms of temporomandibular disorders and orthodontic treatment: a cross-sectional study. *The Angle Orthodontist*, Vol. 73, pp. (411-417), ISSN 0003-3219

Egermark, I; Magnusson, T; Carlsson, GE. (2003). A 20-year follow up of signs and symtoms of temporomandibular disorders and malocclusions in subjects with and without orthodontic treatment in childhood. *The Angle Orthodontist*, Vol. 73, pp. (109-115), ISSN 0003-3219

Fonseca, DM; Bonfante, G; Valle, AL; Freitas, SFT. (1994). Diagnóstico pela anamnese da disfunção crânio-mandibular. *Revista Gaúcha de Odontologia*, Vol. 42, pp. (23-28), ISSN 1981-8637

Gianelly, AA. (1989). Orthodontics, condylar position, and TMJ status. *American Journal of Orthodontics and Dentofacial Orthopedics*, Vol. 95, pp.(521-523). ISSN 0889-5406

Guichet, NF; Niles, F. *Principle of occlusion – A collection of monographs*. Denar Corporation. California: Anaheim, 1970.

He, SS; Deng, X; Wamalwa, P; Chen, S. (2010). Correlation between centric relation-maximum intercuspation discrepancy and temporomandibular joint dysfunction. *Acta Odontologica Scandinavica*, Vol. 68, pp. (368-376), ISSN 0001-6357

Henrikson, T; Nilner, M. (2003). Temporomandibular disorders, occlusion and orthodontic treatment. *Journal of Orthodontics*, Vol. 30, pp. (129-137), ISSN 1465-3125

Kahn, J; Tallents, RH; Katzberg, RW; Ross, EM; Murphy, WC. (1999). Prevalence of dental occlusal variables and intraarticular temporomandibular disorders: molar relationship, lateral guidance, and nonworking side contacts. *The Journal of Prosthetic Dentistry*, Vol. 82, pp. (410-415), ISSN 0022-3913

Karjalainen, M; Le Bell, Y; Jamsa, T; Karjalainen, S. (1997). Prevention of temporomandibular disorder - related signs and symptoms in orthodontically treated adolescents. *Acta Odontologica Scandinavica*, Vol. 55, pp. (319-324), ISSN 0001-6357

Kundinger, KK; Austin, BP; Christensen, LV; Donegan, SJ; Ferguson, DJ. (1991). An evaluation of temporomandibular joints and jaw muscles after orthodontic treatment involving premolar extractions. *American Journal of Orthodontics and Dentofacial Orthopedics*, Vol. 100, pp. (110-115). ISSN 0889-5406

Lundeen, TF; Levitt, SR; McKinney, MW. (1986). Discriminative ability of the TMJ scale: age and gender differences. *The Journal of Prosthetic Dentistry*, Vol. 56, pp (84-92), ISSN 0022-3913

Mello, JB; Araújo, MAM. (1997). Incidência de disfunção da ATM em relação a ausência de guia anterior. *Revista Odontológica do Brasil Central*, Vol. 6, No.22, pp. (52-55), ISSN 1981-3708

Mohlin, B; Kopp, S. (1978). A clinical study on the relationship between malocclusion, occlusal interferences and mandibular pain and dysfunction. *Swedish Dental Journal*, Vol. 2, pp. (105-112), ISSN 0347-9994

Mongini, F. (1977). Anatomic and clinical evaluation of the relationship between the temporomandibular joint and occlusion. *The Journal of Prosthetic Dentistry*, Vol. 38, pp. (539-551), ISSN 0022-3913

Okeson, JP. *Orofacial pain: guidelines for assessment, diagnosis, and management.* The American Academy of Orofacial Pain. Chicago: Quintessence, 1998: 1-287.

Perry, HT. (1995). Temporomandibular joint and occlusion. *The Angle Orthodontist*, Vol. 46, pp. (205-214), ISSN 0003-3219

Rendell, JK; Norton, LA; Gay, T. (1992). Orthodontic treatment and temporomandibular joint disorders. *American Journal of Orthodontics and Dentofacial Orthopedics*, Vol. 101, pp. (84-87), ISSN 0889-5406

Ricketts, RM. (1966). Clinical implications of the temporomandibular joint. *American Journal of Orthodontics*, Vol. 43, pp. (136-152), ISSN 0002-9416

Roth, RH. (1973). Temporomandibular pain-dysfunction and occlusal relationships. *The Angle Orthodontist*, Vol. 43, pp. (136-153), ISSN 0003-3219

Runge, ME; Sadowsky, C; Sakols, EI; BeGole, EA. (1989). The relationship between temporomandibular joint sounds and malocclusion. *American Journal of Orthodontics and Dentofacial Orthopedics*, Vol. 96, pp. (36-42), ISSN 0889-5406

Sadowsky, C; Begole, EA. (1980). Long term status of temporomandibular joint function and functional occlusion after orthodontic treatment. *American Journal of Orthodontics*, Vol. 78, pp. (201-212), ISSN 0002-9416

Sadowsky, C; Polson, AM. (1984). Temporomandibular disorders and functional occlusion after orthodontic treatment: results of two long-term studies. *American Journal of Orthodontics*, Vol. 86, No. 5, pp. (386-390), ISSN 0002-9416

Salzman, JA. *Orthodontics in daily practice*, Philadelphia: Lippincott, 1974: 621-626.

Schwartz, L; Chayes, CM. (1968). *Facial pain and mandibular dysfunction*. W.B. Saunders Co., Philadelphia.

Seligman, DA; Pullinger, AG; Solberg, WK. (1988). Temporomandibular disorders. Part III: occlusal and articular factors associated with muscle tenderness. *The Journal of Prosthetic Dentistry*, Vol. 59, pp. (483-489), ISSN 0022-3913

Stuart, CE. (1964) Good occlusion for natural teeth. *The Journal of Prosthetic Dentistry*,Vol. 14, pp. (716-724), ISSN 0022-3913

Teixeira, ACB; Marcucci, G; Luz, JGC. (1999). Prevalência das maloclusões e dos índices anamnésicos e clínicos, em pacientes com disfunção da articulação temporomandibular. *Revista de Odontologia Universidade de São Paulo*, Vol. 13, PP. (251-256), ISSN 0103-0663

Valle-Corotti, K; Pinzan, A; Valle, CVM; Nahás, ACR; Corotti, MV. (2007). Assessment of temporomandibular disorder and occlusion in treated class III malocclusion patients. *Journal of Applied Oral Science*, Vol. 15, No. 2, pp. (110-114), ISSN 1678-7757

Vanderas, AP. (1993). Relations between malocclusion and craniomandibular dysfunction in children and adolescents: a review. *Pediatric Dentistry*, Vol. 15, pp. (317-322), ISSN 0164-1263

Wigdorowicz-Makowerowa, N; Grodzki, G; Panek, H; Maslanka, T; Plonka, K; Palacha, A. (1979). Epidemiologic studies on prevalence and etiology of functional disturbances of the masticatory system. *The Journal of Prosthetic Dentistry*, Vol. 41, pp.(76-82), ISSN 0022-3913

Winocur, E; Gavish, A; Finkelstein, T; Halachmi, M; Gazit, E. (2001). Oral habits among adolescents girls and their association with symptoms of temporomandibular disorders. *Journal of Oral Rehabilitation*, Vol. 28, pp. (624-629), ISSN 0305-182X

16

Temporomandibular Disorders and Orthodontic Treatment – A Review with a Reported Clinical Case

Tomislav Badel[1], Miljenko Marotti[2] and Ivana Savić Pavičin[3]
[1]*Department of Prosthodontics, School of Dental Medicine, University of Zagreb*
[2]*Department of Diagnostic and Interventional Radiology, "Sestre Milosrdnice" University Hospital Center, University of Zagreb*
[3]*Department of Dental Anthropology, School of Dental Medicine, University of Zagreb*
Croatia

1. Introduction

Temporomandibular disorders (TMDs) are musculoskeletal disorders affecting the temporomandibular joint (TMJ), the masticatory muscles (myogenic subgroup), or both, and they are the most common cause of orofacial somatic nonodontogenic pain. Osteoarthritis (OA) and disc displacement (DD) of TMJ belong to the arthrogenic subgroup of TMDs (Okeson & de Leeuw, 2011).

The aim of the paper is to evaluate the relationship between malocclusion, orthodontic treatment and development of TMD. The article includes a 5-year follow-up of a female patient who underwent orthodontic treatment instead of TMD treatment.

2. Diagnostics of painful TMDs

The multifactorial etiopathogenic models of TMDs have no practical use at patient level because certain occlusal conditions, exposure to psychological macrotrauma, bruxist behaviour, etc., cannot be associated with TMD symptoms which are exhibited by the patient. Idiopathic (nonspecific) etiology imposes a personalised approach to every single patient during diagnostics, planning and the use of treatment modalities as well as during recall. TMD symptomatology includes the main symptoms such as pain of masticatory muscles and/or TMJ, limited and painful mouth opening as well as pathologic noise in the joints. Pain is the most important symptom in TMDs pathogenesis due to which patients seek treatment and therefore, the main aim of the treatment is pain removal (Jürgens, 2009).

The biopsychosocial component is strongly based on chronification of musculoskeletal pain. The biopsychosocial concept includes a combination of biological and psychological considerations on the etiology of TMDs, particularly those accompanied by chronic pain. Chronic pain has its etiologic basis in somatosensory and psychosocial factors. Patients with chronic pain live with their biological problem (pain activation with or without obvious pathology), which can have a psychological foundation as well as effects on their behaviour. Specific social (interpersonal) relations often have negative effects for patients (Türp, 2000; Giannakopoulos et al., 2010).

The most widespread system of standardised examination of patients and asymptomatic individuals is the use of RDC (Research diagnostic criteria)/TMD, which includes a clinical examination in Axis I, and a psychiatric testing in Axis II (Dworkin & Le Resche, 1992). RDC/TMD system classifies TMDs into three subclasses: muscle disorders, DD, and arthralgia/arthritis/arthropathy. The importance of such a system is that it shows a possibility of defining certain diagnoses of TMDs wherein the diagnosis of one subgroup does not exclude the diagnosis from the other subgroup in the same patient. Nevertheless, there are certain limitations because RDC/TMD does not include a supplementary magnetic resonance imaging (MRI) diagnostics.

2.1 Manual functional analysis

Bumann in collaboration with Groot Landeweer provided an overall system to diagnose TMDs, and, together with Lotzmann, confirmed it by thorough MRI diagnostics of TMJ (Bumann & Lotzmann, 2002). The use of manual functional analysis (MFA) is particularly stressed in the evaluation of the condition of the stomatognathic system prior to major irreversible procedures in order to avoid delayed detection of more or less pronounced clinical signs and symptoms of TMDs which would not be recognized and treated on time in such a case (Figure 1). MFA is a result of collaboration between the orthodontist and physiotherapist and its first purpose was to perform screenings prior to orthodontic treatment (Bumann & Lotzmann, 2002). By including MRI along with prior use of MFA, the less known diagnoses can be established such as partial DD and DD upon excursive movement of TMJ (Badel et al., 2009a).

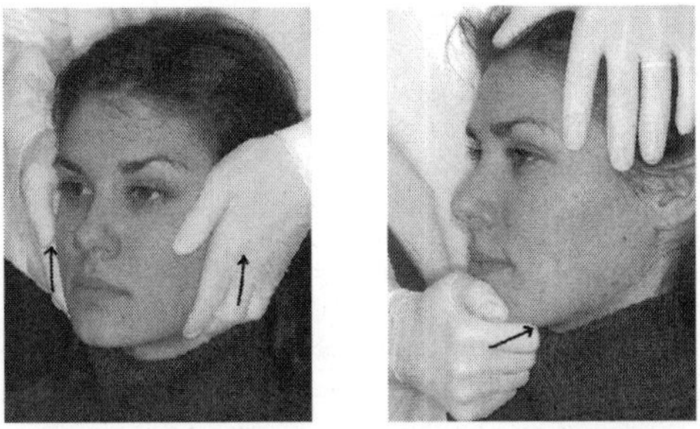

Fig. 1. Dynamic compression starts with the therapist cranially pressuring the distal edge of the mandibular corpus (left), and dorsal passive compression (right).

The main purpose of clinical diagnostics is to determine the pathological condition of masticatory muscles and/or the TMJs. A standard dental examination focusing on dental status and occlusion is insufficient for diagnostics as well as just measuring the mouth opening (Kropmans et al., 2000). Manual diagnostic methods of the stomatognathic system are necessary for (von Piekartz, 2005):

- differential diagnostics of muscular, arthrogenic disorder or both;
- determining the status of the articular disc and the articular surfaces;
- measuring the passive capacity of mouth opening, and
- making specific diagnoses.

2.2 Clinical importance of imaging modalities

A limiting factor in the study of TMDs is radiologic diagnostics, which is often used in dental treatment of teeth and jaw bones. Traditional x-ray images as well as conventional and computed tomography (CT) cannot show all the functional elements of TMJ. The key component in articular biomechanics is the relationship between the articular plate or disc as a cartilaginous structure and the condylar head as an osseous structure. Another factor is the disc-condyle complex relationship with the posterior plane of the articular eminence, across which the articular complex moves simultaneously on mouth opening.

Ahmad et al. (2009) believe that panoramic x-ray and TMJ radiography should not be included into diagnostic procedure at the specialist level. CT is indicated in individuals who have clinical signs of OA and who cannot be exposed to strong magnetic field due to claustrophobia, metal implants or pacemakers. In individuals with such limitations, CT would not be an adequate diagnostic means if they only have DD without any changes in hard osseous tissues. When the MRI finding of OA needs to be confirmed by CT, which is still the gold standard in diagnostics of osseous tissues of joints (Figure 2), one should bear in mind the exposure to x-ray radiation. MRI is a radiologic technique of layered imaging in the desired plane without moving the body and without exposing the patient to ionised radiation. As in the other fields of diagnostics in medicine, MRI is qualitatively better because it enables imaging of soft tissues without invasive effects on the recorded object as opposed to arthrography. Therefore, MRI has become the gold standard of diagnostics and the dominant radiologic technique in diagnostics of TMDs enabling the imaging of cartilaginous articular surfaces and it can successfully show the position of the articular disc (Badel et al., 2009a; Badel et al., 2010a).

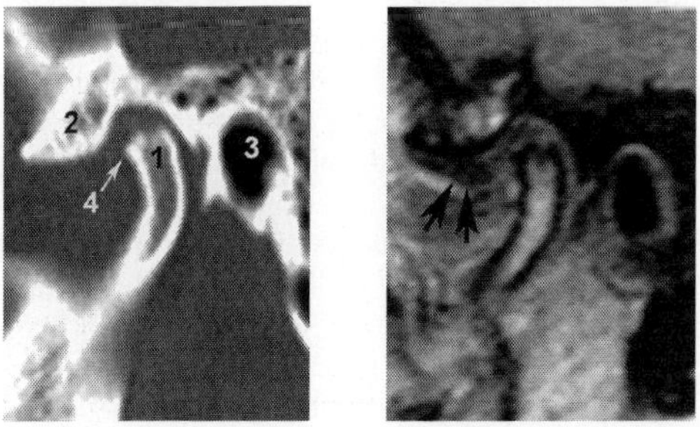

Fig. 2. Computed tomography (left) of temporomandibular joint with degenerative bone changes (1 condyle, 2 articular eminence, 3 external acoustical meatus, 4 osteophyte) and magnetic resonance imaging (right) with anterior displaced disc (arrow).

In orthopedics, the possibilities of manual tests and limitations of traditional radiologic examinations as well as advantages of MRI have already been evaluated. The relationship between pain and diagnostic findings has also been researched, particularly the relationship between the knee and the lumbar region of the spine. Regarding clinical diagnostics, Palla (1998) concluded that certain forms of TMDs do not have specific signs, that is, certain diagnostic tests have low validity and reliability.

3. Epidemiology of TMD and the use of MRI

A high prevalence of symptoms, 25-75%, out of which the major part of the symptoms were pathological noise in the TMJ, was determined in general population by various methods of data gathering (questionnaires, clinical examination, use of radiologic modalities). Although there are some methodological discrepancies which can be hinder the direct comparison of epidemiologic results of TMD, it is certain that temporomandibular pain has a low prevalence, mostly less than 10% of general population, and most often only 5% (Durham, 2008). In an epidemiologic study, Gesch et al. (2004a) determined by a clinical examination of 49.9% of the population that there is at least one clinical sign of TMD, whereas only 2.7% had painful TMJ.

Another issue in the TMD epidemiology is dependence on the age and gender of the patient. Manfredini et al. (2010) differentiated two age peaks (two peaks of greatest incidence) in TMD patients (30-35 and 50-55 years) with female: male ration 5:1, which partly coincides with previous knowledge that the greatest prevalence is in women of reproductive age (that is between 18-45) (Palla, 1998; Badel, 2007a; Durham, 2008). Although osteoarthritis has only partly greater prevalence in elderly people, it is obvious that TMDs do not progress with patients' age. Using MRI, Schmitter et al. (2010) proved that in elderly population, each gender equally, there is a discrepancy of high incidence (70%) of OA signs accompanied by low incidence of clinical signs of TMD (out of 30 subjects only one had painful TMJ). Predominance of females in TMD patients is explained by the effects of female hormones or attribute this to the gender distinction, biological and physiological differences, behavioural characteristics, and genetic factors (Wang et al., 2008).

In order to plan and perform orthodontic treatment, it is important to have all the data regarding TMD symptoms as well as the need to treat them in the population of children and adolescents during the period of growth and the development of jaws and teeth. The issue of orthodontics is related to data gathered within epidemiologic studies of young people. In this way, in a group of adolescents and young adults, Casanova-Rosado et al. (2006) found that 16.55% of them had orthodontic treatment. Some grade of TMD was found by clinical examination in 46.1% of subjects, predominantly females with bruxist behaviour and psychosocial variables (stress and anxiety). However, it is not evident to what extent were the subjects treated orthodontically. Le Resche et al. (2005) pointed to the higher prevalence of pain, including TMD pain (in terms of multiple pain problems) during pubescent development of girls. Pereira et al. (2009) found at least one sign or symptom of TMD in 12.26% of children aged between 4-12 (in 5 boys and 8 girls). Bonjardim et al. (2003) determined a low prevalence of TMD signs and symptoms in children aged between 3 and 5 (primary dentition): 3.03% had TMJ sounds and 4.04% had jaw pain without any gender differences. Köhler et al. (2009) followed the occurrence of signs and symptoms of TMD during 20 years, with the first examination at the age of three. It was determined that TMD symptoms had higher incidence in later examinations (incidence 5-9%) while at the youngest age, there was almost none. However, the need for treatment is particularly low

(1-2%). Huddleston Slater et al. (2007) did a targeted research into prevalence of anterior DD with reduction (accompanied by reciprocal clicking in the TMJ) in children and adolescents which increases with their age, yet there is no statistical difference in prevalence between a subgroup of 18-year-old adolescents and two age groups of adults aged on average 21.9 and 43.5. Prevalence of DD with reduction je rose to 26.6% in adulthood.

MRI diagnostics of a 12-year-old female patient with clinical signs and symptoms of clicking in both jaws was performed as a part of pre-orthodontic treatment. The MRI finding confirmed DD with reduction in the left and without reduction in the right TMJ. The MRI follow-up finding remained unchanged after the treatment of unilateral cross bite. Painless clicking as a compensated condition of TMJ was not sufficient as a symptom which would indicate TMD treatment (Badel et al., 2008a).

In a sample of 40 patients with DD confirmed by MRI, Badel (2007a, 2008b) showed that 25% of them underwent orthodontic treatment (mainly by removable appliances), while in 5 asymptomatic subjects (20%) DD was also determined. Nevertheless, since the asymptomatic group was a population of students of similar age, the share of those with previously performed orthodontic treatments was 40%. Treatment by a fixed appliance was previously performed in an asymptomatic female subject with physiological disc position. Similarly, Katzberg et al. (1996) did not find any correspondence between orthodontic treatment and DD prevalence in patients (77%) and also in asymptomatic subjects (33%).

MRI provides better imaging of soft and hard TMJ structures and since it is not an invasive procedure, it is also used in children of the youngest age. Research has shown that DD is not a congenital disorder and according to Paesani et al. (1999), which has also been confirmed by clinical epidemiologic studies, develops only in older children and adults with the prevalence of as much as 45% (Haiter-Neto et al., 2002). However, studies do not show to what extent is asymptomatic DD related to a possible previous orthodontic treatment (Haiter-Neto et al., 2002).

Numerous studies of TMD patients confirmed the efficiency of MRI use with respect to clinical signs of the disorder (Moen et al., 2010). MRI was very useful in finding or controlling a therapeutic condylar position and its effects on the intraarticular function of TMJ, especially disc position. It has been used in long-term follow-ups of patients without evidence of serious progression of pathological changes in intraarticular structures (de Bont et. al., 1997). Even the subsequent occurrence of osteoarthritic changes in joints of DD patients during the follow-up period did not have clinical manifestations (Kurita et al., 2006). On the other hand, Tominaga et al. (2007) pointed to the changes in disc position with partial displacement occurring in the period of children's growth and development. This stresses the need for thorough analysis of TMJ on three representative layers in an oblique sagittal line in order to avoid doubts about the usefulness of MRI findings (Bumann & Lotzmann, 2002), which still poses a problem of how to interpret the disc image with respect to its physiological position or anterior displacement (Petersson, 2010).

Jensen & Ruf (2007) followed subclinical and clinical symptoms of TMD which were detected and managed by MFA in a group of students. In a period of 2.4 years on average, an increase of those with clinical signs of TMD occurred. Subclinical signs fluctuated a great deal yet one out of three students in the subgroup developed clinically manifested TMD.

4. Occlusion and TMD

Occlusion was considered a possible etiopathogenic factor of TMD but their relationship is complex and still remains partially unexplained. Occlusal treatment is important not only to patients but also to dentists - nearly half of the interviewed Swedish dentists consider that the replacement of molars is necessary due to development of TMD and compromising of masticatory function (Lyka et al., 2001). The importance of occlusion in etiopathogenesis has been redefined by refuting the mechanistic conception which has been present from the beginning of scientific research of TMD. Loss of teeth and/or disorders of occlusion are certainly illnesses by nature but any type of irreversible occlusal treatment cannot be associated with causal treatment of TMD (Slavicek, 2009; Carlsson, 2010).

In an epidemiologic study, Gesch et al. (2004b) found a low incidence of certain variables of malocclusion (unilateral open bite, negative overjet and unilateral cross-bite in men, and edge-to-edge bite in women) with signs or symptoms of TMD. In both genders, anatomically correct occlusion was not significantly associated with TMD compared with malocclusions. By including static and dynamic factors of occlusion, a significant correlation with TMD incidence has been statistically determined but with a low correlation coefficient. Anterior open bite, deep overjet 6 mm or more, unilateral cross-bite and difference between centric relation and maximal intercuspidation amounting to more than 2 mm with more than six posterior teeth to be replaced can be considered increased risk factors for TMD (Pullinger et al., 1993). Conversely, Rammelsberg (1998) offered a review of etiopathogenic model of DD development wherein high abrasion and insufficient restorative procedure on posterior teeth are risk factors causing occlusal instability. In their research, 34% of patients with DD with reduction previously underwent orthodontic treatment. As opposed to that, only 16% of asymptomatic individuals and 14% of patients with DD without reduction were previously orthodontically treated. In order to further confirm the relationship between orthodontic treatment and development of TMD, a follow-up targeted study should be carried out prior to and after orthodontic treatment.

In a population of children, Pereira et al. (2009) did not find any correlation between malocclusion and TMD but they identified bruxism and posterior cross bite as risk factors for TMD. Tecco et al. (2010a) and Tecco & Festa (2011) found a correlation between TMD with painful symptoms in children (5-15 years of age) and unilateral cross bite, but not with TMJ sounds. Myofascial pain was more prevalent in females. Huddleston Slater et al. (2007) found that age, history of orthodontic treatment, overbite and protrusion were significantly associated with DD with reduction. In their study, Badel et al. (2008b) found a significantly higher prevalence of hyperbalance and interference contacts in asymptomatic patients compared to TMD patients. No difference was found between Angle's classes in patients with DD and asymptomatic individuals. There was a statistically significant difference in teeth contact between the maximal intercuspidation and centric positions patients and asymptomatic subjects. Augthun et al. (1998) did not find any correlations between occlusal variables and forms of DD. However, it has been established that the rate of class II increases consecutively depending on the following subjects: asymptomatic subjects, patients with DD with reduction and patients with DD without reduction (14%/33%/52%), while the share of subjects with class I decreases simultaneously (43%/30%/18%).

Taking into account the great number of static and dynamic occlusal variables, it is difficult to comprehend the overall correlation with the development of TMDs due to the often non-standardised studies based on occlusal analysis (John, 1996). According to John et al. (1998), 'complex interaction' is the only but scientifically non-defined link between occlusion and TMDs. Occlusion ensures orthopedic stability of TMJ whereas the occlusal stability is ensured by mutually antagonistic contacts in a position of maximal intercuspidation. When the relationship between the two factors is compromised, it could lead to an overload of articular structures and consequently pose a risk of TMD development. The changes in occlusal relations are pronounced in etiopathogenesis, causing co-contraction of antagonist muscles the purpose of which is to protect the agonists and remove pain. The influence of possible adverse chronic effects can be avoided by the adaptation of muscular activity (Okeson, 2003).

The importance of occlusal interferences was perceived differently regarding the etiopathogenesis of TMDs. Le Bell et al. (2002) found that artificial interferences do not stimulate the development of dysfunctional symptoms in healthy subjects, instead they adapt successfully to them. In patients whose medical histories show TMD interferences stimulate the recurrence of stronger symptoms.

There is a dichotomy between scientific and clinical concepts of occlusion, which can be explained by the concept of integrated neurobiological system (Türp & Schindler, 2003). Occlusion is a basic component of dental restorative procedures, which changes or supplements the compromised or lost occlusal relations in each segment of planning the procedure. Pathogenetic and therapeutic effects of myofascial pain can be explained only as a mutual relationship between occlusion and neuromusculature. The results of La Bella et al. (2002) are explained by the neurobiological hypothesis based on the differentiated activity of the part of the muscle in which increased tension and pain can occur. The changes in occlusal relations cause a mild unloading in painful muscles or within the structures of TMJ which means that different condyle positions during treatment can have the same effect. However, the mutual relationship between occlusal interferences and microtrauma has not been completely explained (Türp & Schindler, 2003).

4.1 Hypervigilance

Reflex response to peripheral stimulus, that is, occlusal interference via periodontal receptors, can be modulated in the central nervous system in such a way that the stimulus causing normal opening in that case causes mouth closing. The hypothalamus and the limbic system mediate in tonus increase in affective conditions and under stress, whereas the reflex response to occlusal stimulus depends on the current state of agitation of those centres. In patients, even the slightest interference can produce the state of high stimulation and muscle hyperactivity, which can cause TMD at a lower level of adaptation. In other individuals with low level of activity of those centres an increase of muscle tonus due to occlusal interference does not occur. Parafunction is initiated only when the occlusal changes turn into a disturbance which leads to an awareness of pathological occlusal relations. A patient does not react to a harmful periodontal stimulus due to disturbed efficiency of behavioural mechanisms by diminishing the parafunction, instead it gains strength. Only in cases of hypervigilance, the occlusal changes will lead to TMD, due to increased awareness of one's own body and intensified activity of emotional motor system such as stress, pain or psychosocially caused parafunction. Hypervigilance is a changed form of observation wherein the harmful nociceptive stimuli are intensified (Hollins et al, 2009; Palla, 1998).

5. Concepts of TMDs treatment

The concept of TMDs treatment procedures is indirectly connected with the already established symptoms and signs from the medical history and clinical examination. Since the exact pathophysiological mechanism of TMDs development has not been fully explained, the main goal of the treatment is the management, reduction and removal of temporomandibular pain. Treatment procedures are divided into reversible and irreversible procedures. Since the treatment is mostly empirical, that is, performed by evaluating the clinical significance if the established symptoms, the reversible procedures are mostly used. Treatment indications, type of treatment procedures and their practical application are based on the existence of a specific form of myogenic and/or arthrogenic disorder in the stomatognathic system accompanied by certain intensity of temporomandibular pain (Gremillion, 2002; Palla, 1998).

The course of development of neuroplastic processes in the central nervous system is prevented by the treatment of acute temporomandibular pain, and those processes result in development of chronic pain (pain present longer than 6 months). The treatment of temporomandibular pain is based on the following (Green, 2006; Palla, 1998, Palla, 2003):

- symptoms and clinical signs have complex features of musculoskeletal disorder;
- the morphofunctional features do not make the TMJ absolutely unique in the human body;
- occlusion is not a crucial etiopathogenic factor;
- patients are successfully treated by simple and non-invasive treatment procedures;
- the patient's psychological reaction should not be in proportion with the somatic pathology;
- the treatment approaches to non-chronic and chronic temporomandibular pain differ;
- the evaluation of the purposefulness and the optimal efficiency of the initial treatment is necessary.

5.1 Aims and forms of the initial treatment

The initial treatment comprises different and to a certain extent, specific procedures and means the main feature of which is to be as non-invasive as possible. The diagnosis should be discussed with the patient as well as its possible etiology and pathophysiology and the prognosis and its possible course of treatment. The patient should understand the diagnosis, especially if it is accompanied by chronic pain. Successfully informing the patient creates a placebo effect thus reducing the secondary induced psychological disorder which can compromise the success of the treatment. The patient is additionally motivated by the good prognosis of treatment. Diet consisting of soft food is recommended as well as instructions on how to change oral activity in the sense of self-observation and self-correction of oral habits and parafunctions (Green, 2006).

Physical and manual therapy plays an important role in treatment of all rheumatic disorders and at the same time it actively involves the patient in the course of the treatment. The aim is to remove musculoskeletal restrictions such as pain removal, detoning and stretching of hypertonic muscles. Therapy is conducted by ultrasound, TENS, laser, kinesiotherapy by Schulte, localised massage, etc. (Badel et al., 2010b). Nonsteroidal anti-rheumatics are indicated in acute pain of different etiologies. Due to systemic side-effects in the gastro-intestinal tract and due to blood circulation disorders in kidneys, it s recommended to prescribe selective inhibitors of the prostaglandin synthesis which should be taken during a longer period of time (Badel et al., 2007b).

The irreversible treatment mostly implies surgical procedures. Arthrocentesis (removal of inflammatory exudate), surgical reposition of articular disc (arthrotomy), discectomy, placement of articular disc implants and condylectomy can be performed on the TMJ. Arthroscopy is a diagnostic-treatment method used for imaging of intraarticular pathologic changes with the possibility of their simultaneous removal (Machon et al., 2010; Palla, 1998).

5.2 Occlusal splints

The occlusal splint is the most common and efficient treatment procedure of arthrogenic and/or myogenic forms of TMDs and bruxism. The occlusal stability is established by specific morphology of the splint which is placed on the teeth alignment of one jaw thus serving as an orthopedic means of TMJ stabilisation (de Leeuw, 2008; Okeson, 2003). The occlusal splint is used as a temporary means of obtaining therapeutic occlusion and as a preparatory stage for definite prosthetic treatment (Badel, 2003).

Depending on the indications of use and treatment effects of the occlusal splint, hyperactivity is reduced, that is, the masticatory muscles are relaxed, the condyle is therapeutically positioned, that is, placed into the centric relation position and the behavioural effects increase awareness about the position, function and parafunction of the mandible thus achieving placebo effect (Dylina, 2001).

5.2.1 Classification of occlusal splints

In occlusal splint treatment the following changes occurred in: biomechanic concepts of their effects, features of their placement and retention on the teeth, morphology of the occlusal plane of the splint and their effect on the position and movements of the mandible.

Relaxation splints are used in the treatment of bruxism as well as in management of arthrogenic and myogenic temporomandibular pain. The Michigan splint (occlusal bite plane stabilisation splint with cuspid rise and freedom in centric) by Ramfjord and Ash is a splint covering all the teeth in the jaw, enabling antagonistic contacts on the flat planes according to occlusal concepts of freedom in centric position. Guiding by canines along the modelled planes of the splint is achieved in each extracentric movement (Ash & Schmieseder, 1999).

Distraction splint (pivot splint) vertically unloads intraarticular structures by condyle distraction and is indicated in arthroses, perforation of articular disc and anterior DD without reductiong. The splint acts as a hypomochlion in individual bilateral contacts in the molar region, by which distraction (decompression) of TMJs is obtained (Okeson, 2003).

Repositioning (protrusion/distraction) splint causes the excentric (anterior) positioning of the mandible and is used for treatment of anterior displacement of the articular disc with repositioning. The aim of the splint treatment is repositioning of the articular disc into the physiological position with respect to the condyle, which is achieved by its occlusal plane. The splint achieves a protrusive (anterior) position of the condyle with a slight distraction effect on the TMJs (Okeson, 2003).

With respect to the variety of design characteristics and the biomechanical effect of occlusal splints, previous concepts of initial treatments have been revised. The effect of anterior displacement/position of the articular disc and subsequent irreversible changes in physiological occlusal relations is questionable. Stabilisation of the mandible in anterior position leads to intraarticular partitioning which can lead to permanent anterior habitual occlusion resulting in malocclusion (back open bite due to extrusion of posterior teeth and orthodontic displacement of anterior teeth) (Brenkert, 2010). In order to avoid irreversible, unwanted changes in the structures of the masticatory system, the Michigan splint is the device of choice due to the proved beneficial effect in alleviation and removal of symptoms TMDs (Badel, 2009b). The occlusal splint, according to the individual case, is combined to a certain extent with other forms of initial treatment of TMDs. In treatment of DD, it is important to consider that repositioning of the articular disc is not satisfactory in as much as 50% of cases and recurrences are possible in 1/3 of the cases (Le Bell & Kirveskari, 1990).

5.3 Implications of orthodontic treatment on TMD

Orthodontic treatment can be viewed from two different points of view: whether orthodontic treatment has a negative impact on development of signs and symptoms of TMDs and what the role of orthodontic treatment is regarding the modality of TMDs treatment. MRI helped with detection, that is, follow-up of the influence of orthodontic treatment on the intraarticular structures of TMJ. In a group of 15 orthodontic patients (aged between 12 and 17) Pancherz et al. (1999) found clinical signs of TMD in two patients (partial DD in one patient and osteoarthritic changes in the other). All orthodontic patients wore a Herbst appliance during 7 months due to Class II malocclusion. In the follow-up period, DD improved (metric evaluation) and in the other patient, the loss of osteoarthritic changes was considered the result of compensatory joint remodelling. Aidar et al. (2006) performed a metric evaluation of the effects of Herbst treatment in adolescents with Class II Division 1 malocclusion. There was no significant influence of orthodontic treatment on DD development.

Tullberg et al. (2001) conducted a research with a follow-up on the correlation between early (children with primary dentition) and late (children with mixed or permanent dentition treatment of unilateral posterior cross-bite. There was no evidence that early treatment, even the later treatment repeated in 11 out of 44 subjects, was related to significant development of signs and symptoms of TMD. Therefore, even in a case of malocclusion as a risk factor, orthodontic treatment could not be related to the development of TMD. Even the first (early) orthodontic treatment could be repeated in older age (as a late treatment) and the subjects aged 19 would not have more significantly manifested TMD. During a 4-month follow-up, Bourzgui et al. (2010) did not find any correlation between development of TMD symptoms and Angle classes. Although the unilateral posterior cross bite is mentioned as a significant variable in DD of TMJ, in a group of children (average age of 9.3 years) their correlation could not be established by MRI analysis (Pellizoni, 2006).

During a long follow-up, Egermark et al. (2003) investigated the relationship between occlusal variables and development of clinical signs and symptoms of TMDs. From a long-term perspective, subjects were very pleased with the orthodontic treatment, and the treatment received in childhood did not increase the risk for TMDs later in life. In some subjects, lateral forced bite between retruded contact position and intercuspal position, as well as unilateral cross bite might be of importance in this respect. Henrikson & Nilner

(2003) followed the clinical signs and symptoms of TMDs during the fixed orthodontic treatment, especially in girls with Class II malocclusion. They were compared with girls who did not receive treatment and controls with normal occlusion. It was observed that signs and symptoms of TMDs equally develop in all three groups and, over time, they fluctuate considerably and unpredictably. A part of patients with Class II and the myogenic form of TMDs even experienced improvement of their condition due to orthodontic treatment. In any case, fixed orthodontic treatment did not particularly aggravate TMDs compared to the pre-treatment period.

Tecco et al. (2010a) compared the efficiency of TMDs treatment by a fixed orthodontic appliance and the anterior repositioning splint. DD was diagnosed by MRI and the effect of both treatments was beneficial to treatment of myogenic and arthrogenic pain, whereas the repositioning splint proved to be more efficient for removal of pathological noise in the joint. Siegmund & Harzer (2002) showed a detailed orthodontic treatment of a patient with DD. Clinical diagnostics was based on MFA and it was supplemented by axiography. The need for pre-treatment diagnostics and treatment planning was stressed which leads to a successful outcome of fixed orthodontic treatment as well as to the avoidance of complications related to possible exacerbation of TMD symptoms.

Jensen & Ruf (2007) showed that during a long-term orthodontic treatment, significant development of TMD is not to be expected. Likewise, the transformation of subclinical signs into clinical signs of TMD can be expected, which should not be associated with the course of possible orthodontic treatment. Although the results of the above mentioned studies reveal that orthodontic treatment does not have a special effect on the condition of TMDs, it should be taken into account that the studies described the treatment which was indicated for entirely orthodontic reasons. However, each treatment, particularly irreversible ones, runs the risk of adverse effects. Condylar resorption is one of the iatrogenic examples of TMDs development possibly related to orthodontic treatment. Orthodontic forces can often cause undesired reactions of partitioning within the alveolar bone. As in the described case, TMD symptoms were not observed on time thus causing the lack of consistent radiological follow-up (Shen et al., 2005).

Idiopathic condyle resorption is the term for the progressive form of OA of TMJ, which is associated with trauma and orthopedic procedure. Although it is an unwanted complication or an independent pathologic process manifested during orthodontic treatment, it certainly gives an impression of failure and of an even worse condition of the stomatognathic system. In the above mentioned study of patients with DD (Badel, 2007a), in the course of the follow-up of intraarticular condition during the treatment by Michigan splint, a rapid osteoarthritic process in a female bruxist patient with unilateral anterior DD without reduction and also malocclusion of Class II division 1 was found by MRI. Condyle resorption resulting in drastically pronounced open bite was not accompanied by exacerbation of TMD symptoms.

6. Clinical case

A 26-year-old female patient, previously under orthodontic treatment, was referred to a prosthodontic specialist, complaining of pain in her right TMJ and clicking in the left one with limited mouth opening. The pain was intensified upon chewing.

Patient's history. Without any particular reason, the patient experienced clicking in her left TMJ and she contacted her dentist, which happened 7 months prior to her visiting the prosthodontist. Her dentist referred her to an orthodontist. She was treated by a bimaxillary removable appliance (bionator) in order to correct a large horizontal overjet (Angle class II/1).

In the course of the orthodontic treatment, the patient still complained about the clicking and after 4 months pain in the right TMJ appeared. She had difficulties opening her mouth, pain appeared upon each movement of the mandible; she had difficulties adjusting to the new occlusal relations established by the orthodontic appliance and had a swelling in the region of the right TMJ. With respect to the above mentioned symptoms, she felt more comfortable in habitual occlusion than in the anterior therapeutic position achieved by the bionator. However, the patient did not realise at first that the pain in the TMJ was not being treated. The orthodontist did not realise that her intention was not to treat the orthodontic anomaly. Since the treatment by bionator obviously did not affect the TMJ symptomatology in that period, and her condition even worsened, the patient realised that her problems were not resolved by the treatment - instead of the TMJ symptoms she was treated for the orthodontic anomaly. According to the patient, the orthodontist realised this and attempted to stop the treatment by bionator without any particular explanation or further counselling with colleagues.

Occlusal analysis. At the first intraoral examination of the patient, two habitual intercuspal positions were detected. Until the lips were spread apart for a detailed dental examination, there was an impression of a physiological relationship between the anterior teeth. However, it was an acquired and forced anterior bite caused by regular wear of the bionator. In this position, the posterior teeth were in non-occlusion (Figure 3).

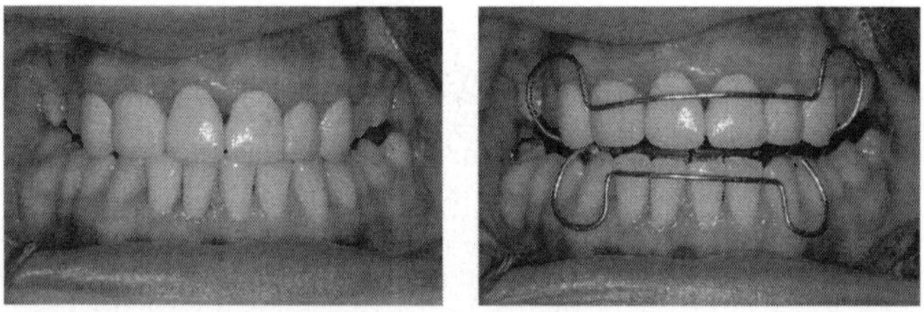

Fig. 3. Occlusion in anterior forced bite without (left) and with inserted bionator (right) in the mouth.

The real anterior-posterior relations between the dental arches were shown in the habitual intercuspal position: Angle Class II/1, an 11 mm horizontal overjet and a 4 mm overbite of upper teeth over the lower ones. In the transversal plane there was a 1 mm displacement of the medial line between lower central incisors to the right compared with the upper central incisors due to the loss of previously extracted first molars, especially of the extracted tooth 46 (Figure 4). In both teeth alignments, there was a crowding of posterior regions. The upper anterior teeth were provided with ceramic crowns. In both lateral movements there was a canine guidance, without balanced contacts or interferences. The teeth did not show any clinical signs of dental abrasion.

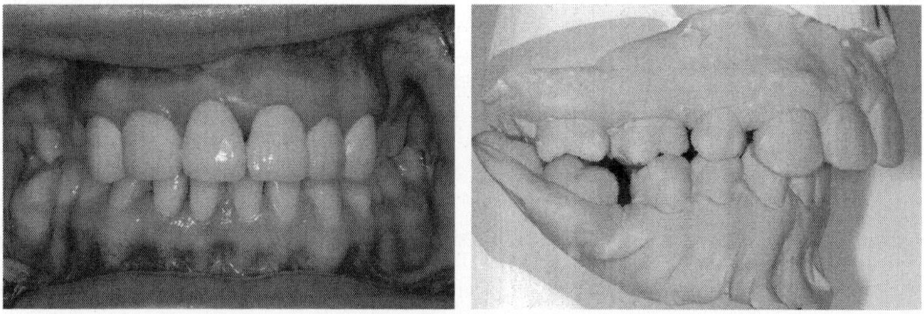

Fig. 4. Habitual occlusion in maximum intercuspidation (left), and lateral view of the model transferred to the articulator. Note: a pronounced horizontal overjet (right).

Clinical diagnostics. Painful right TMJ with limited mouth opening was diagnosed by clinical examination and MFA according to Bumann and Groot Landeweer (Bumann and Lotzmann, 2002). Active mouth opening amounted to 36 mm, whereas passive mouth opening, that is mouth opening by exerting a mild downward passive force on the lower incisors amounted to 41 mm. Protrusive movement amounted to 6 mm, laterotrusion to the right amounted to 8 mm and laterotrusion to the left amounted to 4 mm. The pain intensity on the visual-analogue scale (VAS) (VAS=0-10; 0-10; 0, no pain; 10, the worst pain) was rated 7.4. On mouth opening there was a deviation to the right. On the right and also left laterotrusal movement, the pain appeared only in the right TMJ. Based on clinical findings and according to MFA (painful right TMJ under active and passive compressions) an anterior DD without reduction in the right TMJ was confirmed. Since the clinical signs of the disorder of the left TMJ were not present (the patient stated that she previously experienced reciprocal clicking), a clinical diagnosis of the left TMJ could not be made.

Radiological diagnostics. Panoramic x-ray shows a non-symmetrical relationship between the left and the right condyle: the right condylar head is pointed with a deplaned anterior surface. The bilateral anterior DD was confirmed by MRI. Imaging of both TMJs was performed on a 1T magnetic field device in three different positions: closed mouth position (habitual maximal intercuspidation, anterior position of the mandible caused by orthodontic treatment and open mouth position). The imaging sequences (matrix 256 x 192; 160 x 160 field of view) included the T1 weighted image (TR 450/TE 12), and gradient echo T2 weighted image (TR 760/TE 32), and T2 weighted image (TR 3000/TE 72).

Anterior DD without reduction was confirmed, with collections of inflammatory exudates which are most visible on T2 weighted images (Figure 5). In closed mouth position, the condylar head is anteriorly dislocated (Figure 5a), which is more visible in a forced anterior position (Figure 5b). Further dislocation is minimal (open mouth position) while the disc is constantly anteriorly dislocated and is deformed (Figure 5c). The condyle reaches the peak (zenith) of the articular eminence. Mild osteoarthritic changes in cortical bone of the condylar head in slightly pointed forms without subchondral changes are visible.

The anterior DD with reduction was determined in the left TMJ (Figure 6), which explains the previous symptom of clicking, which vanished in the course of orthodontic treatment. In closed mouth position, the condylar head was centrically placed within the glenoid fossa but in a slightly distraction position resulting in an enlarged intra articular fissure (Figure 6a). The disc was placed anteriorly and remained in this position even when the patient's mandible was in a forced anterior position (Figure 6b). In open mouth position, the disc achieved physiological position with respect to the condyle but it did not reach the peak of the articular eminence (Figure 6c). However, the mobility of the left condyle is more pronounced than in the right joint. The condylar head was slightly pointed with a hint of osteoarthritic changes appearing as a thickened tip of the cortical bone. Subchondral structures had an adequate signal and there was no articular effusion.

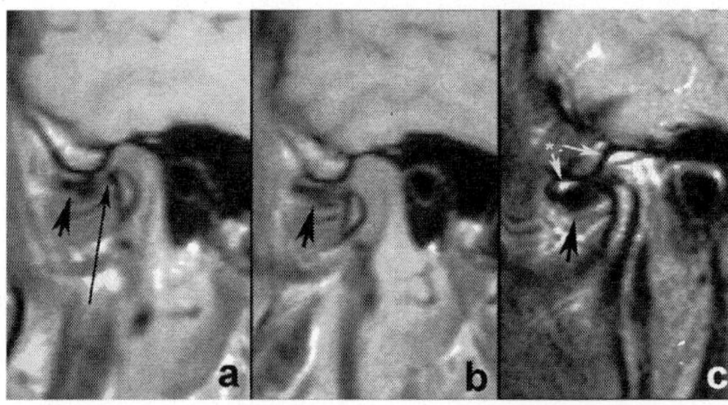

Fig. 5. Magnetic resonance images of the right temporomandibular joint in the position of maximum habitual intercuspidation (a), forced anterior position (b) and open mouth position (c). Note: non-reduced anterior displaced disc (short arrow), joint effusion (marked with *), and degenerative changes of cortical condylar head (long arrow).

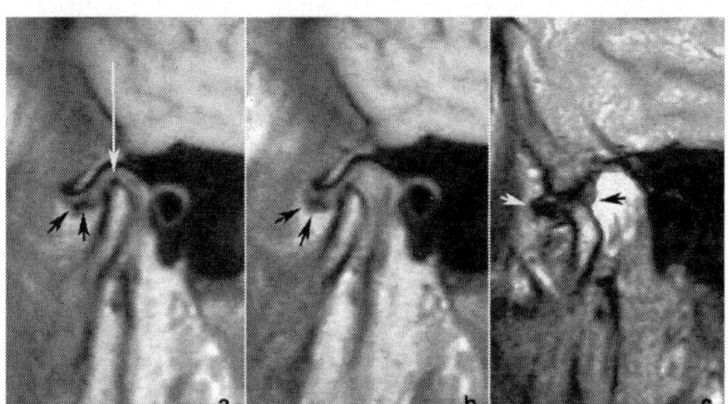

Fig. 6. Magnetic resonance images of the left temporomandibular joint in the position of maximum intercuspidation (a), forced anterior position (b) and open mouth position (c). Note: anterior displaced disc with reduction (short arrows) and degenerative changes of anterior part of cortical condylar head (long arrow).

Treatment. The stabilization splint (according to some authors the Michigan splint) (Badel, 2007a) is indicated for the initial treatment of pain caused by anterior DD (Figure 7). It temporarily provides stable joint position, and in addition, reduces abnormal muscle activity. Both jaw alginate impressions were taken and the splint was fabricated in a new therapeutic position, that is, in a position of centric relation. This was also the best position for stabilization splint fabrication since it ensures a stable position of condyle in the articular fossa. It also enables the removal of the retrodiscal tissue load exerted by the condyle since the articular disc is permanently protruded, that is displaced anteriorly (Badel et al., 2003). The patient was instructed to wear the appliance while sleeping and was asked to come for a check-up in a week.

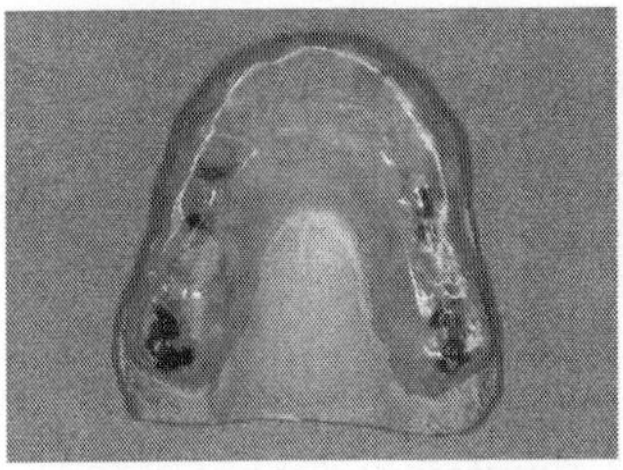
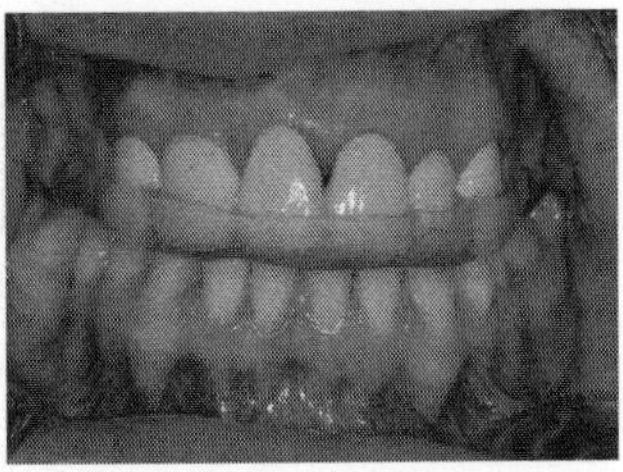

Fig. 7. Michigan splint on a model (left) and the inserted splint in the patient's mouth (right).

In collaboration with a rheumatologist-physiatrist, the patient was referred to physical therapy, which consisted of a routine protocol: TENS (transcutaneous electroneural stimulation), topical non-steroidal analgesic ketoprofen (*Fastum gel*) three times a day and a kinesiotherapy programme by Schulte (Badel et al., 2010b). She continued performing the exercises by Schulte three times a day at home.

Besides stopping the orthodontic treatment, the patient initially wore the Michigan splint for about 5 months. After 6 months, a more significant ability of mouth opening (45 mm) was measured but pain in both joints was still present, particularly upon yawning (VAS=8). While the left joint was painful on wider mouth opening, pain in the right joint was more expressed and accompanied by slight crepitations. The patient was aware of the chronic nature of her pain because, as she stated, she 'got used to' the pain. She stressed the efficiency of oral exercises and topical application of the ketoprofen gel (*Fastum gel*).

Long year follow-up. At a recall 5 years later, the patient did not have pain in the TMJs and only felt discomfort in the right TMJ during wide mouth opening with clinically evidenced minor crepitations. However, she felt discomfort in the right joint on yawning ad sleeping on the right side of her face. When eating an apple and yawning, she sometimes felt pain in the right joint (VAS=4). Also, she mentioned rare occurrences of clicking in the right joint which was also painful. Maximum mouth opening still amounted to 45 mm, which is significant regarding the pre-treatment measurements and equal to the measurements after the initial treatment. Now, she does not have any esthetic or functional needs for orthodontic treatment.

A control MRI taken on the same device showed visible degenerative changes in both TMJs. Significant changes in the sense of OA development occurred in the right joint: the condyle was deplaned and an osteophytic formation on the anterior edge contributed to the unshapely appearance. The disc was deformed with anterior displacement (Figure 8a). Even in the anterior position, the disc still remained in front of the condyle (Figure 8b). In open mouth position, the condyle reached the eminence while the disc remained non-reduced (Figure 8c).

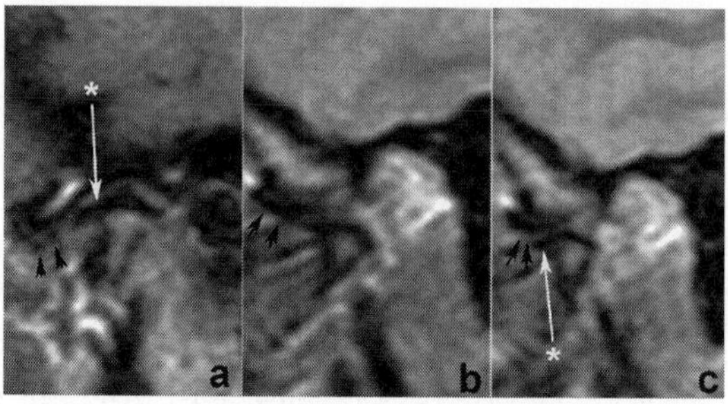

Fig. 8. Follow-up examination of the right temporomandibular joint by magnetic resonance imaging in the position of habitual maximum intercuspidation (a), forced anterior position (b) and open mouth position (c). Note: non-reduced and deformed anterior displaced disc (short arrow) and the osteophyte formation on the anterior edge of the condyle (long arrow).

In closed mouth position (habitual occlusion), a compensatory fibrosation of retrodisc tissue along with the deplaned condylar head of an appropriate size was visible in the left joint (Figure 9a). In the forced anterior position, the greatest part of the disc was placed anteriorly from the condyle (Figure 9b), whereas there was an almost complete reduction of displacement in open mouth position, that is, the disc was almost symmetrically repositioned on the condyle (Figure 9c). The condyle-disc complex almost reached the peak of the eminence when the patient wore the bionator, and also in the position of maximum mouth opening.

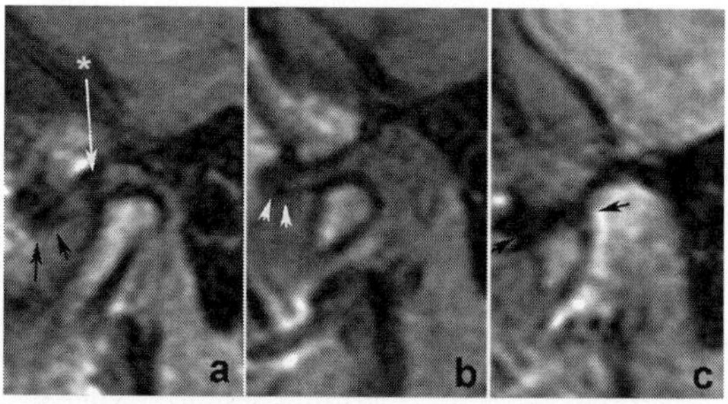

Fig. 9. Follow-up examination of the left temporomandibular joint by magnetic resonance imaging in the position of habitual maximum intercuspidation (a), forced anterior position (b) and open mouth position (c). Note: disc displacement with reduction (arrows), and fibrosation of the retrodisc tissue (marked with *).

7. Discussion and general remarks

Orthodontic treatment should be planned carefully if there are underlying symptoms of TMDs. Clinical importance of certain dysfunctional symptoms has altered the concept of *normal* functioning of the stomatognathic system. A perfected interpretation of certain diagnostic symptoms enables the correct establishing of clinical diagnostic parameters and other diagnostic modalities of TMDs. The approach to patient in the sense of personalised dental medicine gains importance when dealing with patients suffering from certain diagnoses of TMDs. Furthermore, the issue of occlusion in dental medicine has reached a dogmatic level, which in case of TMD patients should not apply, particularly the use of irreversible treatment methods as well as planning of possible preventive procedures (Carlsson, 2010).

As with many other musculoskeletal disorders in the human body, according to modern biomedical beliefs, they are of non-specific etiopathology, that is, they are idiopathic on the level of the individual patient (Green, 2006). Correlating TMDs with numerous etiopathogenic factors does not result in efficient determination of their cause-effect relation. Therefore, current opinion is that TMDs are idiopathic in origin and the correlation with certain etiologic factors cannot be entirely confirmed; on the other hand, the question of chronic musculoskeletal (or non-malignant) pain becomes dominant within the field of pain medicine. Consequently, pain and TMDs cannot be observed only on the level of occlusion, individual patients' wishes regarding esthetic dentistry and relying on scientifically unverified but traditional treatment indications.

Clinical examination, particularly manual examination techniques of patients with TMDs are an indispensable part of diagnostics by which the indication for imaging techniques is determined. MRI has become the gold standard in diagnostics and differential diagnostics of TMDs because it enables imaging of hard and soft tissues of TMJ (primarily the disc) and joint effusion. Although MRI is the gold standard in TMJ diagnostics, there is still no gold standard in diagnostics of temporomandibular pain. Indeed, MRI is not an appropriate screening method but a strictly applied diagnostic and differential-diagnostic method (Ahmad et al., 2009).

TMDs treatment planning can be carried out as the initial treatment and upon reaching a satisfactory degree of recovery, the definitive treatment can be planned as well. This may be applied to all TMDs patients, regardless of their having intact teeth with respect to physiological occlusal relations as well as to patients in need of orthodontic or prosthodontic treatment or even an oral surgical procedure. One should bear in mind the fact that definite treatment should have its indications and should be in accordance with the patient's wishes as well as with the actual state of occlusion and the level of TMDs treatment. In managing of TMDs patients there are always doubts about the indications for definite treatment, if there was a possibility of treating the painful TMD only by reversible treatment modalities, that is, by initial treatment. By recognizing the signs and symptoms of TMDs and by choosing initial methods of treatment as the methods of choice, the excessive use of diagnostics (for example, MRI) as well partial or complete overtreatment modalities are avoided (De Boever, et al., 2008; Türp, 2002).

The possibility of incorrect treatment in cases of TMDs patients can happen as it was shown in the clinical case of the female patient described in this paper, which was contrary to her wishes and individual needs of malocclusion treatment. Excessive, unnecessary and incorrect treatment methods of TMDs patients can have legal repercussions (Manfredini et al., 2011).

The patient has a input in the planning of own treatment and the dentist should consider the patient's wishes, and the current trend is to collaborate with other dental and medical specialists which is a multidisciplinary approach (De Boever et al., 2008).

Since clinical TMDs symptoms range from painless clicking up to severe pain causing problems in basic functioning upon eating and speech, the question arises when TMDs symptoms should be treated. In cases of adolescent patients with an occlusal anomaly there are considerations of whether orthodontic treatment can prevent their exacerbation, particularly pain. Since prevention implies the possibility of affecting causal factors of the disease, there is a lack of scientific facts to support that (Luther, 1998).

The absence of temporomandibular pain and mild functional difficulties caused by remaining TMD symptoms represent the group of passive need for TMD treatment. The idiopathic concept of development of TMDs cannot accept the concept by Kutilla et al. (1996) of active and passive TMD prevention. Preventive measures cannot be planned in patients with unknown etiology. Since the topic of this paper is the relationship between orthodontics and TMDs (although numerous studies are not methodologically coordinated and neither is the sample of patients who are primarily orthodontic or primarily with TMDs), the review papers on this subject constantly reach the conclusion that orthodontics neither treats TMDs nor causes them in particular (Macfarlane et al., 2009). As it happens in every definitive treatment in the stomatognathic system, painful forms of TMDs aggravate orthodontic treatment which was previously planned due to malocclusion rather than TMDs. In the course of orthodontic treatment previously latent symptoms of TMDs may appear (that is why MFA is significant as a clinical screening test) or manifested TMDs symptoms may develop although the patient did not experience such symptoms at any level prior to this. Such a condition particularly aggravates further orthodontic treatment so that it is recommended to temporarily discontinue the orthodontic treatment according to the need and the level of the presence of symptoms (Michelotti & Iodice, 2010). The part of the functional treatment termed initial symptomatic treatment, which should provide a satisfactory degree of painful function of stomatognathic system, should be carried out in order to continue the orthodontic treatment (Badel, 2007a).

In a review of methods of clinical TMD evaluation in population of children and adolescents, Toscano & Defabianis (2009) pointed to a great variability of results which causes problems in their direct possibility of comparison. However, it can be concluded that joint sounds and TMJ symptoms are the most common in that subgroup of population. Bionators initially look like a sort of combined upper and lower Hawley retainer, but do not fasten to the teeth and are not used for post-brace removal treatment. Bionators are held in the mouth within the space that the teeth surround when biting. In the described clinical case, a distinction should be made between short-term wear of bionator and the exacerbation of painful clinical signs and symptoms of TMD as well as manifestation of osteoarthritis with prior DD within a 5-year-follow-up, which was confirmed by MRI. Such long-term effects of MRI imaging of TMJs cannot be ascribed to orthodontic treatment because degenerative changes accompanied by various conditions of DD, according to Kurita et al. (2006) develop even without any clinical symptoms. After all, DD of TMJ can be expected even in asymptomatic subjects (Badel et al., 2008c).

According to the American Academy of Pediatric Dentistry (2010) there are reversible and irreversible methods of TMD treatment. Irreversible methods of treatment include occlusal adjustment, mandibular repositioning (by a repositioning appliance) and also orthodontic treatment, without specific instructions on which group of treatment modalities is recommendable. Regarding the use of reversible treatment methods, there are some positive results obtained by, for example, Tecco et al. (2010) who found a positive effect of a fixed orthodontic appliance and the anterior repositioning splint on TMDs. Arthrocentesis proved to be efficient in combination with the occlusal splint (Machon et al., 2011). The use of the repositioning splint should be controlled and short-term because it can result in development of posterior open bite as a result of partitioning of intraarticular structures of TMJ on forced anterior bite (Türp, 2002; Brenkert, 2010). In such a case the initial treatment can be a failure because repositioning of this kind does not imply moving the anteriorly displaced disc (displacement reduction) but moving the condyle into a position which reduces the displacement thus causing clicking. Asymptomatic causes in non-patients show that DD does not necessarily mean the appearance of symptoms suggesting that such causative treatment is not in accordance with the principle of symptomatic treatment of TMDs (Badel et al, 2008c; Türp, 2002). When choosing the right initial occlusal treatment, permissive and non-invasive occlusal splints, such as the Michigan splint, are given the advantage (Dylina, 2001).

Optimal cost-effectiveness and health care efficiency are achieved by using palliative treatment procedures which cannot result in potentially incorrect, excessive, insufficient or untimely treatment of TMDs (Figure 10).

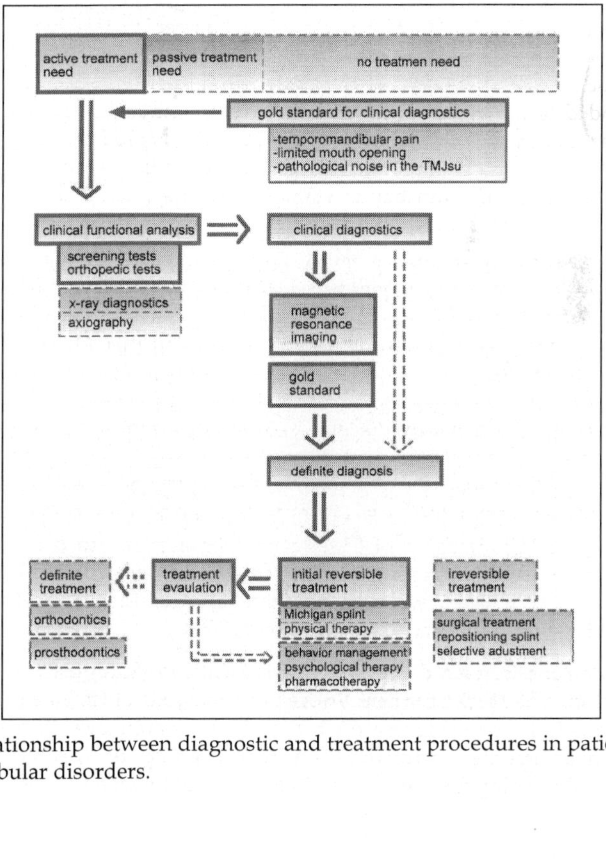

Fig. 10. The relationship between diagnostic and treatment procedures in patients with temporomandibular disorders.

8. Acknowledgment

This paper is a part of the scientific project No. 065-0650445-0441 supported by the Ministry of Science, Education and Sports, Republic of Croatia.

9. References

Aidar, L.A.; Abrahão, M.; Yamashita, H.K. & Dominguez, G.C. (2006). Herbst appliance therapy and temporomandibular joint disc position: a prospective longitudinal magnetic resonance imaging study. *American Journal of Orthodontics and Dentofacial Orthopedics*, Vol.129, No.4, pp. 486-496, ISSN 0889-5406

Ahmad, M.; Hollender, L.; Anderson, Q.; Kartha K.; Ohrbach, R.; Truelove, E.L.; John, M.T. & Schiffman, E. (2009) Research diagnostic criteria for temporomandibular disorders (RDC/TMD): development of image analysis criteria and examiner reliability for image analysis. *Oral Surgery, Oral Medicine, Oral Pathology, Oral Radiology, and Endodontics*, Vol.107, No.6, pp. 844-860, ISSN 1079-2104

American Academy on Pediatric Dentistry Clinical Affairs Committee. (2010) Guideline on acquired temporomandibular disorders in infants, children and adolescents. *Pediatric Dentistry*, Vol.32, No.6, pp. 232-237, ISSN 0164-1263

Ash, M.M. & Schmieseder, J. (1999) *Schienentherapie*. Urban & Fischer, ISBN 3-437-05030-3, München, Germany

Augthun, M.; Müller-Leisse, C.; Bauer, W.; Roth, A. & Speikermann, H. (1998) Anterior disk displacement of the temporomandibular joint. Significance of clinical signs and symptoms in the diagnosis. *Journal of Orofacial Orthopedics*, Vol.59, No.1, pp 39-46, ISSN 1434-5293

Badel, T.; Pandurić, J.; Kraljević, S. & Dulčić, N. (2003) Initial Treatment of Prosthetic Patients with a Michigan Splint. *Acta Stomatologica Croatica*, Vol.36, No.2, pp. 207-210, ISSN 0001-7019

Badel, T.; Kraljević, S.; Pandurić, J. & Marotti, M. (2004) Preprosthetic therapy utilizing a temporary occlusal acrylic splint: A case report. *Quintessence International*, Vol.35, No.5, pp. 401-405, ISSN 0033-6572

Badel, T. (2007a) *Temporomandibularni poremećaji i stomatološka protetika*. Medicinska naklada, ISBN 978-953-176-264-9, Zagreb, Croatia

Badel, T.; Rošin Grget, K.; Krapac, L. & Marotti, M. (2007b) Principi farmakoterapije temporomandibularnih poremećaja. *Medicus*, Vol.16, No.2, pp. 241-250, ISSN 1330-013X

Badel, T.; Lajnert, V.; Marotti, M.; Krolo, I. & Kovačević Pavičić, D. (2008a) Poremećaj čeljusnog zgloba u 12-godišnje pacijentice. *Medicina*. Vol.44, No.1, pp. 91-97, ISSN 0025-7729

Badel, T.; Marotti, M.; Krolo, I.; Kern, J. & Keros, J. (2008b) Occlusion in patients with temporomandibular joint anterior disk displacement. *Acta Clinica Croatica*, Vol.47, No.3, pp. 129-136, ISSN 0353-9466

Badel, T.; Pandurić, J.; Marotti, M.; Kern, J. & Krolo, I (2008c) Metrička analiza temporomandibularnog zgloba magnetskom rezonancijom u asimptomatskih ispitanika. *Acta Medica Croatica*, Vol.62; No.5, pp. 455-460. ISSN 1330-0164

Badel, T.; Marotti, M.; Keros, J.; Kern, J. & Krolo, I. (2009) Magnetic Resonance Imaging Study on Temporomandibular Joint Morphology. *Collegium Antropologicum*, Vol.33, No.2, pp. 455-460, ISSN 0350-6134

Badel, T.; Marotti, M.; Kern, J. & Laškarin, M. (2009) A quantitative analysis of splint therapy of displaced temporomandibular joint disc. *Annals of Anatomy*, Vol.191, No.3, pp. 280-287; ISSN 0940-9602

Badel, T.; Carek, A.; Podoreski, D.; Pavičin, I.S. & Lovko, S.K. (2010a) Temporomandibular joint disorder in a patient with multiple sclerosis--review of literature with a clinical report. *Collegium Antropologicum*, Vol.34, No.3, pp. 1155-1159, ISSN 0350-6134

Badel, T.; Krapac, L. & Marotti , M. (2010b) Dijagnostika i fizikalna terapija osteoartritisa temporomandibularnog zgloba. *Medix*, Vol.16, No.89-90. pp. 214-244, ISSN 1331-3002

Benoliel, R. & Sharav, Y. (2010) Chronic orofacial pain. *Current Pain and Headache Reports*, Vol.14, No.1, pp. 33-40, ISSN 1531-3433

Bonjardim, L.R.; Gaviao, M.B.; Carmagnani, F.G.; Pereira, L.J. & Castelo, P.M. (2003) Signs and symptoms of temporomandibular joint dysfunction in children with primary dentition. *The Journal of Clinical Pediatric Dentistry*, Vol.28, No.1, pp. 53-58, ISSN 1053-4628

Bourzgui, F., Sebbar, M.; Nadour. A. & Hamza, M. (2010) Prevalence of temporomandibular dysfunction in orthodontic treatment. *International Orthodontics*, Vol.8, No.4, pp. 386-398, ISSN 1761-7227

Brenkert, D.R. (2010) Orthodontic treatment for the TMJ patient following splint therapy to stabilize a displaced disk(s): a systemized approach. Part II. *Cranio: the Journal of Craniomandibular Practice*, Vol.28, No.4, pp. 260-265, ISSN 0886-9634

Bumann, A. & Lotzman, U. (2002) *Funktionsdiagnostik und Therapieprinzipien*. Thieme, ISBN 3-13-787501-3, Stuttgart, Germany

Carlsson, G.E. (2010) Some dogmas related to prosthodontics, temporomandibular disorders and occlusion. *Acta Odontologica Scandinavica*, Vol.68, No.6, pp. 313-322, ISSN 0001-6357

Casanova Rosado, J.F.; Medina-Solís, C.E.; Vallejos-Sánchez, A.A.; Casanova-Rosado, A.J.; Hernández-Prado, B. & Avila-Burgos, L. (2006) Prevalence and associated factors for temporomandibular disorders in a group of Mexican adolescents and youth adults. *Clinical Oral Investigations*, Vol.10, No.1, pp. 42-49, ISSN 1432-6981

De Boever, J.A.; Nilner, M.; Orthlieb, J.D. & Steenks, M.H. (2008) Recommendations by the EACD for examination, diagnosis, and management of patients with temporomandibular disorders and orofacial pain by the general dental practitioner. *Journal of Orofacial Pain*, Vol.22, No.3, pp. 268-278, ISSN 1064-6655

de Bont, L.G.; Dijkgraaf, L.C. & Stegenga, B. (1997) Epidemiology and natural progression of articular temporomandibular disorders. *Oral Surgery, Oral Medicine, Oral Pathology, Oral Radiology, and Endodontics*, Vol.83, No.1, pp. 72-76, ISSN 1079-2104

de Leeuw R. (2008) *Temporomandibular disorders. Guidelines for classification, assessment, and management*. 4th ed. Chicago, ISBN 0867154136, Quintessence, USA

Durham, J. (2008) Temporomandibular disorders (TMD): an overview. *Oral Surgery*, Vol.1, No.2, pp. 60-68, ISSN 1752-2471

Dworkin, S.F. & LeResche, L. (1992) Research diagnostic criteria for temporomandibular disorders: Review, criteria, examinations and specifications, critique. *Journal of Craniomandibular Disorders : Facial & Oral Pain*, Vol.6, No.4, pp. 301-355, ISSN 0890-2739

Dylina, T.J. (2001) A common-sence approach to splint therapy. *Journal of Prosthetic Dentistry*, Vol.86, No.5, pp. 539-545, ISSN 0022-3913

Egermark, I.; Magnusson, T. & Carlsson, G.E. (2003) A 20-year follow-up of signs and symptoms of temporomandibular disorders and malocclusions in subjects with and without orthodontic treatment in childhood. *The Angle Orthodontist*, Vo.73, No.2, pp. 109-115, ISSN 0003-3219

Gesch, D.; Bernhardt, O.; Alte, D.; Schwahn, C.; Kocher. T.; John, U. & Hensel, E. (2004a) Prevalence of signs and symptoms of temporomandibular disorders in an urban and rural German population: results of a population-based Study of Health in Pomerania. *Quintessence International*, Vol.35, No.2, pp. 143-50, ISSN 0033-6572

Gesch, D.; Bernhardt, O.; Alte, D.; Kocher, T.; John, U. & Hensel, E. (2004b) Malocclusions and clinical signs or subjective symptoms of temporomandibular disorders (TMD) in adults. Results of the population-based Study of Health in Pomerania (SHIP). *Journal of Orofacial Orthopedics*, Vol. 65, No.2, pp. 88-103, ISSN 1434-5293

Giannakopoulos, N.N.; Keller, L.; Rammelsberg, P.; Kronmüller, K.-T. & Schmitter, M. (2010) Anxiety and depression in patients with chronic temporomandibular pain and controls. *Jouranl of Dentistry*, 2010; Vol.38, No.5, pp. 369-376, ISSN 0300-5712

Green, S.C. (2006) Concepts of TMD Etiology: Effects on Diagnosis and Treatment, In: TMDs. *An Evidence-Based Approach to Diagnosis and Treatment*, Laskin, D.M.; Green, C.S. & Hylander, W.L, pp. 219-228, Quintessence, ISBN 0-86715-447-0, Chicago, USA

Gremillion, H.A. (2002) Multidisciplinary diagnosis and management of orofacial pain. *General Dentistry*, Vol.50, No.2, pp. 178-186, ISSN 0363-6771

Haiter-Neto, F.; Hollender, L.; Barclay, P. & Maravilla, K.R. (2002) Disk position and the bilaminar zone of the temporomandibular joint in asymptomatic young individuals by magnetic resonance imaging. *Oral Surgery, Oral Medicine, Oral Pathology, Oral Radiology, and Endodontics*, Vol.94, No.3, pp. 372-8, ISSN 1079-2104

Henrikson, T. & Nilner, M. (2003) Temporomandibular disorders, occlusion and orthodontic treatment. *Journal of Orthodontics*, Vol.30, No.2, pp. 129-137, ISSN 1465-3125

Hollins, M.; Harper, D.; Gallagher, S.; Owings, E.W.; Lim, P.F.; Miller, V.; Siddiqi, M.Q. & Maixner, W. (2009) Perceived intensity and unpleasantness of cutaneous and auditory stimuli: an evaluation of the generalized hypervigilance hypothesis. *Pain*, Vol.141, No.3, pp. 215-221, ISSN 0304-3959

Huddleston Slater, J.J.; Lobbezoo, F.; Onland-Moret, N.C. & Naeije, M. (2007) Anterior disc displacement with reduction and symptomatic hypermobility in the human temporomandibular joint: prevalence rates and risk factors in children and teenagers. *Journal of Orofacial Pain*, Vol.21, No.1, pp.55-62, ISSN 1064-6655

Katzberg, R.W.; Westesson, P.-L.; Tallents, R.H. & Drake, C.M. (1996) Anatomic Disorders of the Temporomandibular Joint Disc in Asymptomatic Subjects. *Journal of Oral and Maxillofacial Surgery*, Vol.54, No.2, pp. 147-153, ISSN 0278-2391

Köhler, A.A.; Helkimo, A.N.; Magnusson, T. & Hugoson, A. (2009) Prevalence of symptoms and signs indicative of temporomandibular disorders in children and adolescents.

A cross-sectional epidemiological investigation covering two decades. *European Archives of Paediatric Dentistry*, Vol.10, No. Suppl 1, pp.16-25, ISSN 1818-6300

Kropmans, T.; Dijkstra, P.; Stegenga, B.; Steward, R. & de Bont, L. (2000) Smallest detectable difference of maximal mouth opening in patients with painfully restricted temporomandibular joint function. *European Journal of Oral Sciences*, Vol.108, No.1, pp. 9-13, ISSN 0909-8836

Kurita, H.; Uehara, S.; Yokochi, M.; Nakatsuka, A.; Kobayashi, H. & Kurashina, K. (2006) A long-term follow-up study of radiographically evident degenerative changes in the temporomandibular joint with different conditions of disk displacement. International *Journal of Oral and Maxillofacial Surgery*, Vol.35, No.1, pp. 49-54, ISSN 0901-5027

Kuttila, M.; Le Bell, Y. & Alanen, P. (1996) The concepts prevalence, need for treatment, and prevention of temporomandibular disorders: a suggestion for terminology. *Acta Odontologica Scandinavica*, Vol.54, No.5, pp. 332-336, ISSN 0001-6357

Jensen, U. & Ruf, S. (2007) Longitudinal changes in temporomandibular disorders in young adults: indication for systematic temporomandibular joint screening. *Journal of Orofacial Orthopedics*, Vol.68, No.6, pp. 501-509, ISSN 1434-5293

John, M. (1996) Ätiopathogenese von funktionellen Kiefergelenkerkrankungen unter besondere Berücksichtigung der Okklusion. *Deutsche zahnärztliche Zeitschrift*, Vol.51, No.8, pp. 441-447. ISSN 0012-1029

John, M.; Zwijnenburg, A.; Reiber, Th. & Haerting, J. (1998) Okklusale Faktoren bei Patienten mit kraniomandibulären Dysfunktionen (CMD) und symptomfreien Probanden. *Deutsche zahnärztliche Zeitschrift*, Vol.53, No.10, pp. 670-673, ISSN 0012-1029

Jürgens, J. (2009) Sechs Leitsymptome der Kiefergelenkarthropathie. *Deutsche zahnärztliche Zeitschrift*, Vol.64, No.5, pp. 308-317, ISSN 0012-1029

Le Bell, Y. & Kirveskari, P. (1990) Treatment of reciprocal clicking of the temporomandibular joint with a repositioning appliance and occlusal adjustment – results after four and six years. *Proceedings of the Finnish Dental Society*, Vol.86, No.1, pp. 15-21, PFDSAX

Le Bell, Y.; Jämsä, T.; Korri, S.; Niemi, P.M. & Alanen, P. (2002) Effect of artificial occlusal inerferences depends on previous experience of temporomandibular disorders. *Acta Odontologica Scandinavica*, Vol.60, No.4, pp. 219-222, ISSN 0001-6357

LeResche, L., Mancl, L.A.; Drangsholt, M.T.; Saunders, K. & Korff, M.V. (2005) Relationship of pain and symptoms to pubertal development in adolescents. *Pain*, Vol.118, No.1-2, pp. 201-9, ISSN 0304-3959

Luther F. (1998) Orthodontics and the temporomandibular joint: Where are we now? Part 2. Functional occlusion, malocclusion, and TMD. *The Angle Orthodontist*, Vol.68, No.4, pp. 305-318, ISSN 0003-3219

Lyka, I.; Carlsson, G.E.; Wedel, A. & Kiliardis, S. (2001) Dentist's perception of risks for molar without anatagonisten. A questionnaire study of dentists in Sweden. *Swedish Dental Journal*, Vol.25, No.2, pp. 67-73, ISSN 0347-9994

Macfarlane, T.V.; Kenealy, P.; Kingdon, H.A.; Mohlin, B.O.; Pilley, J.R.; Richmond, S. & Shaw. W.C. (2009) Twenty-year cohort study of health gain from orthodontic treatment: temporomandibular disorders. American *Journal of Orthodontics and Dentofacial Orthopedics*, Vol.135, No.6, pp. 692.e1-8, ISSN 1097-6752

Machon, V.; Hirjak, D. & Lukas, J. (2011) Therapy of the osteoarthritis of the temporomandibular joint. *Journal of Cranio-maxillo-facial Surgery*. Vol.39, No.2, pp. 127-130, ISSN 1010-5182

Manfredini, D.; Piccotti. F.; Ferronato, G. & Guarda-Nardini, L. (2010) Age peaks of different RDC/TMD diagnoses in a patient population. *Journal of Dentistry*, Vo.38, No.5, pp. 392-399, ISSN 0300-5172

Manfredini, D.; Bucci, M.B.; Montagna, F. & Guarda-Nardini, L. (2011) *Temporomandibular disorders assessment: medicolegal considerations in the evidence-based era*. Journal of Oral Rehabilitation, Vol.38, No.2, pp. 101-119, ISSN 0305-182X

Michelotti, A. & Iodice, G. (2010) The role of orthodontics in temporomandibular disorders. *Journal of Oral Rehabilitation*, Vol.37, No.6; pp. 411-429, ISSN 0305-182X

Moen, K.; Hellem, S.; Geitung, J.T. & Skartveit, L. (2010) A practical approach to interpretation of MRI of the temporomandibular joint. *Acta Radiologica*, Vol.51, No.9, pp. 1021-1027, ISSN 0284-1851

Okeson, JP. (2003) *Management of Temporomandibular disorders and Occlusion*. Mosby, 5th ed., ISBN 0-323-01477-1; St. Louis, USA

Okeson, J.P. & de Leeuw, R. (2011) Differential diagnosis of temporomandibular disorders and other orofacial pain disorders. *Dental Clinics of North America*, Vol.55, No.1, pp. 105-120, ISSN 0011-8532

Paesani, D.; Salas, E.; Martinez, A. & Isberg, A. (1999) Prevalence of temporomandibular joint disk displacement in infants and young children. *Oral Surgery, Oral Medicine, Oral Pathology, Oral Radiology, and Endodontics*, Vol.87, No1, pp. 15-19, ISSN 1079-2104

Palla, S. (1998) *Myoarthropathien des Kausystems und orofaziale Schmerzen*. ZZMK der Universität Zürich, ISBN 3-9521519-0-4, Zürich, Switzerland

Palla, S. (2003) Myoarthropatischer Schmerz: oft verkannt. *Der Schmerz*, Vol.17, No.6, pp. 425-431, ISSN 0932-433X

Pancherz, H.; Ruf, S. & Thomalske-Faubert, C. (1999) Mandibular articular disk position changes during Herbst treatment: a prospective longitudinal MRI study. *American Journal of Orthodontics and Dentofacial Orthopedics*, Vol.116, No.2, pp. 207-214, ISSN 0889-5406

Pellizoni, S.E.; Salioni, M.A.; Juliano, Y.; Guimarães, A.S. & Alonso, L.G. (2006) Temporomandibular joint disc position and configuration in children with functional unilateral posterior crossbite: a magnetic resonance imaging evaluation. *American Journal of Orthodontics and Dentofacial Orthopedics*, Vol.129, No.6, pp. 785-793, ISSN 0889-5406

Pereira, L.J.; Costa, R.C.; França, J.P.; Pereira, S.M. & Castelo, P.M. (2009) Risk indicators for signs and symptoms of temporomandibular dysfunction in children. *The Journal of Clinical Pediatric Dentistry*, Vol.34, No.1, pp. 81-86, ISSN 1053-4628

Petersson A. What you can and cannot see in TMJ imaging - an overview related to the RDC/TMD diagnostic system. (2010) *Journal of Oral Rehabilitation*, Vol.37, No.10, pp. 771-778, ISSN 0305-182X

von Piekartz H. Physikalische Untersuchung der Dysfunction in der kraniomandibulären Region. In: von Piekartz H (ed). *Kiefer, Gesichts- und Zervikalregion. Neuromuskulskeletale Untersuchung, Therapie und Management*. Stuttgart-New York: Thieme, 2005:122-66. ISBN: 9783131392312

Pullinger, A.G.; Seligman, D.A. & Gornbein, J.A. (1993) A multiple logistic regression analysis of the risk and relative odds of temporomandibular disorders as a function of common occlusal features. *Journal of Dental Research*, Vol.72, No.6, pp. 968-979, ISSN 0022-0345

Rammelsberg, P.(1998) *Untersuchungen über Ätiologie, diagnose und Therapie von Diskopathien des Kiefergelenkes*. Quintessenz, ISBN 3-87652-976-X, Berlin, Germany

Schmitter, M.; Essig, M.; Seneadza, V.; Balke, Z.; Schröder, J. & Rammelsberg, P. (2010) Prevalence of clinical and radiographic signs of osteoarthrosis of the temporomandibular joint in an older persons community. *Dento maxillo facial Radiology*, Vol.39, No.4, pp. 231-234, ISSN 0250-832X

Shen, Y.H.; Chen, Y.K. & Chuang, S.Y. (2005) Condylar resorption during active orthodontic treatment and subsequent therapy: report of a special case dealing with iatrogenic TMD possibly related to orthodontic treatment. *Journal of Oral Rehabilitation*, Vol.32, No.5, pp. 332-336, ISSN 0305-182X

Siegmund, T. & Harzer, W. (2002) Orthodontic diagnostics and treatment planning in adults with temporomandibular disorders a case report. *Journal of Orofacial Orthopedics*, Vol.63, No.5, pp. 435-445, ISSN 1434-5293

Slavicek, G. (2009) Okklusion im Schatten Evidenz basierter Medizin. *Stomatologie*, Vol.106, No.1, pp. 17-22, ISSN 0946-3151

Tecco, S.; Crincoli, V.; Di Bisceglie, B.; Saccucci, M.; MacrÍ, M.; Polimeni, A. & Festa, F. (2011) Signs and symptoms of temporomandibular joint disorders in Caucasian children and adolescents. *Cranio: the Journal of Craniomandibular Practice*, Vol.29, No.1, pp. 71-79, ISSN 0886-9634

Tecco, S. & Festa, F. (2010a) Prevalence of signs and symptoms of temporomandibular disorders in children and adolescents with and without crossbites. *World Journal of Orthodontics*, Vol.11, No.1, pp. 37-42, ISSN 1530-5678

Tecco S, Teté S, Crincoli V, Festa MA, Festa F. (2010b) Fixed orthodontic therapy in temporomandibular disorder (TMD) treatment: an alternative to intraoral splint. *Cranio: the Journal of Craniomandibular Practice*, Vol.28, No.1, pp. 30-42, ISSN 0886-9634

Tominaga K, Konoo T, Morimoto Y, Tanaka T, Habu M, Fukuda J. (2007) Changes in temporomandibular disc position during growth in young Japanese. *Dento maxillo facial Radiology*, Vol.36, No.7, pp. 397-401, ISSN 0250-832X

Toscano, P. & Defabianis, P. (2009) Clinical evaluation of temporomandibular disorders in children and adolescents: a review of the literature. *European Journal of Paediatric Dentistry*, Vol.10, No.4, pp. 188-192, ISSN 1591-996X

Tullberg, M.; Tsarapatsani, P.; Huggare, J. & Kopp S. (2001) Long-term follow-up of early treatment of unilateral forced posterior cross-bite with regard to temporomandibular disorders and associated symptoms. *Acta Odontologica Scandinavica*, Vol.59, No.5, pp. 280-284, ISSN 0001-6357

Türp, J.C. (2000) *Temporomandibular Pain - Clinical Presentation and Impact*. Quintessenz, ISBN 3-87652-648-5, Berlin, Germany

Türp, J.C. (2002) Über- Unter- und Fehlversorgung in der Funktionsdiagnostik und - therapie - Beispiele, Gefahren, Gründe - Teil I. *Schweizer Monatsschrift für Zahnmedizin*, Vol.112, No.8, pp. 819-823, ISSN 1011-4203

Türp, J.C. & Schindler, H.J. (2003) Zum Zusammnehang zwischen Okklusion und Myoarthropathien. Einführung eines integrierenden neurobiologischen Modells. *Schweizer Monatsschrift für Zahnmedizin,* Vol.113, No.9, pp. 965-971, ISSN 1011-4203

Wang, J.; Chao, Y.; Wan, Q. & Zhu, Z. (2008) The possible role of estrogen in the incidence of temporomandibular disorders. *Medical Hypotheses*, Vol.71, No.4, pp. 564-567, ISSN 0306-9877

17

Dentofacial Aspects of the Changes in Body Posture, Investigation Procedures

Emil Segatto and Angyalka Segatto
University of Szeged, Department of Orthodontics and Pediatric Dentistry
Hungary

1. Introduction

The literature exploring the reasons and the development of the orofacial-orthopaedic anomalies and orthodontic deviations deals measurably with the correlation of these deviations and postural disorders. The development of certain pathological curvatures different from the physiological curvatures of the spine is mainly responsible for the majority of the postural deviations present during the pre-puberty. No spinal curvatures are found in the frontal plane at healthy people. In a normal spine there are four types of spinal curvatures (thoracic and sacral kyphosis, and cervical and lumbar lordosis) in the sagittal plane responsible for the upstanding posture. These curvatures become the characteristic attributes of an individual at the age of six-seven (Bellyei, 1995).

During growth the functional disorders at the spinal and body muscles are manifested in poor postures of different severity and directions. These can result in considerable spinal and therefore trunk inclinations in the frontal, the sagittal or both planes. If observed in time the poor or abnormal posture can be corrected with effective muscle strengthening exercises. The failure of the early discovery and of the early started corrective muscle exercises result in the consolidation of the pathological posture and in the development of the spinal deformities. The development of these skeletal problems is associated in many instances by other primary factors of which entire scale has not been disclosed so far. Without reference to the several different causative factors the general characteristic of all spinal deformities is that the active muscle strengthening exercises are not suitable for the fully management though the progression rate can be positively influenced.

The pathological curvature found on any segment of the spine playing a primary role in establishing the static balance induces the apparition of compensating curvatures that many times due to their positional attributes result in abnormal head posture. This way the spinal curvatures found in the frontal plane result in laterally tilted head posture, while the pathological spinal curvatures in the sagittal plane result in forward, respectively backward tilted head posture. In case of compensating spinal deformities the head posture is normal and compensating spinal malformations evolved in lower position level.

The literature studying the deformation of the facial skeletal structures deals with the cause and effect correlations regarding the head posture disorders in several publications (Solow

& Tallgren, 1976; Marcotte, 1981; Solow & Siersbaek-Nielsen, 1986). According to the authors discovering positive relations, the head posture altered in the growth period - through the gravitational effects - induces pathological soft tissue load (Solow & Kreiborg, 1977), that on the basis of the functional matrix theory results in an abnormal development of the cartilage and bone structures concerning the direction and size (Proffit & Fields, 2000).

The literature has disclosed the examination of those subjects suffering from spinal deformities who have scoliosis characterized with curvatures in the frontal plane. There are no detailed data on a comprehensive dentofacial screening at patients with Scheuermann's disease with increased thoracic kyphosis inducing forward tilted head posture. The available researches deal with the dentofacial deviations that can be connected with the examined spinal deformities or with the patients with abnormal head postures. No one research has attempted to specifically examine the previously mentioned two subject groups with congenial methods and in the same time as regards the earlier determined dentofacial deviations, having separated the correlation with the functional and/or structural etiological problems.

The literature presenting the dentofacial aspects of the spinal deformities versus the orofacial orthopaedic examinations at patients with postural disorders does not have a long history. The difficulty of the accurate determination of the postural features was the main reason. The modernization of the posture examining radiation free methods has brought a break-through in this matter, rasterstereography being the most outstanding technology. This examination method enables the calibrated determination of such numerical parameters helping to indirectly describe the spinal curvatures responsible for poor body posture and it can be used for comparison at examinations performed on a large sample. The examination of the dentofacial deviation associated to the postural deformities comprised beside routine orthodontic examination methods functional and radiologic procedures as well. The latter mainly includes the evaluation of the lateral cephalogram, P-A cephalogram and Orthopantomograms (OPG). The P-A cephalogram unlikely the lateral cephalogram and the OPG is not a routine radiologic procedure in orthodontics. As a result of our researches made to decrease the radiation load, the self-developed OPG analysing software is suitable for the expansive topographic asymmetry examinations of the mandible. This way the P-A cephalograms becomes unnecessary.

During our research activity we could amend for the first time the results of the dentofacial examinations of the samples screened by the rasterstereographic method with the results of such a comprehensive examination where the evaluations of the lateral cephalograms were unified with the very detailed data of the mandibular asymmetry examinations. The asymmetry examinations have pointed out results showing close correlation with certain elements of the lateral cephalogram analyses that can substitute during the determination of the dentofacial sample. These findings defines further examination directions for the radiation load reduction with determining such measurements elaborated on OPG's that can replace the performance of the lateral cephalograms in cases that were considered positive during an orthopaedic screening.

The purpose of the chapter is to give a comprehensive vision about the correlation between the dentofacial problems and the changes in body posture which play an etiologic role in their development, with detailed presentation of the specific malformations of both fields, completed with the presentation of the up to date methods of investigation.

2. Factors causing changes in body posture

Among the factors influencing the static body posture - beside the lower limbs structural asymmetries - the structural deviations of the pelvis as well as the malformations of the direction of the spine and the supporting body muscles are present. The structural malformations of the pelvis are relatively rare, and nowadays the disadvantageous effects of the limb asymmetries influencing the body posture are more easily treated with the modern orthopaedic appliances. Due to the earlier mentioned cause and effect correlation among the body posture deviations playing a significant role in the alteration of the head posture, the alterations in the spine and supporting body muscle position deserve more attention because of the frequency indices and the difficult therapeutic treatment. The more severe part of the latter deviation-group is formed by the spinal deformities while the more frequent part by the body muscle morphofunctional deviations.

2.1 Spinal disorders

The common feature of the spinal deformities is the steady, structural deviation of the spine vertebrae which manifests in the pathological curvatures found on the affected spine segment due to the cumulated effects. Based on the frequency indices the two most prevailing spinal deformities are the scoliosis and the Scheuermann's disease, or Scheuermann's kyphosis. While the scoliotic curvature is a lateral curvature in the frontal plane, at Scheuermann's disease the hyperkyphosis developed due to the increase of the physiological thoracic kyphotic curvature. The appearance time and the progression of these deviations can be very diverse. We have to take into consideration that the quick condition decline most frequently is at the beginning of puberty, which - based on the earlier literature - significantly influences the development of the dentofacial deviations (Huggare et al., 1991).

2.1.1 Scoliosis

Scoliosis - its first written records are connected to Hippocrates – is a pathological entity with unknown aetiology. Its characteristic feature is the lateral spinal curvature developed as a result of the asymmetric growth of the vertebrae (Lowe et al., 2000). No spinal deviations are found in the frontal plane at healthy people. With the development of the structural deviations the pathological spinal curvatures become steady later, so the spinal deformity developed this way is called scoliosis. The curvatures found in the frontal plane are accompanied by the rotations measurable at horizontal plane as well as the altered curvatures in the sagittal plane. These deformities most often affect the thoracic and the lumbar segment segregated or entirely affecting such compensating curvatures that are entitled to ease the load and to balance the compression areas.

Scoliosis can be divided upon several aspects. Basically we can talk about primary and secondary scoliosis. The asymmetric growth developed on the spinal vertebral level is the reason of the primary deviation. This can be congenital or acquired. The acquired primary scoliosis can be further divided into idiopathic, traumatic, infectious, neuromuscular, tumorous and degenerative. Scoliosis according to the direction of the curvature can be classified as follows: convex to the right or left, or of double direction. Scoliosis can further be classified by the localization of the curvatures. The curvatures can be structural or functional, as well as compensated or non-compensated. The most frequently examined type is the primary idiopathic scoliosis due to its incidence, its particular clinical feature and its progression. According to when onset occurs scoliosis can be: juvenile and adolescent. While at the juvenile scoliosis 90% of the cases show spontaneous improvement, the adolescent scoliosis is a progressive type deviation and till the age of 25 is constantly worsening in different phases (Herman et al., 1985).

During the examination of the affected spinal segment the morphological features detected on both side of the spinal curvature show correlation with the severity of the curvature. The vertebral bodies broaden on the convex side, the rips are deforming and lifting towards the dorsal while the radius of their curvature is decreasing. On the concave side the vertebral bodies are narrower; the ribs are deformed while losing their normal curvatures they are curving straightforward (Bellyei, 1995). When scoliosis is present, the thoracic kyphosis decreases, straightens or could become lordotic. On the convex side at the apex of the curvature the ribs are heightened because of the spinal torsion, while on the concave side the ribs are sinking. The direction of the ribs deformation on the foreside of the thorax is opposed. The childhood clinical symptoms become localized on the spinal deformity, pains and other complaints are missing. Larger curvatures can be seen due to the postural and the caused structural asymmetries.

The basic conclusions of the researches related to the aetiology of the idiopathic structural scoliosis as regards the development of the scoliosis are the following: correlates to the adolescent growth-spurt; in girls the development of the curvature tends to be of a greater severity; presence of different deformities and genetically inherited (Hadley, 2000). Among the several aetiological factors the most often mentioned are the defect on level of CNS, the failure in the control of the melatonin production, the effect of calmodulin, the collagen abnormality, the altered platelets, as well as several hypothetical genetic inheritance – autosomal dominant inheritance, multi gene inheritance, multi-factorial inheritance and the X-linked dominant inheritance (Wise et al., 2000; Inoue et al., 2002; Parent et al., 2005).

Because of the diversity of world-wide applied early screening protocols, different occurrence data are available. The screenings at school showed such visually detectable body asymmetry at 15% of girls and boys at age 10 and 14, which were later proved by radiological examinations. The international literature data reports a ratio of 10 girls for every one boy (Morissy & Weinstein, 2006). On the basis of the earlier mentioned the classic idiopathic structural scoliosis is a right-curved, dorsal, lateral spinal curvature found at girls between age 10 and 12. The rotation evolved among the affected vertebrae and the presence of the torsion - a shift between certain elements within the vertebrae - is also characteristic features of the disease (Bagnall, 2008). The natural process of scoliosis is basically determined by the etiology and the outline of the curvature. The most frequent symptoms of the untreated scoliosis: the progression of the curvature, back pains, cardiopulmonary complaints and psychosocial problems. Though the mentioned symptoms are present in most of the cases, the effects on the entire organism are various. One single constant adjunct element to the untreated scoliosis, which shows a close correlation with the degree of the curvature, is the decrease of the pulmonary function. This is ascribable to the lateral curvature, the high degree thoracic lordosis, the rotation of the vertebrae and the decreased dynamism of the respiratory muscles. As regards the psychosocial problems, the findings are particularly different. One third of the untreated patients with scoliosis reported that the disease curbed their every day activities (Lin et al., 2001).

2.1.2 Scheuermann's disease

The disease developed with the enlargement of the thoracic kyphosis of the spine and as a result of the structural deviation of the involved spinal segment was named and described as „kyphosis dorsalis juvenilis" by Scheuermann, a Danish radiologist (Ali, 1999). There are several names for the disorder in the literature: M.Scheuermann, osteochondrosis juvenilis dorsi, kyphosis dorsalis juvenilis, Scheuermann's kyphosis, juvenile kyphosis, Calvé's disease (Lowe, 1999). Actually the deformity is considered to be a form of juvenile osteochondrosis of the spine.

The degree of the thoracic kyphosis varies at healthy individuals; the normal curvature of the thoracic spine is between 20 and 40 degrees. The kyphotic curvature of more than 40-45 degrees gives the impression of a humpback, which is sometimes accompanied by the forward tilted head posture. Under the most frequently affected thoracic segment the increased compensatory lordosis of the lumbar part appears. In 25-30 % of the cases a moderate, generally functional dorso-lumbar scoliosis associates the previously mentioned deviations (Lemirre et al., 1996).

According to the localization the Scheuermann's disease can be classified in three main types. The type localized on the thoracic part is the most frequent, it extends on more vertebrae and usually painless. The dorso-lumbar interim type is rare, it covers several vertebrae and pain can be observes. The rarest type is the lumbar localized, it affects only one vertebrae and it is usually accompanied by pain (Bellyei, 1995). The children suffering from Scheurmann's disease are thin, have weak body muscles manifested in poor body posture and in abnormal head posture. In the majority of the cases the increased thoracic kyphosis causes only interim disturbance of growth and lasts till the end of growth with no progression. In a minor number severe progression can be observed, these can hardly be cured with conservative treatments. In these cases the thoracic kyphosis is very increased and the deformity is accompanied by complaints. In general there is no correlation between the onset of the complaints and the severity of the kyphosis - even a severe kyphosis can be painless, and in fact with a mild kyphotic curvature severe pains can be detected.

Similarly as in the case of scoliosis the earlier age the symptoms are present, the more favourable the prognosis is. Progression speeds up at the puberty phase. In this development period the growth of muscles cannot follow the fast grow of the bones. As a result of the endocrine harmonization and the increased stress the severity of deformity develops together with the complaints (Deacon et al., 1985).

The accurate etiology of the disease is still unknown. Some researchers consider the disease as deviations present at the level of the intervertebral discs among the vertebrae; others think that the endochondral ossification disorder of end plates is the causative factor. The notion „insufficientia vertebrae" introduced by Schanz originates the development of the deviation to the balance disorder of the active (muscular) and passive (skeletal) system. Today it is a well-known fact that beside the mechanical factors, weight and height also play an important role. Some researchers proved the presence of the autosomal dominant inheritance - the expected incidence for the repetition of the disorder in the family of the child with Scheuermann's disease is 50 %. Literature sources reports on very diverse incidence values. These vary between 0.4% - 8%, with similar ratio in the two genders (Tribus, 1998).

The most characteristic symptom of the disorder is the increased thoracic kyphosis indicating forward tilted hunchback posture. The compensatory lordosis of the spine segment found caudally from the deformity is less visible similarly to the functional scoliosis present as an accompanying symptom in some of the cases. It is more common the forward tilted head posture as well as the pendulous upper limbs attributable to the myasthenia. The characteristic of the disease is the presence of the "wedging" shape vertebrae developed on the involved spine segment, which makes the kyphotic curvature more increased. The Schmorl's nodes developed as a result of the forces acting through the anterior flattened vertebral discs and the presence of the uneven, attenuated endplate surfaces are very important in the distinctive diagnosis (Bradford, 1981). In case of untreated kyphotic curvature with less than 100 degrees the decrease of the pulmonary function is not common. In case of a kyphotic curvature with more than 100 degrees, with apex of the curve located between 1 and 8 thoracic vertebrae always can be seen restrictive pulmonary disorder (Murray et al., 1993).

2.2 Postural problems

The harmonic spinal curvature system proper to the individual in case of normal static development appears by the age of 6-7. The abnormal or poor body posture develops most frequently due to the spinal deformities in the sagittal plane. When developing beside the lowered load capacity of the spinal and body muscles the lack of will-powers needed for normal body posture as well as psychic factors play a significant role. Postural problems can be divided into three main groups: dorsum rotundum - thoracic kyphosis larger than the normal; dorsum kypholordoticum - increased thoracic kyphosis accompanied by compensatory increased lumbar lordosis and dorsum planum - thoracic kyphosis smaller than the normal. The common feature of postural problems is that they can be corrected by active muscle power. Accompanying symptoms are: loose joints, pes planovagus and vaulted abdomen, procident shoulders and frequent abdominal breathing (Bellyei, 1995).

2.3 Methods of investigation

The examination of the presented postural problems is partly done by physical and partly by instrumental diagnostic examination methods. The use of the clinical examination methods besides the orthopedic consulting-hours is standing orders at school and paediatrician consultation hours. The completion of the instrumental examinations and the result evaluations require specialist background and consulting-room environment.

The observation being used as a first step in the physical examination methods trends to body postures and respectively to the possible asymmetries. The higher-degree pathological spinal curvatures become visible by influencing the body posture. The lateral curvatures higher than 5 degree are responsible for the asymmetric appearance. The increased curvature can be observed laterally on the thoracic segment of the vertebrae with palpation.

The examination of the child's back in forward bend position (Adam's test) follows. At children with scoliosis a rib hump can be seen on the convex side of the curvature, which can be measure by the help of a scoliometer. At children with Scheuermann's disease during the test while the apex of the curvature is pushed down the patient is asked to chase by lifting their arms and head. As opposed to healthy as well as children with postural problems the kyphosis in case of Scheuermann's disease hardly decrease or not at all. As a last step during the examination of the locomotion range of the spine the aim of the trunk bending forward and back and laterally is to detect the restrain, which can be cause by the fixation of the involved spine deformity. At the potential pathological cases screened during testing the performation of an instrumental examination is suggested to confirm the diagnosis (Tribus, 1998).

The most frequent instrumental diagnostic examination methods are the radiological procedures. The methods developed to evaluate the radiograms taken from different sides are of high accuracy, due to their widespread use their evaluations are permeable, they are easily understood both in therapy and researches and can be used by all.

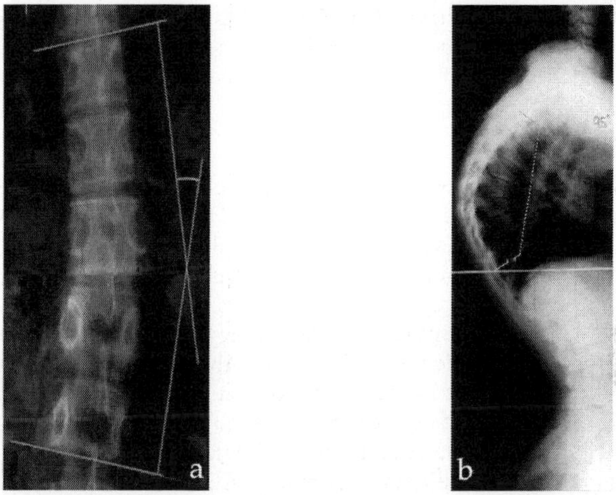

Fig. 1. Measurement of the: scoliotic curvature according to Cobb (a) and kyphotic angle (b).

The most prevailing measure for determining the scoliotic curvatures is the determination of the Cobb angle. These are defined by the adjacent angle of the angle between the lines drawn perpendicular along the superior and inferior end plates of the vertebrae bordering the curvature (Fig.1.a.). Since there is not physiological spinal curvature in the frontal plane the measurable Cobb values unequivocally show the presence of scoliosis. The determination of the kyphotic curvature in degrees in case of Scheuermann's disease happens in the same way using the end plates of the superior and inferior vertebrae of the pathological curvature for the measurements (Fig.1.b.). For a Scheuermann's disease diagnosis the presence of the following x-ray symptoms is essential: khypothic curvature greater than 45°; presence of three or more adjacent "wedging" shape vertebrae; presence of Schmorl's nodes (Ali et al., 1999).

Because of the expansion of the spine the amount of the radiation dosage as well as the more frequent x-ray picture taking explained by the disease process have increasingly highlighted the importance of those attempts, which focused on developing diagnostic examination methods with reduced exposure to radiation. These methods deduce the spinal structural deformities from the morphological features of the surface back contour. During their development period in order to increase the accuracy the most important aspect was the comparability with the reliable radiological parameters. At the beginning the radiation free moiré-topography was the greatest break-through, but because of its efficiency indicator did not work out as a routine application (Kim et al., 2001).

The appearance of the rasterstereography providing more accurate values than the moiré-topography was a milestone (Frobin & Hierholzer, 1981). In the course of the rasterstereography procedure the testing device (Formetric 2, Diers International GmbH, Schlangenbad, Germany) elaborates a 3-D photographic mapping of the patient's back in upright position. For this purpose the device projects a sensitive gridded picture onto the back of the patient positioned at the suitable distance and way.

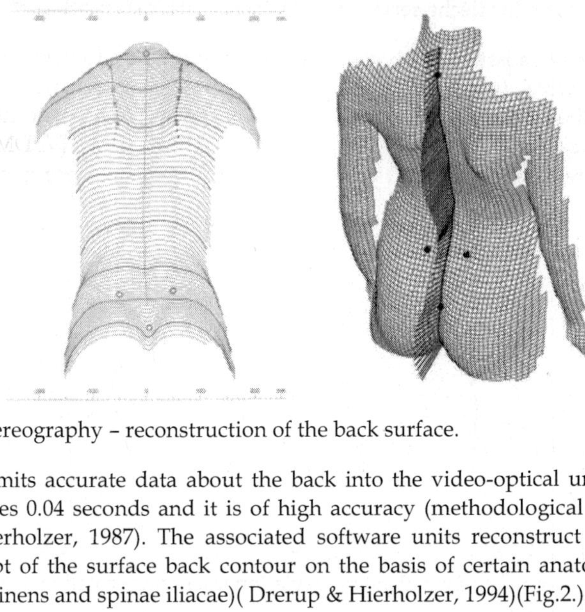

Fig. 2. Rasterstereography – reconstruction of the back surface.

The grid transmits accurate data about the back into the video-optical unit. Mapping the entire back takes 0.04 seconds and it is of high accuracy (methodological error < 0.1 mm) (Drerup & Hierholzer, 1987). The associated software units reconstruct the sagittal and frontal intercept of the surface back contour on the basis of certain anatomical structures (vertebra prominens and spinae iliacae)(Drerup & Hierholzer, 1994)(Fig.2.).

With the usage of mathematical algorithms the visualization of the surface back contour is available from both sagittal and frontal side. The shift of the spine from the real perpendicular can be shown with a mathematical modelling. The curvatures in the sagittal plane can be reproduced with a 2.8° accuracy, those in the frontal plane with a 2° accuracy.

The sagittal curvatures can be characterized with the following measurement from lateral aspect: fléche cervicale and fléche lombaire. Both measurements show the distance of the furthest point of a given area calculated from the tangent lined along the hams and blades, enabling the very accurate approach of the thoracic kyphosis degree (Lippold et al., 2006a)(Fig.3.a.).

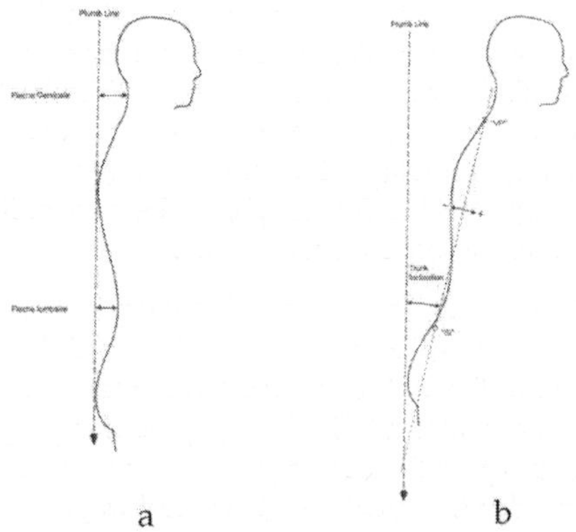

a b

Fig. 3. Rasterstereography: fléche cervicale and fléche lombaire (a) and trunk inclination (b).

The most important measurement related to the body posture from lateral aspect is the trunk inclination, which is described by the angle between the vertical based on the vertebra prominens and the straight line between vertebra prominens and the center point of the straight line between the right and left crista iliaca posterior superior (VPDM line) (Fig.3.b.). Three variables are characteristic for the lateral curvatures from frontal aspect (Fig.4.).

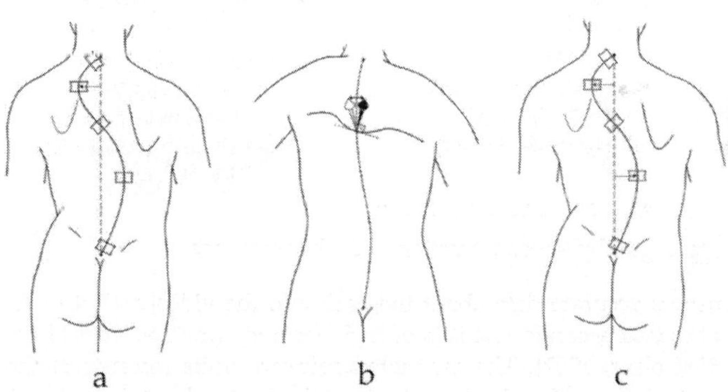

a b c

Fig. 4. Rasterstereography: maximal lateral deviation (a), surface rotational amplitude (b) and lateral amplitude (c).

The maximal lateral deviation shows the distance of the vertebra found at the apex of the greatest curvature in the spinal frontal plane from the VPDM line (Drerup et al., 1997) (Fig.4.a.). The surface rotational amplitude is the angle between the perpendiculars drawn on the vertebrae showing the greatest rotation on the lateral curvature (Fig.4.b.). The lateral amplitude is the sum of the distances measured from the VPDM line of the opposite side curvatures of the apex vertebra found in the frontal plane (Fig.4.c.).

Beside its outstanding reliability the radiation-free aspect of the method makes it favourable for screening the large patient groups for research purposes. Though when developing several instrumental examination methods the main purpose is the accurate, quick and radiation-free diagnostic, these facts are suitable only for determination of the degree of the body posture disorder without x-ray pictures. The rasterstereography procedure is feasible to define the degree of different spinal disorders (Schulte et al., 2008). When compared to some x-ray measurement we obtain results that are closer to the kyphotic curvature values than in the case of the scoliotic curvatures (Weiss & ElObeidi, 2009). To support the diagnosis of the spinal disorders - structural deformed vertebrae - the evaluation of the spine x-rays are still necessary. In diagnosing the postural problems the rasterstereography is suitable for separating three main types, also for accurate localizing and measuring the curves deviated from the normal but not being steady yet. In order to acknowledge these results taking x-ray pictures of differential diagnosis importance is essential, these being suitable for revealing the lack of "wedging" shape vertebrae and Schmorl's nodes.

3. Dentofacial features associated to changes in body posture

3.1 Literature review

In the course of the interdisciplinary researches the investigation of the orthopaedic and orthodontic correlations has an important academic and practical significance concerning the separation of the preventive diagnostic and therapeutic areas within the two specialities. The literature sources reports on several researches that were examining the correlation between certain orthopaedic parameters and certain Angle classes. The results presume possible correlations between the scoliosis and the Angle Class II malocclusion (Huggare et al., 1991) as well as between the poor body posture and Class II malocclusions (Lippold et al., 2003). Similarly the close correlation between the lateral spinal deformity and the unilateral crossbite, as well as the lower midline deviation has been proved in some researches (Huggare, 1998; Ben-Bassat et al., 2006). The cause of the presented malocclusions in majority of the cases is the presence of the skeletal asymmetries. (Sabah, 2002). This is also confirmed by the subgroup of the Angle Class II malocclusion frequently associated with the jaw asymmetry (Ben-Bassat et al., 1993). The registration of the jaw asymmetries related to the scoliosis is due to the tight relation with the adjacent soft tissues and it can be even demonstrated through a simple observation (Korbmacher et al., 2004). The typical deviation of the facial midline and the presence of spinal deformity as a causative agent introduced the naming of facial scoliosis accepted and used in the literature. The findings show a close correlation between the patients with severe scoliosis and the presence of the convergence angle describing the facial scoliosis (U. Hirschfelder & H. Hirschfelder, 1983). The laterally tilted head posture can likely be a cause for the correlation between the facial soft tissue as well as the skeletal asymmetries and the lateral deviation of the spine (Pirttiniemi et al., 1989; Huggare et al., 1991; Huggare, 1998). The pathological symptoms present on the temporomandibular joints level loaded asymmetrical by the abnormal head posture also show a close correlation with the spinal deformities determining the head posture (Kondo & Aoba, 1999). Finally, it is worth mentioning the problems of the dental deformities appearing during the treatment of the scoliosis and as a result of it. This has mainly historic importance since the Milwaukee-brace - which has totally lost ground in the therapeutic practice – played a principal role in the existence of the mentioned dental deformities (Bögi & Nagy, 1970, Paphalmy et al., 1975).

The literature examining the orofacial-orthopaedic deviations beside the orthopaedic disorders deals in details with the deviations observed in the sagittal plane and with the analysis of the pathological spinal deformities possibly allocable to them. Among the orthodontic diagnostic radiologic methods the spread of the lateral cephalograms has launched an extensive research activity aiming at investigation the etiology of the dental and skeletal deviation being measurable this way. These researches enlisted the interest to the correlation between the deviations found in the vertical and sagittal plane and the forward, respectively backward tilted head posture (Yamaguchi & Sueishi, 2003). Various researches revealed close relation between the cervical hyperlordosis and the cl. II malocclusions (Solow & Tallgren, 1976; Huggare, 1998). In average a 2 mm lack of space associates the increased craniocervical angle in the upper or lower frontal regions of the dental arch (Solow & Sonnesen, 1998). Different intra-articular distances were recorded on x-ray pictures taken in with the head in various postures, which is probably a manifestation of differences in mandibular loading in the different head postures (Visscher et al., 2000). In order to explain the precise correlations the demand is to take cephalograms in natural head position (Leitao & Nanda, 2000). The basic criteria of taking cephalograms - the head position which is essential for evaluation - contradict the notion of natural head position, therefore this issue is still unsolved (Raju et al., 2001; Halazonetis, 2002). Contradictory to this the investigations searched the cephalograms taken in the positioned posture related to the true vertical and the true horizontal reference, not taking into account the relationship between natural head position and craniofacial morphology. The cephalograms examined this way enabled accurate measurements, hereby appraisable correlations related to maxilla were possible, while the inaccuracy of the mandibular measurement excluded the use of these methods for scientific purposes. Close correlation with the natural head position is shown only by the following measurement: facial axis, lower facial height and the facial ratios (Leitao & Nanda, 2000). The rasterstereographic procedures - used with research purpose recently - have a great importance in the head posture determination, but findings related to the connection between the body posture affected by the spine morphology and the head posture are still humble in number. The examination of the orthodontic deviations at children with Scheuermann's disease cannot be found in the qualified literature apart from the publications presenting some partial findings of our researches (Segatto et al., 2006, 2008).

There is a relatively great number of findings in the literature dealing with the relationship between the characteristics of the body posture determined by rasterstereographic procedures and certain orofacial-orthopaedic parameters. During the examination of the dental features the investigation did not show any close correlation between the characteristics of the spine morphology and the overjet (Lippold et al., 2006b). Similarly no close correlation was revealed between the mandibular position and the variables of the kyphotic and the lordotic angle or the pelvic inclination (Lippold et al., 2005). Among the craniofacial skeletal parameters the facial axis, the mandibular plane and the facial depth showed a significant correlation with the degree of the cervical curvature (Murray et al., 1993). Similarly, the facial axis together with the lordotic angle and the pelvic inclination, the inner gonial angle and the mandibular plane with the lordotic angle and the pelvic inclination, as well as the facial depth with the pelvic inclination showed a significant correlation (Lippold et al., 2006b). Finally the examination of the correlation between the pelvic torsion, the facial axis and the facial depth whereby the vertical and the sagittal mandibular parameters are in close correlation with the body posture needs to be mentioned (Lippold et al., 2007).

3.2 Methods of investigation

The examination of the dentofacial feature follows the standard orthodontic intra- and extra-oral examination protocol. Beside the physical functional and morphological examinations the evaluation of the x-ray pictures are paid great attention. The physical tests focused on the measurement of the TMJ condition and the activity of the adjacent muscles. The applied procedures comprise of the determination of the movement ranges and the detection of the differences between the sides. The extra-oral part of the morphological tests focused on the observation of the abnormal facial ration and the registration of the facial asymmetries. During the intraoral test the dental and occlusion features were examined. Vertical features: the frontal open bite and the deep bite as well as the lateral deep bite; sagittal features: the frontal overjet, crossbite, as well as the molar relationship ranged in Angle classes.

For analysing the skeletal features, for mapping the dentoskeletal conditions and for determining the position of the two jaws to each other and to the base of the skull the evaluation of different radiograms are available. During several researches the evaluation of the lateral cephalogram, the postero-anterior cephalogram as well as the orthopantomogram pictures provided the data. The standardized conditions provide the adaptability of the radiograms for researches. The determination of the skeletal features on the lateral and the postero-anterior cephalograms is done with one of the known evaluation methods. The most frequently measured parameters on the postero-anterior cephalogram by Ricketts are as follows: the inclination of the occlusal plane, postural symmetry, maxillary ratio, mandibular ratio, maxillary-mandibular midline; while on the lateral cephalogram: the maxillary depth, the ramus position, the facial axis, the lower facial height and the mandibular plane angle. Beside the determination of the asymmetry of the cranial structures on the postero-anterior cephalogram we used the parameters obtained during the definition of the mandibular asymmetries for our researches. Contrary to the cephalometric measurement when measuring the mandibular asymmetry no evaluation software was available. To overcome the compilation difficulties of the digital x-ray pictures and to evaluate quickly and accurately a large number of radiograms we developed the first mandibular asymmetry evaluating software. The measurements done by AsymmetrixX were based on previously accepted methods, which were modified taking into account the compilation characteristics. The asymmetry index calculation is used for the comparison of the distances of the two mandibular-halves (d) on the basis of the following formula: d asymmetry-index (AI) = $\left| (d_{right} - d_{left})/(d_{right} + d_{left}) \right| \times 100$. The importance of the mandibular asymmetry examination is provided by those findings that confirm that two-third of the asymmetries originates from the lower third of the face, and the size or the positional disorders of the mandible are responsible for their development (Vig & Hewitt, 1975; Farkas & Cheung, 1981).

The application of the Orthopantomogram being part of the orthodontic routine radiograms to the examination of mandibular asymmetries has a long history. In the early period of the application the problem of the reproducibility had to be solved; the solution was the creation of the head position standards (Larheim & Svanaes, 1986). After this, in order to eliminate the distortions emerging as the attribute of taking radiograms those recommendations were created that aimed to exclude certain measurement direction from the calculations (Habets et al., 1987). It proved to be similarly useful the application of the threshold value of 6% in the course of introducing the asymmetry index for substituting the head position deviations (Habets et al., 1988). On the basis of the asymmetry index formula the difference of 6% between the two sides equals to an asymmetry index of 3%. The results vary between 0% (full symmetry) and 100% (full asymmetry), and results below 3% conventionally counts as symmetric.

Several papers dealt with the control of the genuineness of the early protocols and of the reliability of the method (Schulze et al., 2000; Stramotas et al., 2002; Saglam, 2003). A couple of them provide newer measurement and structural methods, too. There were some attempts to determine the mandibular asymmetries on the basis of the soft tissues contour with the help of graphical applications, however, the variedly implemented analysis of the OPG's remained the gold standard (Edler et al., 2003; Good et al., 2006).

In the period of the spread of the mandibular asymmetry measurements the distances to be compared became measurable by re-tracing the OPG's and by compiling the reference points and lines. With the spread of the digital x-rays the compilation of the distances required the use of graphical design programs, which meant a great difficulty for a medical research expert. The awkward compilation procedure assumed a deep knowledge of the design program and the long evaluation procedure suitable for limited data collection did not enable the examination of large patient group. The modern cephalometric procedure in the case of the digital lateral and PA cephalograms enabled the combination of the latter ones and the graphical applications used at the mandibular asymmetry measurements. As a result of this the number of the measurements increased and more accurate analysis are possible.

The analysing program AsymmetrixX developed to satisfy the provided claims were made in Delphi 7 development environment (Fig.5.). The principal accuracy of the measurements is determined by the size of the reference point and the thickness of the compiled added lines, whose size is: 1 pixel = 0.26 mm. Because of the measurement accuracy and the comparability it is important to unify the size of the OPG's to be analysed, which complies with the calibration requirement as well. After setting the adequate sharpness and contrast rates the selection of the OPG can be done by browsing from any paths. Before this the data required by the program for identifying the examined person (name, date of birth, date of taking the OPG) are recorded.

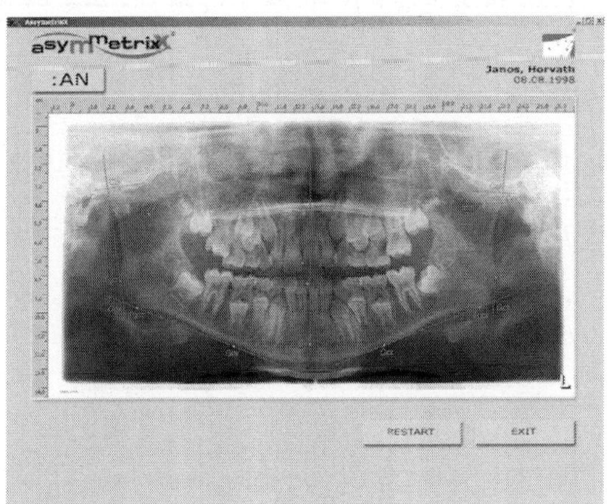

Fig. 5. Drawings performed with AsymmetrixX.

In the first step of the analysis by superposing the moveable Codr - Tgrr line appearing next to the right mandibular ramus to the Codr (Condylion dorsale right) and the Tgrr (Tangent ramus right) points we receive the right ramus tangent. By confirming the movement we determine the Codr point at the meeting of the tangent and the condylion, then the Tgrr point as a next step. After this the moveable Gnr - Tgcr line appears under the mandibular corpus, which we superpose on the Gnr (Gnathion right) and the Tgcr (Tangent corpus right) points, and we receive the right corpus tangent. After the fixation, next to the mentum we determine the Gnr point at the meeting of the tangent and the corpus, then the Tgcr point before the mandibular corner, at the meeting of the tangent and the corpus. Simultaneously with this, on the ramus tangent a slidable added perpendicular line appears; we fix it by moving it up to the top point of the processus condylaris. The next required point is the Cor (Condylion right) determined at the meeting of the fixed added line and the top point of the processus condylaris. By fixing it, the next slidable added line perpendicular to the ramus tangent appears, which we set to the bottom point of the Incisura mandibulae, and the meeting point determines the point Incr (Incisura mandibulae right).

The determination of the aforementioned reference points and lines should be followed by the left counterparts: left ramus tangent, Codl (Condylion dorsale left), Tgrl (Tangent ramus left), left corpus tangent, Gnl (Gnathion left), Tgcl (Tangent corpus left), Col (Condylion left), then Incl (Incisura mandibulae left). After the compilation of the paired measurement points come the unpaired points, which are requested in the following order by the program: the ANS (Anterior nasal spine), the is (incision superior), the ii (incision inferior), then finally the Sy (Symphysis mandibulae). After the fixation of this latter a line compiled from this point appears automatically, which will be perpendicular to the added line linking the meeting points of the bilateral ramus and corpus tangents (Gor - Gonion right and Gol - Gonion left). The program measures the distance of the other three odd points from this line. This way the ANS distance indicates the mentum deviation from the mid-facial reference structures, and the distance of the two dental midlines indicates the deviation thereof from the mandibular midline.

In the course of the compilation we received two important reference lines: the GoL (Gonion line) links the two compiled mandibular angles, and the ML (Midline) perpendicular to this indicates the mandibular midline. The two lines develop such a coordinate system, where the coordinates of the determined measurement points indicate the distance thereof from the adequate lines, in absolute values. Besides the distances measured from the two lines the program determines the distance of the projections of the given measurement points (Cor and Incr as well as Col and Incl) falling to the two ramus tangents. The so received RH (ramus height) = Go-Inc section and CH (condylar height) = Inc-Co section are suitable for the formerly applied mandibular asymmetry measurements. Each of the distances measured on the two halves of the mandible are suitable to be applied in the formerly explained asymmetry index formula.

Besides the indication of the length values the program automatically performs the asymmetry index calculations, and it represents the received 67 variables (51 distance measurements, 16 indices) in a csv file suitable for Excel statistical applications, so the possible errors of the manual data recording are eliminated. The graphic presentation of the major results provides useful help for the fellow professions during the quick orientation among the analysis results. At the same time, the storage of all formats of the results is easily solved; they can be used for comparison with further analyses.

Our attempts get deeper connotations by the principles of the human face asymmetry examinations. In case of apparently symmetric, harmonic faces there are often skeletal asymmetries found which seems to confirm the camouflage ability of the soft tissues (Shah & Joshi, 1978). Due to the lack of the criteria system related to the determination of the asymmetry there is no precise threshold value above which the given measurement is asymmetric. At the same time the more visible an asymmetry is, the more attention deserves since the closer it gets to the pathological condition (Rossi et al., 2003). The asymmetries of the craniofacial area are observed as the size disorders of the two face-halves. The amplitude of the real disorders is often decreased by the well functioning adjacent soft tissues through the camouflage effect (Bishara et al., 1994). The most common method to reveal the skeletal asymmetries being present behind the soft tissues is taking frontal cephalograms (P-A). Taking these postero-anterior cephalograms – due to the unnecessary radiation loading – is needed in the case of one-third of those asymmetries where not the mandibular region is responsible for the deformations. At the examination of the mandibular asymmetries, a further disadvantage is the occlusal position that could result in inaccurate measurements in the case of possible functional deviations.

By developing the AsymmetrixX we aimed at working out such analysing software that is suitable for a simple, quick and very accurate asymmetry analysis of the most widespread - and suitable for large utilization - panoramic radiograms (OPG). Its usage enables the omission of the indication of the postero-anterior cephalograms related to the asymmetry examination, thus decreasing the patients' radiation load.

4. The use of AsymmetrixX to examine the mandibular asymmetries associated with postural deformities

4.1 Aim

The aim of the study is the mandibular asymmetry analysis of the children's orthopantomogram participating in the rasterstereographic surface back contour examination with AsymmetrixX in order to detect the correlations between the surface back contour characteristics and the elements of the topographic patterns of an accurate mandibular asymmetry.

4.2 Subjects and methods

The members of the examination group were selected from 320 children registered at the orthodontic consultations. We used the data of 271 children complied with the selection criteria - spinal deformities neither diagnosed nor treated earlier; dental and orofacial-orthopaedic deviations neither diagnosed nor orthodontically treated earlier; had rasterstereographic back contour analysis, and orthopantomogram done during the consultation – for the examinations. Average age of the group: 11Y8M; min.: 7Y2M; max.: 16Y12M; SD: 2Y0M; distribution of the genders: 42.4% boys, 57.6% girls (Fig.6.).

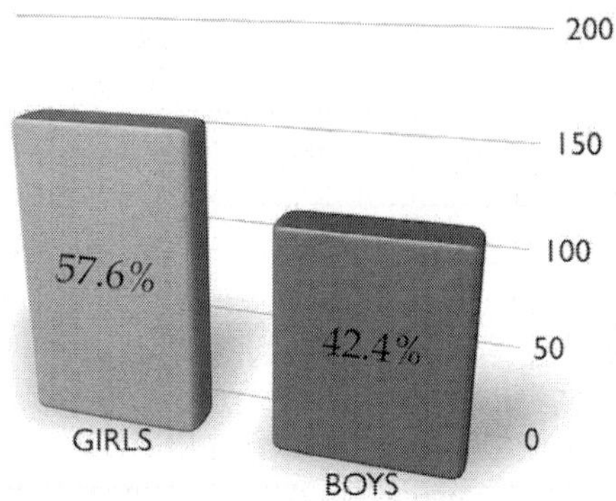

Fig. 6. The distribution of the children participating in the examination by gender.

4.3 Results

After the descriptive statistical analysis of the orthopaedic and dentofacial instrumental testing data, the detailed comparison of these data served the findings of our researches.

4.3.1 The descriptive statistics of the results obtained by the rasterstereographic surface back contour analysis

12 variables are determined during the rasterstereographic procedure, some of them related to the characteristics observed on the sagittal, the other on the frontal plane of the surface back contour. With the help of a multidimensional scaling we place the main components of the 12 variables in 2 dimension so that the heavily correlating ones to be close to each other (distance formula: -ln(abs(Pearson r)). This way the variables are separated into 5 groups, which were reduced to three by the importance concerning the view of the examination. The components being in heavy correlation with each other enabled further reduction, finally this decreased the applied indices to three sagittal and three frontal variables. They are the following:

- fléche cervicale – kyphosis index
- fléche lombaire – lordosis index
- trunk inclination – entire kypholordotic index
- maximal lateral deviation – lateral scoliosis index
- surface rotational amplitude – rotational scoliosis index
- lateral amplitude – entire scoliosis index.

The descriptive statistics of the orthopaedic variables are presented in (Table 1.).

		N	Min.	Max.	Mean	SD
Results of the rasterstereographic analyses	Fléche cervicale	271	0.00mm	138.95mm	53.89	21.28
	Fléche lombaire	271	1.70mm	72.20mm	30.65	13.12
	Trunk inclination	271	-5.65°	11.56°	2.90	3.07
	Maximal lateral deviation	271	-27.92mm	21.53mm	-5.95	8.60
	Surface rotational amplitude	271	1.72°	19.14°	6.79	3.22
	Lateral amplitude	271	3.44mm	34.56mm	11.65	5.19

Table 1. The descriptive statistics of the parameters determined by rasterstereography.

4.3.2 The descriptive statistics of the mandibular asymmetry examination results

The asymmetry examinations of the OPG's of the patient groups were done by the AsymmetrixX analysing software. The program after determining the required tangents and measuring points calculates 67 variables. To reduce these variables we used the 2 dimension projection of the multidimensional scaling of the main components and correlations. This way the variables were classified into three groups, though these groups do not demarcate from each other therefore by further reduction of the heavily correlation variables we did not manage to narrow the number of the measurement suitable for further comparative examination.

Those horizontal linear measurements which due to the inaccuracy of the horizontal lenght measurements characteristics of OPG are omitted from the comparison are not among the applied variables. The remaining 36 variables consist of 6 horizontal and 9 vertical asymmetry indices and 21 vertically oriented distance measurements. The descriptive statistics of the most important vertical mandibular asymmetry variables are presented in (Table 2.).

		N	Min.	Max.	Mean	SD
Results of the analyses performed with AsymmetrixX	Cod-ML index	271	-9.50	29.47	1.78	4.75
	Go-ML index	271	-11.09	30.70	1.05	4.39
	Co-GoL index	271	-11.16	91.69	3.26	15.81
	Tgr-GoL index	271	-80.56	21.42	-4.06	18.21
	CH index	271	-21.07	14.99	-0.29	5.57
	RH index	271	-8.65	11.31	0.48	3.24
	CH+RH index	271	-3.90	7.02	0.29	1.70
	CHr	271	12.74mm	30.29mm	20.67	3.12
	CHl	271	13.72mm	29.66mm	20.74	2.79

Table 2. The descriptive statistics of the main vertical parameters determined by AsymmetrixX.

4.3.3 Comparative examination results

Due to the large number of the comparable variables the examination of correlation between the orthopaedic and dentofacial parameters was done by the stepwise linear regression. In case of the fléche cervicale orthopaedic variable the (CH + RH) mean ($p<0.0005$, coefficient: 1.258), the Tgc-GoL mean ($p=0.024$, coefficient: 0.685), the Gn-GoL mean ($p=0.016$, coefficient: 0.671) and the Tgc-GoL index ($p=0.002$, coefficient: -0.196) seemed to be the significant, absolute linear predictor. The fléche lombaire variable in the linear regression shows correlation only with RH mean ($p=0.011$, coefficient: 0.382). In case of the trunk inclination orthopaedic variable the CH mean ($p=0.034$, coefficient: 0.141) seemed to be the significant, absolute linear predictor.

The maximal lateral deviation, the surface rotational amplitude and the lateral amplitude do not show linear regression correlation with any mandibular asymmetry variables (Table 3.).

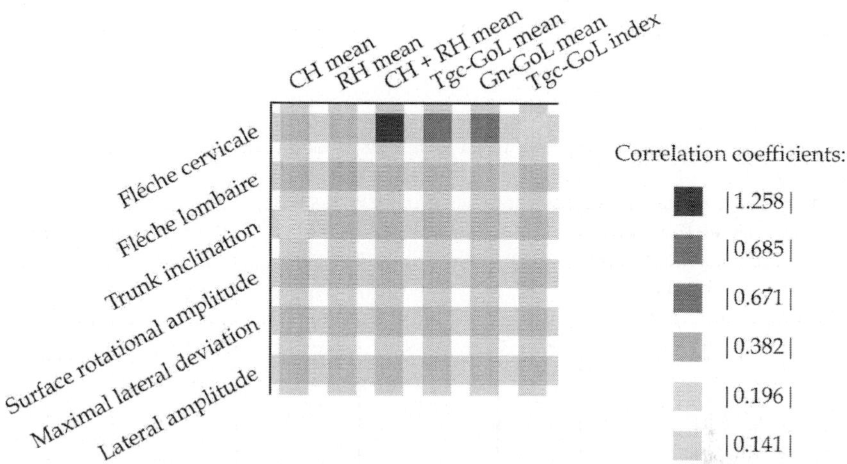

Table 3. The rate of the correlation between the orthopaedic and dentofacial parameters.

4.4 Discussion

The orthopaedic parameters of the examination group were provided by the rasterstereographic analysis. It means that the back contour morphology was mapped through a simultaneous registration of the deviation of different planes, without taking into account the threshold limit values separating the healthy and unhealthy categories. With the help of the statistical methods, out of the 12 measurements we selected 3 determining the sagittal and 3 determining the frontal curvatures and the positional deviations of the spine in the most precise way. For the comparative examinations 36 asymmetry variables measured on OPG's were used.

The fléche cervicale shows close correlation with the entire ramus height as well as the steepness of the inclination of the mandibular corpus out of the asymmetry variables determined on the mandible so the increased ramus height and mandibular base plane accompany the hyperkyphotic back. The fléche lombaire shows a moderately close correlation with the average of the ramus height, thus accentuation of the lumbar lordosis is associated with an increased ramus height. The trunk inclination shows similar correlation with the degree of the condylar height, therefore the forward inclined body posture presumes increase condylar height.

Based on the result of the comparative examination of the maximal lateral deviation, the surface rotational amplitude and the lateral amplitude the distance between the degree of the lateral deviation of the spine, the degree of vertebral rotation being present at the level of scoliotic curvature and the bilateral spinal curvatures is not associated with any of the mandibular asymmetry variables.

The comparative evaluation of the mandibular asymmetry variables obtained at the large number of patient group screened by the rasterstereographic procedure having used the

AsymmetrixX analysing software on examinations brought new results. The asymmetry variables determined with the help of the analysing software show close correlation with the rasterstereographic variables modelling the curvatures on the sagittal plane. The simple, non-invasive examination methods of certain features make possible to explore the given deviations at an early stage and in an interdisciplinary way. The skeletal basis of the postural disorders developing at the same age as well as the early recognition of the mandibular asymmetries showing close correlation therewith should mean the necessity of examining the potentially present joint deviations for the specialists of both fields. The new analysing methods waiting to be introduced are certainly suitable for recognising the features of the asymmetric dentofacial character.

5. Conclusions

The importance of the findings establishing a close correlation between the orthopaedic and orofacial-orthopaedic specialities is described below. The postural problems diagnosed during the pre-puberty as well as the dentofacial problems observed with the spinal deformities adverted to the necessity of the careful and accurate screening in both speciality fields. The prompt orthodontic screening in an early stage of the children diagnosed with spinal deformities can reveal those deviations which can be managed with conservative methods. Similarly to this the joint presence of the dentofacial pattern elements can be a disease-marker from the point of view of revealing a possible orthopaedic background disease.

Our research work focused on the confirmation of the previously listed results and to complement the experienced deficiency accentuating the importance of the identification of such early diseases-markers that can contribute to the formation of already proved associated deformities or to their progression. The early observation methods related to these deformities have to be known by the specialists working in the paediatric field. We have developed the computerized analysing software which significantly simplifies by its accuracy and quickness the early observation of the dentofacial deviations at the mentioned patient groups to help their and the specialists' preventive activity.

The synchronization of the result obtained with the applied examination methods as well as their harmonization with the modern radiologic procedures is a new challenge for the researchers. According to the reviewed detailed information the direction of the researches of this specialty considered to be of high importance has to be determined by the attempts that focus on the elaboration of an automatic classifying system based on the 3D topographic examination of the cranium also contributing to the early orthopaedic diagnosis. On the other hand the work out of those mandibular asymmetry measurements that substitute the disease-marker measurements obtained during the evaluation of the lateral cephalograms and similarly to the rasterstereography further reduce the radiation load of the involved orthopaedic subject is very important.

6. Acknowledgment

I would like to express my gratitude to my colleague Dr. Carsten Lippold for the patients' database provided and to my friend Éva Szász for her help with the translations.

7. References

Ali, RM., Green, DW. & Patel, TC. (1999). Scheuermann's kyphosis. *Curr Opin Pediat.*, 11: 70-75

Bagnall, KM. (2008). Using a synthesis of the research literature related to the aethiology of adolescent idiopathic scoliosis to provide ideas on future directions for success. *Scoliosis*, 3:5

Bellyei, Á. (1995). The diseases of the spine, spinal deformities. In: The book of othopaedics, Vízkelety, T. (1st ed.), 112-159, Semmelweis Publisher, ISBN 963-8154-60-8, Budapest

Ben-Bassat, Y., Yaffe, A., Brin, I., Freeman, J. & Ehrlich, Y. (1993). Functional and morphological-occlusal aspects in children treated for unilateral posterior cross-bite. *Eur J Orthod*, 15: 57-63

Ben-Bassat, Y., Yitschaky, M., Kaplan, L. & Brin, I. (2006). Occlusal patterns in patients with idiopathic scoliosis. *Am J Orthod Dentofacial Orthop*, 130: 629-633

Bishara, SE., Burkey, PS. & Kharouf, JG. (1994). Dental and facial asymmetries: a review. *Angle Orthod*, 64: 89-98

Bradford, DS. (1981). Vertebral osteochondrosis (Scheuermann's kyphosis). *Clin Orthop*, 158: 83-90

Bögi, I. & Nagy, L. (1970). The prevention and management of the denal deformities present as a result of the scoliosis treatment. *Fogorv Sz*, 63: 238-244

Deacon, P., Berkin, CR. & Dickson, RA. (1985). Combined idiopathic kyphosis and scoliosis. *J Bone Joint Surg Br*, 67: 189-192

Drerup, B. & Hierholzer, E. (1987). Automatic localization of anatomical landmarks on the back surface and construction of a body-fixed coordinate system. *J Biomech*, 20: 961-970

Drerup, B. & Hierholzer, E. (1994). Back shape measurement using video rasterstereography and three-dimensional reconstruction of spinal shape. *Clinical Biomechanics*, 9: 28-36

Drerup, B., Hierholzer, E. & Ellger, B. (1997). Shape analysis of the lateral and frontal projection of spine curves assessed from rasterstereographs. In: *Research into Spinal Deformities*, J.A. Sevastik & K.M. Diab, (1st ed.), 271-275, IOS Press, Amsterdam

Edler, R., Wertheim, D., & Greenhill, D. (2003). Comparison of radiographic and photographic measurement of mandibular asymmetry. *Am J Orthod Dentofacial Orthop*, 123: 167-174

Farkas, LG. & Cheung, G. (1981). Facial asymmetry in healthy North American caucasians. *Angle Orthod*, 51: 70-77

Frobin, W. & Hierholzer, E. (1981). Rasterstereography: a photogrammetric method for measurement of body surfaces. *Photogrammetric Engineering and Remote Sensing*, 47: 1717-1724

Good, S., Edler, R., Wertheim, D. & Greenhill, D. (2006). A computerized photographic assessment of the relationship between skeletal discrepancy and mandibular outline asymmetry. *Eur J Orthod*, 28: 97-102

Habets, LLMH., Bezuur, JN., Van Ooij, CP. & Hansson, TL. (1987). The orthopantomogram, an aid in diagnosis of temporomandibular joint problems. I. The factor of vertical magnification. *J Oral Rehabil*, 14: 475-480

Habets, LLMH., Bezuur, JN., Naeiji, M. & Hansson, TL. (1988). The Orthopantomogram®, an aid in diagnosis of temporomandibular joiunt problems. II. The vertical symmetry. *J Oral Rehabil*, 15: 465-471

Hadley, MN. (2000). Spine update: genetics of familiar idiopathic scoliosis. *Spine*, 25: 2416-2418

Halazonetis, DJ. (2002). Estimated natural head position and facial morphology. *Am J Orthod Dentofacial Orthop*, 121: 364-368

Herman, R., Mixon, J., Fischer, A., Maulucci, R. & Stuyck, J. (1985). Idiopathic scoliosis and the central nervous system: a motor control problem. *Spine*, 10: 1-14

Hirschfelder, U. & Hirschfelder, H. (1983). Auswirkungen der Skoliose auf den Gesichtsschädel. *Fortschr Kieferorthop*, 44: 457-467

Huggare, J., Pirttiniemi, P.& Serlo, W. (1991). Head posture and dentofacial morphology in subjects treated for scoliosis. *Proc Finn Dent Soc*, 87: 151-158

Huggare, J. (1998). Postural disorders and dentofacial morphology. *Acta Odontol Scand*, 56: 383-386

Inoue, M., Minami, S., Nakata, Y., Takaso, M., Otsuuka, Y., Kitahara, H., Isobe, K., Kotani, T., Maruta, T. & Moriya, H. (2002). Prediction of curve progression in idiopathic scoliosis from gene polymorphic analysis. *Stud Health Technol Inform*, 91: 90-96

Kim, HS., Ishikawa, S., Ohtsuka, Y., Shimizu, H., Shinomiya, T. & Viergever, MA. (2001). Automatic scoliosis detection based on local centroids evaluation on moiré topographic images of human backs. *IEEE Trans Med Imaging*, 12: 1314-1320

Kondo, E. & Aoba, TJ. (1999). Case report of malocclusion with abnormal head posture and TMJ symptoms. *Am J Orthod Dentofacial Orthop*, 116: 481-493

Korbmacher, H., Eggers-Stroeder, G., Koch, L. & Kahl-Nieke, B. (2004). Correlations between anomalies of the dentition and pathologies of the locomotor system - a literature review. *J Orofac Orthop*, 65: 190-203

Larheim, TA. & Svanaes, DB. (1986). Reproducibility of rotational panoramic radiography: Mandibular linear dimensions and angles. *Am J Orthod Dentofacial Orthop*, 90: 45-51

Leitao, P. & Nanda, RS. (2000). Relationship of natural head position to craniofacial morphology. *Am J Orthod Dentofacial Orthop*, 117: 406-417

Lemirre, JJ., Mierau, DR., Crawford, CM. & Dzus, AK. (1996). Scheuermann's juvenile kyphosis. *J Manipulative Physiol Ther*, 19: 195-201

Lin, MC., Liaw, MY., Chen, WJ., Cheng, PT., Wong, AM. & Chiou, WK. (2001). Pulmonary function and spinal characteristics: their relationships in persons with idiopathic and postpoliomyelitic scoliosis. *Arch Phys Med Rehabil*, 82: 335-341

Lippold, C., van den Bos, L., Hohoff, A., Danesh, G. & Ehmer, U. (2003). Interdisciplinary study of orthopedic and orthodontic findings in pre-school infants. *J Orofac Orthop*, 64: 330-340

Lippold, C., Danesh, G., Schilgen, M., Drerup, B. & Hackenberg, L. (2005). Sagittal jaw position in relation to body posture in adult humans - a rasterstereographic study. *BMC Musculoskeletal Disorders*, 7:8

Lippold, C., Danesh, G., Hoppe, G., Drerup, B. & Hackenberg, L. (2006). Sagittal spinal posture in relation to craniofacial morphology. *Angle Orthod*, 76: 625-631

Lippold, C., Danesh, G., Schilgen, M., Drerup, B. & Hackenberg, L. (2006). Relationship between thoracic, lordotic, and pelvic inclination and craniofacial morphology in adults. *Angle Orthod*, 76: 779-785

Lippold, C., Danesh, G., Hoppe, G., Drerup, B. & Hackenberg, L. (2007). Trunk inclination, pelvic tilt and pelvic rotation in relation to the craniofacial morphology in adults. *Angle Orthod*, 77: 29-35

Lowe, TG. (1999). Scheuermann's disease. *Orthop Clin North Am*, 30: 475-487

Lowe, TG., Edgar, M., Margulies, JY., Miller, NH., Raso, J., Reinker, KA. & Rivard, CH. (2000). Ethiology of idiopathic scoliosis: current trends in research. *J Bone and Joint Surg*, 82-A: 1157-1168

Marcotte, MR. (1981). Head posture and dentofacial proportions. *Angle Orthod*, 51: 208-213

Morissy, RT. & Weinstein, SL. (2006). *Lovell and Winter's Pediatric Orthopedics* (6th ed.), Lippincott-Raven, ISBN 0-7817-5358-9, New York

Murray, PM., Weinstein, SL. & Spratt, KF. (1993). The natural history and long-term follow-up of Scheuermann kyphosis. *J Bone Joint Surg Am*, 75: 236-248

Paphalmy, Zs., Kállay, M. & Tomory, I. (1975). Prevention of the dental deformities appearing durint the treatment of children with scoliosisos. *Fogorv Sz*, 68: 374-376

Parent, S., Newton, PO. & Wenger, DR. (2005). Adolescent idiopathic scoliosis: etiology, anatomy, natural history, and bracing. *Instr Course Lect*, 54: 529-536

Pirttiniemi, P., Lahtela, P., Huggare, J. & Serlo, W. (1989). Head posture and dentofacial asymmetries in surgically treated muscular toricollis patients. *Acta Odontol Scand*, 47: 193-197

Proffit, WR. & Fields, HW Jr. (2000). *Contemporary orthodontics* (3rd ed.), Mosby, ISBN 1-55664-553-8, St.Luis

Raju, NS., Prasad, KG., Jayade, VP. (2001). A modified approach for obtaining cephalograms in the natural head position. *J Orthod*, 28: 25-28

Rossi, M., Ribeiro, E. & Smith, R. (2003). Craniofacial asymmetry in development: An anatomical study. *Angle Orthod*, 73: 381-385

Sabah, ME. (2002). Submentovertex cephalometric analysis of Class II subdivision malocclusion. *Oral Sci*, 44: 125-127

Saglam, AMS. (2003). The condylar asymmetry measurements in different skeletal patterns. *J Oral Rehabil*, 30: 738-742

Schulte, TL., Hierholzer, E., Boerke, A., Lerner, T., Liljenqvist, U., Bullmann, V. & Hackenberg, L. (2008). Raster stereography versus radiography in the long-term follow-up of idiopathic scoliosis. *Journal of spinal disorders & techniques*, 21(1):23-8

Schulze, R., Krummenauer, F., Schalldach, F. & d'Hoedt, B. (2000). Precision and accuracy of measurements in digital panoramic radiography. *Dentomaxillofac Radiol*, 29: 52-56

Segatto, E., Jianu, R., Marschalkó, P. & Végh, A. (2006). Dentofacial features of children diagnosed with scoliosis and Scheuermann's disease. *TMJ*, 56: 259-264

Segatto, E., Lippold, C. & Végh, A. (2008). Craniofacial features of children with spinal deformities. *BMC Musculoskelet Disord*, 9: 169

Shah, SM. & Joshi, MR. (1978), An assessment of asymmetry in the normal craniofacial complex. *Angle Orthod*, 48: 141-148

Solow, B. & Tallgren, A. (1976) Head posture and craniofacial morphology. *Am J Phys Anthropol*, 44: 417-435

Solow, B. & Kreiborg, S. (1977). Soft tissue stretching: a possible control factor in craniofacial morphogenesis. *Scand J Dent Res*, 85: 505-507

Solow, B. & Siersbaek-Nielsen, S. (1986). Growth changes in head posture related to craniofacial development. *Am J Orthod*, 89: 132-140

Solow, B. & Sonnesen, L. (1998). Head posture and malocclusions. *Eur J Orthod*, 20: 685-693

Stramotas, S., Geenty, JP., Petocz, P. & Darendeliler, MA. (2002). Accuracy of linear and angular measurements on panoramic radiographs taken at various positions in vitro. *Eur J Orthod*, 24: 43-52

Tribus, CB. (1998). Scheuermann's kyphosis in adolescents and adults: diagnosis and management. *J Am Acad Orthop Surg*, 6:36-43

Vig, PS. & Hewitt, AB. (1975). Asymmetry of the human facial skeleton. *Angle Orthod*, 45: 125-129

Vissche, CM., Huddleston, S. Jr, Lobbezoo, F. & Naeije, M. (2000), Kinematics of the human mandible for different head postures. *J Oral Rehabil*, 27: 299-305

Weiss, HR. & ElObeidi, N. (2009). Kyphosis angle evaluated by video rasterstereography - relation to X-ray measurements. *Scoliosis*, 4(Suppl 1):O49

Wise, CA., Barnes, R., Gillum, J., Herring, JA., Bowcock, AM. & Lovett, M. (2000). Localization of susceptibility to familial idiopathic scoliosis. *Spine*, 25: 2372-2380

Yamaguchi, H. & Sueishi, K. (2003). Malocclusion associated with abnormal posture. *Bull Tokyo Dent Coll*, 44: 43-54

Part 5

Orthodontics Risks

18

Risks and Complications Associated with Orthodontic Treatment

Cristina Teodora Preoteasa, Ecaterina Ionescu and Elena Preoteasa
Faculty of Dental Medicine, "Carol Davila"
University of Medicine and Pharmacy, Bucharest
Romania

1. Introduction

Orthodontic treatment of malocclusions and craniofacial abnormalities, by ensuring proper alignment of the teeth, harmonious occlusal and jaw relationship, may improve mastication, phonation, facial aesthetics, with beneficial effects on the general and oral health, individual's comfort and self-esteem, having a positive role in improving the quality of life. Therefore, the treatment's objectives are consistent with the aims of medical interventions, namely ensuring health, the "state of complete physical, mental and social well-being", as perceived by the World Health Organization (World Health Organization, 1946).

Like any other medical intervention, orthodontic treatment has, in addition to its benefits, also associated risks and complications. In orthodontics, the risk of "doing harm" is considerably lower compared to other medical interventions, e.g., the surgical ones. However, during the medical act, through usage of various procedures, devices and materials, there might appear unwanted side effects, both local (tooth discolorations, decalcification, root resorption, periodontal complications) and systemic (allergic reactions, chronic fatigue syndrome).

An increased risk of complications may contraindicate the orthodontic therapy or influence its objectives, phases and conduct, aspects directly linked with the quality of the final outcome and prognosis. Generally speaking, the consecutive benefits of the medical intervention must overcome any potential damage. Legal regulations on medical conduct emphases the patient's right, as participant in treatment decision making, to be informed about the benefits and possible risks that might occur. It is recommended to make for each patient a rigorous risk profile analysis, followed by obtaining a signed informed consent. In case side effects appear, the avoidance of informing the patients about possible complications associated with the medical act may lead to malpractice complaints or even lawsuits.

This chapter aims to highlight the main coordinates of risk issues in orthodontics. In this respect, it starts with an analysis of the context in which they occur, followed by a presentation of the main complication linked to orthodontic intervention, and concludes with a general approach of the topic from the perspective of risks management principles

The following information represents a literature review, in the context of the current state of knowledge, combined with data from authors' personal observations and research.

2. Context of the side effects appearance during orthodontic treatment

Side effects associated with orthodontic treatment occur within the interaction between factors related to the patient, medical team and orthodontic technique. These can be perceived as elements belonging to the general therapeutic context, present when medical interventions are delivered, and aspects related to a specific therapeutic context, namely linked to the orthodontic intervention (Table 1). Local and systemic side effects may occur to patients (those receiving the intervention), but also to the medical team members (those managing the intervention, handling various materials and instruments).

CONTEXT OF RISK OCCURRENCE DURING ORTHODONTIC TREATMENT
General therapeutic context • patient's features • orthodontist related factors • doctor-patient relationship
Specific therapeutic context • related to the placement of orthodontic devices • related to the action mechanism of the orthodontic appliances • related to the relation of the orthodontic appliance with the oral structures • related to material properties and technical particularities of the orthodontic appliances

Table 1. Main coordinates of risk occurrence during orthodontic interventions.

2.1 General therapeutic context

During orthodontic therapy complications may be linked to the general context present when medical interventions are delivered, may be appeared in relation to specific patient features, linked to the medical staff responsible for delivering the intervention or associated to a deficient patient-doctor relationship.

There are many variables related to the patient that can influence the risk occurrence during orthodontic therapy. Among these are individual characteristics related to age, gender, environment, physiopathological status, genetic predisposition, psychological type, as well as particularities related to malocclusion (type, etiology, severity) and craniofacial features. In order to reduce the frequency and severity of the complications associated with this type of medical intervention, it is necessary to know the detailed particularities of each case, which need to be integrated within the treatment plan and conduct of the medical care. For example, within various age groups there are specific aspects of the physiopathological status, development and cooperation, which can influence the timing for orthodontic therapy, treatments' objectives, appliances choice, duration of treatment and stability of the outcome. Within young age patients considered appropriate to receive orthodontic intervention, there are mainly those with functional imbalances, anterior or posterior crossbite and those with severe narrow upper dental arch. But there are procedures (like expansion of the lower arch to resolve dental crowding) implemented in the mixed dentition that are sometimes unstable. Therefore, the orthodontic treatment is often instituted into the late mixed dentition, just before loss of the deciduous mandibular second molar, with the benefits of a better collaboration with the patient, the possibility of using the leeway space and influencing the jaw bone growth, with shortening as much as possible the duration of active treatment (DiBiase, 2002). The treatment of the adult patient often requires particularization of the orthodontic intervention due to oral structures changes and modified physiopathological status. More frequently periodontal alterations are present (reduction of the alveolar bone support with the modification of the tooth's rotation center, favoring a faster tooth movement; increased bone density associated with a slower tooth movement), also a higher intensity and duration of pain and increased prevalence of devital teeth (with an uncertain behavior during tooth movement) (Shah & Sandler, 2006). Modified health status may increase the appearance risk of certain complication or interfere with the orthodontic treatment conduct. For example, in case of bisphosphonates usage, among the side effects, the orthodontist should be concerned about the difficulties of achieving a desired tooth movement (long-lasting aspect after drug discontinuation) and also about the slower bone healing rate with the possibility of osteonecrosis appearance (especially important when tooth extractions, implant placement or phases of orthognathic surgery are planned) (Iglesias-Linares et al., 2010).

A good progress of the orthodontic treatment is related also to the patient's understanding and compliance regarding the physician's indications, which aims mainly the oral hygiene and device maintenance, and rigorousity in attending the periodical appointments. Failure to comply with these conditions may result in damaging the components of the orthodontic appliances, damage of the oral structures (risk factor for demineralizations, caries, discolorations, periodontal damage, bad breath), increased duration of the treatment and not achieving the expected result.

The orthodontist has an important role in preventing the complications associated with this type of treatment, being the manager and implementer of the medical intervention delivered. In order to obtain good results and minimize the complications aspects like an appropriate training, knowledge, clinical skills and experience are needed. Being a distinctive specialty within dentistry, orthodontic training has in many countries a particular education system. Usually a 2 to 3 year period of postgraduate study for qualification in this field is done. Over the last decade, there was also observed in this specialty an increased interest for the concept of evidence-based orthodontics. The orthodontist's challenge in the XXI century is to integrate the best scientific evidence into practice, this representing the "gold" standard of the medical care quality, from the perspective of the current state of knowledge (Ackerman, 2004). Also, in order to achieve a high standard of treatment quality, with minimal complication, it is necessary for the orthodontist to have all the necessary means for implementing the optimal considered treatment. For example, in order to include an orthognathic surgical phase it is necessary for the orthodontist to have a professional collaboration with a maxillofacial surgeon, preferably with his practice as close as possible, for an easy patient's access. Generally we can say that complications that occur due to errors of diagnosis, treatment planning or treatment management related to orthodontist's intervention can be avoided through practitioner's appropriate training, good theoretical knowledge and clinical skills and also possession of all necessary elements for implementation of the treatment plan considered optimal.

The doctor-patient relationship is another important key factor in ensuring a high quality medical act, having either positive or negative impact on treatment conduct. When an orthodontic treatment begins the physician, patient and person with the legal authority for minors become a team with a common goal: insuring the health status for identified problems. Communication is a key element in achieving quality results, but difficulties may arise for various reasons like a child patient, a person with disabilities or lack of interest towards the medical aspects. Generally, the most common difficulties are related to the understanding of the medical aspects by the patient, and complementary, the doctor's ability to make himself understood. When the physician is using a specialized medical language, the patient may feel inferior and may avoid requesting additional data, limiting the possibilities of using the received information. In this regard, it is recommended the clear presentation of the medical information to the patient, in a clear language, avoiding the usage of specialized terminology. Frequently, the orthodontically treated patients are children, the cooperation and communication being in general more difficult in younger ages. In their case, the orthodontic appliance is often accepted consecutive to parents' wishes not as a result of a perceived need, unlike adult patients who are usually more motivated. The parents are generally more aware of the orthodontic treatment's necessity and have a more positive attitude than children, but studies show that the doctor-patient relationship is influenced to a small extent by the parents' attitude (Daniels et al., 2009). In order to ensure an optimal treatment conduct it is recommended to evaluate patient's and family's attitude towards the orthodontic intervention before starting the treatment. When dealing with a negative, reticent patient, sometimes it's wise to postpone the treatment, because difficulties in treatment's progression and negative health or even psychological consequences may appear.

2.2 Specific therapeutic context

Part of the complications observed during or after orthodontic treatment can be linked to some specific features of this type of medical intervention. These are mainly related to the placement of orthodontic appliances, to their action mechanism, to the relation of the orthodontic device with the oral structures and linked to material properties and technical particularities of the orthodontic appliances.

Orthodontic devices can be fixed, consisting of elements bonded for the entire period of active treatment (brackets, bands) or removable, being present 2 variants (element removal can be done only by orthodontist - e.g., arch-wire, or also by patient - e.g., removable appliance), with different clinical indications, advantages and disadvantages regarding cleaning, microbial loading, patient's compliance etc. Some components are active, others passive, they can detach or break, causing local or general complications. The orthodontic appliances, fixed or removable, are placed in the oral environment, in relation with the anatomical structures and interfering with dento-maxillary apparatus' functions, being usually used for a long period of time. There is a wide range of materials used for orthodontic devices fabrication and usage (e.g., metal - nickel and titanium-based components, acrylics, cements, composites resins, ceramics, latex), which present different biomechanical characteristics and structure than the oral ones. The components of the orthodontic devices come into contact with the oral tissues and fluids, being submitted to some complex conditions: immersion in saliva and ingested fluids, temperature fluctuations, mechanical loading during chewing and activation of the devices, physical or chemical interactions. Therefore the orthodontic appliances must not contain compounds that may cause a toxic response, not cause allergic reaction or have carcinogenic potential, must be resistant to electrochemical corrosion, should not promote the microbial adherence and development, in general - should present an optimal biocompatibility (Atai & Atai, 2007; Bentahar et al., 2005). In this context, it is recommended to use orthodontic devices with lower nickel content, with a good resistance to corrosion and, in order to avoid corrosion of titanium based components, to limit the use of high concentration fluor-based products (Chaturvedi & Upadhayay, 2010). For an optimal treatment conduct the materials must be resistant to forces that are applied during their usage period, should not fracture and should be suitable for processing in any configuration and shape demanded by their clinical application.

In orthodontics treatment outcome is achieved mainly through orthodontic forces action, delivered against teeth muscles and bones, having as result teeth movement, modification of bone morphology or growth. According to patient's particularities treatments must be individualized, for example orthodontic forces should be dosed in relation to aspects like patient's age and oral structure's health status (e.g. increased force magnitude can be a risk factor for root resorption, ankylosis, pulpal and periodontal damage, pain).

The orthodontic appliances, depending on their type, have a direct contact with various structure of oral cavity like teeth, muco-osseus areas of the palate and alveolar bone, tongue, cheeks, gingiva etc. Sometimes an indirect effect of their placement is present, e.g., temporomandibular joint dysfunction and muscles disorders. Various side effects are linked to the orthodontic device presence, due to modifications in oral structure configuration, special measurements of hygiene requirements, attitudes needed for protection of the soft tissues and ensuring good functionality (for example harmless occlusal contacts). Applying the fixed orthodontic devices is associated with possible irreversible enamel changes, difficulties in oral hygiene maintenance due to decreased self-cleaning and multiple new areas for plaque retention, root resorption presence, discomfort and pain.

3. Classification of risks and complications of orthodontic treatment

During orthodontic treatment management two aspects must be carefully considered, namely the present risks and possible complications. Between these two there is a strong connection, acknowledging them being one of the keys of delivering a safe medical care. A classification, starting from the one presented by Graber (Graber et al., 2004), is the following:

1. based on the condition's localization
   - local effects, with manifestation on dento-maxillary apparatus structures (enamel demineralizations and discolorations, root resorption, gingivitis);
   - systemic effects (allergic reactions to nickel or latex).
2. according to the condition's severity:
   - mild, reversible (gingivitis);
   - moderate, reversible (fracture of a ceramic crown);

- moderate, irreversible (enamel fracture during debonding);
- severe, irreversible (multiples caries and decalcifications, severe root resorption).

3. based on orthodontist's role in the side effect's occurrence:
   - standard inherent complications, being included side effects where the orthodontist's role is irrelevant (enamel changes due to acid etching when resins are used as bonding material);
   - complications related to the patient's particularities (individual susceptibility or disease) not disclosed during evaluation, possibly unknown even to the patient (allergic reaction for which history data was inconclusive; severe root resorption and demineralisations present in association with a metabolic disease unidentified at the initial assessment);
   - conditions arising as a result of a passive operator intervention, associated with a lack of proper monitoring (lack of monitoring and proper prevention methods in cases with severe root resorption or decalcifications);
   - medical errors by wrongful medical objectives and deficient treatment conduct (enamel damage due to improper debonding technique; tooth movement into an area with alveolar bone defect causing severe loss of attachment).

4. Presentation of the main complications linked to orthodontic intervention

Like any other medical intervention, the orthodontic treatment may have, besides the positive effects, also unwanted secondary consequences. In the scientific literature there are numerous conditions to which orthodontic treatment may be associated (Table 2) (Ellis & Benson, 2002; Graber et al., 2004; Lau & Wong, 2006). For most of them a direct cause-efect relation hasn't been proven, but for no reason these aspect should be neglected.

4.1 Dental complications

Linked to orthodontic intervention, there are described numerous side effects present on tooth level. Among the first etiological hypothesis was the one saying that fixed orthodontic technique may induce enamel changes, both quantitatively (enamel loss during bonding and debonding procedures) and qualitatively (discolorations). On root level the most unwanted side effect taken into consideration in the medical literature is severe root resorption, process associated with root shortening that may lead to an insufficient tooth ability to endure the forces present during oral function performance and in extreme cases early tooth loss. Regarding the pulpal reactions, during action of orthodontic forces may appear a decreased oxygenation of pulpal tissue, varying in the same direction with force magnitude and period of action. Usually the inflammatory reactions that appear are transitory, reversible, but severe modifications, like necrosis, sometimes appear. Greater risk of pulpal reactions is present in teeth with a history of severe periodontal injury during certain orthodontic procedures, e.g., during intrusion and extrusion (Bauss et al., 2008; Bauss et al., 2010).

4.1.1 Enamel damage during bonding and debonding of the orthodontic devices

Enamel damage that appears as a side effect of the orthodontic therapy is relatively largely related to the bonding and debonding technique. One of the main preoccupations within the current orthodontics is identifying the ways to obtain, at the end of the treatment, a sound, unmodified enamel surface.

SIDE EFFECTS AND COMPLICATIONS HYPOTHETICALLY LINKED TO ORTHODONTICS
LOCAL EFFECTS
Dental • crown: decalcifications, decays, tooth wear, enamel cracks and fractures; discolorations, deterioration of prosthetic crown (as fracturing a ceramic one during debonding); • root: root resorption, early closure of root apex, ankylosis; • pulp: ischemia, pulpitis, necrosis; **Periodontal** • gingivitis, periodontitis, gingival recession or hypertrophy, alveolar bone loss, dehiscences, fenestrations, interdental fold, dark triangles; **Temporomandibular joint** • condylar resorption, temporomandibular dysfunction; **Soft tissues of the oral and maxillofacial region** • trauma (e.g., long archwires, headgear related), mucosal ulcerations or hyperplasia, chemical burns (e.g., etching related), thermal injuries (e.g., overheated burs), stomatitis, clumsy handling of dental instruments; **Unsatisfactory treatment outcome** • inadequate morpho-functional, aesthetic or functional final result, relapse, failure to complete treatment due to treatment dropout.
SYSTEMIC EFFECTS
Psychological • teasing, behavioral changes of patients and parents; discomfort associated with pain presence and aesthetic look discontents during orthodontic appliance usage; **Gastro-intestinal** • accidental swallowing of small parts of the orthodontic device (tubes, brackets); **Allergies** to nickel or latex; **Cardiac** • infective endocarditis; **Chronic fatigue syndrome;** **Cross infections** • from doctor to patient, patient to doctor, patient to patient.

Table 2. Main risks and complications associated with the orthodontic treatment.

Before applying brackets, tubes and bands, it is recommended to prepare the surface by pumice prophylaxis in order to increase the bond strength, procedure with great importance especially when self-etched adhesives are used as bonding material (Lill et al., 2008). Cleaning and pumicing procedures are accompanied by enamel loss and fissures on its surface, but these alteration present very low severities, neglectable compared to the ones present after debonding (Øgaard & Fjeld, 2010; Hosein et al., 2004).

By current knowledge, bonding of orthodontic appliances may induce irreversible changes of tooth surface. The most severe modifications appear when resins (especially the conventional ones, with a separate etching phase) are used as bonding materials. The bond strength of these materials is directly related to the resin tags formed, that cannot be removed at orthodontic treatment end. The extent of etching depth depends on numerous factors, among those being the acid type and concentration, time of application, enamel surface characteristics (e.g., in the mandibular molars and premolars usually is present aprismatic enamel that is more resistant to etching, aspect that could contribute to the observed higher debonding failure rate of bracket and tubes). Sometimes, after bracket bonding, demineralised enamel remains uncovered by resin, but usually remineralisation occurs, this not being a risk factor for decay appearance. A more recent bonding technique is the one with self-etched adhesive resin, which produces less enamel damage but has the disadvantages of lower bond strength. Resin-modified glass ionomer cement are preferred as bonding materials due to the reduced enamel involvement, fluor releasing properties and bond strength similar to resins. Fjeld, analyzing enamel alteration after 3 variants of bonding materials (conventional resin with 35% phosphoric etching gel and bonding/resin - Transbond XT, 3M Unitek; self-etching adhesives - Transbond Plus, 3M Unitek; resin-modified glass ionomer cement - Fuji ORTHO LC, GC Corporation used after surface conditioning with 10% polyacrylic acid) observes that the most important changes were associated to the first material usage (thick and relative deep – 10-20μm- resign tags accompanied by an increased surface rugosity). Less severe modifications were observed for the second material (smaller, fewer and less profound – 5-10μm- resin tags). When Fuji ORTHO LC was used no resign tags were observed. Authors conclude that by using the last two variants of bonding material advantages in term of fewer irreversible changes of the enamel surface are present (Fjeld & Øgaard, 2006).

During debonding and removal of the residual material there is a risk of tooth damage (enamel loss, cracks), irreversible complication being seen as hard to avoid. Frequency and gravity of enamel loss is usually smaller when metallic braces and bonding materials based on glass ionomer cements are used. More severe modifications were seen when ceramic brackets and adhesive resins were used as bonding materials. The orthodontist has a big role in preventing this irreversible enamel damage by using an appropriate debonding technique. A safe debonding technique aims to break the link between bracket and adhesive, this being preferred especially when adjacent to the bracket base there is softened, demineralised enamel. The residual bonding material is better to be removed with tungsten carbide burs at low speed, followed by surface polishing with pumice or a paste, in order to decrease rugosity and prevent plaque accumulation (Graber et al., 2004). Horizontal enamel cracks present after debonding are associated directly with the orthodontic technique, the vertical ones being present with a high frequency also in the population without previous orthodontic treatment (Øgaard & Fjeld, 2010).

In order to study enamel changes associated with orthodontic treatment we analyzed 2 pairs of upper premolars with a history of orthodontic treatment (treatment duration of 12 and 23 moths), extracted for orthodontic purposes after treatment plan was reassessed. By microscopic analysis, using magnifications till 5X, on the buccal surface there were identified changes in terms of color and roughness, with clear identification of the area where the bracket was applied. The enamel area corresponding to the bracket's base presented a uniform, white aspect. The enamel area corresponding to the margins of the bracket was assessed as having an irregular aspect, with more severe alteration in the gingival region compared to the occlusal one. The enamel lingual area (considered as control) presented an aspect considered as being uniform (Fig. 1). An increased surface roughness was observed at the area correspondent to the bracket's base, this being probably associated with the resin adhesive material used for bracket bonding (Preoteasa et al., 2011a). Using magnifications of 20X, on the buccal tooth surface were observed multiples unordered fissures, caused probably by the bracket debonding and residual material removal technique. The lingual surface presented also cracks, but fewer, this being probable associated to the occlusal contacts. By analyzing the buccal surface of two newly erupted premolars, without history of orthodontic treatment, a uniform aspect, crack and fissure free surface was observed (Fig. 2).

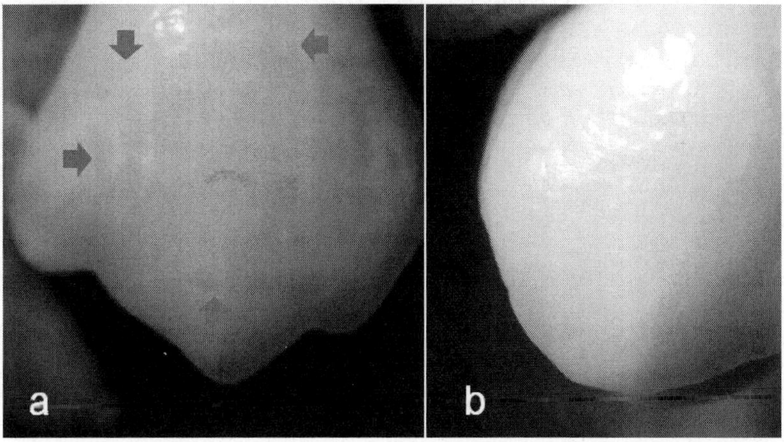

Fig. 1. Microscopic aspect of the enamel surface of a maxillary first premolar with a history of orthodontic treatment - buccal enamel surface (a); lingual enamel surface (b) - magnification 5X.

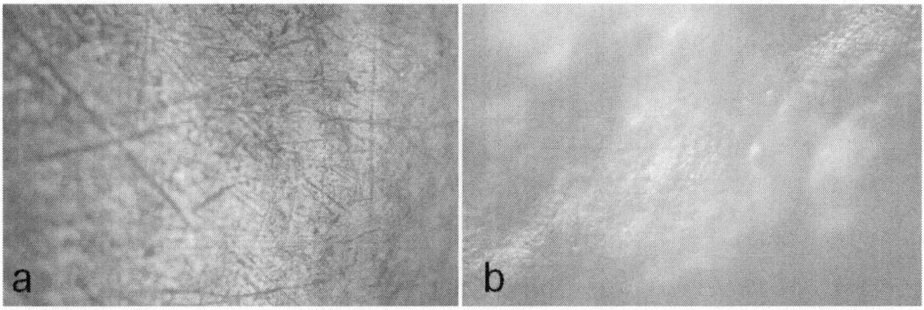

Fig. 2. Microscopic evaluation of buccal enamel surface for two upper first premolars, one with a history of orthodontic treatment (a); one without previous orthodontic treatment (b) - magnification 20X.

4.1.2 Carious complications associated with the orthodontic intervention

As the orthodontic technique developed, concerns regarding tooth damage by carious lesions during treatment increased, this being seen today as one of the most frequent unwanted side effect associated with this particular medical intervention. Decay damage associated with orthodontic technique presents some specific particularities. They appear with increased frequency on the tooth's surface where the bracket is bonded, adjacent to its base, they usually have low severity (most of the times are encountered as white spot lesions, more frequently gingival and distal to the bracket's base than mesial or occlusal) (Fig. 3). Evidence shows that the prevalence of this unwanted side effect is nearby 70% for white spot lesions and less than 5% for cavities (Al Maaitah et al., 2011). According to Chapman's study more than 30% of the maxillary incisors, teeth with the greatest esthetic values, present decalcifications after orthodontic intervention (Chapman et al., 2010).

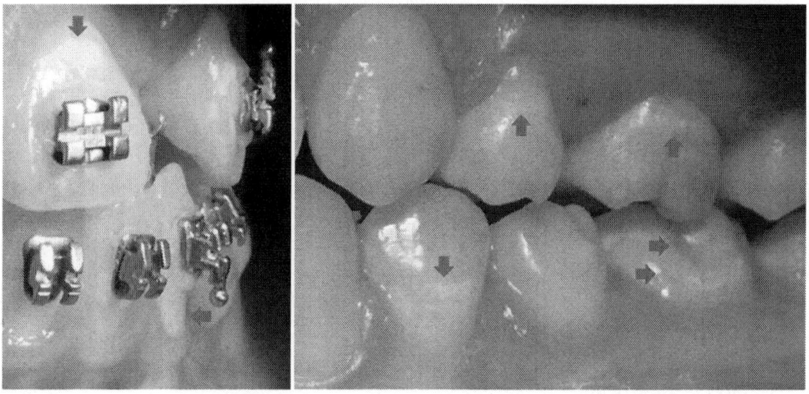

Fig. 3. White spot lesions and cavities related to the presence of orthodontic appliance.

Demineralisations around brackets occur mainly due to improper oral hygiene maintenance. But, in the presence of orthodontic appliance, an increased number of plaque retention areas appear, accompanied by a decrease of the self cleaning. In orthodontic patients plaque coverage is 2 to 3 times higher than the levels present in high plaque forming adults without this type of treatment (Klukowska et al., 2011). It is also observed a decrease of salivary pH and increased level of Streptococcus Mutans and Lactobacillus, elements favoring carioactivity (Vizitiu & Ionescu, 2010). Thus, maintaining a good oral hygiene is mandatory. Also, learning new skills on how to perform oral hygiene and using additional instruments may be needed, e.g., like interdental brush. Consequently, there are higher costs implied, not only financial (the tooth brush wears faster, investments in auxiliary devices like interdental brush or oral shower), but also time-related (more time spent for ensuring a good oral hygiene).

In decay prevention, even if the patient has the main role by maintaining a good oral hygiene, the orthodontist's role isn't neglectable. Before starting the orthodontic therapy it is recommended to evaluate carioactivity and oral hygiene habits, these being sometimes reasons to postpone orthodontic treatment with fixed appliance. Primary prevention methods may be used (e.g., recommendation of how to maintain a good oral hygiene and regarding diet; usage of fluoride releasing materials for bracket bonding and bands cementation). When necessary, secondary prevention methods must be promptly applied (e.g., increasing patient's compliance through operator's active intervention when white spot lesions are observed). One method for decreasing carioactivity, frequently used by orthodontists and dental practitioners, is fluorisation. A systematic review made in 2004 concludes that there is some evidence that supports the hypothesis that daily fluoride mouthrinse or fluoride-containing cement reduces tooth decay during treatment with fixed braces (Benson et al., 2004). A split-mouth study on this theme is the one made by Shungin reported in 2010, with a 12 years follow-up after active treatment ended. Results show that at the end of the treatment a significant increase of white spot lesion frequency was present, this being followed by a significant progressive decreasing. Also, modifications were significantly less severe in all moments when glass ionomer cement was used as bonding material, compared to the acrylic one (Shungin et al., 2010). Different treatment alternatives may be used when white spot lesions are present at treatment end, among these being: waiting for spontaneous remineralisation, usage of fluor or casein phosphopeptide based products, recommendation to chew sugar-free gums. In frontal teeth, when aesthetic complaints are present, microabrasion may be used.

For a better knowledge of orthodontic biomaterials, needed in order to adequate select them, we made an experiment to comparatively evaluate the surface wettability of some orthodontic bonding materials. 4 commercial products were chosen, different 2 by 2 as type of material and as curing method. Surface wettability was assessed by contact angle measurements using KSV Instruments's CAM 101 device (KSV Instruments, 2008). Results showed that for both glass ionomer cements and composite resins curing mechanism influenced wetting properties, the light curing ones presenting lower contact angle values than the self-curing ones. Also, analyzing the materials with the same curing characteristics, acrylic resins presented higher contact angles than the glass ionomer cements (Table 3). Surface wettability is linked to hidrophylicity and microbial adherence. When choosing between materials with the same clinical use, namely bonding of orthodontic brackets, in order to prevent caries apparition, in high risk patients the practitioner may prefer the chemically-cured composite resin, which is more hydrophobic and theoretically predispose less to plaque accumulation. Regarding glass ionomer cements, that are frequently used for band cementation, in time, due to their hydrophilic character and due to the fact that solubilization can take place, it may appear a space which represents a retention zone for the dental plaque, becoming an etiologic agent for decay and periodontitis. Of course, other properties must be analyzed in order to choose the best suited material for each case, but knowing surface properties may help in this direction and also explain some noticed clinical aspects (Preoteasa et al., 2011b).

Commercial product	**Producer**	**Type of material**	**Curing method**	**Contact angle**	
				mean	SD
Resilience	Ortho Technology	composite-based resin	light-cured	48.45°	3.68
Resilience			chemically cured	64.91°	3.40
Fuji Ortho LC	GC Europe	glass ionomer cement	light cured	35.04°	0.81
Fuji PLUS			self cured	56.59°	3.52

Table 3. Contact angle values for some orthodontic materials, with details regarding their characteristics.

4.1.3 Color alterations linked to the orthodontic treatment

Discoloration present after braces removal may have a negative impact on the aesthetics and patient's satisfaction. Karamouzos et al. in a split-mouth study on 26 orthodontic patients reported that teeth's color parameters changed after orthodontic treatment, 80% of the patients presenting at least one tooth with discolorations appreciated by authors as being unacceptable. Time had an aggravating effect on all color parameters evaluated according to the Commission Internationale de l'Eclairage system (L*-lightness; a*-red/green; b*-blue/yellow). There were observed more severe alteration when chemically cured resins were used as bonding material compared to light cured composites (Karamouzos et al., 2010).

Color alterations after orthodontic treatment present a multifactorial etiology, some variables being directly linked to the technique itself. Frequency of these alterations is considerably higher, with increased severity, when fixed appliances are used in comparison with the removable ones. When resins are used for bracket bonding enamel changes are unavoidable (Fig. 4). The resin tags cannot be removed by cleaning procedures without altering considerably the enamel surface. Irreversible changes regarding enamel surface morphology, its rugosity and texture are present, with negative influences on reflection properties, luminosity and optical perception. Evidence shows that adhesives resins used for bracket bonding don't present good color stability in time. Food dyes, ultraviolet light and corrosion products from the orthodontic appliance induce color alterations, with a tendency to modify toward the yellow tones (Faltermeier et al., 2008). In the presence of orthodontic forces that induce variation in pulp vascularization, it is also possible that endogenous discoloration appear, with a premature aging of tooth. Also, if white spots lesions are present, even if remineralisation occurs, most probable the final outcome will be somehow different from the initial enamel structure, the mineral not being identical disposed as in the unaffected enamel, with possible influences on color properties.

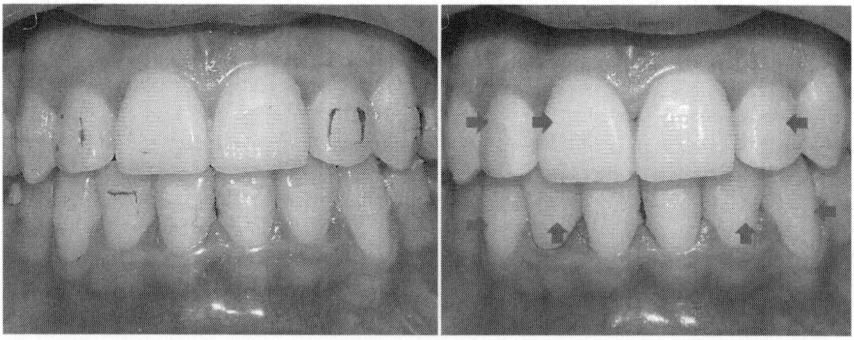

Fig. 4. Color changes integrated to usage of composite resins for bracket bonding.

After bracket removal patients frequently wish to increase their appearance by teeth whitening. This procedure presents particularities especially when resins were used as bonding material, due to the remained resins tags. The residual adhesive behaves different compared to adjacent enamel during whitening, being important to accurately evaluate the situation in order to avoid producing a more unpleasant outcome.

4.1.4 Dental wear associated to the use of orthodontic appliances

Another dental alteration present in the orthodontic patient is tooth wear secondary to the contact between teeth and brackets or tubes. A higher gravity of this process was noticed when ceramic brackets are used, Viazis reporting a severity from 9 to 38 times higher compared to the metallic ones (Lau et al., 2006; Viazis et al., 1990).

It is recommended, especially during certain phases of orthodontic treatment, to avoid usage of ceramic brackets in order to minimize the dental wear, as an irreversible treatment complication. For example, when deep bite is present, ceramic brackets on the lower anterior teeth shouldn't be used until sufficient overjet is created in order not to favor wear of the maxillary incisors, side effect with an increase negative impact on the esthetic dimension of the final result. Precautions must be taken when using the ceramic attachment on canine that are in a class II relationship and also during maxillary incisors retraction (Graber et al., 2004).

4.1.5 External apical root resorption in orthodontic therapy

Apical root resorption is, according to the present knowledge, an unavoidable complication of the orthodontic treatment, microscopic studies showing a prevalence of 100% after the treatment end (Fig. 5 & 6). Segal et al., in a systematic review reported in 2004, using meta-analysis, found a mean value of the root shortening after orthodontic treatment of 1.421 +/- 0.448 mm (Segal et al., 2004). Usually, the process severity is low, root shortening beyond 2mm being present in 5-18% of cases, and beyond 4mm or 1/3 of tooth length in 1-5% of the cases (Lopatiene & Dumbravaite, 2008).

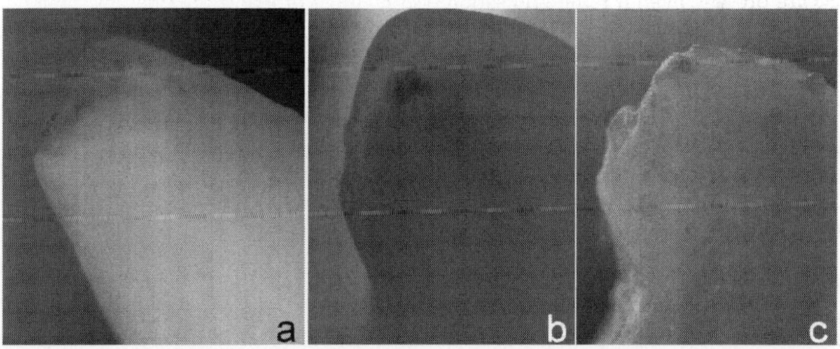

Fig. 5. Aspect of apical third of root of a newly erupted premolar (a), an included molar (b) and a premolar extracted for orthodontic purposes (c) - magnification 4X.

Root resorption's signs and symptoms are usually absent, even mobility been rarely higher than 1st degree on the Miller scale. If in the end of the treatment the root resorption's severity is mild or moderate the tooth prognosis doesn't greatly decrease. Kalkwarf demonstrated that 4 mm root shortening due to this pathological aspect is equivalent to 20% loss of the periodontal attachment, and 3 mm loss equivalent to 1 mm loss of the periodontal attachment (Kalkwarf et al, 1986). The high severity forms of root resorption, corresponding to considerable root shortening with influence on tooth prognosis, are one of the most discussed complications in association with the orthodontic therapy, being perceived as an unpredictable consequence with insufficient knowledge about its treatment alternatives and evolution.

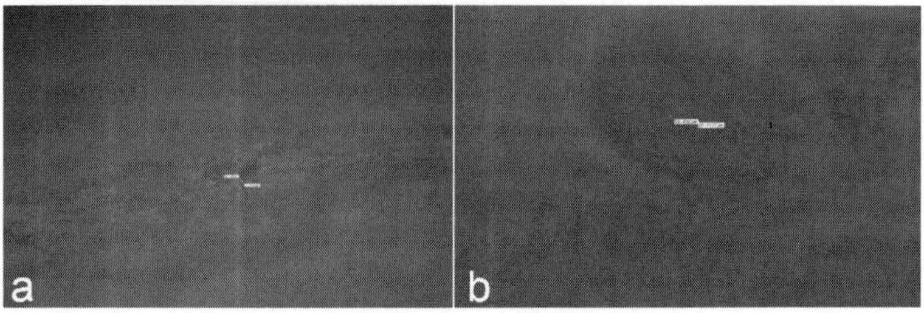

Fig. 6. Resorption lacunae in teeth without (a) and with (b) a history of orthodontic treatment - diameter: (a) 0.72μm; (b) 12.11μm – magnification 20X.

In order to minimize the severity of root resorption a good knowledge of etiopathogenic mechanism is mandatory. Although this aspect presents a series of ambiguities, mainly two categories of factors are incriminated for root resorption appearance, namely related to patient characteristics and to orthodontic technique. Both issues are important to be assessed, the first ones in order to identify high risk patients, and the last ones in order to ensure an orthodontic intervention predisposing at minimum to this unwanted side effect.

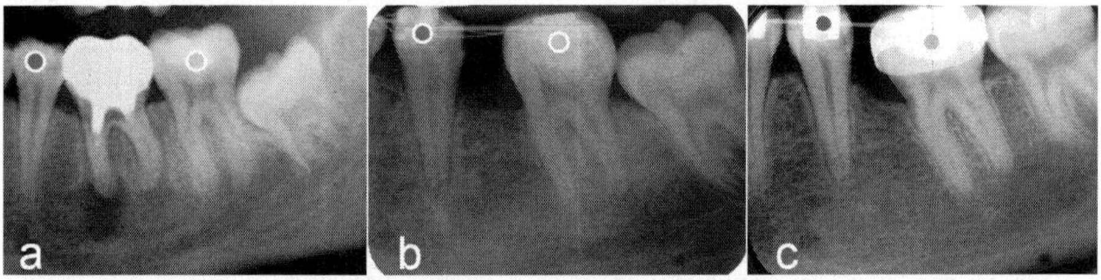

Fig. 7. Patient with identified susceptibility toward root resorption; mandibular first molar with root resorption signs, having as presumed cause incorrect endodontic treatment (a); progressive resorption at the mandibular second molar and premolar after orthodontic intervention was applied (b,c).

By current scientific knowledge, individual susceptibility has the main role in root resorption appearance, aspect difficult to correctly estimate. Indicators of high risk patients may be the signs of root resorption prior to orthodontic therapy, regardless of the presumed cause, and the presence of root resorption in the first degree relatives (Fig. 7). Genetic factors play an important part in root resorption presence, some associations, like the one with the polymorphism of the IL-1beta gene being demonstrated (Bastos Lages et al., 2009). Some study results suggest that this unwanted side effect is different between ethnic groups. Among Asians there is a decreased frequency of root resorption compared to Caucasians or Hispanics (Lopatiene & Dumbravaite, 2008). Modified general health status has been linked to a more severe root resorption process, among the diseases more frequently associated being allergies, asthma, diabetes, arthritis and endocrine disorders (Graber et al., 2004). An increased frequency of root resorption was associated to abnormal eruption path, the mechanism considering the pressure of the included tooth on the adjacent tooth roots. It has been mainly observed as being present in the second molars (produced by pressure of the wisdom teeth) and in the lateral incisor or first premolar (pressure exerted by the canine). Open bite is currently seen as a risk factor for root resorption, arguments being linked to the insufficient development of the periodontal tissue of the interested teeth, being incapable to bear orthodontic and occlusal forces, present during oral functions. Other dental anomalies associated with this particular complication are: hypodontia, class II and III Angle, deep bite and increased overjet (Lopatiene & Dumbravaite, 2008; Preoteasa et al, 2009). One aspect confirmed by many study results is that there is a direct relation between root morphology and root resorption process. A greater risk of root resorption present teeth with long and narrow roots, with abnormal root shape in the apical part of the root, especially eroded, pointed, deviated or bottle shape (Artun et al., 2009; Smale et al., 2005). Depending on the tooth's topography root resorption process presents some variability. Maxillary teeth are more prone to develop root resorption compared to the mandibular ones, and frontal teeth more prone than lateral ones (Brezniak & Wasserstein, 2002). Generally it is said that the more resorbed teeth, in a decreasing sequence, are the following: maxillary lateral incisors, maxillary central incisors, lower incisors, maxillary canines, first molars, lower second premolars and maxillary second premolars (Lopatiene & Dumbravaite, 2008). Also teeth with trauma history present a higher risk of root resorption (Artun et al., 2009).

Among risk factors of root resorption related directly to orthodontic technique the most important seem to be: treatment time, the amount of root apex displacement, the type and amount of orthodontic force, and also the type of orthodontic appliance used (Fox, 2005; Segal et al., 2004). Most study results indicate that one of the most important factor in root resorption appearance is treatment duration, an optimal period in order to prevent severe root resorption being less than 1½ years (Apajalahti & Peltola, 2007). A higher frequency of root resorption was linked to intrusion, expecialy when vestibular coronal torque was associated. Heavy and continuous forces are correlated with significantly more root resorption. Type of used orthodontic appliance influences root resorption process, being less severe in treatment delivered by removable orthodontic devices and higher when disjunction and extraoral appliances are used. Current knowledge indicates that bracket prescription and type (e.g., standard edgewise or straight wire technique, conventional or self-ligating) doesn't influence root resorption severity (Weltman et al., 2010.).

Considering the negative impact of severe root resorption it is recommended that the orthodontist take the necessary measures in order to prevent it from happening. During the initial evaluation, the patients with a high risk to develop root resorption should be identified, by considering previous signs of root resorption and local and systemic risk factors. If a patient with a high risk of root resorption is identified, reassessing the treatment objectives is recommended (whenever possible is best to avoid teeth extractions, heavy and continuous forces, disjunction, long treatment duration). In all cases it is recommended, at approximately 6 month after placement of orthodontic appliance, to acknowledge if root resorption signs appeared by analyzing periapical radiographs, at least for the frontal teeth. If, by that moment, there aren't signs of root resorption, the risk of presenting severe risk resorption at the end of the treatment is usually minimal. If, at that moment, sign of root resorption are present most likely during treatment some progressive modification will appear. Evidence shows that 2-3 months pause in orthodontic treatment, with passive wires, decreases the total amount of root resorption (Weltman et al., 2010). If severe signs of root resorption are present the treatment plan must be reassessed. Treatment alternatives may include prosthodontic solution for space closing, striping instead of extractions, sometimes even discontinuing orthodontic therapy. If severe root resorption is present after the active phase ended it is recommended radiological monitoring till process stabilizes. If a progressive evolution is noticed, frequently factors like occlusal trauma or retention devices that continue to develop orthodontic forces are associated, being necessary to address these items.

In order to study some aspects related to the etiology of root resorption, the authors designed and implemented a cross-sectional study who aimed to see if there is a correlation between root resorption's severity and some of the individual particularities that can be assessed before treatment start. A convenience sample of 55 orthodontic patients (74.5% - n=41 females and 25.5% - n=14 males) treated in the Department of Orthodontics and dentofacial orthopedics from the Faculty of Dental Medicine, Bucharest, from October 2005-October 2009, was used. Inclusion criteria were: orthodontic patients with fixed metallic appliance, standard edgewise or straight-wire technique, applied bimaxillary for at least 6 months. Patients with previous orthognathic interventions, disjunction, radiological signs of root resorption before treatment start, missing or endodontically treated incisors were excluded. Root resorption was assessed by measurements on panoramic radiographs using the Linge and Linge formula and Adobe Photoshop software, version 6.0 (Linge & Linge, 1991). In order to quantify the extent of root resorption for each patient included in the sample, two indices were used: average root resorption (mean value of root resorption registered for the 8 measured incisors in each patient, registered in mm) and the maximum root resorption (maximum value of root resorption from the 8 measured incisors in each patient, registered in mm). Data collection for the study variables was made using patient's file, photographs, study casts and cephalometric evaluation on teleradiographs. For data analysis STATA statistical software, version 11, was used. The sample presented mostly mild or moderate apical root resorption, with an average value of 1.31mm (standard deviation 0.60). The study evidenced a moderately positive statistically-significant correlation between average root resorption and the value of FMA angle, suggesting that patients with hyperdivergent facial pattern have a more pronounce tendency to develop root resorption after the orthodontic intervention, compared to the hypodivergent ones. Also our results suggest that patients with skeletal open bite tend to be more severely affected by external root resorption (Table 4). By comparing data regarding the root resorption among subgroups (made according to the normal and, respectively abnormal values of the parameters registered from their cephalometric assessment and dental evaluation) some additional information were obtained. Within the subgroups made according to the values of the parameters that evaluate the sagittal skeletal relations, the mean values of root resorption indices evidenced a more severe process in patients with values different from the average. The difference between groups was not statistically significant. Analysis of the subgroups constituted according to the value of the parameters selected for vertical skeletal relations evidenced the tendency of a more severe modification in the cases with higher values than the average (Preoteasa & Ionescu, 2011). Patients with Angle class II or III malocclusion presented more severe modifications than those belonging to class I (Table 5). In conclusion we can say that the pathological process of external root resorption is a reality accompanying frequently the orthodontic intervention, its severity

Cephalometric parameter	Mean root resorption		Root resorption with maximum severity	
	Correlation coefficient	p-value	Correlation coefficient	p-value
SNA[1]	-0.082	NS	-0.128	NS
SNB[1]	-0.058	NS	-0.127	NS
ANB[2]	-0.008	NS	0.040	NS
FMA[1]	0.303	0.024*	0.316	0.019*
SNA-SNP/Go-Gn[2]	0.228	NS	0.275	0.042*
Z-angle[1]	-0.180	NS	-0.219	NS
Total chin[2]	0.282	0.037*	0.276	0.041*
[1] Pearson	* - $p<0.05$			
[2] Spearman	NS – not significant			

Table 4. Correlations between root resorption and craniofacial particularities.

Parameter	Group	Mean root resorption			Root resorption with maximum severity		
		Mean(SD)	Test	p-value	Mean(SD)	Test	p-value
SNA	<80	1.44(0.66)	1	NS	3.11 (1.32)	1	NS
	80-84	1.18 (0.48)			2.40 (0.88)		
	>84	1.38 (1.00)			2.63 (1.68)		
SNB	<78	1.37 (0.65)	1	NS	2.89 (1.26)	1	NS
	78-82	1.15 (0.53)			2.43 (1.04)		
	>82	1.64 (0.55)			2.85 (1.11)		
ANB	<0	1.31 (0.47)	1	NS	2.64 (1.08)	2	NS
	0-4	1.23 (0.57)			2.54 (1.05)		
	>0	1.51 (0.74)			3.11(1.42)		
FMA	<22	1.05 (0.56)	1	NS	2.29 (0.91)	2	0.040*
	22-28	1.34 (0.58)			2.57 (1.02)		
	>28	1.52 (0.62)			3.26 (1.37)		
SNA-SNP/ Go-Gn	<19	1.04 (0.55)	1	NS	2.32(0.95)	2	0.004*
	19-31	1.30 (0.50)			2.49 (0.90)		
	>31	1.62 (0.78)			3.64(1.51)		
Z-angle	<70	1.39 (0.67)	1	NS	2.87 (1.33)	1	NS
	70-80	1.29 (0.55)			2.63 (1.11)		
	>80	1.16 (0.58)			2.50 (0.85)		
Angle class	I	1.14 (0.69)	1	NS	2.34 (1.96)	1	NS
	II	1.30 (0.49)			2.73 (1.05)		
	III	1.57 (0.62)			3.15 (1.25)		
[1] Kruskal Wallis				* - $p<0.05$			
[2] Anova				NS – not significant			

Table 5. Root resorption among groups of patients structured according to the normality of investigated parameters.

being associated at some extent with the individual morphological characteristics. A good knowledge on the variables associated to severe root resorption is essential for the identification of the high risk patients, as well as for the selection of the best suited treatment alternative in terms of low probability of root resorption occurrence.

4.2 Periodontal complications

Periodontal complications are one of the most actual side effects linked to the orthodontics, not rarely being the reason for malpractice complaints. It can be found in various forms, from gingivitis to periodontitis, dehiscence, fenestrations, interdental fold, gingival recession or overgrowth, black triangles (Fig. 8). Severe damage can considerably interfere with the teeth prognosis. Etiopathogeny is complex, involving factors related to the patient (e.g., previous condition present, increased susceptibility, poor oral hygiene) and to orthodontic technique.

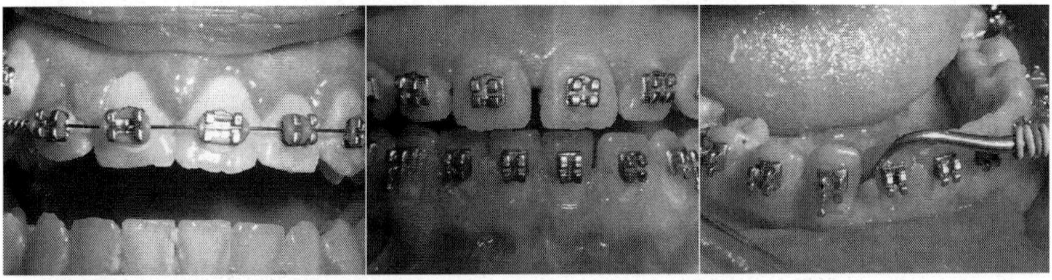

Fig. 8. Periodontal alteration present during orthodontic treatment.

Gingivitis usually occurs due to the incorrect maintenance of the oral hygiene, in the presence of the orthodontic appliance, that seems to favor plaque accumulation. Their frequency is increased in some particular situations, like in the presence of orthodontic bands that usually are placed subgingival, accompanied sometime by the solubilisation of luting agent, favoring the gingival overgrowth by mechanical trauma and existence of retention space for plaque accumulation. This is why, in order to ensure a safer medical care, bondable tubes are more indicated than bands. Even so, research has shown that during orthodontic therapy gingival enlargement occurs, but approximately 3 month after the removal of the appliance, in most cases, the gingiva presents a similar aspect as before treatment (Kouraki et al., 2005).

Careful management of orthodontic treatment is recommended when previous periodontal alterations are identified. Orthodontic intervention may aggravate a previous condition, which may lead to severe disease form, sometimes difficult to control. In these cases is best to postpone the treatment till a very good oral hygiene is present and the periodontal disease is stable. During the initial assessment, patients with factors that predispose to worsening the periodontal condition (e.g., presence of diabetes or epilepsy treated with drugs that induce gingival enlargement) need to be identified. During orthodontic therapy it is recommended to insist on the importance of maintaining a good oral hygiene, to monitories the periodontal status (at least every three month to do an examination and dental cleaning) and to take the necessary measures in order to control the risk factors. Also orthodontic therapy should be particularized, e.g., by choosing the treatment alternative who favors less accumulation of plaque, devices as simpler as possible and developing small orthodontic forces. In this regard it is recommended to avoid as much as possible hooks, elastic ligatures and chains, bands being preferable to tubes, and metallic ligatures to elastomeric ones.

During some particular orthodontic interventions an increased frequency of periodontal complications was noticed. For example, within extraction treatment after space closure, a higher frequency of periodontal interdental folds, associated sometimes with gingival enlargement, were observed (Fig. 9). Also after moving teeth in the buccal-lingual direction, as in the expansion or intermaxillary disjunction, the risk of fenestrations and dehiscences is higher. In this context it is recommended to choose the treatment alternative that predisposes as little as possible to these impairments.

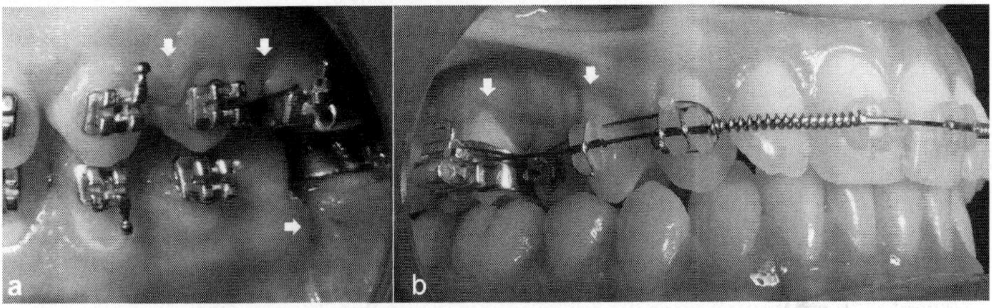

Fig. 9. Periodontal complications - gingival enlargement, interdental fold - present during orthodontic therapy (a); Gingival recessions associated with crossbite malocclusion, not linked to the orthodontic appliance's presence (b).

4.3 Soft tissue alterations

During orthodontic treatment intra- and extraoral (face and neck) soft tissue alterations may appear. For the oral lesions, the etiological mechanism involves the direct contact of gingiva and mucosa with brackets, bands, tubes and arches, and it is also related to the incorrect handling of the orthodontic instruments. The outcome usually consists in erosions and ulcerations on the buccal, labial, lingual or gingival mucosa. Pain and discomfort are associated, but by using orthodontic wax it may be possible to ameliorate to some extent the symptoms. Improper hygiene of the removable orthodontic appliances is sometimes associated with stomatitis appearance, which may sometimes be overinfected with Candida albicans (Shah & Sandler, 2006). Headgear appliance was linked to facial and intraoral trauma, appearing accidentally during game, sleep or incorrect handling. Blum-Hareuveni reports a case of a 12 year old boy who presented an ocular trauma by the external headgear arm, during sleep. He developed an intraocular infection (endophthalmitis), the final outcome being severe, decreased visual acuity. The author observes that in 10 out of 11 cases (the ones identified in the medical literature till that point) the consequences were dramatic, visual acuity decreasing to hand movement perception or less (Blum-Hareuveni et al., 2004; Blum-Hareuveni et al., 2006). After several cases of trauma associated with headgear devices were reported, modifications of its design were made in order to prevent this severe possible complication.

4.4 Temporomandibular joint disorders

Postorthodontically temoporomandibular disorders are usually part of the cranio-mandibular dysfunction, which includes beside joint modifications also muscle and dental impairments. By the current research knowledge, it isn't clearly elucidated the relation between temporomandibular alterations and orthodontic intervention, usually being found contradictory opinions, explication varying. Some sustain that, by the state of morpho-functional equilibrium present after orthodontic intervention, optimal conditions for this side effects prevention are created. Other believe that, because of the premature occlusal contacts present during therapy, there is a greater risk for this complication to appear (Bourzgui et al., 2010; Gebeile-Chauty et al. 2010).

Before starting orthodontic treatment every patient must be examined in order to detect previous temporomandibular disorders and identify high risk patients. Aspects like inflammatory bone and muscular disorders (reumathoid arthritis), head and neck trauma, chronic head pain or high stress level must be taken into account. If signs and symptoms of temporomandibular disorders are present reaching a diagnosis is mandatory and also establishing its degree of severity. It isn't recommended to start an orthodontic therapy if the patient presents acute or severe signs of pain belonging to the temporomandibular disfunction. If severe modifications are observed during treatment, depending on case's particularities, it might be decided the correction of the abnormal occlusal contacts, referral to an orthopedic surgeon, or even treatment discontinuing. For patient who presented signs of temporomandibular disorder after active orthodontic treatment phase, it is recommended to take the necessary measures in order to prevent the relapse, the maintenance of a good morpho-functional equilibrium being essential. In some cases mouth guards as retention device may help in reducing the symptoms and facilitate healing (Graber et al., 2004).

4.5 Allergic reactions

One hypothetical reaction linked to the orthodontic treatment is the allergic one. Hypersensitivity reactions can occur associated to the well known allergens like nickel, cobalt, chromium, latex and polymers. The most frequent form is the contact dermatitis of the face and neck, but lesions can appear also on the oral mucosa and gingiva, and rarely even systemic reactions may occur.

Nickel allergies are the most frequent ones in the industrialized countries, manifesting usually as a type IV hypersensitivity reaction. Orthodontic devices contain approximately 8% nickel and the nickel-titanium alloy near 70% nickel (Leite & Bell, 2004). The allergic signs may vary from small rash on skin or mucosa, to generalized dermatitis. In high severity cases the manifestations may lead to discontinuation of the orthodontic treatment.

Another allergen taken into consideration when orthodontic treatment is performed is latex (from medical gloves, elastomeric ligatures, elastic chain, rubber dam etc). Prevalence of latex related allergies is reported as being lower than 1% in the general population, but greater than 5% among dental professionals (Leite, 2004). Associated to it, types I and IV hypersensitivity reactions may appear, the most severe one, type I, being life threatening. In order to ensure a safe medical treatment it is important to identify allergic patients before starting the intervention. Higher risk present people with a history of complex or repeated surgical interventions (prolonged contact with rubber drains and tubes), those with spina bifida, and of course those who reported presence of itching and redness from contact to rubber objects and having allergies or contact dermatitis. A definitive diagnosis is established by combining the anamnestic data with the clinical data and hipersensibility tests. When allergic reaction to latex is identified, alternative latex-free devices should be used, and it is also recommended to avoid nickel-based components (Kolokitha, 2008).

4.6 Infective endocarditis

Infective endocarditis is rarely associated with the orthodontic interventions, but if it does, it can present severe complications that can be life threatening. The American Heart Association recommends prophylactic methods in order to prevent infectious endocarditis appearance if the patient presents prosthetic cardiac valve, previous infective endocarditis, congenital heart disease and cardiac transplantation with cardiac valvulopathy. The prophylaxis is mainly indicated in dental procedures that belong to oral and maxillofacial surgery, endodontics and periodontics, routinely in orthodontics being no need to implement it. Prophylactique therapy may be indicated in some particular orthodontic phases, where bleeding during interventions occur (e.g., teeth extraction, mini-implant placement used for anchorage control, interventions of orthognathic surgery and sometimes during placement and removal of orthodontic bands) (Wilson et al., 2007).

5. Applications of the risk management principles within orthodontics

Orthodontic treatment is a complex medical intervention, carried out over a long period of time, during which risks (seen as unplanned events) may materialize as complications. Their presence is linked to several factors like orthodontic technique, medical knowledge in this field, but also to patient's individual particularities (e.g., general and oral health). The outcome can include one or several side effects, generally, but not always, presenting low severity, appeared after initiation of orthodontic therapy or by aggravating some previous conditions. In order to ensure a high quality of the medical care, from the treatment planning phase, the risks must be considered, evaluated and communicated to the patient. This conduct promotes an optimal treatment period with lower risk of disagreements that may lead to malpractice complaint and even lawsuits.

One method for risks assessment may be to follow the methodology described in Risk Management, using the risk matrix (Table 6). This approach includes proactive management items (measures for avoiding and preventing the risk), as well as reactive elements (actions taken for minimizing damage after occurrence of the adverse effect). The use of risk management plan can't guarantee a health care intervention without side effects but, by controlling risks, it may considerably decrease the associated complications, ensuring a better prognosis.

At first it is necessary to identify the risks that are associated with the medical intervention that is going to be applied. By the current medical knowledge there are a great number of complications that are hypothetically linked to the orthodontic treatment. Their occurrence depends on numerous factors, from orthodontic technique (e.g., appliance type) to patient related variables (e.g., oral hygiene habits). These must be considered even from the start because it might influence treatment's objectives, phases and sometimes may even postpone the medical intervention. To identify the risks, it may be helpful for the orthodontist to ask himself the basics question "what may appear? why? how? when?".

RISK MANAGEMENT	
1.	**Risks identification** • what may appear? why? how? when?
2.	**Risks assessment → RISK MATRIX** • value for probability (measures the extent to which risk can become real) • value for impact (measures the effect of a particular risk on the outcome quality) • establishing priorities
3.	**Risk response planning** • risk avoidance • risk mitigation • risk acceptance • risk transfer

Table 6. Risk management phases.

After identifying the risks, the next step is their assessment. The identified risks are analyzed by the probability of appearance (e.g., likelihood; almost certain; likely; possible; unlikely; rare) and impact on the quality of healthcare intervention (e.g., severe; major; moderate; minor; insignificant) in conjunction. An ergonomic method to do this is to give scores to the items investigated and introduce the identified risks in a 2X2 table, this being known as a risk matrix analysis. For example, risk of severe root resorption can be differently assessed depending on case particularities. Generally, it is evaluated as being unlikely to appear, but if it does, it can have a major impact on tooth prognosis. But if, before beginning the orthodontic treatment, there can be detected signs of idiopathic root resorption, the probability of occurrence increases, transforming this risk into a priority issue, needed to be carefully considered when treatment plan is developed.

After that, the risk response is planned for those complications which, corresponding to the previous analysis, present the best chances to negatively influence the treatment outcome. In risk management there are described several techniques that can be applied individual or in conjunction (Piney, 2002). By risk avoidance there are addressed the measurements taken into consideration in order to minimize the situational risk as much as possible. For example in a high risk root resorption case, if it is possible, the treatment objectives should be minimized so treatment duration delivered by the orthodontist will be as short as possible and these means do not favor the side effects appearance. Risk mitigation refers to the actions taken in order to reduce the probability or the impact of the risk event. This type of measure can be integrated to the primary, secondary or tertiary prevention methods described for many pathological medical aspects (Ionescu et al., 2008). For example, in orthodontics there are described various procedures for minimizing enamel demineralization associated with bad oral hygiene habits, from motivating the patient and parents to indicating auxiliary devices (single-tuft brushes, oral irrigators) and fluoride-based products. Risk acceptance suggests the decision to accept the possibility of the event appearance. Acceptance can be passive, when the impact presents a minor impact on the outcome. In orthodontics this can be seen in the acceptance of minor root resorption process, a side effect present with a high frequency after this type of medical interventions, but with insignificant impact on outcome quality. Acceptance can be active; this means that, if the risks occur, the planned methods to minimize its consequences must be implemented. This is the case of infection risk, present in any medical surgical act (e.g., tooth extraction for orthodontic purposes, mini-implants placement, orthognathic surgery phases). Usually, it presents low frequency, but if it occurs, prompt response measurements must be taken. Risk transfer implies a 3rd part that will bear partially or totally the risks if they appear. This type of risk response can be seen in contemporary medical field by the usage of informed consent. Patients are informed about the possible risks and complications of the medical intervention, by signing the informed consent, which certifies the understanding of the aspects mentioned and assume the possibility of side effects occurrence.

6. Conclusions

In conclusion, the risks associated with orthodontic treatment are a reality, complications being a result of a multifactorial process, including aspects related to patient, orthodontist and the technical features of orthodontic appliances and procedures. These can be prevented or limited through identification and implementation of best treatment alternative for each individual case. Patient's compliance is an important factor that can contribute to a high standard outcome, with minimum side effects.

7. References

Ackerman, M. (2004). Evidence-based orthodontics for the 21st century. *Journal of the American Dental Association*, Vol.135, No.2, pp. 162-167, ISSN 0002-8177

Al Maaitah, E.F., Adeyemi, A.A., Higham, S.M., Pender, N. & Harrison, J.E. (2011). Factors affecting demineralization during orthodontic treatment: a post-hoc analysis of RCT recruits. *American Journal of Orthodontics and Dentofacial Orthopedics*, Vol.139, No.2, pp. 181-191, ISSN 0889-5406

Apajalahti, S. & Peltola, J.S. (2007). Apical root resorption after orthodontic treatment - a retrospective study. *European Journal of Orthodontics*, Vol.29, No.4, pp.408-412, ISSN 0141-5387

Artun, J., Van 't Hullenaar, R., Doppel, D. & Kuijpers-Jagtman, A.M. (2009). Identification of orthodontic patients at risk of severe apical root resorption. *American Journal of Orthodontics and Dentofacial Orthopedics*, Vol.135, No.4, pp. 448-455, ISSN 0889-5406

Atai, Z. & Atai, M. (2007). Side Effects and Complications of Dental Materials on Oral Cavity. *American Journal of Applied Sciences*, Vol.4, No.11, pp. 946-949, ISSN 1554-3641

Bastos Lages, E.M., Drummond, A.F., Pretti, H., Costa, F.O., Lages, E.J., Gontijo, A.I., Miranda Cota, L.O. & Brito, R.B. (2009). Association of functional gene polymorphism IL-1beta in patients with external apical root resorption. *American Journal of Orthodontics and Dentofacial Orthopedics*, Vol.136, No.4, pp. 542-546, ISSN 0889-5406

Bauss, O., Röhling, J., Sadat-Khonsari, R. & Kiliaridis, S. (2008). Influence of orthodontic intrusion on pulpal vitality of previously traumatized maxillary permanent incisors. *American Journal of Orthodontics and Dentofacial Orthopedics*, Vol.134, No.1, pp. 12-17, ISSN 0889-5406

Benson, P.E., Parkin, N., Millett, D.T., Dyer, F., Vine, S. & Shah, A. (2004). Fluorides for the prevention of white spots on teeth during fixed brace treatment. *Cochrane Database of Systematic Reviews*, No.3, CD003809. DOI: 10.1002/14651858.CD003809

Bentahar, Z., Bourzgui, F., Zertoubi, M., EL Adioui- Joundy, S. & Morgan, G. (2005). Dégradation électrochimique des matériaux métalliques utilisés en orthodontie. *International Orthodontics*, Vol. 3, No.5, pp. 5–17, ISSN 1761-7227

Blum-Hareuveni, T., Rehany, U. & Rumelt, S. (2004). Blinding endophthalmitis from orthodontic headgear. *New England Journal of Medicine*, Vol.351, No.26, pp.2774-2775, ISSN 0028-4793

Blum-Hareuveni, T., Rehany, U. & Rumelt, S. (2006). Devastating endophthalmitis following penetrating ocular injury during night sleep from orthodontic headgear: case report and literature review. *Graefes Archive for Clinical and Experimental Ophthalmology*, Vol.244, No.2, pp.253-258, ISSN 0721-832X

Bourzgui, F., Sebbar, M., Nadour, A. & Hamza, M. (2010). Prevalence of temporomandibular dysfunction in orthodontic treatment. *International Orthodontics*, Vol.8, No.4, pp. 386-398, ISSN 1761-7227

Brezniak, N. & Wasserstein, A. (2002). Orthodontically Induced Inflammatory Root Resorption. Part I: The Basic Science Aspects. *Angle Orthodontist*, Vol.72, No.2, pp. 175-179, ISSN 0003-3219

Chapman, J.A., Roberts, W.E., Eckert, G.J., Kula, K.S. & González-Cabezas, C. (2010). Risk factors for incidence and severity of white spot lesions during treatment with fixed orthodontic appliances. *American Journal of Orthodontics and Dentofacial Orthopedics*, Vol.138, No.2, pp. 188-194, ISSN 0889-5406

Chaturvedi, T.P. & Upadhayay, S.N. (2010). An overview of orthodontic material degradation in oral cavity. *Indian Journal of Dental Research*, Vol.21, No.2, pp. 275-284, ISSN 0970-9290

Daniels, A.S., Seacat, J.D. & Inglehart, M.R. (2009). Orthodontic treatment motivation and cooperation: a cross-sectional analysis of adolescent patients' and parents' responses. *American Journal of Orthodontics and Dentofacial Orthopedics*, Vol.136, No.6, pp. 780-787, ISSN 0889-5406

DiBiase, A. (2002). The timing of orthodontic treatment. *Dental Update*, Vol.29, No.9, pp. 434-441, ISSN 0305-5000

Ellis, P.E. & Benson, P.E. (2002). Potential Hazards of Orthodontic Treatment - What Your Patient Should Know. *Dental Update*, Vol.29, No.10, pp. 492-496, ISSN 0305-5000

Faltermeier, A., Rosentritt, M., Reicheneder, C. & Behr, M. (2008). Discolouration of orthodontic adhesives caused by food dyes and ultraviolet light. *European Journal of Orthodontics*, Vol.30, No.1, pp. 89-93, ISSN 0141-5387

Fjeld, M. & Øgaard, B. (2006). Scanning electron microscopic evaluation of enamel surfaces exposed to 3 orthodontic bonding systems. *American Journal of Orthodontics and Dentofacial Orthopedics*, Vol.130, No.5, pp. 575-581, ISSN 0889-5406

Gebeile-Chauty, S., Robin, O., Messaoudi, Y. & Aknin, J.J. (2010). Can orthodontic treatment generate temporomandibular disorders and pain? A review. *L'Orthodontie Francaise*, Vol.81, No.1, pp.85-93, ISSN 0078-6608

Graber, T., Eliades, T. & Athanasiou, A.E. (2004). *Risk Management in Orthodontics: Expers' Guide to Malpractice*, Quintessence Publishing Co, Inc, ISBN 0-86715-431-4, Chicago

Hosein, I., Sherriff, M. & Ireland, A.J. (2004). Enamel loss during bonding, debonding, and cleanup with use of a self-etching primer. *American Journal of Orthodontics and Dentofacial Orthopedics*, Vol.126, No.6, pp. 717-724, ISSN 0889-5406

Iglesias-Linares, A., Yáñez-Vico, R.M., Solano-Reina, E., Torres-Lagares, D. & González Moles, M.A. (2010). Influence of bisphosphonates in orthodontic therapy: Systematic review. *Journal of Dentistry*, Vol.38, No.8, pp. 603-611, ISSN 0300-5712

Ionescu, E., Teodorescu, E., Badarau, A., Grigore, R. & Popa, M. (2008). Prevention perspective in orthodontics and dento-facial orthopedics. *Journal of Medicine and Life*, Vol.1, No.4, pp.397-402, ISSN 1884-122x

Kalkwarf, K.L., Krejci, R.F. & Pao, Y.C. (1986). Effect of apical root resorption on periodontal support. Journal of Prosthetic Dentistry. Vol.56, No.3, pp. 317-319, ISSN 0022-3913

Karamouzos, A., Athanasiou, A.E., Papadopoulos, M.A.& Kolokithas, G. (2010). Tooth-color assessment after orthodontic treatment: a prospective clinical trial. *American Journal of Orthodontics and Dentofacial Orthopedics,* Vol.138, No.5, pp. 537.e1-8, ISSN 1097-6752

Kolokitha, O.E. & Chatzistavrou, E. (2008). Allergic reactions to nickel-containing orthodontic appliances: clinical signs and treatment alternatives. *World Journal of Orthod*ontics, Vol.9, No.4, pp.399-406, ISSN 1530-5678

Kouraki, E., Bissada, N.F., Palomo, J.M., Ficara, A.J. (2005). Gingival enlargement and resolution during and after orthodontic treatment. *New York State Dental Journal*, Vol.71, No.4, pp. 34-37, ISSN 0028-7571

Klukowska, M., Bader, A., Erbe, C., Bellamy, P., White, D.J., Anastasia, M.K. & Wehrbein, H. (2011). Plaque levels of patients with fixed orthodontic appliances measured by digital plaque image analysis. *American Journal of Orthodontics and Dentofacial Orthopedics,* Vol.139, No.5, pp. 463-470, ISSN 1097-6752

KSV Instruments. (2008). *Operating Manual for Contact Angle and Surface Tension Determination* (2nd edition), Helsinki

Lau, P.Y. & Wong, R.W.K. (2006). Risks and complications in orthodontic treatment. *Hong Kong Dental Journal*, Vol.3, No.1, pp. 15-22, ISSN 1727-2300

Leite, L.P. & Bell R.A. (2004). Adverse Hypersensitivity Reactions in Orthodontics. *Seminars in Orthodontics,* Vol.10, No. 4, pp. 240-243, ISSN 1073-8746

Lill, D.J., Lindauer, S.J., Tüfekçi, E. & Shroff, B. (2008). Importance of pumice prophylaxis for bonding with self-etch primer. *American Journal of Orthodontics and Dentofacial Orthopedics,* Vol.133, No.3, pp. 423-426, ISSN 0889-5406

Linge, L. & Linge B.O. (1991). Patient Characteristics and treatment variables associated with apical root resorption during orthodontic treatment. *American Journal of Orthodontics and Dentofacial Orthopedics,* Vol.99, No.1, pp. 35-43, ISSN, ISSN 0889-5406

Lopatiene, K. & Dumbravaite, A. (2008). Risk factors of root resorption after orthodontic treatment. *Stomatologija, Baltic Dental and Maxillofacial Journal,* Vol.10, No.3, pp. 89-95, ISSN 1392-8589

Øgaard, B. & Fjeld, M. (2010). The Enamel Surface and Bonding in Orthodontics. *Seminars in Orthodontics,* Vol.16, No.1, pp. 37-48, ISSN 1073-8746

Piney, Crispin. (2003). Risk response planning: selecting the right strategy. *Proceedings of Fifth European Project Management Conference*, Cannes, France, June 2002

Preoteasa, C.T., Ionescu, E., Preoteasa, E., Comes, C.A., Buzea, M.C. & Grămescu, A. (2009). Orthodontically induced root resorption correlated with morphological characteristics. *Romanian Journal of Morphology and Embryology*, Vol.50, No.2, pp. 257-262, ISSN 1220-0522

Preoteasa, C.T. & Ionescu, E. (2011). Link between skeletal relations and root resorption in orthodontic patients. *International Journal of Medical Dentistry,* Vol.1, No.3, pp. 267-271, ISSN 2066-6063

Preoteasa, C.T., Ionescu, E., Didilescu, A.C., Melescanu-Imre, M., Bencze, M.A. & Preoteasa, E. (2011a) Undesirable dental hard tissue effects hypothetically linked to orthodontics - a microscopic study. *Romanian Journal of Morphology and Embryology,* Vol.52, No.3, pp. 937-941, ISSN 1220-0522

Preoteasa, C.T., Nabil Sultan, A., Popa, L., Ionescu, E., Iosif, L., Ghica, M.V. & Preoteasa, E. (2011b). Wettability of some dental materials. *Optoelectronics And Advanced Materials - Rapid Communications,* Vol.5, No.8, pp. 874-878,ISSN 1842-6573

Segal, G.R., Schiffman, P.H.& Tuncay, O.C. (2004). Meta analysis of the treatment-related factors of external apical root resorption. *Orthodontics and Craniofacial Research,* Vol.7, No.2, pp. 71-78, ISSN 1601-6335

Shah, A.A. & Sandler, J. (2006). Limiting factors in orthodontic treatment: 1. Factors related to patient, operator and orthodontic appliances. *Dental Update,* Vol.33, No.1, pp. 43-44, 46-48, 51-52, ISSN 0305-5000

Shungin, D., Olsson, A.I. & Persson, M. (2010). Orthodontic treatment-related white spot lesions: a 14-year prospective quantitative follow-up, including bonding material assessment. *American Journal of Orthodontics and Dentofacial Orthopedics,* Vol.138, No.2, pp. 1-8, ISSN 1097-6752

Smale, I., Artun, J., Behbehani, F., Doppel, D., van't Hof, M. & Kuijpers-Jagtman, A.M. (2005). Apical root resorption 6 months after initiation of fixed orthodontic appliance therapy. *American Journal of Orthodontics and Dentofacial Orthopedics,* Vol.128, No.1, pp. 57-67, ISSN 0889-5406

Viazis, A.D., DeLong, R., Bevis, R.R., Rudney, J.D.& Pintado, M.R. (1990). Enamel abrasion from ceramic orthodontic brackets under an artificial oral environment. *American Journal of Orthodontics and Dentofacial Orthopedics,* Vol.98, No. 2, pp. 103-109, ISSN 0889-5406

Vizitiu, T. C.& Ionescu, E. (2010). Microbiological changes in orthodontically treated patients. *Therapeutics, Pharmacology and Clinical Toxicology,* Vol.14, No.4, pp. 283-286, ISSN 1583-0012

Weltman, B., Vig, K.W., Fields, H.W., Shanker, S.& Kaizar, E.E. (2010) Root resorption associated with orthodontic tooth movement: A Systematic Review *American Journal of Orthodontics and Dentofacial Orthopedics,* Vol.137, No.4, pp. 462-476, ISSN 0889-5406

Wilson, W., Taubert, K. A., Gewitz, M., Lockhart, P. B., Baddour, L. M., Levison, M., Bolger, A., Cabell, C. H., Takahashi, M., Baltimore, R. S., Newburger, J. W., Strom, B. L., Tani, L. Y., Gerber, M., Bonow, R. O., Pallasch, T., Shulman, S. T., Rowley, A. H., Burns, J. C., Ferrieri, P., Gardner, T., Goff, D. & Durack, D. T. (2007). Prevention of infective endocarditis: guidelines from the American Heart Association, *Journal of the American Dental Association,* Vol.138, No.6, pp. 739–745,747-760, ISSN 0002-8177

World Health Organization. (1946). Preamble to the Constitution of the World Health Organization as adopted by the International Health Conference in 1946, In: *Basic Documents,* 24.08.2011, Available from:
http://www.who.int/governance/eb/who_constitution_en.pdf

19

Root Resorption in Orthodontics: An Evidence-Based Approach

Leandro Silva Marques[1], Paulo Antônio Martins-Júnior[1], Maria Letícia Ramos-Jorge[1] and Saul Martins Paiva[2]

[1]*Federal University of Vales do Jequitinhonha e Mucuri*
[2]*Federal University of Minas Gerais*
Brazil

1. Introduction

Root resorption is a pathological process that causes a shortening of the dental root. Although this condition is generally asymptomatic and missed in diagnosis, it may result in tooth mobility and even tooth loss if not diagnosed and treated early (Ahangari et al., 2010). In orthodontics, induced inflammatory root resorption is a form of pathologic root resorption related to the removal of hyalinized areas of the periodontal ligament following the application of orthodontic forces and is considered an undesirable but unavoidable iatrogenic consequence of orthodontic treatment (Brezniak & Wasserstein, 2002a; Brezniak & Wasserstein, 2002b).

The root resorption may compromise the continued existence and functional capacity of the affected tooth, depending on their magnitude (Brezniak & Wasserstein, 1993a, Brezniak & Wasserstein, 1993b), since the root structure (volume and contour) is changed (Consolaro, 2002). However, as the process of root resorption during orthodontic treatment is usually smooth and ends when the force is removed (Brezniak & Wasserstein, 1993, Levander et al., 1994) some authors have pointed out that the aesthetic and functional improvements justify the risks (Brezniak & Wasserstein, 1993).

1.1 Aims of the chapter

The aims of this chapter are to give a detailed description of root resorption, how it begins, the mechanisms involved in this condition and how the risk factors described in the literature contribute toward the development of root resorption related to orthodontic treatment. The importance of a thorough patient history and early diagnosis are also discussed. The value of high-quality research, such as longitudinal cohort and prospective studies, randomized clinical trials, systematic reviews and meta-analysis, is stressed in light of the current emphasis on evidence-based dentistry. Care and recommendations, legal implications and a case description of a patient with root resorption following orthodontic treatment are also presented.

2. Etiology of root resorption

Determining the cause of root resorption requires a thorough history, rescuing the previous dental history, addiction, accidentes, previous treatment, associated diseases and other details relevant to pathogenesis, but not always remembered by patients and identified by orthodontists. Several authors have pointed out that the multifactor etiology of root resorption is complex, but the condition appears to result from a combination of individual biologic variability, genetic predisposition and the effect of mechanical factors (Bartley et al., 2011; Weltman et al., 2010; Zahrowski & Jeske, 2011). However, no definitive conclusion has been drawn as to whether sex (Harris et al., 1997; Hendrix et al., 1994; Sameshina & Sinclair, 2001), age (Baumrind et al., 1996; Costopoulos & Nanda, 1996; Harris et al., 1997; Harris & Baker, 1990; Owmann-Moll et al., 1995), tooth extractions (Baumrind et al., 1996; Blake et al., 1995; Hendrix et al., 1994; McNab et al., 2000) and duration of active treatment (Baumrind et al., 1996; Beck & Harris, 1994; Harris et al., 1997; Kaley & Phillips, 1991; Kurol et al., 1996; Mirabella & Artun, 1995; Sameshina & Sinclair, 2001) are risk factors for root resorption. Conflicting data are reported on the relationship between root resorption and hypodontia or partial anodontia (Artun, 2000; Kjaer, 1995, 2000; Lee et al., 1999) and ectopic teeth (Kjaer, 2000; Lee et al., 1999).

2.1 How root resorption begins?

Orthodontic tooth movement is based on force-induced periodontal ligament and alveolar bone remodeling (Abuabara, 2007). So, orthodontic forces represent a physical agent capable of inducing inflammatory reaction in the periodontium (Giannopoulou et al., 2008). When a tooth moves, a necrosis of periodontal ligament on the pressure side with formation of a cell-free hyaline zone occurs. This event is followed by osteoclast resorption of the neighbouring alveolar bone and bone apposition by osteoblasts on the tension side (Abuabara, 2007). The resorption process of dental hard tissues seems to be triggered by the activity of some cytokines as well as that of bone. Immune cells migrate out of the capillaries in the periodontal ligament and interact with locally residing cells by elaborating a large array of signal molecules (Jäger et al., 2005). According Consolaro et al. (2011), the causes of root resorption should be related to the loss of root surface cementoblasts.

2.2 Orthodontic treatment-related factors

The ideal force for tooth movement would mimic a physiologic balance between tooth movement and bony adaptation (Paetyangkul et al., 2009). Schwarz (1932) advocated the optimal force level for tooth movement between 7 and 26 g per square centimeter. He also stated that, when force exceeded this threshold, root resorption occurs. When pressure decreases below this limit, root resorption ceases (Owman Moll et al., 1996). This was later confirmed by King and Fischlschweiger (1982), who found that light forces produced insignificant root resorption, whereas intermediate or heavy forces resulted in substantial crater formation.

In this context, several aspects have been related to induce root resorption during orthodontic treatment. This aspects are as follows: treatment duration (Casa et al., 2001; Fox, 2005; Levander & Malmgren, 1988; Otis et al., 2004; Paetyangkul et al., 2011; Sameshima & Sinclair, 2004; Segal et al., 2004), magnitude of the applied forces (Barbagallo et al., 2008; Bartley et al., 2011; Casa et al., 2001; Chan et al., 2005; Harris et al., 2006; Paetyangkul et al.,

2011), direction of tooth movement (Barbagallo et al., 2008; Han et al., 2005) amount of apical displacement (Fox, 2005; Segal et al., 2004), force application method (continuous vs. intermittent) (Brezniak & Wasserstein, 2002; Faltin et al., 2001), type of appliance (Brezniak & Wasserstein, 1993; Pandis et al., 2008) and treatment technique (Bartley et al., 2011; Beck & Harris, 1994; Janson et al., 1999; Marques et al., 2010; Pandis et al., 2008; Parker & Harris, 1998; Scott et al., 2008).

2.2.1 Treatment duration, force application method and magnitude of the applied forces

In a study, Acar et al. (1999) compared a 100-g force with elastics in either an interrupted (12 hours per day) or a continuous (24 hours per day) application. Group who has teeth experiencing orthodontic movement had significantly more root resorption than the control group. Besides that, continuous force produced significantly more root resorption than discontinuous force application.

Later, Ballard et al. (2009) conducted a prospective randomized clinical trial to compare root resorption with two force application patterns (continuous and intermittent) and they concluded that the application of intermittent orthodontic forces of 225 cN for 8 weeks (14 days of force application, 3 days of rest, then 4 days of force application repeated for 6 weeks) caused less root resorption than continuous forces of 225 cN for 8 weeks. The authors stated that, although it might not be clinically practical, compared with continuous forces, intermittent forces might be a safer method to prevent significant root resorption.

More recently, Paetyangkul et al. (2011) investigated the amounts of root resorption volumetrically after the application of controlled light and heavy forces in the buccal direction for 4, 8, and 12 weeks. They found significant differences in the extent of root resorption between 4, 8, and 12 weeks of force application ($P < 0.001$), with substantially more severe resorption in the longer force duration groups. The light force produced significantly less root resorption than did the heavy force. The authors argued that the duration of force application appears to be an important factor in orthodontic root resorption. Even though the application of light orthodontic forces did not show a significant difference between 4 and 8 weeks of buccal force application, the amount of root resorption increased significantly from 8 to 12 weeks of force application. So the duration of orthodontic force application caused more root resorption even when light forces of 25 g were used. This finding agrees with others studies published by Vardimon et al. (1991) and Gonzales et al. (2008). Paetyangkul et al. (2011) affirmed that this might be due to the increased osteoclastic activity around 8 weeks of force application.

In another study, Chan and Darendeliler (2006) found that the mean volume of the resorption craters was 11.59 times greater in the heavy-force group than in the control group. Barbagallo et al. (2008), in a prospective randomized clinical trial compared forces applied with removable thermoplastic appliances (TA) and fixed orthodontic appliances. The results showed that teeth experiencing orthodontic movement had significantly more root resorption than did the control teeth. They also found that heavy force produced significantly more root resorptions (9 times greater than the control) than light force (5 times greater than the control).

In this context, Harris et al. (2006) conducted a prospective randomized clinical trial to quantify the amount of root resorption when controlled light and heavy intrusive forces were applied to human premolars and to establish the sites where root resorption is more prevalent. They found that the volume of the root resorption craters after intrusion was directly proportional to the magnitude of the intrusive force applied. The findings showed that the control group had fewer and smaller root resorption craters, the light force group had more and larger root resorption craters than the control group, and the heavy force group had the most and the largest root resorption craters of all groups. A trend of linear increase in the volume of the root resorption craters was observed from control to light to heavy groups, and these differences were statistically significant. The mean volumes of the resorption craters in the light and heavy force groups were 2 and 4 times greater than in the control groups, respectively. The mesial and distal surfaces had the greatest resorption volume, with no statistically significant difference between the 2 surfaces.

2.2.2 Direction of tooth movement

Evaluating the direction of tooth movement (intrusive vs. extrusive force), Han et al. (2005) found that root resorption from extrusive force was not significantly different from the control group. Intrusive force significantly increased the percentage of resorbed root area (4 fold). The correlation between intrusion or extrusion and root resorption in the same patient was $r = 0.774$ ($P = 0.024$).

2.2.3 Amount of apical displacement

In orthodontics, total apical displacement might represent a better marker for overall treatment activation. A tooth that is moved greater distances through bone is subjected to longer durations of activation. There is no way to move a tooth between two points with fixed appliances, without causing hyalinization. Perhaps, this is why maxillary incisors are most likely to exhibit severe levels of root resorption (Segal et al., 2004). Segal et al. (2004) conducted a meta-analysis to elucidate possible treatment-related etiological factors - such as, duration of treatment and apical displacement – for external root resorption and they found that mean apical root resorption was strongly correlated with total apical displacement ($r = 0.822$) and treatment duration ($r = 0.852$). In 2005, Fox also found that treatment-related root resorption is correlated with the distance the apex moves and the length of time the treatment took.

2.2.4 Archwire sequence

Mandall et al. (2006) compared 3 orthodontic archwire sequences in terms of: (1) patient discomfort, (2) root resorption, and (3) time to working archwire. In that study, all patients were treated with maxillary and mandibular preadjusted edgewise appliances (0.022-in slot), and all archwires were manufactured by the same manufacturer. The results showed that there was no statistically significant difference between archwire sequences, for maxillary left central incisor root resorption (F ratio, $P = 0.58$). There was also no statistically significant difference between the proportion of patients with and without root resorption between archwire sequence groups ($P = 0.8$).

2.2.5 Type of appliance

Reukers et al. (1998) compared the prevalence and severity of root resorption after treatment with a fully programmed edgewise appliance (FPA) and a partly programmed edgewise appliance (PPA). All FPA patients were treated with 0.022-in slot Roth prescription ("A" Company, San Diego, Calif), and misplaced brackets were rebonded. All PPA patients were treated with 0.018-in slot Microloc brackets (GAC, Central Islip, NY), and the archwires were adjusted for misplaced brackets. They found no statistically significant differences in the amount of tooth root loss (FPA, 8.2%; PPA, 7.5%) or prevalence of root resorption (FPA, 75%; PPA, 55%) between the groups.

More recently, Scott et al. (2008) investigated the effect of either Damon3 self-ligating brackets or a conventional orthodontic bracket system on mandibular incisor root resorption. Patients were treated with Damon3 self-ligating or Synthesis (both, Ormco, Glendora, Calif) conventionally ligated brackets with identical archwires and sequencing in all patients. The results showed that mandibular incisor root resorption was not statistically different (Damon3, 2.26 mm, SD 2.63; Syn-thesis, 1.21 mm, SD 3.39) between systems.

2.2.6 Treatment technique

Brin et al. (2003) examined the effect of 2-phase vs 1-phase Class II treatment on the incidence and severity of root resorption. The results showed that children treated in 2 phases with a bionator followed by fixed appliances had the fewest incisors with moderate to severe root resorption, whereas children treated in 1 phase with fixed appliances had the most resorption. However, the difference was not statistically significant. As treatment time increased, the odds of root resorption also increased (P = 0.04). The odds of a tooth experiencing severe root resorption were greater with a large reduction in overjet during phase 2.

2.3 Patient-related risk factors

Possible patient-related risk factors include a previous history of root resorption (Brezniak & Wasserstein, 1993; Hartsfield et al., 2004; Marques et al., 2010), tooth/root morphology, length and roots with developmental abnormalities (Brin et al., 2003; Fox, 2005; ; Marques et al., 2010; Sameshima & Sinclair, 2001, 2004; Smale et al., 2005), genetic influences (Al-Qawasmi et al., 2003; Bollen, 2002; Hartsfield et al., 2004; Ngan et al., 2004; Sameshima & Sinclair, 2001), systemic factors (Adachi et al., 1994; Igarashi et al., 1996), including drugs (nabumetone) (Villa et al., 2005), hormone deficiency, hypothyroidism, hypopituitarism (Loberg & Engstrom, 1994; Poumpros et al., 1994), asthma (Brezniak & Wasserstein, 2002; McNab et al., 1999), proximity of root to cortical bone (Horiuchi et al., 1998; Kaley & Phillips, 1991; Otis et al., 2004), alveolar bone density (Midgett et al., 1981; Otis et al., 2004), previous trauma (Brezniak & Wasserstein, 2002; Brin et al., 2003; Hartsfield et al., 2004; Mandall et al., 2006), endodontic treatment (Brezniak & Wasserstein, 2002; Hamilton et al., 1999), severity and type of malocclusion (Brin et al., 2003; Sameshima & Sinclair, 2001; Segal et al., 2004), patient age (Bishara et al., 1999; Fox, 2005; Harris et al., 1993; Levander & Malmgren, 1998; Mavragani et al., 2002) and gender (Chan & Darendeliler, 2006; Fox, 2005; Harris et al., 1997; Sameshima & Sinclair, 2001).

2.3.1 Genetic influences

Although several studies proved that there is a relationship between orthodontic force and root resorption, individual susceptibility also appears to influence the occurrence of root resorption. Since mechanical forces and other environmental factors do not adequately explain the variation seen among individual expressions of root resorption, interest has increased on genetic factors influencing the susceptibility to root resorptions (Hartsfield, 2009). The reaction to orthodontic force, including rate of tooth movement, can differ depending on the individual's genetic background (Abass & Hartsfield, 2007; Iwasaki et al., 2008).

In this context, pro-inflammatory cytokines like interleukin-1 (IL-1) and tumour necrosis factor (TNF) are known to induce synthesis of various proteins that, in turn, elicit acute or chronic inflammation. Al-Qawasmi et al. (2003) identified linkage disequilibrium between the IL-1B gene and root resorption in orthodontically treated individuals. The polymorphism variation was found to account for 15% of the variation in root resorption in that sample. Persons in their sample homozygous for the IL-1B allele 1 had a 5.6 fold (95 % CI 1.9–21.2) increased risk of root resorption greater than 2 mm as compared with those who are not homozygous for the IL-1 beta allele 1. Data indicate that allele 1 at the IL-1B gene, known to decrease the production of IL-1 cytokine in vivo (Pociot et al., 1992), significantly increases the risk of root resorption (Al-Qawasmi et al., 2003).

2.3.2 Systemic factors

A study conducted by Nishioka et al. (2006) determined whether there is an association between excessive root resorption and immune system factors. The prevalence of root resorption found was 10.3%. Allergy, abnormalities in root morphology and asthma showed be high risk factors for the development of excessive root resorption during orthodontic tooth movement. The modifying effect of several pharmacological agents on orthodontic root resorption also has been examined. Among them, L-thyroxine has been shown to have an inhibitory effect and clinical application has been attempted (Shirazi et al., 1999). Studies have been published describing anti-inflammatory properties of tetracyclines (and their chemically modified analogues) unrelated to their antimicrobial effect. A significant reduction in the number of mononucleated cells on the root surface was observed. Such cells have been related to root resorption (Mavragani et al., 2005).

Some authors have pointed that bone turnover has an important influence during orthodontic treatment. High bone turnover, found in patients with hyperthyroidism, can increase the amount of tooth movement compared with the normal or low bone turnover state and adult patients. Low bone turnover, found in patients with hypothyroidism, can result more root resorption, suggesting that in subjects where a decreased bone turnover rate is expected, the risk of root resorption could be increased (Verna et al., 2003). Bisphosphonates, potent inhibitors of bone resorption, causes a significant dose-dependent inhibition of root resorption in rats after force application. These results prompt that a thorough case history regarding possible pathophysiological conditions influencing bone metabolism should be performed on an individual patient basis. In subjects where increased bone turnover rates are expected, the reactivation of the appliance could be performed more frequently. However, in patients where decreased bone turnover rates are expected, the reactivation should be carried out less frequently and the risk of root resorption should be carefully evaluated (Verna et al., 2003).

Most studies agree that patients who have extractions during orthodontic treatment have greater chances of severe resorption than those treated without extractions (Beck & Harris,

1994; Harris & Baker, 1990; Hendrix et al., 1994; McNab et al., 2000). One possible explanation for this could be the increased movement and retraction of the apex to close extraction spaces.

Another risk factor for severe root resorption is triangular roots (Marques et al., 2010). The geometric form of dental roots influences the distribution of forces on the alveolar bone and the dent al structure itself. Blunt roots and pipette-shaped apices (triangular) tend to concentrate the forces in a smaller area than roots with a normal shape (Marques et al., 2010). Most studies agree that pointed roots undergo resorption more frequently than those with normal shape (Hartsfield et al., 2004; Nigul & Jagomagi, 2006; Ng'ang'a & Ng'ang'a, 2003; Sameshima & Sinclair, 2001; Smale et al., 2005; Stenvik & Mjor, 1970).

2.4 How root resorption is repaired?

The transition of active root resorption into a process of repair is associated with the invasion of fibroblast-like cells from the circumference of the resorption crater into the active root resorption site even with a light force. The formation of new tooth-supporting structures is seen in the pheriphery of the resorption lacunae, whereas active resorption by multinucleated odontoclast-like cells took place in the central parts. When orthodontic force is discontinued, the reparative process is similar to early cementogenesis during tooth development (Brudvik & Rygh, 1995a, Brudvik & Rygh, 1995b). It has been suggested that the epithelial cell rests of Malassez might have a significant role in mediating repair cementogenesis (Brice et al., 1991; Hasegawa et al., 2003). The resorptive defects are repaired by the deposition of new cementum and the reestablishment of new periodontal ligament (Andreasen, 1973; Barber & Sims, 1981; Brice et al., 1991; Brudvik & Rygh, 1995b; Langford & Sims, 1982; Reitan, 1974).

3. Quality of research

Most of the studies cited in this chapter offer a low amount of scientific evidence and therefore do not yet allow the precise prediction of the interaction between orthodontic treatment, genetic/systemic factors and root resorption. Part of this insufficient evidence may be explained by the different methodological criteria employed, different sample sizes and the heterogeneity of the study populations. Thus, the findings have been conflicting, which compromises both the credibility and clinical application of the results. Also, the current state of knowledge does not allow orthodontists to identify which patients are vulnerable. In a recent systematic review, Weltman et al. (2010) stated that "only 11 trials were considered appropriate for inclusion in this review, and their protocols were too variable to proceed with a quantitative synthesis. This reflects the state of the published scientific research on this topic."

Furthermore, although severe root resorption can have drastic consequences to both treatment and patient health, there is only one study that specifically addresses the risk factors for this condition (Marques et al., 2010). The main factors directly involved in severe root resorption are extraction of first premolars, triangle-shaped roots and root resorption before treatment. In cases of extensive root resorption induced by orthodontic movement, there might be flaws in the predictability, prevention, and early diagnosis of this condition.

It is therefore important to determine the magnitude and prevalence of root resorption in various populations as well as related risk factors (Marques et al., 2010).

However, some challenging situations may appear to the orthodontist during orthodontic treatments. For example, in the study published by Marques et al. (2010), they found an excessive percentage of patients (6%) that experienced pauses in the mechanical treatment, there was a severe root resorption at the end of the treatment. This finding suggests the influence of genetic factors and further increases the responsibility of orthodontists with regard to this issue. If severe root resorption is identified, the treatment plan should be reassessed with the patient. Alternative options might include prosthetic solutions to close spaces, releasing teeth from active archwires if possible, stripping instead of extracting, and early fixation of resorbed teeth (Brezniak & Wasserstein, 2002).

4. Care and recommendations

Determining the cause of root resorption requires a thorough medical history, including the past history of the tooth involved as well as vices, accidents, types of sports practiced, previous treatment and associated diseases. Relevant details, such as mild trauma (concussion and subluxation) should be analyzed in detail (Consolaro et al., 2011).

As root resorption is often asymptomatic, radiographic images constitute the best way to detect the condition and measure its severity in order to establish an early diagnosis (Eraso et al., 2007), especially control radiographs obtained after six to 12 months of orthodontic treatment (Artun et al., 2009; Weltman et al., 2010). Digital radiography (DR) and digital subtraction radiography (DSR) can be used for the detection of apical root resorption as small as 0.5 mm and lingual resorption of 1 mm or more. In this context, DSR frequently performs better than DR (Ono et al., 2011).

When an orthodontist identifies root resorption in a patient, the severity of the condition is decreased with a pause in active orthodontic movement for two to three months with a use of a passive archwire (Weltman et al., 2010; Zahrowski & Jeske, 2011). However, if the resorption is severe, the orthodontist and patient should reassess the treatment plan (Weltman et al., 2010). Alternative options include prosthetic solutions to close spaces, releasing teeth from active archwires when possible, stripping instead of extracting and early fixation of resorbed teeth (Brezniak & Wasserstein, 2002). If root resorption is diagnosed on the final radiographs after treatment, follow-up radiographic examinations are recommended until the resorption has stabilized (Weltman et al., 2010). However, if it continues, sequential root canal therapy with calcium hydroxide may be considered (Pizzo et al., 2007).

There is little evidence that previous trauma (with no history of root resorption) and unusual tooth morphology play roles in increasing root resorption (Weltman et al., 2010). Caution should be used when retaining the teeth with fixed appliances, as occlusal trauma to the fixed teeth or segments may lead to extreme root resorption (Brezniak & Wasserstein, 2002). As the magnitude of force has been documented to be directly correlated with the severity of root resorption (Casa et al., 2001; Darendeliler et al., 2004; Faltin et al., 2001; Harris et al., 2006), the ideal force for dental movement would mimic a physiologic balance between tooth movement and bone adaptation (Paetyangkul et al.,

2011). It is therefore recommended to employ light forces, especially for intrusive movements (Weltman et al., 2010).

5. Case report

The case described below illustrates an atypical situation, since with only four months of treatment using alignment and leveling wires (0.14 and 0.16), a severe root resorption was detected. This situation led the orthodontist to stop the orthodontic treatment. Fortunately, the case had low complexity and did not involve extensive tooth movements. In such cases, the orthodontist should be aware of the systematic radiological examinations.

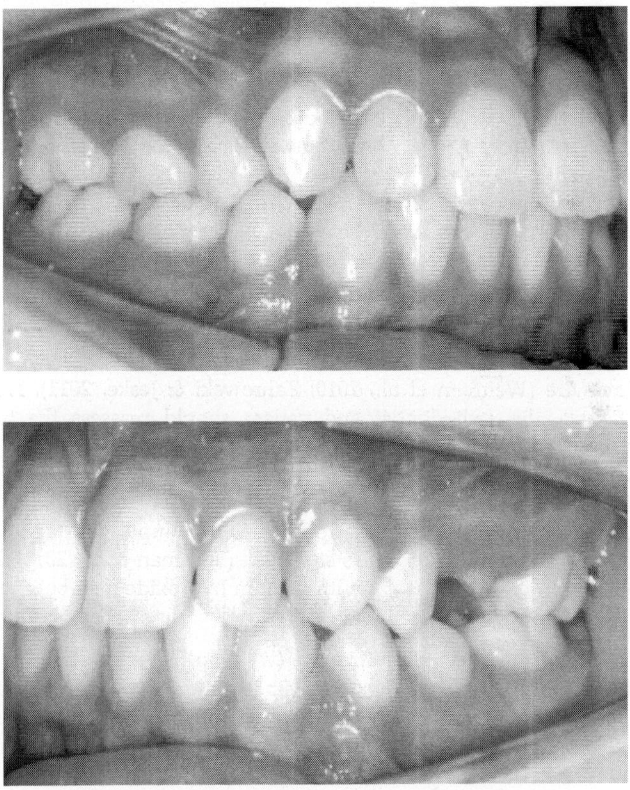

Fig. 1. Initial situation of the patient.

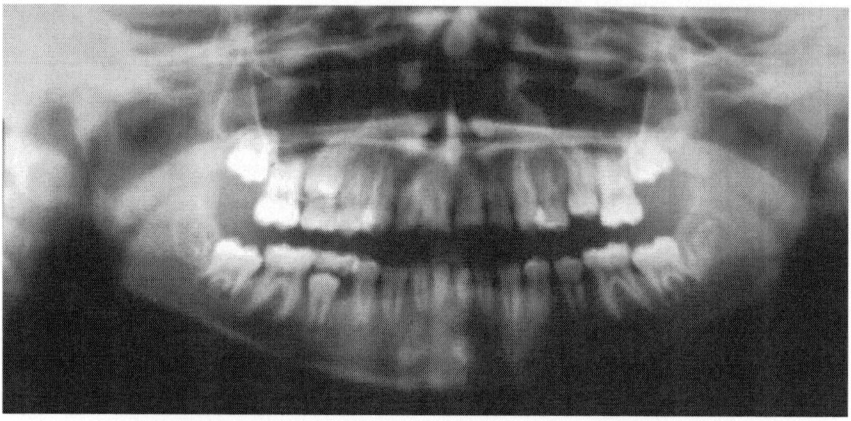

Fig. 2. Panoramic radiograph.

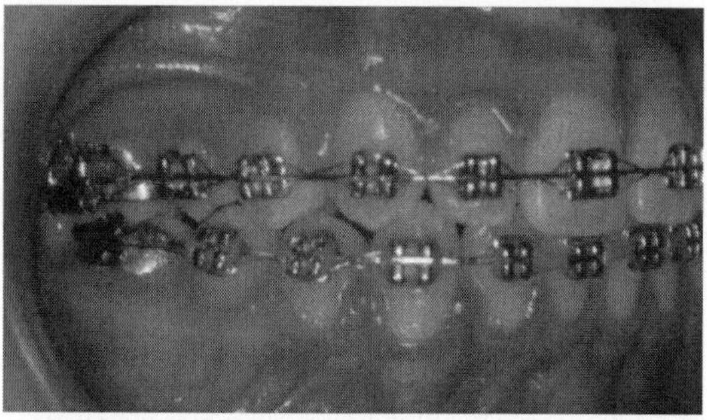

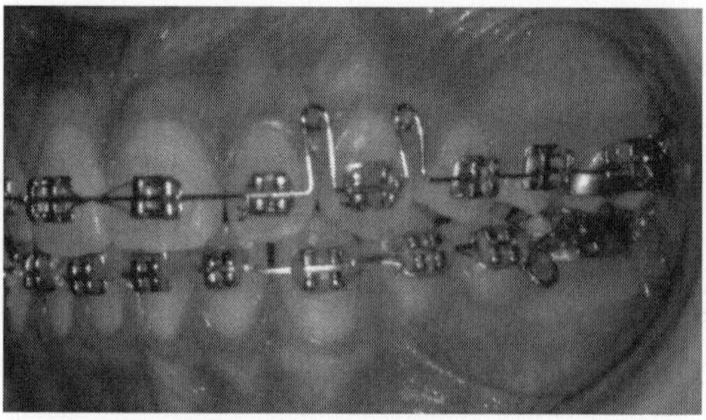

Fig. 3. (a, b). Alignament using wire 0.14.

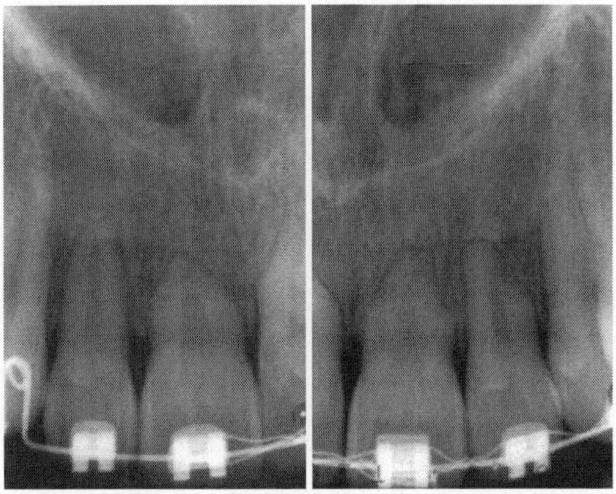

Fig. 4. (a, b). Periapical radiographs showing root resorption of superior incisors.

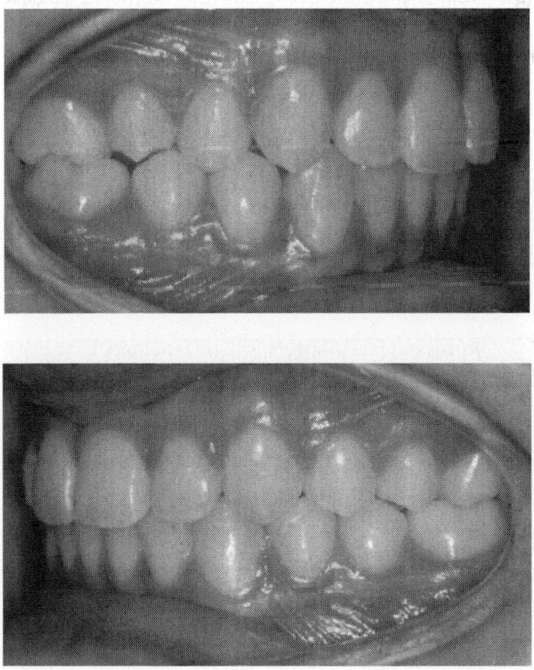

Fig. 5. (a, b). Final aspect of treatment.

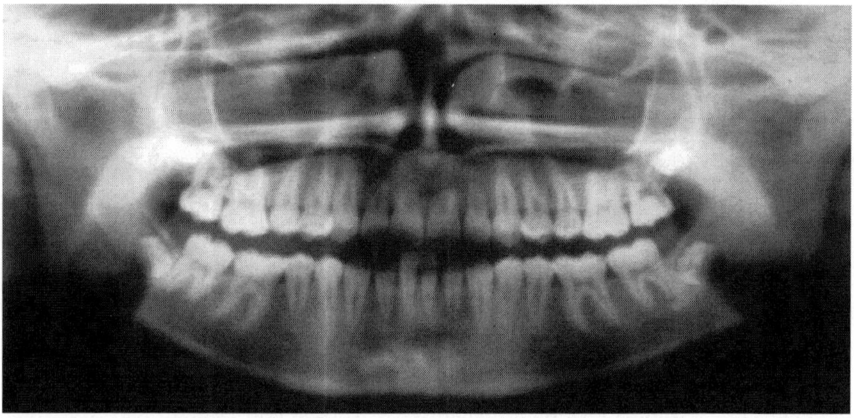

Fig. 6. Final panoramic radiograph.

6. Conclusions

While science provides no consistent evidence for the precise identification of the orthodontic patient that will develop root resorption, orthodontists should keep in mind the various indicators known and promote systematic radiographic to monitor their patients. Individualize the diagnosis and treatment plan could mean the difference between the success and failure of orthodontic treatment.

7. Acknowledgments

The authors thank the Coordenação de Aperfeiçoamento de Pessoal de Nível Superior (CAPES) for financial support to carry out this research.

8. References

Abass, S.K.; Hartsfield, J.K. Jr. (2007) Orthodontics and external apical root resorption. *Semin Orthod*, 13, 246-56.

Abuabara, A. (2007). Biomechanical aspects of external root resorption in orthodontic therapy. *Med Oral Patol Oral Cir Bucal*, 12, 8, E610-3.

Acar, A.; Canyurek, U.; Kocaaga, M.; Erverdi, N. (1999). Continuous vs. dis-continuous force application and root resorption. *Angle Orthod*, 69, 159-63.

Adachi, H.; Igarashi, K.; Mitani, H.; Shinoda, H.; (1994). Effects of topical administration of a bisphosphonate (risedronate) on orthodontic tooth movement in rats. *J Dent Res*, 73, 1478-86.

Ahangari, Z.; Nasser, M.; Mahdia, M.; Fedorowicz, Z.; Marchesan, M.A. (201). Interventions for the management of external root resorption. *Cochrane Database Syst Rev*, Jun 16, 6, CD008003.

Al-Qawasmi, R.A.; Hartsfield, J.K. Jr, Everett, E.T. et al. (2003). Genetic predisposition to external apical root resorption in orthodontic patients: linkage of chromo-some-18 marker. *J Dent Res*, 82, 356-60.

Andreasen, J.O. (1973). Cementum repair after apicoectomy in humans. *Acta Odontol Scand*, 31, 211-21.

Årtun, J.; Van 't Hullenaar, R.; Doppel, D.; Kuijpers-Jagtman, A.M. (2009) Identification of orthodontic patients at risk of severe apical root resorption. *Am J Orthod Dentofacial Orthop*, 135, 4, 448-55.

Årtun, J. (2000). Revisiting root resorption. *Am J Orthod DentofacialOrthop*, 118, 3, 14A.

Ballard, D.J.; Jones, A.S;. Petocz, P.; Darendeliler, M.A. (2009). Physical properties of root cementum: part 11. Continuous vs intermittent controlled orthodontic forces on root resorption. A microcomputed tomography study. *Am J Orthod Dentofacial Orthop*, 136, 1, 8.e1-8, discussion 8-9.

Barbagallo, L.J.; Jones, A.S.; Petocz, P.; Darendeliler, M.A. (2008). Physical properties of root cementum: part 10. Comparison of the effects of invisible removable thermoplastic appliances with light and heavy orthodontic forces on premolar cementum. A microcomputed-tomography study. *Am J Orthod Dentofacial Orthop*, 133, 218-27.

Barber, A.F.; Sims, M.R. (1981). Rapid maxillary expansion and external root resorption in man: a scanning electron microscope study. *Am J Orthod*, 79, 630-52.

Bartley, N.; Türk, T.; Colak, C.; Elekdağ-Türk, S.; Jones, A.; Petocz, P.; Darendeliler, M.A. (2011). Physical properties of root cementum: Part 17. Root resorption after the application of 2.5° and 15° of buccal root torque for 4 weeks: a microcomputed tomography study. *Am J Orthod Dentofacial Orthop*, 139, 4, e353-60.

Baumrind, S.; Korn, E.L.; Boyd, R.L. (1996). Apical root resorption in orthodontically treated adults. *Am J Orthod Dentofacial Orthop*, 110, 311-20.

Beck, B.W.; Harris, E.F. (1994). Apical root resorption in orthodontically treated subjects: analysis of edgewise and light wire mechanics. *Am J Orthod Dentofacial Orthop*, 105, 350-61.

Blake, M.; Woodside, D.G.; Pharoah, M.J. (1995). A radiographic comparison of apical root resorption after orthodontic treatment with the edge-wise and Speed appliances. *Am J Orthod Dentofacial Orthop*, 108, 76-84.

Bishara, S.E.; Vonwald, L.; Jakobsen, J.R. (1999). Changes in root length from early to mid-adulthood: resorption or apposition? *Am J Orthod Dentofacial Orthop*, 115, 563-8.

Bollen, A.M. (2002). Large overjet and longer teeth are associated with more root resorption when treated orthodontically. *J Evid Based Dent Pract*, 2, 44-5.

Brezniak, N.; Wasserstein, A. (1993). Root resorption after orthodontic treatment: Part 1. Literature review. *Am J Orthod Dentofacial Orthop*, 103, 1, 62-6.

Brezniak, N.; Wasserstein, A. (1993). Root resorption after orthodontic treatment: Part 2. Literature review. *Am J Orthod Dentofacial Orthop*, 103, 2, 138-46.

Brezniak, N.; Wasserstein, A. (2002). Orthodontically induced inflammatory root resorption. Part I: The basic science aspects. *Angle Orthod*, 72, 2, 175-9.

Brezniak, N.; Wasserstein, A. (2002). Orthodontically induced inflammatory root resorption. Part II: the clinical aspects. *Angle Orthod*, 72, 180-4.

Brice, G.L.; Sampson, W.J; Sims, M.R. (1991). An ultrastructural evaluation of the relationship between epithelial rests of Malassez and orthodontic root resorption and repair in man. *Aust Orthod J*, 12, 90-4.

Brin, I.; Tulloch, J.F.; Koroluk, L.; Philips, C. (2003). External apical root resorption in Class II malocclusion: a retrospective review of 1- versus 2-phase treatment. *Am J Orthod Dentofacial Orthop*, 124, 2, 151-6.

Brudvik, P.; Rygh, P. (1995). The repair of orthodontic root resorption: an ultrastructural study. *Eur J Orthod*, 17, 189-98.

Brudvik, P.; Rygh, P. (1995). Transition and determinants of orthodontic root resorption-repair sequence. *Eur J Orthod*, 17, 177-88.

Casa, M.A.; Faltin, R.M.; Faltin, K.; Sander, F.G.; Arana Chavez, V.E. (2001). Root resorptions in upper first premolars after application of continuous torque moment. Intra-individual study. *J Orofac Orthop*, 62, 285-95.

Chan, E.; Darendeliler, M.A. (2005). Physical properties of root cemen-tum: part 5. Volumetric analysis of root resorption craters after application of light and heavy orthodontic forces. *Am J Orthod Dentofacial Orthop*, 127, 186-95.

Chan, E.; Darendeliler, M.A. (2006). Physical properties of root cementum: part 7. Extent of root resorption under areas of compression and tension. *Am J Orthod Dentofacial Orthop*, 129, 4, 504-10.

Consolaro, A. (2002). Reabsorções dentária na movimentação ortodôntica. In: *Reabsorções dentárias nas especialidades clínicas*. Dental Press Editora pp. 259-289, Maringá.

Consolaro, A.; Franscischone, T.R.G.; Furquim, L.Z. (2011). As reabsorções As múltiplas ou severas não estão relacionadas a fatores sistêmicos, suscetibilidade individual, tendência familiar e predisposição individual. *Dent Press J Orthod*, 16,1, 17-21.

Costopoulos, G.; Nanda, R. (1996). An evaluation of root resorption incident to orthodontic intrusion. *Am J Orthod Dentofacial Orthop*, 109,543-8.

Darendeliler, M.A.; Kharbanda, OP.; Chan, E.K.M et al. (2004). Root resorption and its association with alterations in physical properties, mineral contents and resorption craters in human premolars following application of light and heavy con-trolled orthodontics forces. *Orthod Craniofac Res*, 7, 79-97.

Eraso, F.E.; Parks, E.T.; Roberts, W.E.; Hohlt, W.F.; Ofner. S. (2007). Density value means in the evaluation of external apical root resorption: an in vitro study for early detection in orthodontic case simulations. *Dentomaxillofac Radiol*, 36, 3, 130-7.

Faltin, R.M.; Faltin, K.; Sander, F.G.; Arana Chavez, V.E. (2001). Ultrastructure of cementum and periodontal ligament after continuous intrusion in humans: a transmission electron microscopy study. *Eur J Orthod*, 23, 35-49.

Fox, N. (2005). Longer orthodontic treatment may result in greater external apical root resorption. *Evid Based Dent*, 6, 1, 21.

Giannopoulou, C.; Dudic, A.; Montet, X.; Kiliaridis, S.; Mombelli, A. (2008). Periodontal parameters and cervical root resorption during orthodontic tooth movement. *J Clin Periodontol*, 35, 6, 501-6.

Gonzales, C.; Hotokezaka, H.; Yoshimatsu, M.; Yozgatian, J.H.; Darendeliler, M.A.; Yoshida, N. (2008). Force magnitude and duration effects on amount of tooth movement and root resorption in the rat molar. *Angle Orthod*, 78, 502-9.

Han, G.; Huang, S.; Von den Hoff, J.W.; Zeng, X.; Kuijpers-Jagtman, A.M. (2005). Root resorption after orthodontic intrusion and extrusion: an intraindividual study. *Angle Orthod*, 75, 912-8.

Hamilton, R.S.; Gutmann, J.L. (1999). Endodontic-orthodontic relation-ships: a review of integrated treatment planning challenges. *Int Endod J*, 32, 343-60.

Harris, D.A.; Jones, A.S,. Darendeliler, M.A. (2006). Physical properties of root cementum: part 8. Volumetric analysis of root resorption craters after application of controlled intrusive light and heavy orthodontic forces: a microcomputed tomography scan study. *Am J Orthod Dentofacial Orthop*, 130, 639-47.

Harris, E.F.; Baker, W.C. (1990). Loss of root length and crestal bone height before and during treatment in adolescent and adult orthodontic patients. *Am J Orthod Dentofacial Orthop*, 98, 463-9.

Harris, E.F.; Kineret, S.E.; Tolley, E.A. (1997). A heritable component for external apical root resorption in patients treated orthodontically. *Am J Orthod Dentofacial Orthop*, 111, 301-9.

Hartsfield, J.K. Jr.; Everett, E.T.; Al-Qawasmi, R.A. (2004). Genetic factors in external apical root resorption and orthodontic treatment. *Crit Rev Oral Biol Med*, 15: 115-22.

Hartsfield, J.K. Jr. (2009). Pathways in external apical root resorption associated with orthodontia. *Orthod Craniofac Res*, 12, 3, 236-42.

Hasegawa, N.; Kawaguchi, H.; Ogawa, T.; Uchida, T.; Kurihara. H. (2003). Immunohistochemical characteristics of epithelial cell rests of Malassez during cementum repair. *J Periodontal Res*, 38, 51-6.

Hendrix, I.; Carels, C.; Kuijpers-Jagtman, A.M,; Van 'T Hof. M. (994). A radiographic study of posterior apical root resorption in orthodontic patients. *Am J Orthod Dentofacial Orthop*, 105, 345-9.

Horiuchi, A.; Hotokezaka, H.; Kobayashi, K. (1998). Correlation between cortical plate proximity and apical root resorption. *Am J Orthod Dentofacial Orthop*, 114, 311-8.

Igarashi, K.; Adachi, H.; Mitani, H.; Shinoda, H. (1996). Inhibitory effect of topical administration of a bisphosphonate (risedronate) on root resorption incident to orthodontic tooth movement in rats. *J Dent Res*, 75, 1644-9.

Iwasaki, L.R.; Crouch, L.D.; Nickel, J.C. (2008). Genetic factors and tooth movement. *Semin Orthod*, 14, 135–45.

Janson, G.R.; De Luca Canto, G.; Martins, D.R.; Henriques, J.F.; De Freitas, M.R. (1999). A radiographic comparison of apical root resorption after orthodontic treatment with 3 different fixed appliance techniques. *Am J Orthod Dentofacial Orthop*, 118, 262-73.

Jäger, A.; Zhang, D.; Kawarizadeh, A.; Tolba, R.; Braumann, B.; Lossdörfer, S.; Götz, W. (2005). Soluble cytokine receptor treatment in experimental orthodontic tooth movement in the rat. *Eur J Orthod*, 27, 1, 1-11.

Kaley, J.; Phillips, C. (1991). Factors related to root resorption in edgewise practice. *Angle Orthod*, 61, 125-32.

King, G.J.; Fischlschweiger, W. (1982). The effect of force magnitude on extractable bone resorptive activity and cemental cratering in orthodontic tooth movement. *J Dent Res*, 61, 775-9.

Kjaer, I. (1995). Morphological characteristics of dentitions developing excessive root resorption during orthodontic treatment. *Eur J Orthod*, 17, 25-34.

Kjaer, I. (2000). Revisiting root resorption. *Am J Orthod Dentofaci al Orthop*, 117, 4, 23A.

Kurol, J.; Owman-Moll, P.; Lundgren, D. (1996). Time-related root resorption after application of a controlled continuous orthodontic force. *Am J Orthod Dentofacial Orthop*, 110, 303-10.

Langford, S.R.; Sims, M.R. (1982). Root surface resorption, repair, and periodontal attachment following rapid maxillary expansion in man. *Am J Orthod*, 81, 108-15.

Lee, R.Y.; Årtun, J.; Alonzo, T.A. (1999). Are dental anomalies risk factors for apical root resorption in orthodontic patients? *Am J Orthod Dentofacial Orthop*, 116, 187-95.

Levander, E.; Malmgren, O.; Eliasson, S. (1994). Evaluation of root resorption in relation to two orthodontic treatment regimes. A clinical experimental study. *Eur J Orthod*, 16, 3, 223-8.

Levander, E.; Malmgren, O.; Stenback, K. (1998). Apical root resorption during orthodontic treatment of patients with multiple aplasia: a study of maxillary incisors. *Eur J Orthod*, 20, 427-34.

Loberg, E.L.; Engstrom, C. (1994). Thyroid administration to reduce root resorption. *Angle Orthod*, 64, 395-9.

Mandall, N.; Lowe, C.; Worthington, H. et al. (2006). Which orthodontic archwire sequence? A randomized clinical trial. *Eur J Orthod*, 28, 6, 61-6.

Marques, L.S.; Chaves, K.C.; Rey, A.C.; Pereira, L.J.; Ruellas, A.C. (2011). Severe root resorption and orthodontic treatment: clinical implications after 25 years of follow-up. *Am J Orthod Dentofacial Orthop*, 139, 4 , S166-9.

Mavragani, M.; Boe, O.E.; Wisth, P.J.; Selvig, K.A. (2002). Changes in root length during orthodontic treatment: advantages for immature teeth. *Eur J Orthod*, 24, 91-7.

Mavragani, M,. Brudvik, P.; Selvig, K.A. (2005). Orthodontically induced root and alveolar bone resorption: inhibitory effect of systemic doxycycline administration in rats. *Eur J Orthod*, 27, 3, 215-25.

McNab, S.; Battistutta, D.; Taverne, A.; Symons, A.L. (1999). External apical root resorption of posterior teeth in asthmatics after orthodontic treatment. *Am J Orthod Dentofacial Orthop*, 116, 545-51.

McNab, S.; Battistutta, D.; Taverne, A.; Symons, A.L. (2000). External apical root resorption following orthodontic treatment. *Angle Orthod*, 70, 227-32

Midgett, R.J.; Shaye, R.; Fruge, J.F. Jr. (1981). The effect of altered bone metabolism on orthodontic tooth movement. *Am J Orthod*, 80, 256-62.

Mirabella, A.D.; Årtun. J. (1995). Risk factors for apical root resorption of maxillary anterior teeth in adult orthodontic patients. *Am J Orthod Dentofacial Orthop*, 108, 48-55.

Ng'ang'a, P.M.; Ng'ang'a, R.N. (2003). Maxillary incisor root forms in orthodontic patients in Nairobi, Kenya. *East Afr Med J*, 80, 101-4.

Ngan, D.C.S.; Kharbanda, O.P.; Byloff, F.K.; Darendeliler, M.A. (2004). The genetic contribution to orthodontic root resorption: a retrospec-tive twin study. *Aust Orthod J*, 20, 1-9.

Nigul, K.; Jagomagi, T. (2006). Factors related to apical root resorption of maxillary incisors in orthodontic patients. *Stomatologija*, 8, 76-9.

Nishioka, M.; Ioi. H.; Nakata, S.; Nakasima. A.; Counts. A. (2006). Root resorption and immune system factors in the Japanese. *Angle Orthod*, 76, 1, 103-8.

Ono, E.; Medici Filho, E.; Faig Leite, H.; Tanaka, J.L.; De Moraes, M.E.; De Melo Castilho. J.C. (2011). Evaluation of simulated external root resorptions with digital radiography and digital subtraction radiography. *Am J Orthod Dentofacial Orthop*, 139, 3, 324-33.

Otis, L.; Hong, J.; Tuncay, O. (2004). Bone structure effect on root resorption. *Orthod Craniofac Res*, 21, 165-77.

Owman-Moll, P.; Kurol, J.; Lundgren, D. (1995). Continuous versus interrupted continuous orthodontic force related to early tooth movement and root resorption. *Angle Orthod*, 65, 395-401.

Owman-Moll, P.; Kurol, J.; Lundgren, D. (1996). The effects of a four-fold increased orthodontic force magnitude on tooth movement and root resorptions. An intra-individual study in adolescents. *Eur J Orthod*, 1996, 18, 287-94.

Paetyangkul, A.; Türk, T.; Elekdağ-Türk, S.; Jones, A.S.; Petocz, P.; Darendeliler, M.A. (2009). Physical properties of root cementum: part 14. The amount of root resorption after force application for 12 weeks on maxillary and mandibular premolars: a microcomputed-tomography study. *Am J Orthod Dentofacial Orthop*, 136, 4, 492.e1-9.

Pandis, N.; Nasika, M.; Polychronopoulou, A.; Eliades, T. (2008). External apical root resorption in patients treated with conventional and self-ligating brackets. *Am J Orthod Dentofacial Orthop*, 134, 646-51.

Parker, R.J.; Harris, E.F. (1998). Directions of orthodontic tooth movements associated with external apical root resorption of the maxillary central incisor. *Am J Orthod Dentofacial Orthop*, 114, 672-83.

Pizzo, G.; Licata, M.E.; Guiglia, R.; Giuliana, G. (2007). Root resorption and orthodontic treatment. Review of the literature. *Minerva Stomatol*, 56, 1-2, 31-44.

Pociot, F.; Mølvig, J.; Wogensen, L.; Worsaae, H.; Nerup, J. (1992). A TaqI polymorphism in the human interleukin-1 beta (IL-1 beta) gene correlates with IL-1 beta secretion in vitro. *Eur J Clin Invest*, 22, 6, 396-402.

Poumpros, E.; Loberg, E.; Engstrom, C. (1994). Thyroid function and root resorption. *Angle Orthod*, 64, 389-93.

Reitan, K. (1974). Initial tissue behavior during apical root resorption. *Angle Orthod*, 44, 68-82.

Reukers, E.A.; Sanderink, G.C.; Kuijpers-Jagtman, A.M.; van't Hof, M.A. (1998). Radiographic evaluation of apical root resorption with 2 different types of edgewise appliances. Results of a randomized clinical trial. *J Orofac Orthop*, 59, 2, 100-9. Erratum in: *J Orofac Orthop*, 59, 4, 251.

Sameshima, G.T.; Sinclair, P.M. (2001). Predicting and preventing root resorption: part I. Diagnostic factors. *Am J Orthod Dentofacial Orthop*, 119, 505-10.

Sameshima, G.T.; Sinclair, P.M. (2004). Characteristics of patients with severe root resorption. *Orthod Craniofac Res*, 7, 2, 108-14.

Scott, P.; DiBiase, A.T.; Sherriff, M.; Cobourne, M.T. (2008). Alignment efficiency of Damon3 self-ligating and conventional orthodontic bracket systems: a randomized clinical trial. *Am J Orthod Dentofacial Orthop*, 134, 470.e1-8.

Schwarz, A.M. (1932). Tissue changes incidental to orthodontic tooth movement. *Int J Orthod*, 18, 331-52.

Segal, G.; Schiffman, P.; Tuncay, O. (2004). Meta analysis of the treatment-related factors of external apical root resorption. *Orthod Craniofac Res*, 7, 71-8.

Shirazi, M.; Dehpour, A.R.; Jafari, F. (1999). The effect of thyroid hormone on orthodontic tooth movement in rats. *J Clin Pediatr Dent*, 23, 3, 259-64.

Smale, I.; Artun, J.; Behbehani, F.; Doppel, D.; van't Hof, M.; Kuijpers-Jagtman, A.M. (2005). Apical root resorption 6 months after initiation of fixed orthodontic appliance therapy. *Am J Orthod Dentofacial Orthop*, 128, 1, 57-67.

Stenvik, A.; Mjor, I.A. (1970). Pulp and dentine reactions to experimental tooth intrusion. A histologic study of the initial changes. *Am J Orthod*, 57, 370-85.

Vardimon, A.D.; Graber, T.M.; Voss, L.R.; Lenke, J. (1991). Determinants control-ling iatrogenic external root resorption and repair during and after palatal expansion. *Angle Orthod*, 61, 113-22.

Verna, C.; Dalstra, M.; Melsen, B. (2003). Bone turnover rate in rats does not influence root resorption induced by orthodontic treatment. *Eur J Orthod*, 25, 4, 359-63.

Villa, P.A.; Oberti, G.; Moncada, C.A. et al. (2005). Pulp-dentine complex changes and root resorption during intrusive orthodontic tooth movement in patients prescribed nabumetone. *J Endod*, 31, 61-6.

Weltman. B.; Vig, K.W.; Fields, H.W.; Shanker, S.; Kaizar, E.E. (2010). Root resorption associated with orthodontic tooth movement: a systematic review. *Am J Orthod Dentofacial Orthop*, 137, 4, 462-76, discussion 12A.

Zahrowski, J.; Jeske, A. (2011). Apical root resorption is associated with comprehensive orthodontic treatment but not clearly dependent on prior tooth characteristics or orthodontic techniques. *J Am Dent Assoc*, 142, 1, 66-8.